Handbook of ICU Therapy

Third edition

Handbook of ICU Therapy

Third edition

Edited by

John Fuller MD FRCPC

Professor in the Department of Anesthesia and Perioperative Medicine, and Division of Critical Care (Department of Medicine),
Western University, London, ON, Canada

Jeff Granton MD FRCPC

Associate Professor in the Department of Anesthesia and Perioperative Medicine, Division of Critical Care (Department of Medicine),
Western University, London, ON, Canada

Ian McConachie MB ChB FRCA FRCPC

Associate Professor in the Department of Anesthesia and Perioperative Medicine, Division of Critical Care (Department of Medicine),
Western University, London, ON, Canada

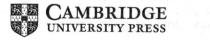
CAMBRIDGE
UNIVERSITY PRESS

CAMBRIDGE
UNIVERSITY PRESS

University Printing House, Cambridge CB2 8BS, United Kingdom

Cambridge University Press is part of the University of Cambridge.

It furthers the University's mission by disseminating knowledge in the pursuit of education, learning and research at the highest international levels of excellence.

www.cambridge.org
Information on this title: www.cambridge.org/9781107641907

© Cambridge University Press 2015

First published 1998
Second edition 2006
Third edition 2015

A catalogue record for this publication is available from the British Library

Library of Congress Cataloguing in Publication data
Handbook of ICU therapy / edited by John Fuller, Jeff Granton, Ian McConachie. – Third edition.
p. ; cm.
Includes bibliographical references and index.
ISBN 978-1-107-64190-7 (Paperback)
I. Fuller, John, 1955-editor. II. Granton, Jeff, editor.
III. McConachie, Ian, editor.
[DNLM: 1. Intensive Care–methods–Handbooks. WX 39]
RC86.8
616.02'8–dc23   2014018828

ISBN 978-1-107-64190-7 Paperback

Contents

Section 1 – Basic principles

Contributors

Mowaffaq Almikhlafi MD FRCPC
Fellow, Critical Care Western, Schulich School of Medicine and Dentistry, Western University, London Health Sciences Centre, London, Ontario, Canada

Osama Al-muslim MD, MRCP (UK)
Critical Care Consultant, Director of Life Support Training Center, King Fahad Specialist Hospital, Dammam, Saudi Arabia

Robert Arntfield MD FRCPC FCCP FACEP
Assistant Professor, Schulich School of Medicine and Dentistry, Western University, Director, Critical Care Ultrasound, Division of Critical Care (Department of Medicine), London Health Sciences Centre and St. Joseph's Healthcare London, London, Ontario, Canada

Ian M Ball MD DABEM FCCP FRCPC
Assistant Professor, Queen's University, Kingston, Department of Emergency Medicine, Department of Biomedical and Molecular Sciences, Program in Critical Care Medicine, Consultant Toxicologist, Ontario Poison Information, Kingston General Hospital, Kingston, Ontario, Canada

Sue Berney PhD PT
Associate Professor, Department of Physiotherapy, Melbourne School of Health Sciences, The University of Melbourne, Parkville, Victoria, Australia

Mohit Bhutani MD FRCPC FCCP
Associate Professor, Division of Pulmonary Medicine, Department of Medicine, University of Alberta, Edmonton, Alberta, Canada

Clay A Block MD
Associate Professor, Department of Medicine (Nephrology section), Geisel School of Medicine, Dartmouth, NH, USA

Ken Blonde MD
Critical Care Fellow, Faculty of Medicine, University of Calgary, Calgary, Alberta, Canada

Rudi Brits MB ChB FRCA FICM
Consultant Anaesthetist, Tygerberg Hospital, Cape Town, South Africa

Ron Butler MD FRCPC
Associate Professor, Department of Anesthesia and Perioperative Medicine and Division of Critical Care (Department of Medicine), Schulich School of Medicine and Dentistry, Western University, London Health Sciences Centre and St. Joseph's Healthcare London, London, Ontario, Canada

Lois Champion MD FRCPC
Professor, Department of Anesthesia and Perioperative Medicine and Division of Critical Care (Department of Medicine), Schulich School of Medicine and Dentistry, Western University, London Health Sciences Centre and St. Joseph's Healthcare London, London, Ontario, Canada

Chris Clarke FRCA
Consultant in Anaesthesia and Critical Care, Blackpool Teaching Hospitals NHS Foundation Trust, Blackpool, UK

Linda Denehy PhD PT
Professor and Head, Department of Physiotherapy, Melbourne School of Health Sciences, The University of Melbourne, Parkville, Victoria, Australia

Joseph Dreier MD
Department of Medicine (Nephrology section), Geisel School of Medicine, Dartmouth, NH, USA

A Ebersohn MB ChB, DA, Dip Obs
Department of Anaesthesia, Tygerberg Hospital, Cape Town, South Africa

Shane W English BSc MSc MD FRCPC
Assistant Professor, Dept of Medicine (Critical Care), University of Ottawa, Clinical Associate, Dept of Critical Care, The Ottawa Hospital, Associate Scientist, Ottawa Hospital Research Institute, Centre for Transfusion Research, Clinical Epidemiology Program, Ottawa, Canada

Ari Ercole MB BChir MA PhD FRCA FFICM
Consultant in Neurocritical Care, Neurosciences Critical Care Unit, Cambridge University Hospitals NHS Foundation Trust, Cambridge, UK

Darren H Freed MD PhD FRCSC
Associate Professor of Surgery and Physiology, Head, Surgical Heart Failure Program, Cardiac Sciences Program, St. Boniface Hospital, Winnipeg, Manitoba, Canada

John Fuller MD FRCPC
Professor, Department of Anesthesia and Perioperative Medicine and Division of Critical Care (Department of Medicine), Schulich School of Medicine and Dentistry, Western University, London Health Sciences Centre and St. Joseph's Healthcare London, London, Ontario, Canada

Julio P Zavala Georffino MD
Department of Medicine (Nephrology section), Geisel School of Medicine, Dartmouth, NH, USA

RT Noel Gibney MB FRCPC
Professor, Division of Critical Care Medicine, Faculty of Medicine and Dentistry, University of Alberta, Edmonton, Alberta, Canada

Jeff Granton MD FRCPC
Associate Professor, Department of Anesthesia and Perioperative Medicine and Division of Critical Care (Department of Medicine), Schulich School of Medicine and Dentistry, Western University, London Health Sciences Centre and St. Joseph's Healthcare London, London, Ontario, Canada

Donald EG Griesdale MD MPH FRCPC
Assistant Professor, Department of Anesthesia, Pharmacology and Therapeutics, Department of Medicine, Division of Critical Care Medicine, University of British Columbia, Vancouver, British Columbia, Canada

Arun K Gupta MBBS MA PhD FFICM FRCA FHEA
Director of Postgraduate Education, Academic Health Sciences Centre, Cambridge University Health Partners, Consultant in Anaesthesia and Neurointensive Care, Cambridge University Hospitals NHS Foundation Trust, Cambridge, UK

Wael Haddara BSc MD FRCPC
Associate Professor, Department of Medicine, (Division of Endocrinology and Metabolism and Division of Critical Care Medicine), Schulich School of Medicine and Dentistry, Western University, London, Ontario, Canada

Ahmed F Hegazy
Assistant Professor, Department of Anesthesia and Perioperative Medicine, Schulich School of Medicine and Dentistry, Western University, London Health Sciences Centre and St. Joseph's Healthcare London, London, Ontario, Canada

Umjeet Singh Jolly BSc MD FRCPC
Cardiology Fellow, Schulich School of Medicine and Dentistry, Western University, Division of Cardiology (Department of Medicine), University Hospital, London Health Sciences Centre, London, Ontario, Canada

Philip M Jones MD FRCPC
Associate Professor, Department of Anesthesia and Perioperative Medicine and Division of Critical Care (Department of Medicine), and Department of Epidemiology & Biostatistics, Schulich School of Medicine and Dentistry, Western University, London Health Sciences Centre and St. Joseph's Healthcare London, London, Ontario, Canada

Ilya Kagan MD
Senior Physician, General Intensive Care Department, Rabin Medical Centre, Beilinson Campus, Petah Tikva, Israel

Kala Kathirgamanathan MD FRCPC
Division of Cardiology, Department of Medicine, Schulich School of Medicine and Dentistry, Western University, London, Ontario, Canada

Harneet Kaur MD
Department of Medicine (Nephrology Section), Geisel School of Medicine, Dartmouth, NH, USA

John Kellett MD FRCPI
Consultant Physician, Nenagh Hospital, Nenagh, County Tipperary, Ireland

Bhupesh Khadka MD
Department of Medicine (Nephrology section), Geisel School of Medicine, Dartmouth, NH, USA

Biniam Kidane MD MSc FRCSC
Thoracic Surgery Fellow, Department of Surgery, University of Toronto, Toronto, Ontario, Canada

Carlos Kidel MB ChB FRCA
Obstetric Anaesthetic Fellow, Department of Anaesthesia, Royal Free Hospital, London, UK

Anand Kumar MD FRCPC
Professor, Departments of Medicine, Medical Microbiology and Pharmacology/ Therapeutics, University of Manitoba, Winnipeg, Manitoba, Canada

Alejandro Lazo-Langner MD MSc
Assistant Professor of Medicine, Oncology, and Epidemiology and Biostatistics, Schulich School of Medicine and Dentistry, Western University, London Health Sciences Centre and St. Joseph's Healthcare London, London, Ontario, Canada

David Leasa MD FRCPC
Professor of Medicine, Schulich School of Medicine and Dentistry, Western University, Consultant, Divisions of Critical Care Medicine and Respirology, Department of Medicine and Critical Care, London Health Sciences Centre, London, Ontario, Canada

W Robert Leeper MD FRCSC
Trauma and Acute Care Surgery Johns Hopkins Hospital, Baltimore, MD, USA

Stephen Y Liang MD
Instructor, Divisions of Infectious Diseases and Emergency Medicine, Washington University School of Medicine, St. Louis, Missouri, USA

Tania Ligori BSc MD FRCPC
Assistant Clinical Professor, Department of Anesthesia and Department of Critical Care, St Joseph's Healthcare, Hamilton, McMaster University, Hamilton, Ontario, Canada

Jaimie Manlucu MD, FRCPC
Assistant Professor, Schulich School of Medicine and Dentistry, Western University, Clinical Cardiac Electrophysiologist, Division of Cardiology (Department of Medicine), University Hospital, London Health Sciences Centre, London, Ontario, Canada

Janet Martin PharmD, MSC(HTA&M), PhD
Director, Medical Evidence | Decision Integrity | Clinical Impact (MEDICI),

Co-Director, Evidence-Based Perioperative Clinical Outcomes Research (EPiCOR), Assistant Professor, Department of Anesthesia and Perioperative Medicine and Department of Epidemiology and Biostatistics, Schulich School of Medicine and Dentistry, Western University, London, Ontario, Canada

Ian McConachie MB ChB FRCA FRCPC
Associate Professor, Department of Anesthesia and Perioperative Medicine, Schulich School of Medicine and Dentistry, Western University, London Health Sciences Centre and St. Joseph's Healthcare London, London, Ontario, Canada

Alan McGlennan MB BS FRCA
Consultant Anaesthetist, Department of Anaesthesia, Royal Free Hospital, London, UK

Lauralyn McIntyre MD MSc FRCPC
Assistant Professor, Department of Medicine (Critical Care), Ottawa Hospital, Scientist, Ottawa Hospital Research Institute, Centre for Transfusion and Critical Care Research, Adjunct Scientist, Canadian Blood Services, Ottawa, Canada

Tina Mele MD, PhD FRCSC
Assistant Professor, Department of Surgery and Division of Critical Care (Department of Medicine), Schulich School of Medicine and Dentistry, Western University, London Health Sciences Centre and St. Joseph's Healthcare London, London, Ontario, Canada

MJ Naisbitt FRCA FFICM DICM
Consultant in Critical Care, Salford Royal Foundation Trust, Salford, UK

Raj Nichani FRCA
Consultant in Anaesthesia and Critical Care, Blackpool Teaching Hospitals NHS Foundation Trust, Blackpool, UK

Daniel H Ovakim MD MSc FRCPC
Critical Care Medicine, Vancouver Health Island Health Authority, Victoria, British Columbia, Canada; Medical Toxicology, British Columbia Drug and Poison Information Center Vancouver, British Columbia, Canada

Neil Parry MD FRCSC
General Surgery, Trauma and Critical Care, Director of Trauma, LHSC, Associate Professor of Surgery, Western University, London Health Sciences Centre and St. Joseph's Healthcare London, London, Ontario, Canada

Daniel Castro Pereira MD
Department of Medicine (Nephrology section), Geisel School of Medicine, Dartmouth, NH, USA

Thomas Piraino RRT
Assistant Clinical Professor (Adjunct), Department of Anesthesia (Critical Care), Faculty of Health Sciences, McMaster University, Best Practice Clinical Educator, Respiratory Therapy Services, St. Joseph's Healthcare, Hamilton, Ontario, Canada

Brian Pollard BPharm MB ChB MD FRCA MEWI
Professor of Anaesthesia, Manchester Medical School, The University of Manchester, Consultant in Anaesthesia and Intensive Care, Manchester Royal Infirmary, Manchester, UK

Valerie Schulz MD FRCPC MPH
Associate Professor, Department of Anesthesia and Perioperative Medicine, Schulich School of Medicine and Dentistry, Western University, Director of Palliative Care, London Health Sciences Centre and St. Joseph's Healthcare London, London, Ontario, Canada

Michael D Sharpe MD FRCPC
Professor, Department of Anesthesia and Perioperative Medicine and Division of

Critical Care (Department of Medicine), Schulich School of Medicine and Dentistry, Western University, London Health Sciences Centre, London, Ontario, Canada

Rohit K Singal MD MSc FRCSC
Assistant Professor of Surgery, Cardiac Sciences Program, St. Boniface Hospital, Winnipeg, Manitoba, Canada

Pierre Singer MD
Professor, Director General Intensive Care Department, Rabin Medical Center, Beilinson Campus, Petah Tikva, Israel

Mark Soth MD FRCPC
Associate Professor, Department of Medicine, McMaster University, Chief, Department of Critical Care, St Joseph's Healthcare, Hamilton, Ontario, Canada

Christian P Subbe DM FRCP
Senior Clinical Lecturer, School of Medical Sciences, Bangor University, Consultant Acute, Respiratory and Critical Care Medicine, Ysbyty Gwynedd, Bangor, UK

Jaffer Syed MD, MEd, FRCPC
Division of Cardiology, Department of Medicine, McMaster University, Hamilton, Ontario, Canada

Ravi Taneja FFARCSI, FRCA, FRCPC
Associate Professor, Department of Anesthesia and Perioperative Medicine and Division of Critical Care (Department of Medicine), Schulich School of Medicine and Dentistry, Western University, London Health Sciences Centre and St. Joseph's Healthcare London, London, Ontario, Canada

Tom Varughese MD
Department of Anesthesia and Perioperative Medicine and Division of Critical Care (Department of Medicine), Schulich School of Medicine and Dentistry, Western University, London Health Sciences Centre and St. Joseph's Healthcare London, London, Ontario, Canada

Jennifer Vergel Del Dios MD
Department of Anesthesia and Perioperative Medicine and Division of Critical Care (Department of Medicine), Schulich School of Medicine and Dentistry, Western University, London Health Sciences Centre and St. Joseph's Healthcare London, London, Ontario, Canada

Jessie R Welbourne MB ChB FRCA
Consultant in Intensive Care Medicine, Derriford Hospital, Plymouth Hospitals NHS Trust, Plymouth, UK

Christopher W White MD
Cardiac Sciences Program, St. Boniface Hospital, Winnipeg, Manitoba, Canada

Rebecca P Winsett PhD RN
Nurse Scientist, St. Mary's Medical Center, Evansville, IN, USA

Titus C Yeung MD FRCPC
Department of Medicine, Division of Critical Care Medicine, University of British Columbia, Vancouver British Columbia, Canada

G Bryan Young MD, FRCPC
Departments of Clinical Neurological Sciences and Medicine (Critical Care), Schulich School of Medicine and Dentistry, Western University, London, Ontario, Canada

Shelley R Zieroth MD FRCPC
Assistant Professor of Medicine, Director, St. Boniface Hospital Heart Failure and Transplant Clinics, Head, Medical Heart Failure Program, Cardiac Sciences Program, St. Boniface Hospital, Winnipeg, Manitoba, Canada

Preface to the third edition

- This text is aimed primarily at trainees working in intensive care – especially multidisciplinary trainees being exposed to the intensive care unit (ICU) for the first time. It may also be of interest to ICU nurses looking for information on modern medical (in the strictest sense) approaches to ICU therapy. A basic knowledge of physiology and pharmacology is assumed, as well as either a medical background or advanced nursing experience in intensive care.
- It may also be a useful "aide memoire" for specialist ICU examinations.
- The editors have enlisted a multinational team of contributors active in both practice and training from institutions on both sides of the Atlantic and beyond. The aim has therefore been to produce a text of international relevance.
- The authors are all either experienced ICU practitioners or invited experts on specialist issues. Being involved in ICU research was not a pre-requisite although many of the authors have been or are involved in ICU research.
- This text aims to provide practical information on the management of common and/or important problems in the critically ill patient, as well as sufficient background information to enable understanding of the principles and rationale behind their therapy. We hope it will prove useful at the bedside, but we would like to emphasize that this, or any other book, is no substitute for experienced supervision, support and training.
- Throughout, the importance of cardiac function is emphasized.
- This text does not aim to cover all of ICU practice and is not a substitute to the major ICU reference textbooks. For example, practical aspects of monitoring techniques are not covered (best learnt at the bedside), but the philosophy of monitoring is covered where necessary to illustrate important management points. Similarly, pathophysiology is included to help understand management principles.
- The third edition contains several new chapters on topical aspects of ICU therapy, as well as revisions of older chapters – many have been completely rewritten.
- The format is designed to provide easy access to information presented in a concise manner. We have tried to eliminate all superfluous material. Selected important or controversial references are presented, as well as suggestions for further reading.

Oxygen delivery, cardiac function and monitoring

Lois Champion

Oxygen delivery

The purpose of the circulatory system is ultimately the delivery of oxygen and nutrients to cells, with removal of waste and carbon dioxide. Oxygen delivery depends on blood flow (cardiac output) and the amount of oxygen in the blood.

Oxygen delivery = cardiac output × oxygen content in arterial blood

Oxygen is carried in the blood in two forms:
1. Bound to hemoglobin (the amount of oxygen bound to hemoglobin depends on oxygen saturation)
2. Dissolved in plasma (the amount of oxygen dissolved in plasma depends on the arterial partial pressure of oxygen (PaO_2) and the solubility of oxygen)

Arterial oxygen content = oxygen bound to hemoglobin + oxygen dissolved in plasma

Most of the oxygen in blood is carried bound to hemoglobin, and only a small fraction is dissolved. Clinically, this means that an arterial oxygen saturation of 90% (corresponding to a PaO_2 of ~60 mmHg) provides essentially normal arterial oxygen content. Oxygen saturation is measured noninvasively using pulse oximetry.

Arterial oxygen content = oxygen bound to hemoglobin + oxygen dissolved in plasma

$$\text{Arterial oxygen content } (CaO_2) = (\text{hemoglobin})(\text{oxygen saturation}) (1.34) + (PaO_2) (0.031)$$

The usual arterial oxygen saturation is close to 100%, and PaO_2 is approximately 90 mmHg. Arterial blood normally contains approximately 200 mL of oxygen per liter of blood. If we assume a cardiac output of ~5 L/min then this is an oxygen delivery of ~1 L/min.

Oxygen consumption

Oxygen is carried to the tissues and delivered to cells via the capillaries, where oxygen is taken up (consumed) by cells, so that venous blood contains less oxygen (and more carbon dioxide) than arterial blood. The partial pressure of oxygen in the venous blood (PvO_2) is, on average, ~40 mmHg (this corresponds to an oxygen saturation of ~70–75% in the venous blood).

Handbook of ICU Therapy, third edition, ed. John Fuller, Jeff Granton and Ian McConachie. Published by Cambridge University Press. © Cambridge University Press 2015.

The overall oxygen content of venous blood is ~150 mL of oxygen/liter of blood. Overall oxygen consumption is ~250 mL of oxygen per minute; if delivery is ~1 L/min this means we usually extract about 25% of the oxygen delivered.

- Oxygen consumption (demand) will increase with exercise or fever
- Sedation, paralysis and hypothermia decrease oxygen consumption.

Venous oxygen saturation

Venous oxygen saturation (SvO_2) reflects oxygen supply and demand; venous oxygen saturation will decrease if there is a decrease in oxygen delivery or an increase in oxygen consumption, because cells will extract more oxygen from the blood to meet demand [1].

Venous oxygen saturation can be monitored either:

- Intermittently, with blood gas sampling from a central venous catheter in the superior vena cava, or from the pulmonary artery using a pulmonary artery catheter.

Or

- Continuously, using a central venous or pulmonary artery catheter designed to continuously measure venous oxygen saturation.
- Note that measuring venous oxygen saturation from a femoral venous catheter is not reliable as an indicator of global perfusion since it reflects oxygen supply and demand only from the lower extremity [2].

A decrease in venous oxygen saturation below the usual value of ~70–75% suggests increased oxygen extraction and an oxygen supply/demand imbalance. Increasing oxygen delivery with inotropic support, or red blood cell transfusion if the hemoglobin is low, may improve patient outcomes in sepsis [3].

- A normal SvO_2, however, does not necessarily reflect normal oxygen delivery because venous oxygenation is a flow-weighted average of venous blood (no flow in means no flow out of tissues).
- In some clinical situations, in particular sepsis, there is maldistribution of flow at the microvascular level. A normal or high venous oxygen saturation may be associated with a worse prognosis in these patients [4].

Lactic acid is a by-product of anaerobic metabolism. Monitoring lactate levels as an indicator of tissue ischemia and anaerobic metabolism may also be used to monitor response to therapy [5–7].

Cardiac function
Cardiac output

Cardiac output (CO) is the volume the heart ejects over time (usually expressed as L/min), a normal cardiac output is about 5 L/min. Normal cardiac output varies with the size of a patient (you would expect a 200 kg patient to have a higher cardiac output than a 50 kg patient because of the increased body mass that must be perfused). In order to standardize measurements cardiac output is divided by a patient's body surface area (BSA) to calculate the cardiac index (CI). The normal CI is 2.5–4 L/min/m^2.

Cardiac index (CI) = CO/BSA

Stroke volume (SV) is the volume of blood ejected with a single contraction (because the right and left ventricle are in series, it follows that the stroke volume of the right ventricle must be the same as the left ventricle). Cardiac output over a minute therefore is the stroke volume multiplied by the number of beats per minute (or heart rate).

CO = SV × HR

Stroke volume is determined by:

1. Preload – the end-diastolic volume of the ventricle
2. Afterload – the wall tension the ventricle must develop to eject blood
3. Contractility (or inotropy) – the intrinsic performance of the heart at a given preload and afterload.

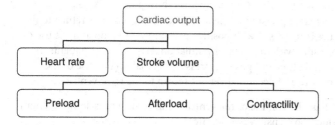

Heart rate

Since cardiac output depends on heart rate it follows that a low heart rate (bradycardia) can contribute to low cardiac output.

- An increase in heart rate increases the force of ventricular contraction (this is known as the treppe phenomenon). This effect, however, is minimal or absent in a failing ventricle with poor systolic function.
- An increase in heart rate increases myocardial oxygen demand, which may precipitate cardiac ischemia, and decreases the time available for diastolic filling.

Overall, the optimal heart rate is determined by a combination of the treppe phenomenon and the need for diastolic filling time, as well as other factors in individual patients such as intrinsic contractility, and valvular or ischemic heart disease.

Stroke volume

The normal ventricle ejects approximately 70 mL of blood with each beat – this is the stroke volume (SV). The ventricles do not empty completely with contraction, there is some residual volume remaining at the end of systole (end-systolic volume). During diastole the ventricles fill; a normal end-diastolic volume (EDV) is approximately 120 mL.

Ejection fraction

Ejection fraction is defined as the ratio of SV/EDV. A normal ejection fraction is 60–65%.

Preload

Preload is defined as the end-diastolic volume (EDV) of the left ventricle.

The determinants of preload include:

- Circulating blood volume – more volume increases preload.
- Venous tone – venoconstriction increases preload. Venous tone determines venous capacitance (the veins are the major reservoir for blood volume).
- Ventricular compliance – a more compliant ventricle can hold more blood at a given pressure than a noncompliant (stiff) ventricle.
- Afterload – if afterload is increased acutely, less blood is pumped out with ventricular contraction, which leaves more residual blood to add on to end-diastolic volume. Preload therefore is increased (this is one of the acute compensatory responses to an increase in afterload).
- Atrial contraction – especially in patients with stiff noncompliant ventricles, by forcing some additional blood into the ventricles from the atria during late diastole.
- Intrathoracic pressure – increased pressure in the thorax can reduce venous return to the heart; intrathoracic pressure is increased with positive-pressure ventilation and the use of positive end-expiratory pressure with mechanical ventilation. Hypovolemic patients may become hypotensive with intubation and positive-pressure ventilation because of the increased intrathoracic pressure and decreased venous return to the right ventricle.

An increase in preload (end-diastolic volume of the ventricle) and hence muscle-fiber length increases resting tension, velocity of tension development and peak tension:

- This allows for greater stroke volume and therefore cardiac output. This is the Frank–Starling relationship.
- Excessive ventricular volume, however, will eventually overwhelm the ventricle's capacity to pump blood forward, and lead to decompensation. As well, a ventricle with poor systolic function has less capacity to improve contractility with an increase in preload.

Clinically we cannot easily measure preload. Central venous pressure or pulmonary capillary wedge pressure measurements provide information about ventricular filling pressures; however, correlation with intravascular and intraventricular volume depends on many factors, such as vascular tone and ventricular compliance.

Afterload

Afterload is the wall tension or stress the ventricle must develop to eject blood. The law of Laplace states that tension is proportional to both the pressure and radius of a sphere, divided by twice the wall thickness. This equation assumes that the ventricles are spheres. Although the ventricles are not true spheres, pressure, radius and wall thickness contribute to ventricular afterload.

Tension ~ (pressure × radius)/(wall thickness × 2)

- Afterload will therefore be increased if the ventricle generates higher pressures or becomes larger (dilates). This means that the afterload for the left ventricle is normally higher than for the right ventricle – it is larger and develops much higher pressures. This is offset somewhat by the fact that the left ventricle is more muscular, with a thicker wall than the right ventricle.

- Afterload to the ventricle includes a component of preload (ventricular size or radius), therefore afterload and preload are interdependent.
- In a normal heart, changes in afterload do not impact stroke volume until extreme values are reached; however, a ventricle with decreased contractility (a "failing ventricle") is very sensitive to an increase in afterload.

Clinically, we often simplify the concept of afterload to refer to the pressure the ventricle generates; we can measure blood pressure quite easily, but it is much more difficult to quantify the size of a ventricle or its wall thickness.

- Typical conditions that will increase the afterload of the left ventricle are hypertension and aortic stenosis (aortic stenosis produces a pressure gradient between the left ventricle and aorta).
- Examples of diseases that increase afterload to the right ventricle include pulmonary hypertension and pulmonary embolism.
- A chronic increase in afterload leads to compensatory ventricular hypertrophy. An acute increase in afterload can cause acute cardiac dilatation.
- A clinical example is acute massive pulmonary embolism leading to increased pulmonary artery pressures and acute right ventricular dilatation seen on echocardiography.

Compliance

Compliance is the relationship between volume and pressure.

Compliance = Δ volume/Δ pressure

The concept of compliance applies to the heart and diastolic function.

- Ventricular volume can be increased in the normal ventricle with little change in pressure, but as ventricular end-diastolic volume increases further, the diastolic intraventricular pressure will increase.
- With a less compliant (stiffer or less distensible) ventricle, the same end-diastolic volume is associated with a higher left-ventricular diastolic pressure.

Contractility

Inotropy or contractility is the intrinsic ability of cardiac muscle cells to shorten in response to a stimulus (the stimulus is an action potential); shortening of cardiac muscle tissue results in ejection of blood. An increase in contractility results in a higher stroke volume.

Inotropy can be acutely (myocardial infarction) or chronically (systolic heart failure) reduced. Clinically this is seen as a reduction in ejection fraction of the left ventricle. The autonomic nervous system is responsible for controlling the inotropic state of the heart.

- Increased levels of circulating catecholamines result in greater contractility and an increase in heart rate (mediated by the adrenergic β-receptors), as well as increased vascular resistance (vasoconstriction mediated by the adrenergic α-receptors).
- Inotropic medications (such as dopamine, dobutamine or epinephrine) can be given as intravenous infusions to increase cardiac contractility.
- These medications, however, may cause tachycardia, arrhythmias and increased myocardial oxygen consumption predisposing to myocardial ischemia [8].

The right and left ventricles: similar but different

The right ventricle (RV) pumps blood to the relatively low-pressure, low-resistance pulmonary system. Pulmonary hypertension is defined as a mean pulmonary artery pressure of >25 mmHg, or a pulmonary vascular resistance of >3 Wood's units); the left ventricle generates higher pressures (the normal systemic mean arterial pressure is ~65 mmHg or more).

- The normal right ventricle is less muscular than the left ventricle (LV) anatomically. The right ventricle may hypertrophy over time (for example in patients with chronic pulmonary hypertension), just as the left ventricle may hypertrophy when faced with an increase in afterload.
- The right ventricle may acutely dilate with a sudden increase in afterload. For example, in a patient with acute pulmonary embolism a sudden increase in pulmonary artery pressure can lead to acute right ventricular dilation and RV failure.
- With severe RV dilation the RV may "push" the interventricular septum over toward the LV, impacting left ventricular diastolic filling, compliance and systolic function. This phenomenon is known as "ventricular interdependence" [9].

Coronary blood flow to the right ventricle occurs throughout the cardiac cycle – during both systole and diastole – because the right ventricle systolic pressures are not high enough to compress the coronary blood vessels. Maximal coronary blood flow to the left ventricle, however, occurs during early diastole. With the left ventricle there is actually a brief reversal of coronary flow during systole, as the muscular left ventricle contracts and generates high systolic pressures.

- Right heart failure is associated with an increase in right-sided pressures – clinically this is seen as elevated jugular venous pressure or central venous pressure – this pressure may be transmitted downstream causing congestion of the liver, ascites formation and peripheral edema.
- Patients can have biventricular failure (both right and left ventricular failure), pure right-sided heart failure (for example, with chronic pulmonary hypertension), or left-sided failure.
- Note, however, that with chronic left-heart failure the left-sided pressures will be increased, and the right ventricle will have to pump against these higher pressures, eventually causing the right ventricle to fail also; in fact the most common cause of right-sided failure is chronic left-heart failure.

Monitoring

Monitoring may be described as the intermittent or continuous observation of a patient using clinical examination and appropriate equipment to assess progress of the condition:

- The most useful and reproducible monitor remains a thorough and repeated clinical examination by the doctor.
- Not all critical care environments are the same, and all models of monitoring equipment are slightly different. The clinician must take time to become familiar with the equipment in his or her own hospital.

Monitoring may allow us to:

- intervene therapeutically in emergency situations,
- guide and plan future therapy,

- establish diagnoses,
- establish prognosis.

Monitoring, however, is not a therapy in itself; in order for monitoring to improve outcome it must be correctly interpreted and acted upon, and done with the minimum of complications.

Oxygen saturation monitoring (pulse oximetry)

Oxygen saturation monitors (pulse oximetry) use two different wavelengths of light in the red and infrared spectrum, which are absorbed differentially by oxyhemoglobin and deoxyhemoglobin. The pulse oximeter separates the pulsatile component of the absorption signal from the nonpulsatile component – the assumption being that the pulsatile component represents arterial blood.

- If a patient is hypotensive or severely vasoconstricted, the pulse oximeter may not be able to detect an accurate signal.
- The pulse oximeter shines the light through tissue (usually a finger, but earlobe, nose etc. can be used) and then determines how much of each wavelength was absorbed – and calculates the oxygen saturation.
- Since the absorption spectrum of carboxyhemoglobin (COHb) and oxyhemoglobin with the light wavelengths used in pulse oximetry are similar, the oximeter will give a falsely high oxygen saturation reading with carbon monoxide poisoning. Similarly methemoglobinemia may interfere with accurate pulse oximetry [10].

Noninvasive blood pressure monitoring

NIBP stands for noninvasive blood pressure and uses a blood pressure cuff, with a machine that automatically inflates and deflates the cuff. Noninvasive blood pressure devices provide systolic, diastolic and mean arterial pressure, as well as an audible alarm system, and can be programmed to measure BP as often as required clinically (as often as every minute in an unstable patient). The measurement is based on oscillometry; variations in the pressure in the BP cuff due to arterial pulsations are sensed by the monitor (if you take a blood pressure manually you will note these oscillations yourself as small deflections in the sphygmomanometer as you deflate the cuff). The pressure at which oscillations are maximal correlates with mean arterial pressure; systolic and diastolic pressures are calculated using a formula based on the peak of the oscillations.

- Automated NIBP measurements correlate closely with directly measured BP (standards require that error be less than 5 ± 8 mmHg with respect to reference standard); in severely hypotensive patients it may be impossible to measure BP using NIBP.
- Noninvasive blood pressure measurements will be less accurate (just as manual BP measurement is) if the BP cuff is the incorrect size.
- Complications of NIBP measurement that have been described include petechiae, bruising, and neuropathy (if the cuff compresses a nerve).

Direct arterial blood pressure measurement

- The insertion of a small (common sizes are 20 or 22 gauge) teflon-coated catheter into an artery (usually the radial, ulnar, brachial, dorsalis pedis or femoral are used) allows direct beat-to-beat assessment of the systemic BP [11]. This may be required in patients with hemodynamic instability, or with the use of inotrope or vasopressor infusions.

- The presence of an arterial line also provides access for the measurement of arterial blood gas samples.
- Complications include local bleeding and infection. Serious complications include thrombosis and development of arterio-venous (AV) fistulas.
- Accurate pressure measurement requires zeroing of the transducer (opening the transducer to atmospheric pressure and identifying that as a pressure of "zero").
- In addition, the height of the transducer relative to the patient is important – the transducer should be positioned at the level of the mid-axillary line, 4th intercostal space of the patient (at the level of the heart). If the transducer was inadvertently raised to 14 cm above the patient, for example, the pressure reading would be ~ 10 mmHg lower than the true reading.
- Other reasons for inaccuracy of invasive pressure monitoring include damping or under-damping of the pressure trace. The pressure waveform may be "damped" if the catheter is kinked, or with blood or air within the catheter. It is also possible for the pressure waveform to be "under-damped" – typically recognized as a rapid, spiked upstroke in the waveform with a systolic pressure overshoot. This occurs when the pressure waveform in the catheter causes the transducer to reverberate at its own harmonic frequency. Typically, mean pressures are more accurate in the presence of under-damped system.

Central venous pressure (CVP) monitoring

Central venous catheters may be used to:
- Monitor central venous pressure.
- Provide central venous access for infusions of potent vasoconstrictors or hypersosmolar solutions such as total parenteral nutrition or both.
- Central venous pressure (pressure in the superior vena cava) may be monitored with jugular, subclavian or peripherally inserted central venous catheters [12].
- Femoral venous catheters are not useful for monitoring of central venous pressure.
- Accurate measurement of CVP requires that the catheter be zeroed, and the transducer leveled at the mid-axillary fourth intercostal space (as for arterial catheters) [13].

In addition CVP will fluctuate with changes in intrathoracic pressure:
- In a spontaneously breathing patient the CVP will decrease on inspiration as intrathoracic pressure decreases; with positive-pressure ventilation the CVP will increase on inspiration due to increased intrathoracic pressure.
- The actual filling pressure (transmural pressure) for the right ventricle is the CVP measured when intrathoracic pressure is zero – this will tend to be at end-expiration.
- For patients on positive end-expiratory pressure (PEEP), particularly levels over 10 cm H_2O, the CVP will be increased relative to the true filling pressure; the actual amount of increase can only be measured using a measurement of intrathoracic pressure (such as a pleural or esophageal pressure manometer).

CVP is often used as a guide for fluid management:

- A protocol for therapy in patients with early sepsis (within 6 hours), which included a goal of CVP of 8–12 mmHg, and additional fluid resuscitation to meet the target CVP, was associated with improved outcome [3].
- Ongoing aggressive fluid resuscitation after the initial early resuscitation, however, may not be beneficial [14, 15].

CVP is not an accurate surrogate for intravascular volume. The CVP depends on many factors:

- Patients may have a low CVP with a normal intravascular volume (for example with vasodilation, or a compliant right ventricle).
- Patients may have a higher than normal CVP and have a low intravascular volume, or benefit from additional fluid challenge (for example, with vasoconstriction, high intrathoracic pressure due to positive end-expiratory pressure, cardiac tamponade, or pulmonary hypertension and right-heart failure).

Clinically, patient assessment for intravascular volume status should include heart rate, blood pressure, capillary refill, urine output, response to previous fluid challenges, inotrope and vasopressor requirements, and overall fluid balance, venous oxygen saturation, lactate levels etc., as well as any trends in monitored parameters.

Other ways to assess cardiac function and intravascular volume

Pulse pressure variation (PPV)

- Pulse pressure variation is the cyclic variation in pulse pressure and systolic blood pressure with respiration due to changes in intrathoracic pressure; pulse pressure will be maximal at the end of inspiration and minimal during exhalation (in a mechanically ventilated patient); the PPV response is exaggerated in patients with "preload reserve" [16, 17].
- Pulse pressure variation can be used to predict response to fluid challenge (volume responsiveness).

Limitations of PPV monitoring include:

- Requires patients to be on positive-pressure ventilation; spontaneous breathing attempts (including triggering) will lead to changes in venous return and make PPV analysis inaccurate.
- Patients must be in sinus rhythm.
- PPV may be less accurate in patients with elevated filling pressures [17].
- Tidal volume is important – a small tidal volume (resulting in smaller changes in intrathoracic pressure) will make PPV inaccurate; a tidal volume of at least 8 mL/kg PBW is required [17].

Echocardiogram

- Echocardiography can provide information about ventricular size, ejection fraction and also identify pericardial fluid.

- Visualization of the inferior vena cava (IVC) as it enters the right atrium provides information about the size of the IVC, and in spontaneously breathing patients "collapse" of the IVC (or a decrease in diameter of over 30%) on inspiration suggests preload responsiveness.
- Cyclic variation in IVC volume/diameter may predict fluid responsiveness in a mechanically ventilated patient; however, large tidal volumes (at least 8 mL/kg PBW are required, even temporarily) and spontaneous breathing attempts are required for this assessment [18].

Pulmonary artery catheters

Pulmonary artery catheters (PAC) are catheters that use a distal balloon filled with 1.5 mL of air to "float" the catheter:

- from the central vein into the **right atrium** (pressure measured from the tip of the catheter will show a typical venous waveform), then
- across the **tricuspid valve** and into
- the **right ventricle** (as the catheter enters the right ventricle the waveform will show an increase in systolic pressure with the diastolic pressure approximately equal to the venous and atrial pressure). Typical RV pressure, in the absence of pulmonary hypertension is ~ 20–25 mmHg/0–8 mmHg. The catheter will then float across the pulmonic valve and into
- the **pulmonary artery**. As the catheter crosses the pulmonic valve the waveform of the systolic pressure will be unchanged, but the diastolic pressure will increase – typically to 10–15 mmHg. If the balloon is left inflated the catheter will continue to float along the pulmonary artery until it "wedges" and cannot float any further distally. At this point the pressure monitored from the tip of the catheter will be
- the **pulmonary wedge pressure** – this pressure reflects left atrial pressure (since there is an uninterrupted column of blood from the tip of the catheter to the left atrium, and a zero flow state since the catheter is occluding flow). This pressure is sometimes also called pulmonary artery occlusion pressure.

Pulmonary artery catheters have the ability to measure CVP (from the CVP port which is ~ 30 cm proximal to the catheter tip) as well as pulmonary artery pressure and the pulmonary wedge pressure.

Pulmonary artery catheters can also measure cardiac output using a principle known as thermodilution. There is a thermistor (temperature monitor) at the tip of the PAC. If a known quantity of fluid (typically 10 mL) at a known temperature (typically room temperature or ice-cold saline is used) is injected proximal to the thermistor (through the CVP port) the distal thermistor will detect a decrease in temperature relative to the baseline pulmonary artery temperature. In patients with a high cardiac output the relatively cold bolus of saline will be "diluted" by the large volume of blood flowing by and the temperature change will be small and short-lived. In a patient with a low cardiac output the temperature decrease will be larger and last longer. A computer is used to integrate the area under the temperature change curve and calculate the cardiac output.

Note that cardiac output measurements will not be accurate in patients with tricuspid regurgitation; other causes of cardiac output measurement error include: malpositioning of the catheter, rapid infusion of cold solutions (for example blood products) at the time of thermodilution, cardiac output measurement, injection of an inaccurate volume or temperature of the injectate, uneven or slow injection rate.

Although the ability to monitor cardiac output and left-sided filling pressures is intuitively appealing, this does not necessarily translate to benefit for the patient.

- A number of studies have shown that use of a pulmonary artery catheter monitor is not associated with improved outcome in high-risk surgery patients, heart-failure patients, septic patients or patients with acute respiratory distress syndrome [19–21].
- The utilization of PACs has decreased over the past two decades as a result [22].

References

1. Walley K. Use of central venous oxygen saturation to guide therapy. *Am J Resp Crit Care Med* 2011; 184 : 514–20.

2. Davison DL, Chawla LS, Selassie L et al. Femoral-based central venous oxygen saturation not a reliable substitute. *Chest* 2010; 138 : 76–83.

3. Rivers E, Nguyen B, Havstad S et al. Early goal-directed therapy in the treatment of severe sepsis and septic shock. *NEJM* 2001; 345 : 1368–77.

4. Pope JV, Gaieski DF, Trzeciak S, Shapiro NI. Multicenter study of central venous oxygen saturation (ScvO2) as a predictor of mortality in patients with sepsis. *Ann Emerg Med* 2010; 55 : 40–6.

5. Jones AE, Shapiro NI, Trzeciak S et al. Lactate clearance vs central venous oxygen saturation as goals. *JAMA* 2010; 303 : 739–46.

6. Jackson AE. Point: Should lactate clearance be substituted for central venous oxygen saturation as goals of early severe sepsis and septic shock therapy? Yes. *Chest* 2011; 140 : 1406–08.

7. Rivers EP, Elkin R, Cannon CM. Counterpoint: Should lactate clearance be substituted for central venous oxygen saturation as goals of early severe sepsis and septic shock? No. *Chest* 2011; 140 : 1408–13.

8. DeBacker D, Biston P, Devriendt J et al. Comparison of dopamine and norepinephrine in the treatment of shock. *N Engl J Med* 2010; 362 : 779–89.

9. Castillo C, Tapson VF. Right ventricular responses to massive and submassive pulmonary embolism. *Cardiol Clin* 2012; 30 : 233–41.

10. Ortega R, Hansen CJ, Ellerman K, Woo A. Videos in clinical medicine. Pulse Oximetry. *N Engl J Med* 2011; 364 : e33.

11. Tegtmeyer K, Brady G, Lai S, Hodo R, Braner D. Placement of an arterial line. *N Engl J Med* 2006; 354 : e13.

12. Braner D, Lai S, Eman S, Tegtmeyer K. Videos in Clinidal Medicine. Central Venous Catheterization – Subclavian Vein. *N Engl J Med* 2007; 357 : e26.

13. Gelman, S. Venous function and central venous pressure: a physiologic story. *Anesthesiology* 2008; 108 : 735–48.

14. Vincent JL, Weil MH. Fluid challenge revisited. *Crit Care Med* 2006; 34 : 1333–7.

15. Durairaj L, Schmidt GA. Fluid therapy in resuscitated sepsis: less is more. *Chest* 2008; 133 : 252–63.

16. Marik PE, Monnet X, Teboul J. Hemodynamic parameters to guide fluid therapy. *Annals Int Care* 2011; 1 : 1–9.

17. Cannesson M, Aboy M, Hofer C, Rehman M. Pulse pressure variation: where are we today? *J of Clin Monit Comp* 2011; 1 : 45–56.

18. Schmidt GA, Koenig S, Mayo PH. Shock: ultrasound guide to diagnosis and therapy. *Chest* 2012; 142 : 1042–8.

19. ESCAPE Investigators. Evaluation study of congestive heart failure and pulmonary artery catheterization effectiveness: the ESCAPE trial. *JAMA* 2005; 294 : 1625–33.

20. Sandham JD, Hull RD, Brant RF et al. A randomized, controlled trial of the use of pulmonary artery catheters in high-risk surgical patients. *N Engl J Med* 2003; 348 : 5–14.

21. National Heart, Lung and Blood Institute Acute Respiratory Distress Syndrome Clinical Trials Network. Pulmonary-artery versus central venous catheter to guide treatment of acute lung injury. *N Engl J Med* 2006; 354 : 2213–24.

22. Weinder RS, Welch G. Trends in the use of the pulmonary artery catheter in the United States, 1993–2004. *JAMA* 2007; 298 : 423–429.

Chapter

2

Shock

Philip M Jones

"Shock" is a very imprecise term for a common, life-threatening condition. It affects about one-third of ICU patients [1]. It is associated with a high mortality rate and requires a rapid clinical assessment and intervention if significant complications are to be avoided.

- Shock can be defined as a clinical state in which tissue blood flow is inadequate for tissue requirements (insufficient oxygen delivery), there is maldistribution of oxygen delivery, or when cellular oxygen utilization is impaired.
- At the cellular level, shock is a state of acute nutritional insufficiency for oxygen and other essential substrates, resulting in cellular anoxia, cellular dysfunction, and, eventually, cell death.

Pathophysiology

- Although it is common, and in many ways appropriate, to think of shock in hemodynamic terms (see below), shock is simultaneously a systemic and a cellular disease leading ultimately to decreased adenosine triphosphate (ATP) production, cell-membrane dysfunction, cellular swelling and cell death.
- Once cellular swelling occurs, restoration of local tissue perfusion may not be possible, leading to progressive secondary ischemia.
- Damage to other organs such as the lungs results from leukocyte sequestration and deposition in the pulmonary capillaries – leading to increased pulmonary dead space and increased capillary permeability from the release of inflammatory mediators.
- The reticulo-endothelial system function is depressed, which decreases clearance of toxic materials (e.g. endotoxin, foreign proteins, immune complexes and platelet aggregates).
- It is therefore clear how an initial insult to one organ system may quickly result in multisystem organ failure.

Types of shock

There are four types of shock:

Type of shock	Clinical Examples	Comments
Hypovolemic (decreased blood volume)	Trauma, surgical bleeding, gastrointestinal bleeding, burns or severe diarrhea.	With volume depletion, left ventricular pre-load is too low to support adequate stroke volume. Compensatory mechanisms

---

Handbook of ICU Therapy, third edition, ed. John Fuller, Jeff Granton and Ian McConachie. Published by Cambridge University Press. © Cambridge University Press 2015.

(cont.)

Type of shock	Clinical Examples	Comments
		begin, including tachycardia, increased venous tone, increased vascular resistance, increased myocardial contractility, decreased urine output and sodium reabsorption. However, compensation can only go so far, and hypovolemic shock develops when blood loss exceeds 20–25% of normal circulating volume. Prolonged hypovolemic shock leads to metabolic acidosis and secondary cardiogenic shock.
Distributive (abnormal vascular tone)	Sepsis, anaphylaxis or acute spinal-cord injury.	Usually involves a hyperdynamic state with high cardiac output, normal-to-low filling pressures, decreased total peripheral resistance and a mixed venous oxygen saturation that is normal or even increased. The most common cause of distributive shock in the ICU is sepsis. It is important to remember that septic shock sometimes involves myocardial depression, and, in this case, patients may not present with distributive shock (rather they may have cardiogenic shock).
Obstructive (obstructed flow of blood)	Cardiac tamponade, severe pulmonary embolism or tension pneumothorax.	This type of shock involves impaired diastolic filling of the heart (such as with cardiac tamponade) and/or increased right or left ventricular afterload (such as with severe pulmonary embolism or tension pneumothorax).
Cardiogenic (abnormal pump function)	Acute myocardial infarction, severe valvular disease, end-stage cardiomyopathy, severe dysrhythmias or myocarditis.	Cardiogenic shock results in reduced cardiac output due to a problem with one or more of: the myocardium, the heart valves or heart rhythm.

The shock cycle

Various shock states may inter-relate clinically to produce a mixed picture.

- For example, hypovolemic shock may lead to acidosis and result in secondary cardiogenic shock, whilst septic shock commonly leads to hypovolemia as a result of microbial toxins and cytokines, which result in increased capillary permeability and leaking of fluid into the interstitial space.
- Clinicians must be cognizant of these secondary manifestations of the primary clinical problem.
- When left under-treated, many types of shock will result in hypothermia, coagulopathy, acid–base disturbances, electrolyte abnormalities, cellular injury, multisystem organ failure and, ultimately, death.

Clinical presentation

Shock commonly presents with:

Problem	Manifestation
Hypotension	Systolic blood pressure <90 mmHg or mean arterial pressure <60 mmHg
Tissue hypoperfusion	Oliguria <0.5 mL/kg/h Pale, cool and clammy skin (due to vasoconstriction) Rapid, thready pulse Altered level of consciousness
Inadequate oxygen delivery to tissue	Lactic acidosis (due to anaerobic glycolysis under conditions of low oxygen tension)

Although not all patients with shock present with arterial hypotension (one can have shock without hypotension and one can have hypotension without shock), hypotension is common enough that analyzing the individual determinants of blood pressure provides a useful schema to think about shock. Since blood pressure is equal to the cardiac output multiplied by the total peripheral resistance, all types of shock will involve a problem with one or more of pre-load, myocardial contractility, afterload, heart rate (or rhythm) or total peripheral resistance. For example, Figure 2.1 shows the reason why a patient with a large acute myocardial infarction (loss of myocardial contractile function) will have hypotension and shock.

Monitoring
General

All patients should be monitored with continuous ECG and pulse oximetry. An arterial cannula is mandatory in most cases of moderate or severe shock, to have blood pressure measured beat-to-beat, as well as to facilitate serial measurements of blood gases and lactate concentration.

- It is reasonable to target a mean arterial pressure of over 60–65 mmHg in most cases of shock.

Serial lactate concentrations

Following serial lactate concentrations allows the clinician to assess the efficacy of interventions taken to treat shock.

- When therapy is effective, the lactate concentration should fall over a matter of hours.

It must be kept in mind, however, that liver dysfunction occurring concurrently with shock will potentially slow the clearance of lactate from the blood, as the reaction occurring in the liver (converting lactate to pyruvate – the Cori cycle) will occur more slowly.

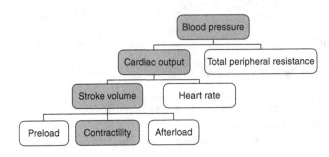

Figure 2.1 Determinants of blood pressure. The boxes shaded gray are implicated in shock in a patient with a large myocardial infarction.

$$SvO_2 = SaO_2 - \frac{VO_2}{CO \times Hb \times 1.34}$$

Figure 2.2 Equation for mixed venous oxygen saturation. SvO_2 denotes mixed venous oxygen saturation, SaO_2 is arterial oxygen saturation, VO_2 is oxygen consumption, CO is cardiac output, and Hb is hemoglobin concentration.

Central venous cannulation

The severity of shock (except for distributive shock) can be initially assessed and followed using the mixed venous oxygen saturation (SvO_2) of blood taken from the distal port of a pulmonary artery catheter.

- The normal oxygen saturation of this blood is about 75%, but the saturation will be lower in most shock states.

The SvO_2 is completely determined by only four variables (Figure 2.2).

Out of the four variables, two are easily measurable and correctable (arterial saturation using a pulse oximeter and hemoglobin concentration with a full blood count), leaving only two pertinent variables to consider in most patients: oxygen consumption and cardiac output. Therefore, in a patient with low SvO_2, whose arterial oxygen saturation is normal and whose hemoglobin concentration is normal, the only way for a decreased SvO_2 to occur is via either an increase in oxygen consumption or a decrease in cardiac output. The latter is by far the most common reason for decreased SvO_2 in hypovolemic, obstructive and cardiogenic shock.

- This provides the rationale for using fluids and vasoactive agents in shock (as appropriate for the diagnosis), and it provides a mechanism to monitor the effectiveness of interventions taken.

The central venous oxygen saturation ($ScvO_2$ – taken from a central line in the superior vena cava) in healthy volunteers is usually slightly less than the SvO_2, but in critically ill patients with shock, it may be higher than the SvO_2.

- The $ScvO_2$ has been shown to be useful in early goal-directed therapy of septic shock [2] and may be a reasonable substitute for a true SvO_2 in other types of shock [3]. This is important, as the pulmonary artery catheter is used infrequently in modern ICU practice.

Management of shock

Unfortunately, our knowledge of the pathophysiological cellular events in shock outweigh our ability to modify these events. Therapy is still largely "macroscopic" (i.e. restoration of tissue perfusion), not "microscopic." As well as general management, it is important to provide specific therapy according to cause.

Timing

It is very important to aggressively treat shock states, as the pathological changes seen at a microcirculatory level can become irreversible after a certain point. The earlier treatment begins, the less likely multisystem organ failure will occur. Resuscitation should start while concurrent investigation of the underlying cause of shock is undertaken.

Airway, oxygenation and ventilation

The threshold for tracheal intubation and mechanical ventilation of patients with shock should be low since:

- Patients are likely to have a decreased level of consciousness and therefore are unlikely to be able to protect their airway. Aspiration is a risk.
- Mechanical ventilation reduces the work of breathing and oxygen consumption, and it helps to compensate for a metabolic acidosis.
- In cardiogenic shock due to myocardial dysfunction, the addition of positive end-expiratory pressure can help with cardiac performance by reducing LV afterload.

Circulatory support

It is necessary to tailor circulatory support to each patient, using Figure 2.1 as a guide and treating the underlying cause.

- A fluid challenge is appropriate in virtually all patients, unless obviously suffering from gross congestive cardiac failure.
- Fluids must be given, but should be given carefully to avoid adverse effects.
- At the start of a resuscitation of a patient in shock, fluids should be given rapidly and the response of the patient to a fluid challenge (300–500 mL over 20–30 minutes) should be assessed.
- If no desirable response is obtained (increase in blood pressure, improved urine output or decrease in heart rate), aggressive fluid therapy should be stopped in favor of providing maintenance fluid requirements only, to prevent fluid overload.
- If the central venous pressure rises more than a few millimetres of mercury above baseline, this is a warning sign of potential fluid overload [1].

Increasingly, bedside transthoracic or transesophageal echocardiography is used to guide the diagnosis and therapy of shock.

- For instance, in a patient with suspected hypovolemic shock, seeing a low left ventricular end-diastolic diameter (LVEDD), a collapsed inferior vena cava, no evidence of pericardial effusion and normal LV systolic function confirms the diagnosis, rules out other potential diagnoses (such as cardiac tamponade) and provides direct evidence of response to therapy (increasing LVEDD with fluid transfusion).

- Stroke volume can be followed with serial measurements of the aortic velocity–time integral.
- For cardiogenic shock due to cardiomyopathy, evidence of poor LV systolic function will be present, and inotropic/vasopressor support can be dynamically titrated to the echocardiographic results in addition to standard resuscitative endpoints, such as improving mental status, raised blood pressure and increasing urine output.

Vasoactive support :

- For many shock states, the vasoactive agent of choice is noradrenaline (norepinephrine), since it has both α- and β1-agonist activity and can theoretically limit the reduction in cardiac output caused by pure α-agonists such as phenylephrine.
- Dopamine is not recommended as a first-line agent since it does not reduce renal failure and is associated with a significant incidence of dysrhythmias.
- Adrenaline (epinephrine) is an effective inotropic agent, but it is associated with an increase in blood lactate concentrations, even when cardiac output is normal. This can confound the assessment of response to therapy in many shock states, and is therefore recommended only as a second-line agent.
- Dobutamine is useful in cardiogenic shock due to cardiomyopathy.

Vasoactive agents are discussed more fully in their own chapter.

Intra-aortic balloon pump support used to be recommended for many types of cardiogenic shock, such as acute myocardial infarction. However, evidence from a large randomized clinical trial published in 2012 suggests that there is no mortality benefit to this intervention [4].

Anaphylactic shock

In anaphylactic shock the trigger stimulus causes release of histamine, serotonin, tryptase, leukotrienes, prostaglandins, kinins and other vasoactive materials, mainly from mast cells. These substances act primarily on smooth muscle, leading to peripheral and airway edema (stridor may not appear until 80% of the airway is obstructed), bronchospasm, vasodilatation and capillary leakage. Some of the mediators may also act directly on the myocardium. Management includes:

- Withdrawing the trigger stimulus, and then basic life support and cardiopulmonary resuscitation (CPR).
- Oxygen therapy.
- Laryngeal edema may require intubation or cricothyrotomy or may settle with nebulized adrenaline in less severe reactions.
- IV fluids should be administered to restore plasma volume at an initial dose of 20 mL/kg.
- **The agent of choice in severe reactions is adrenaline (epinephrine).** The initial dose should be given IM if no IV access is yet available. Infusions may be required after the initial treatment, especially following reactions to agents with a long elimination half-life. In addition to its beneficial cardiac effects it is a specific antidote, as it blocks mediator release from mast cells.

- Antihistamines are given as a second-line treatment after initial resuscitation. The evidence supporting antihistamines in anaphylaxis is weak, but logical reasons exist to give them. Agents of choice include chlorphenamine or diphenhydramine. Using H_2-antagonists such as ranitidine is no longer recommended.
- Steroids such as hydrocortisone are usually administered after the initial resuscitation, but take several hours to have an effect.
- Inhaled salbutamol may help to treat bronchospasm.

References

1. Vincent JL, De Backer D. Circulatory shock. *N Engl J Med* 2013; 369 : 1726–34.

2. Rivers E, Nguyen B, Havstad S *et al.* Early goal-directed therapy in the treatment of severe sepsis and septic shock. *N Engl J Med* 2001; 345 : 1368–77.

3. Walley KR. Use of central venous oxygen saturation to guide therapy. *Am J Respir Crit Care Med* 2011; 184 : 514–20.

4. Thiele H, Zeymer U, Neumann FJ *et al.* Intraaortic balloon support for myocardial infarction with cardiogenic shock. *N Engl J Med* 2012; 367 : 1287–96.

Oxygen therapy

3

Ahmed F Hegazy and Ian McConachie

"Oxygen lack not only stops the machine but wrecks the machinery"
JS Haldane (1860–1936)

Oxygen is the molecule of life. A vast array of intensive care interventions aim to improve oxygen delivery to end-organs. In this chapter, we focus on oxygen delivery to the lungs, the various oxygen delivery devices (in non-intubated patients), and some of the side effects of oxygen therapy. Long-term oxygen therapy is beyond the scope of this chapter.

In simple terms, the amount of oxygen transferred from the lungs into the blood stream can be increased in one of two ways:

- Increasing the inspired oxygen concentration (FiO_2)
- Increasing the mean airway pressure.

Increases in mean airway pressure can be achieved by:

- Increasing tidal volume (but high tidal volumes can be detrimental, as discussed in other chapters in this text).
- Lengthening the I:E ratio
- Adding or increasing positive end-expiratory pressure (PEEP).

Increasing PEEP is arguably the best way to increase mean airway pressure, especially in view of the other beneficial effects of PEEP.

Inspired oxygen concentrations can also be easily manipulated by changing the FiO_2 on the ventilator or by using different oxygen delivery devices. Knowledge of certain physiologic principles, oxygen delivery devices and pathological conditions that may impair oxygen delivery is paramount.

Physiology and pathology

At the cellular level, oxygen is required by mitochondria for the aerobic formation of ATP. Before reaching the mitochondria, however, oxygen needs to cross multiple barriers and exist in different phases. Dry atmospheric air at sea level has an oxygen partial pressure (PO_2) of 159 mmHg. After passing through the alveoli, arterial blood, capillary circulation and the interstitium, it eventually reaches the mitochondria with a PO_2 of 4 to 22 mmHg. This series of partial pressure reductions is called the oxygen cascade. Administering higher inspired oxygen concentrations aims at preventing tissue hypoxia, although this may be only one of a myriad of interventions necessary to achieve this goal.

Handbook of ICU Therapy, third edition, ed. John Fuller, Jeff Granton and Ian McConachie. Published by Cambridge University Press. © Cambridge University Press 2015.

Hypoxia can be detrimental at both the tissue and organ system levels. The brain seems to be the most vulnerable organ to the effects of acute hypoxia. Acute reductions in arterial oxyhemogblobin saturation, to values below 80%, can cause confusion and agitation, even in healthy subjects. At the tissue level, lack of oxygen delivery can lead to the anaerobic formation of ATP, a process that involves the generation of lactic acid and may lead to metabolic acidosis.

Causes of tissue hypoxia can be classified into four main categories:

1. **Hypoxemic hypoxia** results from low levels of dissolved oxygen in the blood. Low inspired oxygen concentrations (e.g. at high altitudes), respiratory failure and V/Q shunts can all cause hypoxemic hypoxia.

2. **Anemic hypoxia** is usually caused by low hemoglobin levels limiting the amount of chemically bound oxygen that can be delivered to the tissues. Carbon monoxide poisoning can also reduce the amounts of hemoglobin able to carry oxygen to the tissues leading to a form of anemic hypoxia.

3. **Stagnant hypoxia** occurs when the oxygen content of blood is normal, but lack of adequate blood flow results in decreased oxygen delivery. This can be regional (e.g. secondary to peripheral vascular disease) or global (in cases of low cardiac output).

4. **Histotoxic hypoxia** occurs when oxygen delivery is normal, but the cellular organelles and mitochondria are unable to utilize oxygen normally. Cyanide poisoning is the classical example of this form of hypoxia.

Delivery devices

As with most drugs, oxygen administration requires titration. Prolonged periods of excessive oxygen administration can be detrimental. Titrating oxygen therapy to an SpO_2 of 94 to 98% is recommended in the general ICU population [1]. Certain patient populations, however, require different target ranges, as discussed later.

During normal tidal breathing, peak inspiratory flow rates can be as high as 60 L/min. At times of respiratory distress, however, flow rates exceeding 100 L/min are commonly encountered. The amount of oxygen delivered to the trachea with various oxygen delivery devices depends on the patient's peak inspiratory flow rate and the flow capacity of the device. If device flow rates are lower than the patient's peak inspiratory flow, air will be entrained into the trachea, diluting the delivered oxygen. Using high-flow masks, adding a reservoir bag and delivering oxygen with a mask seal (e.g. CPAP masks) are all ways with which delivered oxygen concentrations can be increased.

Nasal cannulae

Oxygen concentrations delivered by nasal cannulae depend on the set oxygen flow rate and the patient's own inspiratory flows. As a general approximation, each increase in the oxygen flow rate by 1 L/min, will increase the FiO_2 by around 4% above room air. An oxygen flow rate of 6 L/min will deliver the maximal FiO_2 achievable by nasal prongs, usually in the range of 40 to 50%. Nasal prongs are very well tolerated by patients and are therefore more likely to be kept on. Flow rates in excess of 4–5 L/min can, however, cause nasal dryness, irritation and discomfort, and should generally be avoided.

Simple face masks

Side holes in simple face masks allow entrainment of air with high inspiratory flow rates leading to variable delivered FiO_2. Increasing oxygen flows from 5 to 10 L/min will raise the delivered oxygen concentrations from approximately 40 to 60%. It is not recommended to reduce oxygen flows below 5 L/min while using simple face masks, as low flows will not effectively flush CO_2 from the mask and rebreathing might result.

Venturi masks

Specific air entrainment (Venturi) adapters can deliver oxygen concentrations ranging from 24 to 50% with fair accuracy. These adapters are designed to entrain air with a specific ratio to maintain a constant FiO_2. Increasing oxygen flows will entrain more air and increase the total delivered gas flow without altering oxygen concentrations. Increased minute ventilation or hyperventilation will decrease the oxygen concentration delivered to the trachea [2]. Venturi masks are useful when precisely controlled, low-concentration oxygen supplementation is required, e.g. in COPD patients.

Non-rebreathing masks

Non-rebreathing masks are equipped with a reservoir bag that is continuously being filled with the oxygen supply. When patients inhale they draw on the high oxygen content of the reservoir bag. A one-way valve situated at the bag's entrance prevents exhaled CO_2 from entering. Oxygen flows of 10 to 15 L/min are required to maintain bag inflation. Non-rebreathing masks are capable of delivering oxygen concentrations in the range of 60 to 90%.

Tracheostomy masks

As their name implies, these allow supplemental oxygen delivery to spontaneously breathing patients with a tracheostomy. The delivered oxygen bypasses the upper airway and so humidification is preferable with any prolonged use. Oxygen flows are usually adjusted to achieve target oxyhemoglobin saturation ranges.

Continuous positive airway pressure (CPAP) masks

Continuous positive airway pressure masks improve oxygenation through two mechanisms: by increasing the mean airway pressures and by reliably delivering high FiO_2s. A tight-fitting full-face mask or nasal mask can be used and a fixed level of continuous positive airway pressure and FiO_2 are prescribed. In the expiratory phase, airway pressures are not allowed to return to baseline, in a manner very similar to PEEP, with invasive mechanical ventilation and EPAP (expiratory positive airway pressure) with noninvasive ventilation.

- This increases the functional residual capacity and helps recruit more alveoli for gas exchange.
- Other beneficial effects of CPAP include reducing the work of breathing, relief of dynamic upper airway obstruction, decreasing preload and afterload, and decreasing the pulmonary vascular resistance [3].

Continuous positive airway pressure is indicated in the treatment of hypoxemia secondary to obstructive sleep apnea and acute heart failure. If patients present with significant hypercapnia, however, noninvasive ventilation might be a better option. Other situations where CPAP may be beneficial include respiratory failure secondary to splinting following major abdominal surgery and in cases of chest-wall trauma. It should be noted, however, that some people will not tolerate the tight-fitting mask and that prolonged application might lead to local pressure effects on the nasal bridge.

Oxygen therapy in specific illnesses

Supplemental oxygen should be administered with caution to certain patient populations.

Chronic obstructive pulmonary disease (COPD)

Patients at risk for hypercapnic respiratory failure, e.g. those with COPD (but also patients with chronic neuromuscular disease or obesity hypoventilation syndrome) may exhibit a further rise in their arterial CO_2 levels with excessive oxygen therapy [1].

- In the past, this was thought to be largely the result of an improvement in arterial oxygenation causing a reduction in the hypoxic ventilatory drive.
- More recently however, it has been demonstrated that worsening ventilation perfusion (V/Q) mismatching is likely the main reason for this phenomenon. The observed V/Q mismatch might be secondary to an exaggerated release of hypoxic pulmonary vasoconstriction when high-flow supplemental oxygen is administered. This in turn might cause a maldistribution of pulmonary blood flow, leading to an overall increase in alveolar dead space and a rise in arterial CO_2.
- Oxygen-induced reduction of hypoxic drive and the Haldane effect (increased ability of deoxygenated hemoglobin to carry CO_2) in COPD may also play a role in increasing arterial CO_2 in these patients, though their contribution is likely not as significant as previously thought [4].
- Patients presenting with acute exacerbations of COPD will have significantly increased work of breathing. It is important to recognize that an increase in arterial pCO_2 may represent fatigue and impending respiratory arrest.

In patients presenting with acute COPD exacerbations, current guidelines suggest initiating oxygen therapy with a 24% Venturi mask at an O_2 flow of 4 L/min if they are not in extremis [1]. Aiming for a target arterial oxyhemoglobin saturation in the range of 88–92% is recommended with frequent clinical, blood gas and oxyhemoglobin saturation monitor assessment. In a prehospital, paramedic randomized study of COPD patients, controlled oxygen therapy was associated with significantly improved survival overall, compared to noncontrolled, high-flow oxygen therapy [5].

Patients with COPD presenting critically ill or in peri-arrest conditions, however, should receive much higher levels of supplemental O_2 aiming for higher saturations during their initial resuscitation phase. In these situations, invasive or noninvasive ventilation maybe indicated. Once more stable, oxygen titration to lower oxyhemoglobin saturation targets (88–92%) should be resumed. It is important to note that profound hypoxemia is a more imminent threat to life than hypercapnia, and that the effects of prolonged severe hypoxia can be much more devastating in the critically ill.

Acute coronary syndromes

Classically, oxygen therapy has been a first-line treatment for patients presenting with an acute coronary syndrome. Although this makes sense in the setting of myocardial ischemia, it has been recently suggested that there may be no benefit and a potential for harm with this practice. Routine oxygen administration has been associated with increased infarct size, likely secondary to coronary vasoconstriction [6]. This is still controversial and further, ongoing studies are eagerly awaited [7]. At present, patients presenting with an acute coronary syndrome should not be given supplemental oxygen unless hypoxic.

Acute stroke

A similar controversy exists regarding oxygen therapy in acute stroke with, again, studies suggesting a potential worse outcome when oxygen therapy is routinely administered [8].

Shock

Oxygen administration has long been advocated during the treatment of shocked patients. There is some evidence from animal studies that 100% oxygen during treatment of hemorrhagic shock maintains blood pressure and prolongs survival compared to controls [9]. It is thought that oxygen inhalation may reduce the work of breathing in shocked patients – certainly increased work of breathing may cause diaphragmatic fatigue and animal studies suggest that respiratory arrest may be the mode of dying in shocked patients [10].

Cardiac arrest

Hyperoxia has long been known to be detrimental during neonatal resuscitation (see below for adverse ocular effects), but recently it has been suggested that hyperoxia may also result in worse outcomes following resuscitation after adult cardiac arrest [11]. This is likely secondary to increases in reactive oxygen species during brain reperfusion.

Hazards of oxygen therapy

Oxygen therapy is not without risk. In general, the potential hazards of oxygen therapy include its biologic toxic effects and its potential for physical hazards, e.g. fires. Excessive oxygen administration has been associated with adverse effects involving several organ systems.

Central nervous system (CNS)

Exposure to hyperbaric oxygen at more than 2 atmospheres of pressure may cause generalized tonic-clonic (grand mal) seizures. This is the Paul Bert effect – first described in the nineteenth century. Higher oxygen pressures can induce seizures with shorter durations of exposure. This side effect constitutes the main limitation to increasing oxygen pressures in hyperbaric chambers [12]. The mechanism by which hyperbaric oxygen induces seizures is unclear. Other CNS manifestations of oxygen toxicity include dizziness, nausea, headaches, disorientation, tinnitus, paresthesias and facial twitching.

Ocular

Neonatal exposure to high oxygen concentrations can lead to retinopathy of prematurity (ROP). The risk seems to be greatest in the premature and continues up to 44 weeks of post-conceptual age. Oxygen therapy in neonates at risk should therefore be very tightly controlled and their saturations should never be allowed to exceed 95%. The mechanism for development of ROP in the immature retina seems to be related to hyperoxia-induced retinal vasoconstriction, followed by abnormal vasoproliferation. In its most severe forms, it could result in retinal detachment and blindness.

Pulmonary

Hyperoxia-induced lung injury has long been recognized as a major limitation to the liberal administration of oxygen in the world of critical care. Breathing 100% oxygen over prolonged periods of time can adversely affect the entire respiratory tract.

- Atelectasis is increased due to denitrogenation and alveolar absorption.
- Acute tracheobronchitis may be the earliest manifestation of oxygen toxicity, generally appearing after 4 to 22 hours of breathing 100% oxygen at one atmospheric pressure.
- Diffuse alveolar damage (DAD) develops soon thereafter, starting after 48 hours of inspiring FiO$_2$s greater than 60%.
- With prolonged hyperoxia, ARDS-like changes are observed at the alveolar level and capillary endothelial damage takes place resulting in interstitial edema.
- The long-term effects of oxygen toxicity are similar to those of ARDS with pulmonary fibrosis, emphysema and worsening gas exchange being the end-result.
- Retrospective studies suggest that survivors of ARDS who received more than 24 hours of an inspired oxygen concentration >60%, may have worsened lung diffusion capacity at 1 year follow-up [13].

The toxic effects of hyperoxia are thought to be related to the formation of reactive oxygen species (ROS) that are in excess of the capacity of the endogenous detoxifying enzyme systems. These oxygen free radicals injure cell structures at multiple levels. Cell membranes, mitochondria and other organelles seem to sustain damage with prolonged hyperoxia. Animal studies suggest that it is possible that tolerance to these ROS may occur because of increases in superoxide dismutase activity and/or administration of antioxidants.

To avoid pulmonary oxygen toxicity, it is important for the clinician to try to minimize any time periods during which patients are exposed to FiO$_2$s greater than 50%. Increasing PEEP or changing ventilation strategies could be of value in reducing FiO2s to more acceptable levels.

Drug-induced potentiation of pulmonary oxygen toxicity

Some chemotherapy agents – the classic example being bleomycin – enhance pulmonary oxygen toxicity. The mechanisms for bleomycin-induced pulmonary oxygen toxicity are unclear, but may include oxidative damage, inflammatory responses and, possibly, a genetic predisposition. Interestingly, there are reports of delayed bleomycin-induced pulmonary oxygen toxicity after chemotherapy has ceased [14]. There are no randomized trials in this area and, thus, there is no known maximum "safe" level of inspired oxygen in these patients. It is generally advised, however, to reduce the FiO$_2$ to the lowest level that will maintain an SpO$_2$ in the range of 88 to 92% when providing care for these patients.

Other chemotherapy agents may have similar effects, but there is less evidence for these, apart from animal studies. Other drugs, e.g. amiodarone, are known to cause pulmonary toxicity, but via other mechanisms.

Permissive hypoxemia

It is questionable whether traditional oxygenation targets are appropriate for all critically ill patients. Some authorities propose individualizing oxygenation targets such that lower arterial pO_2 may be appropriate in selected patients. This is known as permissive hypoxemia [15]. This concept stems partly from the potential for harm with hyperoxia, excessively high ventilator pressures and high FiO_2s. Moreover, we still lack the understanding of what exactly constitutes optimum arterial pO_2 in critically ill patients. Permissive hypoxemia as a concept still requires further study.

Key points

- Acute hypoxia can be very detrimental and its immediate treatment should never be delayed out of fear of the harmful effects of oxygen therapy.
- Certain aspects of oxygen delivery devices will dictate how suitable they are for the situation. Their use to target specific oxyhemoglobin saturation ranges is recommended.
- An oxyhemoglobin saturation of 94 to 98% might be reasonable for most patients. Lower targets are indicated, however, for those at risk for hypercapnic respiratory failure.
- After patient stabilization, it is important to limit the FiO_2 administered to avoid oxygen-induced pulmonary toxicity.

References

1. O'Driscoll BR, Howard LS, Davison AG. BTS guideline for emergency oxygen use in adult patients. *Thorax* 2008; 63 Suppl 6 : vi1–68.

2. Gibson RL, Comer PB, Beckham RW, Mcgraw CP. Actual tracheal oxygen concentrations with commonly used oxygen equipment. *Anesthesiology* 1976; 44: 73

3. British Thoracic Society Standards of Care Committee. Non-invasive ventilation in acute respiratory failure. *Thorax* 2002; 57 : 192–211.

4. Budinger GR, Mutlu GM. Balancing the risks and benefits of oxygen therapy in critically ill adults. *Chest* 2013; 143 : 1151–62.

5. Austin MA, Wills KE, Blizzard L et al. Effect of high flow oxygen on mortality in chronic obstructive pulmonary disease patients in prehospital setting: randomised controlled trial. *BMJ* 2010; 341 : c5462.

6. Wijesinghe M, Perrin K, Ranchord A, et al. Routine use of oxygen in the treatment of myocardial infarction: systematic review. *Heart* 2009; 95: 198–202.

7. Stub D, Smith K, Bernard S et al. A randomized controlled trial of oxygen therapy in acute myocardial infarction Air Verses Oxygen In myocarDial infarction study (AVOID Study). *Am Heart J* 2012; 163 : 339–345.

8. Rønning OM, Guldvog B: Should stroke victims routinely receive supplemental oxygen? A quasi-randomized controlled trial. *Stroke* 1999; 30 : 2033–2037.

9. Bitterman H, Reissman P, Bitterman N et al. Oxygen therapy in hemorrhagic shock. *Circ Shock.* 1991; 33 : 183–91.

10. Aubier M, Trippenbach T, Roussos C. Respiratory muscle fatigue during cardiogenic shock. *J Appl Physiol Respir Environ Exerc Physiol* 1981; 51 : 499–508.

11. Kilgannon JH, Jones AE, Shapiro NI et al; Emergency Medicine Shock Research Network (EMShockNet) Investigators. Association between arterial hyperoxia following resuscitation from cardiac arrest and in-hospital mortality. *JAMA* 2010; 303 : 2165–2171.

12. Bitterman H. Bench-to-bedside review: oxygen as a drug. *Crit Care* 2009; 13(1) : 205.

13. Elliott CG, Rasmusson BY, Crapo RO *et al.* Prediction of pulmonary function abnormalities after adult respiratory distress syndrome (ARDS). *Am Rev Respir Dis* 1987; 135 : 634–8.

14. Gilson AJ, Sahn SA. Reactivation of bleomycin lung toxicity following oxygen administration: a second response to corticosteroids. *Chest* 1985; 88 : 304–6.

15. Martin DS, Grocott MP. Oxygen therapy in critical illness: precise control of arterial oxygenation and permissive hypoxemia. *Crit Care Med* 2013; 41 : 423–32.

Chapter

4

Central venous access

Ken Blonde and Robert Arntfield

Over 5 million central venous catheters (CVCs) are inserted in the United States each year and many of these are either inserted or cared for in the intensive care setting [1].

Indications

Typical indications for CVCs include:

- Hemodynamic monitoring
- Large volume fluid resuscitation
- Infusion of vasoactive drugs
- Total parenteral nutrition (TPN)
- Renal replacement therapy
- Failure to achieve peripheral access
- Transvenous pacing.

Insertion sites

The most common sites for CVC insertion are:

- Internal jugular vein (IJV)
- Subclavian vein (SV)
- Femoral vein (FV)
- Upper extremity veins (basilic, cephalic, brachial) for peripherally inserted central catheter (PICC).

The skilled clinician possesses knowledge of each site and its advantages, disadvantages and clinical scenarios that may favor one site over another.

Catheter characteristics

Many different catheters are available for use in the ICU. Variation in catheter characteristics allows for the selection of the most appropriate CVC for a given clinical condition. These characteristics are:

- Length: shorter catheters allow more rapid rates of infusion. Longer catheters are more appropriate for certain anatomical sites such as upper extremity veins (PICC) and the femoral site.

Handbook of ICU Therapy, third edition, ed. John Fuller, Jeff Granton and Ian McConachie. Published by Cambridge University Press. © Cambridge University Press 2015.

- Gauge: catheters with larger diameters allow more rapid rates of infusion. In the traditional French system, higher French catheters are wider (1 F = 1/3 mm).
- Number of lumens: single lumen catheters typically allow more rapid infusion rates, making them ideal for large-volume resuscitations. Multilumen catheters can be used for the multiple, simultaneous infusions frequently required in those with multiple organ failures.

For initial resuscitation of a critically ill patient, a large gauge, short, single-lumen catheter is therefore often the most appropriate CVC.

Insertion technique

In 1953 Dr. Sven Seldinger first described his now universal method of vascular access utilizing catheter-over-guidewire exchange [2]. Application of Seldinger's technique for CVC insertion traditionally relies on established anatomical landmarks for procedural guidance. The landmark method is limited by uncertainty of the underlying anatomy; the IJV, for instance, does not follow traditional landmarks in up to 10–20% of patients [3,4]. This uncertainty reduces the likelihood of success and increases the chance of complications. This has led to the rise of ultrasound (US) guidance for the insertion of CVCs.

Three meta-analyses have demonstrated the superiority of real-time ultrasound-guided insertion over the landmark method in CVC insertion [5–7]. Although the majority of the studies included in the most recent meta-analysis were looking at the IJV, there was still benefit for US guidance in SCV and FV.

Established advantages of US for CVC include [7]:

- Reduction in cannulation failure
- Fewer arterial punctures
- Reduced rates of hematomas
- Reduced rates of pneumothorax
- Reduced rates of hemothorax.

Other studies have shown that US guidance can also reduce time to cannulation and the number of punctures required for IJV insertion [8]. Although the benefits of US guidance are less robust in SCV and FV, there are prospective, randomized data demonstrating improved performance for these sites as well [9,10].

On the strength of this evidence, many professional society guidelines have formally endorsed ultrasound for CVC insertion [11–13]. In the hands of an appropriately trained operator, most CVC insertions should take place under ultrasound guidance.

Complications of CVCs

Adverse events may occur from the insertion and maintenance of a CVC; these can lead to increased morbidity, mortality, length of hospitalization and cost. Knowledge of the important complications of CVCs will allow for their prompt recognition and management when they occur. Major complications of CVCs are mechanical, infectious and thrombotic and are summarized in Table 4.1.

Table 4.1 Major complications and associated risk factors for central venous catheterization. Percentages indicate estimated incidence of the complication [7,14–20]. CRBSI = Catheter-related bloodstream infection; BMI = body mass index; VTE = venous thromboembolism.

	Risk factors
Mechanical (1–19%)	
Arterial puncture	Inexperience
Pneumothorax	Multiple attempts at cannulation
Hematoma	Failure to use ultrasound guidance
Hemothorax	Hypovolemia
Catheter misplacement	Previous radiation, scar or surgery
Arrhythmia	Previous central venous catheters
Wire embolism	Coagulopathy
AV fistula	Very low or very high BMI
Infectious (1.5–25%)	
CRBSI	Prolonged catheter use
Catheter colonization	Multilumen catheters
Local infection	Femoral vein catheters
	Failure to use full sterile insertion technique
	Hemodialysis catheters
Thrombotic (6.5–21.5%)	
Deep-vein thrombosis	History of VTE
Vascular stenosis	Malignancy
Pulmonary embolism	Incorrect catheter placement
	Large gauge catheters
	Multiple attempts at cannulation
	Infection
	Multiple lumens
	Femoral vein catheter

Mechanical CVC complications

Catheter misplacement

Central venous catheters should be positioned parallel to the long axis of a large central vein (IVC or SVC, depending on site chosen) as close to the right atrium as possible [18].

- A chest X-ray can confirm CVC positioning if the catheter tip is seen at the level of the carina, although this method has some limitations [21].
- Misplacement of the catheter can increase the risk of complications; placing the catheter too high can lead to increased risk of thrombosis, whereas placement too far into the right atrium can lead to arrhythmias and the often feared cardiac puncture and tamponade [18,22,23].
- The true incidence of cardiac tamponade from CVC is unknown since it is an extremely rare event limited to case series where the reported mortality is as high as 100% [24]. With modern use of soft-tipped catheters, the actual risk of cardiac tamponade is very small, and efforts to ensure correct catheter placement may reduce this risk even further [25].

A CVC placed in the correct position should allow for easy withdrawal of nonpulsatile venous blood through all catheter lumens. Transduction will demonstrate normal venous waveforms and pressures. If concern for arterial placement exists, advanced imaging and consultation with a vascular specialist should be considered.

Arterial puncture and hematoma

Arterial puncture can produce significant bleeding, hematoma, patient discomfort, AV fistulas or pseudoaneurysms.

- A recent meta-analysis found that the overall incidence of arterial puncture in CVC insertion was 5.7%, although this varied considerably by anatomic site [7].
- Arterial puncture is more common in IJV and FV catheterization than SCV.
- Punctures can be reduced with the use of ultrasound and decreasing the number of cannulation attempts [7].
- Arterial puncture should be suspected on the basis of aspiration of bright red pulsatile blood.
- Basic management includes withdrawal of the needle and application of firm pressure to the affected area. Fortunately the carotid and femoral arteries are both readily compressible in the event of puncture and hematoma, although the subclavian artery is not.
- If the artery has been dilated and a catheter inserted, leave the catheter in place and consult with a vascular surgeon or interventional radiologist for appropriate management [15].

Pneumothorax

Pneumothorax, the introduction of air into the pleural space, is a frequent complication of CVC insertion with an incidence of 0–3% [7].

- It is more common with SV than IJV catheterization [17].
- Symptoms of pneumothorax include dyspnea, cough and pleuritic chest pain, but the patient may progress to obstructive shock.
- Aspiration of air into the finder needle during CVC insertion should raise suspicion of a pneumothorax.
- Like many mechanical complications, the incidence of pneumothorax is reduced with the use of US guidance and minimizing the number of cannulation attempts[7].
- In patients with severe respiratory failure it may be prudent to use an IJV or FV approach to minimize the risk of introducing a pneumothorax.
- Pneumothorax may be diagnosed on plain chest radiography, although there is a growing role for bedside thoracic ultrasound [26].

Thrombotic CVC complications
Catheter-related thrombosis

Catheter-related thrombosis (CRT) refers to venous thrombosis of a vein containing a catheter.

- CRTs occur in 6.5–21.5% of CVCs and they represent 70–80% of all upper extremity deep-venous thromboses (DVTs) [27].
- Many patients with CRT are asymptomatic, while others may present with local symptoms such as pain, swelling, redness and dilated superficial veins [20].
- Pulmonary embolism occurs in roughly 6% of CRTs of the upper extremity [27].
- The post-thrombotic syndrome of chronic limb pain, heaviness and swelling may occur as a consequence of CRT [28].
- In addition to thromboembolic events, CRT can also produce blocked catheters and may increase the risk of developing sepsis.

There are many identified risk factors for CRT, although the majority of studies were conducted in cancer patients with long-term CVC.

- The FV has the highest rate of CRT, while studies vary on the comparative rate of thrombosis between SCV and IJV [19,20,27].
- Left-sided IJV and SCV are more likely to develop CRT.
- Longer, larger catheters with multiple lumens are at an increased risk of CRT, particularly if they are not well placed near the IVC.
- Patient factors such as a history of venous thromboembolism (VTE), malignancy or thrombophilia all increase the risk of CRT [20,27].

Once suspected, the diagnosis of CRT can be made with the use of compression or Doppler ultrasonography. Management of CRT is largely extrapolated from studies of symptomatic lower-extremity DVT and depends on the degree of symptoms, catheter function and the need for ongoing central access.

- Routine catheter removal is not recommended; however, in the face of suspected sepsis, persistent symptomatic DVT, despite anticoagulation, or catheter failure, the CVC should be removed.
- Although practice patterns vary, a general recommendation for treatment would be initiation of therapeutic low-molecular-weight heparin transitioned to oral warfarin targeted to an International Normalized Ratio (INR) of 2–3 for a minimum of three months [27,29].

Preventing CRT with prophylactic systemic anticoagulation is an intuitive consideration for those with indwelling CVCs and has, in fact, been studied. At this time, however, there is insufficient evidence to support the routine use of warfarin, heparin or the novel oral anticoagulants for prevention of CRT [29,30].

Infectious CVC complications

Catheter-related infections

There are a variety of infectious complications associated with CVC including [31]:

- Catheter colonization: Growth of $\geq$15 colony-forming units (cfu) of a microorganism in a quantitative or semi-quantitative culture of a catheter tip, hub or subcutaneous segment.
- Exit-site infection: Exudate, tenderness and erythema at the catheter exit site or associated catheter tunnel or pocket.

- Catheter-related bloodstream infection (CRBSI): Bacteremia or fungemia in a patient with a catheter, a positive peripheral vein blood culture and no other suspected source for infection.

Of these, CRBSI is the most serious complication.

- Roughly 80 000 CVC-related bloodstream infections occur in American intensive care units every year.
- These infections have an estimated mortality of 12–25% and are associated with both increased cost and duration of hospitalization [31,32].

Microbiology of CRBSI

From most to least common, the typical organisms cultured in CRBSI are (33,34):

1. Coagulase-negative *Staphylococci*
2. *Staphylococcus aureus*, including methicillin-sensitive and methicillin-resistant species (MRSA). Roughly 50% of *S. aureus* isolates obtained in ICUs are MRSA.
3. *Candida* species, including *C. albicans, C. glabrata* and *C. kruseii*.
4. Enteric Gram-negative bacilli: *E. coli, K. pneumonia, P. aeruginosa, Enterobacter* species, *A. baumannii* and *Serratia* species.

Catheters can become infected from a variety of routes.

- Migration of skin flora along the catheter tract to the catheter tip is the most common method for acquiring CRBSI.
- Alternatively, direct contamination of the catheter may occur from non-sterile manipulation or hematogenous seeding from a distal source such as infective endocarditis, osteomyelitis or septic arthritis.

Diagnosis of CRBSI

Detailed guidelines for the diagnosis and management of CRBSI are available through the Infectious Diseases Society of America [31].

- In general, CRBSI should be suspected in any patient with a CVC who has signs or symptoms of infection.
- It is important to remember to draw blood cultures *before* the initiation of antibiotic therapy in order to maximize the chance of obtaining a positive culture for determining antimicrobial susceptibility.

A diagnosis of CRBSI can be made when the following criteria are met:

1. Signs or symptoms of infection
2. Positive peripheral vein-blood cultures
3. Cultures drawn through the catheter match the peripheral cultures and at least one of the following is present:
   - ≥15 cfu growth from cultured catheter tip
   - Simultaneous quantitative cultures from catheter and peripheral culture grow in a 3:1 ratio
   - Positive quantitative catheter culture 2 hours before peripheral culture.

Management of CRBSI

Antimicrobial coverage for CRBSI is usually initiated empirically. The choice of antibiotics will depend on your local resistance patterns, patient characteristics and disease severity, as well as cost and availability. Important considerations in the management of CRBSI include:

- **Catheter removal**: a CVC should be removed if it is no longer needed and if the patient has severe sepsis, endocarditis, or persistent bacteremia. CVCs should also be removed when the cultured organism is MRSA, *P. aeruginosa* or *Candida* species. A trial of systemic antibiotics without catheter removal is reasonable for certain long-term catheters, like dialysis lines and tunneled catheters for chemotherapy (31).
- **Antimicrobial selection**: for most patients in an intensive care setting, empiric antibiotic selection should cover for MRSA and the possibility of multidrug-resistant Gram-negative organisms. Reasonable choices would include vancomycin plus an antipseudomonal cephalosporin, carbapenem or a β-lactam/β-lactamase inhibitor combination [31].
- **Special populations**: patients receiving chemotherapy, dialysis, total parenteral nutrition or with a history of transplantation or immunosuppression are at risk for invasive fungal infections with *Candida* species. Treatment of CRBSI in this population should include an azole antifungal, unless there is a high local incidence of *C. glabrata*, in which case an echinocandin antifungal is preferred, due to increasing azole resistance [31].
- **Duration of treatment**: is determined by the pathogen isolated and clinical response to treatment, as well as potential complications of bacteremia. Uncomplicated coagulase-negative *Staphyloccocus* can be treated with 7 days of antibiotics if the catheter is removed. On the other hand, MRSA usually requires 4–6 weeks of therapy [31].
- **Hematogenous spread**: CRBSIs have the potential to seed multiple sites in the body, leading to endophthalmitis, endocarditis, septic arthritis or osteomyelitis. In one series, the incidence of infective endocarditis in patients with MRSA bacteremia was nearly 20% [35]. Careful physical exam and appropriate investigations can identify the complications of CRBSI.

Ultimately the management of CRBSI in the intensive care unit is a multidisciplinary task best tackled by combining the expertise of local microbiologists, infectious disease consultants and pharmacists.

Prevention of CRBSI

Given their high morbidity, mortality and cost, interventions to reduce the incidence of CRBSI have become a priority for many healthcare bodies. The United States Centers for Disease Control (CDC) publishes clinical guidelines on the prevention of intravascular catheter-related infections [34]. Fortunately, these interventions appear to be working, as a 2011 report from the CDC demonstrated a 58% reduction in CRBSI in American ICUs between 2001 and 2009 [32]. Effective preventative measures include:

- **Education**: a focused educational module about CRBSI for nurses and physicians in a community ICU resulted in a nearly 60% relative risk reduction of infection [36].
- **Access site**: the IJV and SCV have historically been associated with a reduced risk of infection when compared to the FV, although a recent meta-analysis would suggest that the overall risk with FV is not as high as previously reported [16,19].

- **Ultrasound guidance:** a randomized controlled trial comparing US-guided to landmark insertion of IJ CVC in critically ill patients showed a 5.6% absolute risk reduction in CRBSI with ultrasound [8].
- **Hand washing:** hand washing with soap and water or alcohol-based hand sanitizers before and after utilizing a CVC reduces rates of infection [34].
- **Full barrier precautions:** while inserting CVCs, maximum barrier precautions should be maintained with a cap, mask and sterile gloves, gown and full-body drape [37].
- **Chlorhexidine skin preparation:** sterilizing of skin with a >0.5% chlorhexidine solution prior to CVC insertion is superior to povidone-iodine [38].
- **Removing unnecessary catheters:** risk of infection increases with duration of catheterization, so prompt removal of CVCs when indicated is critical.

These interventions are most successful when applied together [39,40]. Continued success in reducing CRBSI will require ongoing quality control and application of evidence-based preventative initiatives to our intensive care units.

Summary

Central venous catheterization is an important and life-sustaining therapy in the modern intensive care unit. Consequently safe, skillful access of central veins and introduction of an appropriately selected catheter is a critical skill for any intensive care provider. Ultrasound guidance provides numerous advantages, with compelling evidence to support its use as the standard of care when accessible. Our increasing understanding and awareness of the major complications of CVCs have allowed us to develop effective strategies for mitigating the risk and/or managing the consequences of this invasive procedure.

References

1. Mermel LA, Farr BM, Sherertz RJ et al. Guidelines for the management of intravascular catheter-related infections. Clin Infect Dis 2001; 32 : 1249–1272.

2. Seldinger SI. Catheter replacement of the needle in percutaneous arteriography: a new technique. Acta Radiol 1953; 39 : 368–376.

3. Gordon AC, Saliken JC, Johns D et al. US-guided puncture of the internal jugular vein: complications and anatomic considerations. J Vasc Interv Radiol 1998; 9 : 333–338.

4. Maecken T, Marcon C, Bomas S et al. Relationship of the internal jugular vein to the common carotid artery: implications for ultrasound-guided vascular access. Eur J Anaesthesiol 2011; 28 : 351–355.

5. Randolph AG, Cook DJ, Gonzales CA, Pribble CG. Ultrasound guidance for placement of central venous catheters: a meta-analysis of the literature. Crit Care Med 1996; 24 : 2053–2058.

6. Hind D, Calvert N, McWilliams R et al. Ultrasonic locating devices for central venous cannulation: meta-analysis. BMJ 2003; 327 : 361.

7. Wu SY, Ling Q, Cao LH et al. Real-time two-dimensional ultrasound guidance for central venous cannulation: a meta-analysis. Anesthesiology 2013; 118 : 361–375.

8. Karakitsos D, Labropoulos N, De Groot E et al. Real-time ultrasound-guided catheterisation of the internal jugular vein: a prospective comparison with the landmark technique in critical care patients. Crit Care 2006; 10 : R162.

9. Prabhu MV, Juneja D, Gopal PB et al. Ultrasound-guided femoral dialysis access placement: a single-center randomized trial. Clin J Am Soc Nephrol 2010; 5: 235–239.

10. Fragou M, Gravvanis A, Dimitriou V *et al.* Real-time ultrasound-guided subclavian vein cannulation versus the landmark method in critical care patients: a prospective randomized study. *Crit Care Med* 2011; 39 : 1607–1612.

11. Troianos CA, Hartman GS, Glas KE *et al.* Guidelines for performing ultrasound guided vascular cannulation: recommendations of the American Society of Echocardiography and the Society of Cardiovascular Anesthesiologists. *J Am Soc Echocardiogr* 2011; 24 : 1291–1318.

12. Lamperti M, Bodenham AR, Pittiruti M *et al.* International evidence-based recommendations on ultrasound-guided vascular access. *Intensive Care Med* 2012; 38 : 1105–1117.

13. National Institute for Clinical Excellence. Technology Appraisal No 49. Guidance on the use of ultrasonic locating devices for placing central venous catheters. 2005; Available at: http://www.nice.org.uk/ nicemedia/pdf/ Ultrasound_49_GUIDANCE.pdf (accessed April 20, 2013).

14. O'Grady NP, Alexander M, Dellinger EP *et al.* Guidelines for the prevention of intravascular catheter-related infections. Centers for Disease Control and Prevention. *MMWR Recomm Rep* 2002; 51 : 1–29.

15. Kusminsky RE. Complications of central venous catheterization. *J Am Coll Surg* 2007; 204 : 681–696.

16. Marik PE, Flemmer M, Harrison W. The risk of catheter-related bloodstream infection with femoral venous catheters as compared to subclavian and internal jugular venous catheters: a systematic review of the literature and meta-analysis. *Crit Care Med* 2012; 40 : 2479–2485.

17. McGee DC, Gould MK. Preventing complications of central venous catheterization. *N Engl J Med* 2003; 348 : 1123–1133.

18. Gibson F, Bodenham A. Misplaced central venous catheters: applied anatomy and practical management. *Br J Anaesth* 2013; 110 : 333–346.

19. Ge X, Cavallazzi R, Li C, Pan SM, Wang YW, Wang FL. Central venous access sites for the prevention of venous thrombosis, stenosis and infection. *Cochrane Database Syst Rev* 2012; 3 : CD004084.

20. Lee AY, Kamphuisen PW. Epidemiology and prevention of catheter-related thrombosis in patients with cancer. *J Thromb Haemost* 2012; 10 : 1491–1499.

21. Albrecht K, Nave H, Breitmeier D *et al.* Applied anatomy of the superior vena cava-the carina as a landmark to guide central venous catheter placement. *Br J Anaesth* 2004; 92 : 75–77.

22. Boersma RS, Jie KS, Verbon A *et al.* Thrombotic and infectious complications of central venous catheters in patients with hematological malignancies. *Ann Oncol* 2008; 19 : 433–442.

23. Cadman A, Lawrance JA, Fitzsimmons L *et al.* To clot or not to clot? That is the question in central venous catheters. *Clin Radiol* 2004; 59 : 349–355.

24. Collier PE, Blocker SH, Graff DM, Doyle P. Cardiac tamponade from central venous catheters. *Am J Surg* 1998; 176 : 212–214.

25. Shamir MY, Bruce LJ. Central venous catheter-induced cardiac tamponade: a preventable complication. *Anesth Analg* 2011; 112 : 1280–1282.

26. Rowan KR, Kirkpatrick AW, Liu D *et al.* Traumatic pneumothorax detection with thoracic US: correlation with chest radiography and CT–initial experience. *Radiology* 2002; 225 : 210–214.

27. Kucher N. Clinical practice. Deep-vein thrombosis of the upper extremities. *N Engl J Med* 2011; 364 : 861–869.

28. Elman EE, Kahn SR. The post-thrombotic syndrome after upper extremity deep venous thrombosis in adults: a systematic review. *Thromb Res* 2006; 117 : 609–614.

29. Kearon C, Akl EA, Comerota AJ *et al.* Antithrombotic therapy for VTE disease: Antithrombotic Therapy and Prevention of Thrombosis, 9th ed: American College of Chest Physicians Evidence-Based Clinical Practice Guidelines. *Chest* 2012; 141 : e419S–94S.

30. Akl EA, Vasireddi SR, Gunukula S *et al.*
Anticoagulation for patients with cancer
and central venous catheters. *Cochrane
Database Syst Rev* 2011; 16 : CD006468.

31. Mermel LA, Allon M, Bouza E *et al.*
Clinical practice guidelines for the
diagnosis and management of intravascular
catheter-related infection: 2009 Update by
the Infectious Diseases Society of America.
Clin Infect Dis 2009; 49 : 1–45.

32. Centers for Disease Control and Prevention
(CDC). Vital signs: central line-associated
blood stream infections – United States,
2001, 2008, and 2009. *MMWR Morb
Mortal Wkly Rep* 2011; 60 : 243–248.

33. Wisplinghoff H, Bischoff T, Tallent SM
et al. Nosocomial bloodstream infections in
US hospitals: analysis of 24,179 cases from
a prospective nationwide surveillance
study. *Clin Infect Dis* 2004; 39 : 309–317.

34. O'Grady NP, Alexander M, Burns LA *et al.*
Guidelines for the prevention of
intravascular catheter-related infections.
Clin Infect Dis 2011; 52 : e162–193.

35. Abraham J, Mansour C, Veledar E *et al.*
Staphylococcus aureus bacteremia
and endocarditis: the Grady
Memorial Hospital experience with
methicillin-sensitive *S aureus* and
methicillin-resistant *S aureus* bacteremia.
Am Heart J 2004; 147 : 536–539.

36. Warren DK, Zack JE, Cox MJ *et al.* An
educational intervention to prevent
catheter-associated bloodstream infections
in a nonteaching, community medical
center. *Crit Care Med* 2003; 31 : 1959–1963.

37. Raad II, Hohn DC, Gilbreath BJ *et al.*
Prevention of central venous catheter-
related infections by using maximal sterile
barrier precautions during insertion. *Infect
Control Hosp Epidemiol* 1994; 5 : 231–238.

38. Mimoz O, Pieroni L, Lawrence C *et al.*
Prospective, randomized trial of two
antiseptic solutions for prevention of
central venous or arterial catheter
colonization and infection in intensive care
unit patients. *Crit Care Med* 1996; 24 :
1818–1823.

39. Pronovost P, Needham D, Berenholtz S
et al. An intervention to decrease catheter-
related bloodstream infections in the ICU.
N Engl J Med 2006; 355 : 2725–2732.

40. Marsteller JA, Sexton JB, Hsu YJ *et al.*
A multicenter, phased, cluster-randomized
controlled trial to reduce central line-
associated bloodstream infections in
intensive care units. *Crit Care Med* 2012;
40 : 2933–2939.

Chapter 5

Fluid therapy in ICU

Janet Martin, John Fuller and Ian McConachie

Maintenance of appropriate hydration and electrolyte composition is essential in ICU and surgery patients. However, the ideal balance between under- and overhydration remains poorly understood across patient scenarios:

- "Volume loading" may be important for cardiovascular management and remains a cornerstone for selected surgical and trauma patients.
- Conversely, bolus challenges and "positive fluid balance" may contribute to poor clinical outcomes in ICU and surgical patients.

Decisions to initiate, maintain and discontinue IV fluids requires careful assessment to minimize risk of:

- Insufficient or excess administration of fluids
- Electrolyte abnormalities such as hypo- or hypernatremia, hypo- or hyperkalemia and hyperchloremic acidosis.

Consequences of fluid mismanagement may include:

- Organ dysfunction, such as renal dysfunction (and risk of renal replacement therapy), pulmonary edema (reduced oxygenation, risk of pneumonia), cardiac arrhythmias and ischemia (and risk of myocardial infarction and heart failure), reduced GI function (and risk of ileus), neurologic decline (decreased consciousness, coma) and increased risk of death.
- Peripheral and sacral pitting edema (reduced tissue oxygenation; potential for skin-related ulceration) if extracellular fluid is expanded by 2–3 L.

Body fluid compartments

- Water comprises approximately 60% of body weight (2/3 intracellular fluid and 1/3 extracellular fluid).
- Extracellular fluid is mainly interstitial fluid, with only 15–20% consisting of blood and plasma.
- Critically ill patients may experience "leaky vasculature" with increased extracellular fluid and edema.

Type of fluid is recommended according to which target body fluid compartment needs to be resuscitated or maintained:

- Intracellular space – deficits mainly due to H_2O loss.
- Interstitial space – deficits mainly due to H_2O and electrolyte loss.
- Intravascular space – deficits of plasma volume and/or red blood cells (RBC).

Fluid balance

The balance between total intake of fluid and electrolytes (enteral and IV) versus the combined output (from kidneys, GI tract and insensible losses through skin, and lungs) determines overall fluid and electrolyte balance.

Intake

- Average required daily intake for healthy adults is: water 25–35 mL/kg/day; sodium ~1 mmol/kg/day; potassium ~1 mmol/kg/day.
- When estimating intake, remember to include concomitant IV medication fluids (i.e. from antibiotics, steroids, inotropes, etc.)

Output

Ongoing losses may occur from:

- Kidney losses (obligatory volume to excrete solute load and maintain renal function is ~500 mL in healthy adults):
  - Kidneys are the main regulator for fluid and electrolyte elimination and metabolism
  - Polyuria indicates potential excessive renal losses of water, sodium and potassium
  - Obligatory volume increases during critical illness, surgery and catabolic conditions.
- Gastrointestinal losses (normally 100–500 mL/day in the stool in healthy adults):
  - Vomiting and NG loss – excessive losses of K^+ and Cl^- may cause hypochloremic (hypokalemic) metabolic alkalosis
  - Biliary drainage, pancreatic drainage or fistula
  - Ileal or jejunal loss via stoma or fistula
  - Diarrhea or excess colostomy loss.
- Insensible losses (normally 0.5–1 L/day from skin and lungs in healthy adults):
  - Pure water loss (i.e. low in electrolyte contents) through skin and lungs
  - Increased by fever, sweating, hyperventilation and burns.
- Blood loss:
  - Blood is an important source of fluid, and losses during surgery, or due to internal hemorrhage, GI hemorrhage or melena should be considered.

Types of fluids

The two main classes of fluids for resuscitation, replacement and maintenance purposes are crystalloids and colloids.

Table 5.1 summarizes characteristics of available fluids.

Table 5.1 IV fluids – comparative characteristics

Fluid	Na⁺ (mmol/L)	K⁺ (mmol/L)	Cl⁻ (mmol/L)	Mg²⁺ (mmol/L)	Ca²⁺ (mmol/L)	Lactate/Bircarb/ Acetate/Gluconate/ Malate/Octanoate (L/B/A/G/M/Oc)	Osmolarity (mOsm/L)	MWt (kD)	Duration of effect	Risks
Human Plasma										
Plasma	135–145	4.5–5.0	94–111	0.8–1.0	2.2–2.6	L: 1–2 B: 23–27	280–300	–	–	–
Crystalloids										
0.9% Saline ("normal" saline)	154	0	154	–	–	–	287	–	10–15min	Hyperchloremic acidosis (dose-related)
0.45% Saline ("half normal" saline)	77	0	77	–	–	–	144	–	10–15min	Hyperchloremic acidosis (dose-related)
Ringer's lactate, Hartmann's solution	131	5.0	111	1.0	2.0	L: 29	273	–	10–15min	Hyponatremia and respiratory acidosis (dose-related) Note: Contains calcium, and citrated blood *should not be mixed* in the same IV set[a]
Plasma-Lyte 148	140	5.0	98	3.0	–	A: 27; G: 23	294	–	10–15min	Unknown risks (absence of clinical trials of clinically relevant outcomes)

	Na	K	Cl	Ca	Mg		Osmolality	MW	Duration	Notes
Sterofundin	140	4.0	127	1.0	2.5	A: 24, M: 5	309	–	10–15min	Unknown risks (absence of clinical trials of clinically relevant outcomes) Note: Contains calcium, and citrated blood *should not be mixed* in the same IV set[a]
Natural Colloids										
4% Albumin	140–160	<2.0	128			Oc: 6.4	250	68 000	2–4 hrs	Source: Human plasma, therefore, theoretical risk of BSE transmission (heat treatment prevents HIV transmission)
20% Albumin	48–100	Varies	Varies			Oc: 32	130	68 000	2–4 hrs	
Synthetic Colloids										
Gelatin 4% (ie, Hemaccel, Gelofusin, Geloplasma, Plasmion, Polygeline, Gelifundol) Note: Composition differs by product	145–154	4.0–5.1	105–145	1.0	–	Ac: 24 (varies by product)	270	5 to 50 000 (mean: 30 000)	1–2 hrs	↑ blood loss ↑ RBC transfusion Note: Gelatin products containing calcium (i.e. Hemaccel), and citrated blood *should not be mixed* in the same IV set[a] Source: Bovine bone (BSE/prion disease a potential concern; though very rare)

Table 5.1 (cont.)

Fluid	Na$^+$ (mmol/L)	K$^+$ (mmol/L)	Cl$^-$ (mmol/L)	Mg^{2+} (mmol/L)	Ca^{2+} (mmol/L)	Lactate/Bircarb/Acetate/Gluconate/Malate/Octanoate (L/B/A/G/M/Oc)	Osmolarity (mOsm/L)	MWt (kD)	Duration of effect	Risks
Voluven (6% HES 130/0.4, maize starch)	154	–	154	–	–	–	308	130 000	4–8 hrs	↑ blood loss ↑ RBC transfusion ↑ renal failure, dialysis ↑ death
Volulyte (6% HES 140/0.4, maize starch)	137	4.0	110	1.5	–	A: 34	286	130 000	4–8 hrs	Pruritis (delayed onset) Anaphylaxis (rare)
Venofundin (6% HES 130/0.42, Potato starch)	154	–	154	–	–	–	308	130 000	4–8 hrs	Note: Products containing calcium may react with citrated blood and *should not be mixed*
Tetraspan (6% HES 130/0.42, Potato starch)	140	4.0	114	1.0	2.5	A:24 M:5	296	130 000	4–8 hrs	in the same IV set as citrated blood[a]
PlasmaVolume (6% HES 130/ 0.42, Potato starch)	130	5.4	112	1.0	0.9	A:27	300	130 000	4–8 hrs	Blackbox warning, contraindicated in sepsis, renal failure. Withdrawn from market in some countries due
10% HES 200/0.5	154	0	154	–	–	–	308	200 000	6–12 hrs	to risks of bleeding, RF, and death.
6% HES 450/0.6	154	0	154	–	–	–	308	450 000	24–48 hrs	
Dextran 40	–	–	–	–	–	–		40 000	6–8 hrs	

Dextran 70	may be in saline or glucose				70 000	Anaphylaxis is a *significant* risk. ↑ blood loss (dose-related) Interferes with bilirubin assay and blood glucose tests. ***Interferes with cross-matching.***
Other IV fluids (NOT suitable for resuscitation)						
Dextrose 5%	0	0	–	–	278	NOT for primary resuscitation. May be useful when reserved for difficult cases such as in hypernatremia.
Dextrose 4%, Saline 0.18%	20	0	30	–	–	278

ᵃ Caution for all IV fluids that contain Ca^{2+} – can cause problems if administered with stored blood. It is possible for the Ca^{2+} in IV solutions to complex with citrate (the anticoagulant used in stored blood), and cause clotting of blood in the infusion tubing, particularly if the blood is given slowly or the tubing contains reservoir areas (e.g. as in pump sets). For this reason, it is standard practice to administer normal saline before and after a blood transfusion to prevent blood and Ca^{2+} mixing in the infusion tubing. Solutions which contain Mg^{2+} instead of Ca^{2+} can be administered with stored blood without causing this problem.

Crystalloids

- H_2O with electrolytes approximating the composition and osmolality of plasma.
- Inexpensive, and easy to store.
- Traditionally, saline has been suggested to expand blood volume by 25–30% of the volume infused, with the remainder shifting to the interstitial space. However, this is based on physiologic studies, largely from healthy volunteers [1–4].
- In large double-blind RCTs of synthetic colloids (HES or albumin) versus crystalloids in hypovolemic critically ill patients the effective intravascular volume expansion is greater than that expected by physiologic prediction alone, with ratios of crystalloid to colloid volume ranging from 1.3:1 to 1.4:1 [5–8]. Nevertheless, these trials did not specifically assess the earliest phase of resuscitation, and while small clinical trials have shown faster hemodynamic response to colloids than crystalloids for acute resuscitation, none of these trials has measured clinically important outcomes such as organ failure and survival [9,10].
- Theoretically, it has been suggested that saline results in greater **edema** than colloids. In practice, **both colloids and crystalloids increase risk of edema**, and studies have not proven whether the differences are clinically relevant, especially for critically ill patients (i.e. sepsis), where decreased vascular integrity increases transvasation of any fluid (colloid or crystalloid) into the interstitial space, and where the classic laws of diffusion are revised [11–16].

Saline

- "Normal saline" is not "normal" at all (its chloride concentration is 154 mmol/L, which is higher than serum chloride concentrations of 100–110 mmol/L).
- Sodium chloride 0.9% (with or without added potassium) is the most commonly used IV fluid.
- Excess sodium and chloride may be beneficial in chloride-wasting syndromes (excess GI or renal losses). However, ability to clear excess sodium and chloride may be impaired in critical illness, and may lead to hyperchloremia.
- Hyperchloremia may increase risk of hyperchloremic acidosis, impaired renal blood flow and reduced glomerular filtration, and GI acidosis-induced ileus [1,2].
- It may lead to hyperchloremic acidosis (dose-dependent and rate-dependent risk), which may increase risk of renal dysfunction [17–19].
  - However, the clinical significance of this acidosis is debatable since large randomized trials of crystalloids versus colloids in critical care and surgery have reported a favorable balance of clinical outcomes, including renal function with saline relative to colloids, and clinically relevant acidosis has not been reported in these trials. [7,8,20].
  - On the other hand, large retrospective observational studies have suggested increased risk of morbidity and mortality in patients who experience hyperchloremia after surgery due to chloride-liberal fluid administration [17,18]. This remains to be confirmed in head-to-head randomized trials since, to date, existing randomized comparisons of saline versus Ringer's lactate or Ringer's acetate (or chloride-liberal

versus chloride-restrictive fluid-replacement strategies) have
been severely underpowered to detect clinically relevant differences
(see "Saline versus balanced solutions" below).

Balanced (or "physiologic") crystalloid solutions

- Solutions with electrolytes (containing sodium, potassium, calcium, magnesium and with significantly lower concentration of chloride than saline solutions) have been suggested to provide a potentially safer alternative to saline since they more closely resemble normal plasma electrolyte concentrations.
- Balanced solutions such as Ringer's lactate (Hartmann's solution) or Plasma-Lyte provide similar volume expansion and similar distribution into ECF.
- Balanced crystalloid solutions may be more costly than saline (but less costly than colloids).

Saline versus "balanced" crystalloid solutions

At least in principle, the balanced or buffered solutions (in which lactate or acetate buffers the chloride) may have a lesser risk of hyperchloremic acidosis.

- As a result, some have suggested "balanced" or "buffered" solutions such as Ringer's lactate are preferred over "unbalanced" saline for use as a routine fluid [17,18,21].
- However, adequately powered randomized evidence that measures clinically important outcomes are awaited to determine which crystalloid is best (see below), and it is important to note that even balanced solutions bring risks [22]. For example, infusion of large volumes of Ringer's lactate during surgery may cause hyponatremia and respiratory acidosis [23].

Studies that directly compare chloride-rich versus chloride-poor fluid management have been observational or retrospective, and subject to bias:

- A non-randomized time series study (n=1533) suggested that switching from chloride-rich fluid management (by phasing out the use of 0.9% saline, 5% gelatin, 4% albumin) to a chloride-restrictive strategy (use of Ringer's lactate, chloride-poor 20% albumin, or Plasma-Lyte 148) in the ICU was associated with a significant decrease in the incidence of acute kidney injury and need for renal replacement therapy. [17]
- A propensity-matched cohort analysis of non-cardiac surgical patients (n=8532) reported that hyperchloremia after surgery was associated with increased morbidity and mortality. [19]
- In elderly surgical patients, the use of crystalloids and colloids containing balanced electrolyte solutions prevented the development of hyperchloremic metabolic acidosis and improved indices of gastric mucosal perfusion (surrogate outcome) compared with saline-based crystalloid and colloid fluids; however, hard endpoints were not measured [19].

In conclusion, excessive volumes of any type of fluid, regardless of whether chloride-rich or more physiologically "balanced," are associated with benefits and risks, and the balance effects of saline versus Ringer's lactate have not been studied sufficiently to recommend one over the other. Adequately powered randomized trials that evaluate clinically important outcomes rather than only physiologic or hemodynamic parameters will be required to resolve the saline versus "balanced" crystalloids controversy for ICU and surgery settings [23].

Glucose and glucose/salines

- 5% glucose and glucose/saline are not truly "crystalloids" and are NOT intended for resuscitation or replacement of electrolyte losses.
- Glucose solutions provide free water, and may be useful for treating simple dehydration if intravascular expansion is not required (once glucose is metabolized, the free water is distributed through total body water with a negligible and transient effect on blood volume).
- Glucose solutions alone increase the risk of hyponatremia (a dose-related and administration-rate-related risk), especially in children, the elderly and patients on diuretics or with SIADH.

Colloids

Colloids (starch, gelatin, dextran, albumin):
- Contain larger particles (synthetic or natural) suspended in crystalloid solution
- More expensive, and often more difficult to store than crystalloids
- Colloids have traditionally been thought to remain in the intravascular space longer, achieve faster circulatory stabilization and require lower amount of fluid for resuscitation compared with crystalloids; however, recent evidence has called these claims into question, especially in the setting of sepsis, since similar volumes of crystalloid and colloid (~1.3:1 or 1.4:1) were required in large-scale double-blind randomized trials [5–8,20].
- All synthetic colloids have dose-related side effects, including coagulopathy, renal failure and tissue storage (pruritis) [24,25].
- None of the colloids have been shown to improve clinically relevant outcomes compared with crystalloids in critical care.
- Resuscitation with colloids has not been shown to reduce risk of death compared to resuscitation with crystalloids, in patients with trauma, burns or following surgery. Furthermore, the use of hydroxyethyl starch might increase mortality, particularly in critically ill or septic patients [14,15, 26–30].
- For this reason, crystalloids remain the fluid of first choice for critical care [31] (see "Surviving Sepsis Guidelines" below).

Albumin

- Albumin is a natural colloid derived from pooled human plasma (heat-treated to reduce viral transmission, but still carries theoretical risk of BSE transmission).
- It is very expensive relative to other fluids, and is in limited supply in some countries.
- Concentrated sodium-poor albumin (20–25% albumin) may theoretically be useful in patients with edema from sodium overload and who still have low plasma volumes, or in liver failure with ascites. However, this strategy remains to be tested in clinical trials [34].
- While the use of 4–5% albumin has been surrounded by controversy, the SAFE trial (albumin versus saline) and subsequent meta-analyses (albumin versus

crystalloids, or versus other colloids) now provide greater clarity for the recommended place of albumin in practice [8,34].

- The SAFE trial (n = 7000) showed no significant difference in clinical outcomes for critically ill patients randomized to 4–5% albumin or saline. The difference in volume administered was 1.4:1 for saline:albumin.

  - Subgroup analysis of patients with sepsis in the SAFE trial suggested albumin might improve survival compared with saline; however, this is based on post hoc subanalysis, and remains to be confirmed prospectively. Since meta-analyses (see below) have not confirmed this result, the potential for survival advantage in sepsis subgroups remains to be confirmed in prospective RCTs [32,34].

  - Subgroup analysis of patients with traumatic brain injury in the SAFE trial showed a higher risk of death with albumin versus saline. Until proven otherwise, albumin is not recommended for resuscitation in patients with traumatic brain injury. [35]

- Meta-analyses of albumin versus crystalloids in critically ill patients with hypovolemia concluded that that albumin does not reduce mortality when compared with cheaper alternatives such as crystalloids. The possibility that there may be highly selected populations of critically ill patients who may benefit remains open to further study [30,32].

- Since albumin results in similar clinical outcomes to crystalloids, has no proven mortality benefit and is more costly than crystalloids, it should be reserved as a second-line after crystalloids for fluid management in ICU [30,31,34].

- The International Surviving Sepsis Campaign recommend [31]:

  - Crystalloids as the initial fluid of choice for the resuscitation of patients with severe sepsis.

  - Albumin is recommended only when "substantial amounts" of crystalloid have been administered with unsatisfactory effect.

  - See also NICE Guidelines from the UK, which provide similar recommendations [32].

Gelatins

- Relatively cheap and widely used in a number of countries.
- Gelatins may also increase risk for bleeding or transfusion. Whether coagulation effects are due to hemodilution or inherent pharmacologic effects remains undetermined.
- In contrast to hydroxyethyl starches, large-scale clinical trials of gelatins have not been conducted. Therefore, it is not known whether they are safer than other IV fluids, such as albumin or crystalloids [30].

Dextrans

- Higher-molecular-weight dextrans (dextran 70 000 kD) are effective plasma volume expanders.

In general, dextrans have fallen out of favor because:
- They interfere with cross-matching
- They may induce coagulopathy (dose-dependent)

- Anaphylaxis is a significant risk
- Some practitioners make use of their antithromboembolic and antisludging properties in situations where peripheral perfusion is compromised.

Starches (Hydroxyethyl starches, HES)

Hydroxyethylstarch products have fallen out of favor for use in critically ill patients:

- HES has no proven benefit over crystalloids [5–7,14,15,20] or compared with other colloids [30].
  - . In randomized studies, HES did not result in much difference in volume administered versus crystalloid (1.4:1 for crystalloid versus HES) [5–7].
- All HES products increase bleeding, blood transfusion, renal failure and all-cause mortality [5–7,14,15,20]. These risks have been most clearly proven in sepsis and critically ill patients [26–30]; however, safety in surgical patients has been inadequately studied and it is questionable whether surgical patients would be exempt from the risks of bleeding, renal failure and death [16,28,30]:
  - . Albeit a limitation of the existing trials of HES versus crystalloid is that patients were usually not recruited into the study until after admission to ICU, which in some cases will be after the initial period of fluid resuscitation has already occurred. Nevertheless, post hoc analyses by timing of HES did not show that patients receiving starches during acute resuscitation were spared of the adverse effects, relative to crystalloids [34].
- While older high-molecular-weight HES products have the highest magnitude of risk for bleeding and renal failure, even the newest low-molecular-weight HES products (HES 130/0.4) still increase the risks of transfusion, renal failure and death, when compared with crystalloids in critically ill patients [14,26–30].
- Regulatory agencies have issued severe warnings not to use HES in sepsis or in patients who are critically ill [37,38], and some countries have recently withdrawn all HES products from the market [39,40].
- This is a complex, long-standing debate, but the conclusion of no benefit and increased risk of harm from colloids (especially starches) is best summed up by a recent Cochrane review [37]: "There is no evidence from randomized controlled trials that resuscitation with colloids reduces the risk of death, compared to resuscitation with crystalloids, in patients with trauma, burns or following surgery. Furthermore, the use of hydroxyethyl starch might increase mortality."

Positive fluid balance, or liberal versus restrictive fluids

- During critical illness, the patient's weight may increase due to fluid retention, possibly reflecting increased endothelial permeability ("leaky vessels"), as well as excessive administration of fluids.
- This is associated with a poor outcome [41,42]. Whether intervening to remove this extra fluid can *reverse* this excess risk back to "normal" is less certain. Certainly, the balance of opinion for ventilated patients with acute respiratory distress syndrome (ARDS) has shifted towards "keeping the patient dry" (as long as organ perfusion is well maintained) [43].

- Clinical trials suggest a positive fluid balance in sepsis or shock [41] and ARDS [43] may reduce mortality.
- In surgical patients, clinical trials suggest improved outcomes with restrictive instead of liberal fluid management; however, further large-scale trials are warranted to establish the most appropriate definition of "restricted."

Surviving Sepsis Guidelines

Based on best available evidence, the International Surviving Sepsis Campaign recommends for severe sepsis [31]:

1. Crystalloids should be initial fluid of choice in the resuscitation of severe sepsis and septic shock (grade 1B).
2. Hydroxyethyl starches (HES) *should not be used* for fluid resuscitation of severe sepsis and septic shock (grade 1B).
3. Albumin may be used in the fluid resuscitation of severe sepsis and septic shock when patients require substantial amounts of crystalloids (grade 2C).
4. Initial fluid challenge should be administered to patients with sepsis-induced tissue hypoperfusion with suspicion of hypovolemia to achieve a minimum of 30 mL/kg of crystalloids (a portion of this may be albumin equivalent). More rapid administration and greater amounts of fluid may be needed in some patients (grade 1C).
5. Fluid challenge technique should be applied wherein fluid administration is continued as long as there is hemodynamic improvement, either based on dynamic (e.g. change in pulse pressure, stroke volume variation) or static (e.g. arterial pressure, heart rate) variables (UG).

Fluid therapy for resuscitation in sepsis is further discussed in Chapter 28.

Additional practical points

- Weighing the patient daily is important.
- Minimize fluids required to administer medications.
- Once patient is established on nutritional support they may not require "routine" maintenance crystalloids.
- Dramatic weight gain due to fluid overload may respond to judicious use of low-dose diuretics *if* hemodynamically tolerated.

References

1. Chowdhury AH, Cox EF, Francis ST, Lobo DN. A randomized, controlled, double-blind crossover study on the effects of 2-L infusions of 0.9% saline and plasma-lyte® 148 on renal blood flow velocity and renal cortical tissue perfusion in healthy volunteers. *Ann Surg* 2012; 256 : 18–24.

2. Lobo DN, Stana Z, Simpson JA *et al.* Dilution and redistribution effects of rapid 2-litre infusions of 0.9% (w/v) saline and 5% (w/v) dextrose on haematological parameters and serum biochemistry in normal subjects: a double-blind crossover study. *Clin Sci* 2001; 101 : 173–9.

3. Lobo DN, Stanga Z, Aloysius MM *et al.* Effects of volume loading with 1 liter intravenous infusions of 0.9% saline, 4% succinylated gelatine (Gelofusine) and 6% hydroxyethyl starch (Voluven) on blood volume and endocrine responses: a

randomized, three-way crossover study in healthy volunteers. *Crit Care Med* 2010; 38 : 464–70.

4. Reid F, Lobo DN, Williams RN *et al.* (Ab)normal saline and physiological Hartmann's solution: a randomized double-blind crossover study. *Clin Sci* 2003; 104 : 17–24.

5. Brunkhorst FM, Engel C, Bloos F, *et al.* Intensive insulin therapy and pentastarch resuscitation in severe sepsis. *N Engl J Med* 2008; 358 : 125–39.

6. Perner A, Haase N, Guttormsen AB, *et al.* Hydroxyethyl starch 130/0.42 versus Ringer's acetate in severe sepsis. *N Engl J Med* 2012; 367 : 124–34.

7. Myburgh JA, Finfer S, Bellomo R, *et al.* Hydroxyethyl starch or saline for fluid resuscitation in intensive care. *N Engl J Med* 2012; 367 : 1901–11.

8. Finfer S, Bellomo R, Boyce N *et al.* A comparison of albumin and saline for fluid resuscitation in the intensive care unit. *N Engl J Med* 2004; 350 : 2247–56.

9. Verheij J, van Lingen A, Beishuizen A *et al.* Cardiac response is greater for colloid than saline fluid loading after cardiac or vascular surgery. *Intensive Care Med* 2006; 32 : 1030–8.

10. van der Heijden M, Verheij J, van Nieuw Amerongen GP, Groeneveld AB. Crystalloid or colloid fluid loading and pulmonary permeability, edema, and injury in septic and nonseptic critically ill patients with hypovolemia. *Crit Care Med* 2009; 37 : 1275–81.

11. Levick JF, Michel CC. Microvascular fluid exchange and the revised Starling principle. *Cardiovasc Res* 2010; 87 : 198–210.

12. Goldenberg NM, Steinberg BE, Slutsky AS, Lee WL. Broken barriers: a new take on sepsis pathogenesis. *Sci Transl Med* 2011; 3 (88) : ps25.

13. Myburgh JA, Mythen MG. Resuscitation fluids. *N Engl J Med* 2013; 369 : 1243–51.

14. Zarychanski R, Abou-Setta AM, Turgeon AF, *et al.* Association of hydroxyethyl starch administration with mortality and acute kidney injury in critically ill patients requiring volume resuscitation: a systematic review and meta-analysis. *JAMA* 2013; 309 : 678–88.

15. Haase N, Perner A, Hennings LI, *et al.* Hydroxyethyl starch 130/0.38–0.45 versus crystalloid or albumin in patients with sepsis: systematic review with meta-analysis and trial sequential analysis. *Br Med J* 2013; 346 : f839.

16. Hartog C, Reinhart K. CONTRA: Hydroxeythyl starch solutions are unsafe in critically ill patients. *Intensive Care Med* 2009; 25 : 1337–42.

17. Yunos NM, Bellomo R, Hegarty C *et al.* Association between a chloride-liberal vs chloride-restrictive intravenous fluid administration strategy and kidney injury in critically ill adults. *JAMA* 2012; 308 : 1566–72.

18. McCluskey SA *et al.* Hyperchloremia after noncardiac surgery is independently associated with increased morbidity and mortality: a propensity-matched cohort study. *Anesth Analg* 2013; 117 : 412–21.

19. Wilkes NJ, Woolf R, Mutch M, Mallett SV *et al.* The effects of balanced versus saline-based hetastarch and crystalloid solutions on acid-base and electrolyte status and gastric mucosal perfusion in elderly surgical patients. *Anesth Analg* 2001; 93 : 811–6.

20. Guidet B, Martinet O, Boulain T *et al.* Assessment of hemodynamic efficacy and safety of 6% hydroxyethylstarch 130/0.4 vs. 0.9% NaCl fluid replacement in patients with severe sepsis: The CRYSTMAS study. *Crit Care* 2012; 16 : R94.

21. Powell-Tuck J, Gosling P, Lobo DN *et al.* British consensus guidelines on intravenous fluid therapy for adult surgical Patients, GIFTASUP. Available at http://www.bapen.org.uk/pdfs/bapen_pubs/giftasup.pdf (accessed June 2014).

22. Takil A, Eti Z, Irmak P, Yilmaz Gogus F. Early postoperative respiratory acidosis after large intravascular volume infusion of lactated ringer's solution during major spine surgery. *Anesth Analg* 2002; 95 : 294–8.

23. Burdett E, Dushianthan A, Bennett-Guerrero E *et al.* Perioperative buffered versus non-buffered fluid administration for surgery in adults. *Cochrane Database Syst Rev* 2012; 12 : CD004089.

24. Hartog CS, *et al.* Fluid replacement with hydroxyethyl starch in critical care – a reassessment. *Dtsch Arztebl Int* 2013;110:443–50.

25. Bork K. Pruritis precipitated by hydroxyethyll starch: a review. *Br J Dermatol* 2005; 152 : 3–12.

26. Patel A, Waheed U, Brett SJ. Randomised trials of 6% tetrastarch (hydroxyethyl starch 130/0.4 or 0.42) for severe sepsis reporting mortality: systematic review and meta-analysis. *Intensive Care Med* 2013; 39 : 811–22.

27. Gattas DJ, Dan A, Myburgh J *et al.* Fluid resuscitation with 6% hydroxyethyl starch (130/0.4 and 130/0.42) in acutely ill patients: systematic review of effects on mortality and treatment with renal replacement therapy. *Intensive Care Med* 2013; 39 : 558–68.

28. Gillies MA, Habicher M, Jhanji S *et al.* Incidence of post-operative death and acute kidney injury associated with intravenous 6% hydroxyethyl starch use: systematic review and meta-analysis. *Br J Anaesth* 2014; 112 : 25–34.

29. Bunn F, Trivedi D. Colloid solutions for fluid resuscitation. *Cochrane Database Syst Rev* 2012; 7 : CD001319.

30. Perel P, Roberts I, Ker K. Colloids versus crystalloids for fluid resuscitation in critically ill patients. *Cochrane Database Syst Rev* 2013; 2 : CD000567.

31. Dellinger RP, Levy MM, Rhodes A, *et al.* Surviving sepsis campaign: international guidelines for management of severe sepsis and septic shock: 2012. *Crit Care Med* 2013; 41 : 580–637.

32. National Institute for Health and Care Excellence. Intravenous fluid therapy: Intravenous fluid therapy in adults in hospital. Clinical Guideline: Methods, evidence and recommendations, May 14, 2013. Available at http://www.nice.org.uk/nicemedia/live/13298/63879/63879.pdf (accessed June 2014).

33. Allison SP, Lobo Dn. Debate: albumin administration should not be avoided. *Crit Care* 2000; 4 : 147–50.

34. Roberts I, Blackhall K, Alderson P *et al.* Human albumin solution for resuscitation and volume expansion in critically ill patients. *Cochrane Database Syst Rev* 2011; 11 : CD001208.

35. Myburgh J, Cooper DJ, Finfer S, *et al.* Saline or albumin for fluid resuscitation in patients with traumatic brain injury. *N Engl J Med* 2007; 357 : 874–84.

36. Muller RG, Haase N, Wetterslev J, Perner. Effects of hydroxyethylstarch in subgroups of patients with severe sepsis: exploratory post-hoc analyses of a randomised trial. *Intensive Care Med.* 2013; 39 : 1963–71.

37. Medicines and US Food and Drugs Agency. FDA Safety Communication: Boxed Warning on increased mortality and severe renal injury, and additional warning on risk of bleeding, for use of hydroxyethyl starch solutions in some settings, June 24, 2013. Available from http://www.fda.gov/biologicsbloodvaccines/safetyavailability/ucm358271.htm (accessed June 2014).

38. Government of Canada, Health Protection Branch. Voluven and Volulyte (hydroxyethyl starch (HES)) – Increased Mortality and Severe Renal Injury – Notice to Hospitals. http://healthycanadians.gc.ca/recall-alert-rappel-avis/hc-sc/2013/34697a-eng.php (accessed June 2014).

39. Pharmacovigilance Risk Assessment Committee of the European Medicines Agency. PRAC recommends suspending marketing authorisations for infusion solutions containing hydroxyethyl-starch. Available from http://www.ema.europa.eu/docs/en_GB/document_library/Press_release/2013/06/WC500144446.pdf (accessed July 2013).

40. Medicines and Health Care Healthcare Products Regulatory Agency. Class 2 drug alert (action within 48 hours): hydroxyethyl starch (HES) products—B Braun Melsungen AG and Fresenius Kabi Limited

(EL (13)A/18). Available from http://www.
mhra.gov.uk/Publications/Safetywarnings/
DrugAlerts/CON287025 (accessed July
2013).

41. Boyd JH, Forbes J, Nakada T *et al.*
Fluid resuscitation in septic shock:
a positive fluid balance and elevated central
venous pressure are associated
with increased mortality. *Crit Care Med*
2011; 29 : 259–65.

42. Doherty M, Buggy DJ. Intraoperative
fluids: how much is too much? *Br
J Anaesthesia* 2012; 109 : 69–79.

43. National Heart, Lung, and Blood Institute
Acute Respiratory Distress Syndrome
(ARDS) Clinical Trials Network;
Wiedemann HP, Wheeler AP, Bernard GR,
et al. Comparison of two fluid-
management strategies in acute lung injury.
N Engl J Med 2006; 354 : 2564–75.

Anemia and blood transfusion

Shane W English and Lauralyn McIntyre

Red blood cells comprise almost 50% of blood volume in the average healthy adult. Integral to its vital function of transporting oxygen to and carbon dioxide away from the organs and tissues of the body is the hemoglobin (Hb) contained within its cytoplasm. The average healthy adult hemoglobin level measures between 140–180 g/L in males and 130–160 g/L in females.

- Although the strictest definition of anemia describes a hemoglobin level that falls below this threshold, the WHO set the criteria as <130 g/L and <120 g/L for men and women, respectively [1].
- Practically speaking, in the ICU literature, anemia is considered important when moderate and is typically restricted to describe a hemoglobin of less than or equal to 100 g/L [2].

Amongst critically ill adult patients, anemia is an extremely common occurrence and in many instances will lead to a blood transfusion. Our understanding of the effects of anemia and how it is tolerated amongst ICU patients, the indications for, benefits and risks of blood transfusion has grown over the last several years. This chapter will focus on these aspects of anemia and blood transfusion in a nonacutely bleeding adult critically ill population. Although not comprehensive, it should provide an overall sense of what is known from the literature to guide a practical clinical approach and will conclude with suggested further reading.

Epidemiology and etiology of anemia in adult intensive care units

Anemia is extremely common amongst critically ill patients, whether as a direct result of their admission diagnosis, as a complication of their stay in intensive care, or from iatrogenic causes:

- As many as 30% of critically ill patients have been anemic at some point during their admission [3].
- In an observational study of 1023 sequential Scottish ICU admissions [4], anemia (Hb <130 g/L in men, <115 g/L in women) was prevalent in 87% and 80% of male and female survivors, respectively. Hb <90 g/L at ICU discharge occurred in 24% and 28% of men and women, respectively.
- The CRIT study (an American observational study of 4892 patients) [5] demonstrated anemia (Hb <120 g/L) in 70% of patients by 48 hours of ICU admission, with half having an Hb <100 g/L

Handbook of ICU Therapy, third edition, ed. John Fuller, Jeff Granton and Ian McConachie. Published by Cambridge University Press. © Cambridge University Press 2015.

- In nonbleeding ICU patients the average fall in Hb concentration has been shown in one study to be 5.2 g/L/day. The decline was larger for the first three days than later days and was greater in septic patients [6].

Many factors are involved in the etiology of anemia in the critically ill and include:
- Surgical and traumatic blood loss
- A blunted erythropoietin (EPO) response in critical illness [7], which is further reduced in the context of renal failure
- Diagnostic blood sampling: a large multicenter observational study of 1136 ICU patients demonstrated the average volume per blood draw was 10.6 ml, resulting in approximately 40 mL of blood loss per day [6]
- Gastrointestinal blood loss; either as the admission diagnosis or occurring as a complication of critical illness
- Spillage during vascular cannulation
- Coagulopathy and hemolysis
- Renal failure: demonstrated to be an independent risk factor for anemia in critical illness [4]. (In part may relate to need for renal replacement therapy and blood losses associated with anticoagulation and filter changes)
- Other factors (e.g. iron, B_{12} and folate availability).

Physiologic effects of anemia

Chapter 1 has shown the role of Hb in overall oxygen delivery (DO_2). Oxygen delivery to vital organs can be expressed by the equation $DO_2 = CO \times ([Hb] \times SaO_2 + 0.0031 \times PaO_2)$, where DO_2 is oxygen delivery in mL/min, CO is cardiac output in ml/min, Hb is hemoglobin in g/L and PaO_2 is partial pressure of arterial oxygen. Thus, DO_2 is dependent predominantly upon cardiac output, hemoglobin concentration and oxygen saturation [8].

- Under normal physiologic circumstances, a partial pressure of oxygen of 27 mmHg results in 50% oxygen saturation of Hb. A right shift of the curve, or decreased oxygen affinity, is observed with increased temperature, CO_2, increased 2,3-DPG levels or a decreased pH. A left shift, or increased oxygen affinity, is observed with lower temperature, lower CO_2, decreased 2,3-DPG levels or a higher pH.
- Given a normal cardiac output and high oxygen saturation, the variable most easily manipulated to increase oxygen delivery is hemoglobin concentration.
- It is on this premise that RBCs are often transfused.

One must distinguish between the effects of anemia and those of hypovolemia – especially with acute blood loss. There is no doubt that hypovolemia is less well tolerated than anemia. Thus, where hypovolemia is present, restoration of blood volume and cardiac output is the first priority.

In the normovolemic patient a rapid fall in Hb brings about certain compensatory changes:
- The decrease in plasma viscosity improves peripheral blood flow and thus enhances venous return to the right atrium. The reduced viscosity also reduces afterload, which may be an important mechanism in maintaining or increasing cardiac output [9].

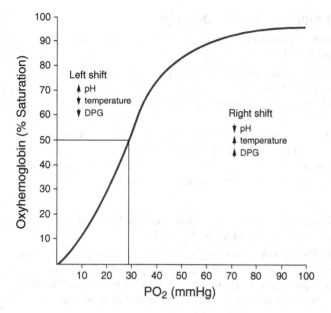

Figure 6.1 Factors affecting the oxyhemoglobin dissociation curve

- A rightward shift in the oxyhemoglobin dissociation curve (ODC) is seen, which increases the O_2 unloading by Hb at the tissues for a given blood PO_2 – thus increasing oxygen availability to the tissues. The primary reason for this rightward shift is the increased red cell 2,3-diphosphoglycerate (DPG) synthesis seen during anemia.
- Conversely, old transfused blood may have reduced DPG levels, theoretically shifting the oxyhemoglobin dissociation curve to the left, increasing the affinity of Hb for oxygen and potentially reducing oxygen availability to the tissues.
- Figure 6.1 shows the influence of pH, temperature and DPG levels on the ODC.

Whether or not these compensatory mechanisms are as successful in maintaining oxygen consumption (VO_2) during critical illness as they are during other anemic states is unknown.

Although it is clear that RBC transfusion may improve oxygen delivery in the critically ill, its effect on oxygen consumption is less clear:

- In an early systematic review of 13 studies evaluating the impact of RBC transfusion on O_2 kinetics, a consistent increase in O_2 delivery was observed post-transfusion but a change in O_2 consumption occurred in less than half [10].
- In a more recent prospective observational study of 44 anemic critically ill patients in Belgium, muscle-tissue oxygen consumption, as determined with near-infrared spectroscopy, was globally unaltered by RBC transfusion [11].
- Another prospective observational study of 51 cardiovascular surgical patients with nadir Hb of 75–85 g/L demonstrated no increased oxygen consumption following transfusion of 1–2 units of RBC [12]. It is important to note that although this was once a frequently cited paper, it has since been retracted.

The role of anemia in morbidity and mortality

Following a review of the literature, Hébert *et al.* concluded that in young healthy patients, perioperative survival is possible with Hb as low as 50 g/L [13].

- However, both critical illness and anemia put stress on the myocardium to increase cardiac output and hence global DO_2.
- To do so, myocardial DO_2 must increase to meet its own increased O_2 demand (MVO_2).
- As normal myocardial O_2 extraction runs at between 75% and 80%, any increase in MVO_2 must be met primarily by an increase in coronary flow.
- The presence of fixed coronary stenoses (e.g. coronary artery disease) may prevent any increase in myocardial flow, thus limiting myocardial DO_2 (and creating a "supply and demand" issue).

During anemia, the demands of an increased cardiac output may result in cardiac ischemia with, at least the potential for, increased morbidity and mortality:

- A retrospective analysis by Carson [14], involving patients who had a religious objection to blood undergoing surgery, demonstrated a significantly higher morbidity and mortality in patients with a pre-operative Hb of <60 g/L. This effect was substantially more significant in patients with pre-existing cardiac disease and in those who had a larger blood loss.
- A similar, more recent study [15] found that the risk of death was low in patients with post-operative Hb levels of 71–80 g/L. As post-operative anemia worsened, the risk of mortality rises and becomes extremely high below 50–60 g/L.
- A large observational study found that elderly anemic patients with myocardial infarction have a higher mortality rate [16], even when other factors have been taken into account.

Although there is little doubt that moderate to severe anemia may be associated with adverse consequences, it is less clear at what level to transfuse and in whom a red blood cell transfusion may be beneficial in the nonacutely bleeding critically ill patient.

The following section will discuss the management of anemia in the critically ill.

Management of anemia in the critically ill

Prevention

Strategies to reduce blood loss and/or prevent anemia are well described in the perioperative literature. A detailed account of these strategies is outside the scope of this text, but some directly apply to the critically ill patient, including: improved interventional techniques assisted by enhanced imaging or minimally invasive approaches (e.g. use of bedside ultrasonography, percutaneous tracheostomy and gastroscopy tubes) and the use of hemostatic agents to reduce bleeding (e.g. use of tourniquets, vasoconstrictors and antifibrinolytics). In addition, and perhaps more specific to the ICU setting, strategies to reduce and or prevent anemia include:

- Blood-loss reduction associated with diagnostic testing (e.g. inline waste reservoirs, use of microanalyzer systems for blood testing and other "point-of-care" laboratory systems, indwelling continuous oximetry and pH sensors).

- Improved membrane biocompatibility of extracorporeal technologies, including those used for renal replacement therapy or cardiac bypass (e.g. improved removal of erythropoiesis inhibitors and endotoxins, improved iron utilization and erythropoietin response) [17].
- The routine use of pulse oximetry (reducing the need for arterial blood gas sampling).
- Preservation of gut mucosal integrity.

It has been demonstrated that critically ill patients with low levels of endogenous EPO can respond to exogenous EPO by increasing reticulocytes [18].

- Early evidence suggested that prophylactic administration of EPO may be of value, but a large multicenter blinded randomized controlled trial involving 1460 patients failed to demonstrate a decrease in either the number of patients transfused or the mean number of RBC units transfused between the two groups (weekly subcutaneous injections of 40 000 units of EPO (max. 3 weeks) versus placebo). Despite a trend in decreased 29- and 140-day mortality amongst the EPO group (adjusted HR 0.79, 95% CI 0.56 to 1.10; and adjusted HR 0.86, 95% CI 0.65 to 1.13, respectively), they observed a significant increase in thrombotic events amongst the intervention group (HR 1.41, 95% CI 1.06 to 1.86).
- Further, a meta-analysis of nine RCTs [19] (including the above trial) demonstrated a decreased transfusion rate amongst those patients treated with erythropoietin-receptor agonists (OR 0.73, 95% CI 0.64 to 0.84), but no change in overall mortality (OR 0.86, 95% CI 0.71 to 1.05).

Erythropoietin therapy is expensive and the benefits are, so far, controversial at best, with evidence of potential harm. Thus its routine use has fallen out of favor.

Similarly, there remains significant interest in blood alternatives (e.g. diaspirin cross-linked hemoglobin (DCLB), polymerized human Hb, bovine Hb, etc).

- However, none are commonplace in the ICU setting and are of limited access to date, as there is no definitive evidence demonstrating benefit.
- In fact, several large multicenter trials testing such products have been prematurely terminated due to safety concerns and as such there is no current role for these alternatives in everyday practice in the ICU.

Transfusion in critically ill patients

It is not surprising, given the frequency of anemia in the critically ill, that red blood cell (RBC) transfusion is also common:

- In the previously described Scottish observational study (1023 sequential ICU admissions) 39.5% of patients received an RBC transfusion [4].
- The CRIT study (4892 patients) [5] had an ICU RBC transfusion rate of 44%, with length of ICU stay related to proportion transfused and number of units received.
- In the European ABC study [3] quoted above, 37% of ICU patients received one or more units during their ICU stay. Older patients and those with a longer ICU stay received more transfusions.

Based on examination of practice, the most common reason for administering an RBC transfusion to an ICU patient, aside from an acute bleed, is to improve oxygen delivery [20].

Although the benefit of maintaining and/or improving tissue oxygenation through RBC transfusion can be life-saving in the context of acute blood loss or severe anemia, its potential benefit in the mildly/moderately anemic, critically ill patient is less clear. Certainly oxygen delivery improves with RBC transfusion; however, oxygen consumption at the tissue level does not necessarily increase [9,13]. In balance with the real risks associated with transfusion, the indication for RBC transfusion is becoming more and more restrictive.

- In the CRIT study (4892 patients) [5], the most common reasons for RBC transfusion included low hemoglobin (90%), active bleeding (24%) and hemodynamic instability/hypotension (21%).
- The most common reasons for transfusion in the ABC study [3] included active bleeding (56%) and low hemoglobin, with one of diminished physiologic reserves, altered tissue perfusion or coronary artery disease (28%, 17% and 8%, respectively).

Effect of transfusion on oxygen transport

It has been assumed that an increase in global DO_2 (e.g. by red-cell transfusion) would result in an increase in VO_2 in critical illness:

- However, Dietrich [21] studied the increase of DO_2 by red-cell transfusion in non-surgical intensive care patients. After volume resuscitation, patients were transfused if their Hb was <100 g/L. He showed neither an increase in VO_2 nor a decrease in blood lactate levels in any patient and concluded that the shock state of this patient group was not improved by red-cell transfusion.
- In post-cardiac-surgery patients, the oxygen transport responses to transfusion vary. Even in anemic patients there is no consistent VO_2 response to transfusion [22].

Several studies have addressed this issue in patients with sepsis and septic shock:

- Conrad [23] studied augmentation of DO_2 by blood transfusion in septic patients. Transfusion resulted in a significant increase in Hb and DO_2. However, despite the increase in DO_2, there was no increase in VO_2 or decrease in lactate. Subset analysis showed that a pre-transfusion oxygen extraction ratio (OER) <24% was associated with an increase in VO_2. It was concluded that only in the subset of septic shock patients with a low OER may an improvement in VO_2 be seen with transfusion, which may represent a different microcirculatory disturbance.
- Numerous small prospective studies in severe sepsis have demonstrated increased DO_2 with RBC transfusion, but no increase in O_2 utilization [24]. For example, Marik [25] prospectively examined the effect of RBC transfusion on whole-body oxygen uptake (measured by indirect calorimeter) GI perfusion and found no evidence of improved VO_2.
- Steffes [26] further studied the role of lactic acidosis (implying tissue hypoxia) as a predictor of response to augmenting DO_2 with transfusion. In patients with normal lactic acid, both DO_2 and VO_2 increased. However, in patients with lactic acidosis VO_2 did not significantly change after transfusion, despite increased DO_2. He concluded that lactic acidosis may predict patients who will not respond to transfusion. It was suggested

Table 6.1 Infectious complications of RBC transfusion

Infection	Risk per 1 unit RBC transfused
HIV/AIDS	1:7 800 000
Hepatitis A	1:2 000 000
Hepatitis B	1:153 000
Hepatitis C	1:2 300 000
HTLV	1:4 300 000
Sepsis	1:250 000
Bacterial contamination	1:50 000
Parasitic infection	1:4 000 000
Prions	Exceedingly rare

Reproduced with permission from McIntyre L *et al*. Blood component transfusion in the critically ill. *Curr Opin Crit Care* 2013; 19 : 326–33.

that patients with lactic acidosis may have a peripheral oxygen utilization defect that prevents improvement in VO_2 with increasing DO_2.

Thus, red-cell transfusion for the purposes of increasing DO_2 may not be of benefit since VO_2 is not consistently increased and hence may expose the patient to possible harmful effects of blood transfusion.

Harmful effects of blood transfusion

Massive blood transfusion imparts its own set of important potential complications, including hyperkalemia, hypocalcemia, metabolic acidosis, hypothermia, dilutional coagulopathy and citrate toxicity. This will not be discussed further in this text.

Risks otherwise associated with RBC transfusion are best considered under the categories of "infectious" and "noninfectious."

Infectious complications of RBC transfusion

Fortunately, due to significant advances in the screening and testing of blood donors and products, respectively, infectious complications of RBC transfusion are rare (see Table 6.1).

Noninfectious complications of RBC transfusion

Noninfectious complications of RBC transfusion are significantly more common (see Table 6.2) and have varying degrees of impact on patient morbidity and mortality. The mechanisms of these potential complications are not entirely understood, but may reflect immune and inflammatory responses, as well as red-cell storage lesion (effects of biochemical changes in RBCs or effects from the mediators they release over time or related to the medium in which they are stored).

It is thought that cytokines, such as interleukins and tumor necrosis factor, and antibodies, either from donor blood [27,28] or activated neutrophils [29], play a significant

Table 6.2 Noninfectious complications of RBC transfusion

Complication	Risk per 1 unit RBC transfused
Urticarial Reaction	1:100
Febrile nonhemolytic reaction	1:300
Transfusion-associated cardiac overload (TACO)	1:700
Transfusion-related acute lung injury (TRALI)	1:5000–10 000
Delayed hemolytic transfusion reaction	1:7 000
Acute hemolytic transfusion reaction	1:40 000
Anaphylactic reaction	1:40 000
Post-transfusion purpura	Rare

Reproduced with permission from McIntyre L *et al*. Blood component transfusion in the critically ill. *Curr Opin Crit Care* 2013; 19 : 326–33.

role in immune-mediated transfusion reactions. With the significant improvements in screening and testing processes around blood donation, infectious complications are now uncommon. Transfusion-related acute lung injury (TRALI) is now the leading cause of transfusion-related morbidity and mortality [28,30].

Transfusion-related acute lung injury (TRALI)

Acute lung injury following blood transfusion is thought to result from the activation of recipient neutrophils by donor antibodies (human leukocyte antibodies and human neutrophil antibodies) [30] and donor RBC-derived membrane lipids. Such neutrophil activation increases endothelial permeability with extravasation of inflammatory mediators and fluid. The resultant clinical picture is indistinguishable from acute respiratory distress syndrome (ARDS).

- In the perioperative or critically ill patient there are often other factors that could explain why a patient should develop ARDS and so the incidence of TRALI is probably underestimated.
- Epidemiologic studies have demonstrated significant association with risk of TRALI and the transfusion of blood product with female donor plasma, particularly post-pregnancy [30,31]. The increased human leukocyte or human neutrophil antibodies, which are more frequent in the immunized post-pregnancy female population, are thought to be central to the pathophysiologic process. Reduction in the use of plasma from this donor pool has led to reduced incidence of TRALI [32].

Transfusion-related immune modulation (TRIM)

Although the immunosuppressive effects of allogenic blood transfusion have been well described in the literature, [28,32], the exact mechanisms and effect on clinical outcomes remains unclear. Transfused leukocytes are believed to play a role, and ultimately induce a relative immunosuppression predisposing to infection and possible cancer recurrence. These hypotheses remain controversial and debated.

- Nonetheless, leukoreduction or depletion of RBC units has been proposed as a method to reduce the risk of TRIM.
- Universal leukoreduction programs have been adopted by many countries, including Canada, the UK and several other European nations, and by the American Red Cross.

Age of blood

The series of biochemical and biomechanical changes that occur as a result of RBC storage are collectively called "storage lesion."

- Biochemical changes occurring in stored RBCs include depletion of 2,3-DPG, ATP and S-nitroso-hemoglobin, as well as calcium and metabolic modulation.
- Biomechanical changes include membrane phospholipid redistribution, microvesiculation and loss, protein oxidation and lipid peroxidation, and release of free Hb [33,34].

The exact clinical significance of aged blood as a result of these changes and their physiologic effects are still debated:

- As mentioned previously, stored blood has reduced levels of 2,3-DPG causing a leftward shift in the ODC and a reduced unloading of O_2 from Hb (see Figure 6.1).
- The reduced membrane deformability of red cells, as a result of morphological changes from biconcave RBCs to irreversibly deformed spheroechinocytes [34], brought about through their storage, is thought to impede their passage through the narrow confines of a capillary bed with potential implications for ischemic organs and tissues. The high hematocrit of packed red cells may increase blood viscosity and further threaten perfusion of such areas.
- A small retrospective study of patients with severe sepsis found that the age of the stored transfused RBC was directly associated with mortality [35].
- Another retrospective study, this time of post-coronary-artery bypass grafting (CABG) patients, showed that the age of the stored blood was associated with the chance of developing pneumonia [36]. However, another study from the same group has found no evidence of increased morbidity in cardiac surgery patients when old blood is transfused [37].
- From a trauma unit database, multivariate analysis has identified that the mean age of blood transfused, number of units older than 14 days, and number of units older than 21 days are independent risk factors for the development of organ failures [38]. They suggest that fresh blood may be more appropriate for the initial resuscitation of trauma patients requiring transfusion.

Several critical care trials are ongoing, which will hopefully more definitively answer the question regarding RBC age and effect on outcome:

- Age of Blood Evaluation (ABLE) trial in the resuscitation of critically ill patients (ISRCTN44878718): Canadian lead multicenter study recruiting 2510 patients to test if the transfusion of fresh (stored <8 days) RBCs will lead to a 5% or greater improvement in 90 day all-cause mortality and clinically important morbidity in critically ill patients.
- TRANSFUSE-RCT (Standard Issue Transfusion versus Fresher Red Blood Cell Use in Intensive Care) (NCT01638416): Australian led multicenter study recruiting

5000 critically ill patients to test if transfusion of the freshest available RBCs versus standard practice (oldest available) decreases 90-day mortality.

Effect of RBC transfusion on outcome

To date, the most rigorous study guiding the use of RBC transfusion in the critical care population remains the influential TRICC trial [39].

- In this randomized, controlled trial of 838 ICU patients with a hemoglobin concentration of ≤90 g/L within 3 days of admission, the authors compared a restrictive versus liberal (70 g/L versus 100 g/L) transfusion threshold strategy and found no significant difference in outcome.
- In fact, those patients managed with a restrictive transfusion strategy trended toward a lower 28-day mortality (18.7 versus 23.3%, p = 0.11) and less organ dysfunction and cardiac complications.

Numerous other studies have been published in this area. However, with the exception of TRICC, in the critically ill population these studies are all observational in nature. As in all observational transfusion studies, they are significantly limited by bias, predominantly confounding by indication in that sicker patients are not only more likely to be anemic, but more likely to receive any and more frequent RBC transfusion.

- In the systematic review by Marik *et al.* (2008) [40] of 45 observational studies in the critically ill, he demonstrated an association between RBC transfusion and increased risk of death, infection, organ dysfunction and acute respiratory distress syndrome.
- A more recent Cochrane Database systematic review [41] has also been published. In this review of 19 RCTs of restrictive versus liberal transfusion strategies in a heterogeneous (medical and surgical) population, the restrictive strategy was associated with a reduction in mortality (hospital), but not with an increase in pneumonia, stroke, cardiac or venous thromboembolic events.

Indications for transfusion

Given the available evidence, for most adult critically ill patients, a management strategy that includes a transfusion trigger of 70 g/L is reasonable. Potential exceptions may apply for certain patient populations, including those with ischemic heart disease, septic shock and acute neurological injuries, and are reviewed below.

Ischemic heart disease

In large observational studies of patients with acute coronary syndromes, anemia has been shown to be associated with additional cardiac events, longer lengths of hospital stay and death [16,42]. However, the association of RBC transfusion thresholds and death in this same group is contradictory.

- In a subgroup analysis from the TRICC trial [43], among patients with cardiovascular disease (n = 357), 30-day mortality was the same between the two groups (restrictive and liberal transfusion arms, 23% versus 23%). However, among the 257 patients with severe ischemic heart disease, there was a trend towards increased mortality in the group randomized to restrictive transfusion (26% versus 21%, p = 0.38).

- A recent small pilot RCT (n = 110) [44] of a liberal transfusion threshold (Hb ≥100 g/L) versus a restrictive threshold (Hb >80 g/L) in patients with acute coronary syndrome or stable angina undergoing cardiac catheterization, demonstrated a decreased risk of the primary outcome (combined death, myocardial infarction or unscheduled revascularization within 30 days) (10.9% versus 25.5%; risk difference = 15.0%, p = 0.054), and death at 30 days (1.8% versus 13.0%, p = 0.032). The authors concluded the need for a definitive trial.
- A large observational study of 2202 patients undergoing coronary-artery bypass surgery [45] demonstrated a significantly increased risk of left ventricular dysfunction and mortality in the high and medium Hct groups (Hct ≥25%) compared to the low Hct group (Hct <25%), suggesting that a restrictive transfusion strategy is better. However, in the TRACS noninferiority RCT [46] (n = 502), a liberal transfusion strategy (goal Hct ≥30%), as compared to a restrictive strategy (Hct ≥24%), following cardiac surgery resulted in noninferior rates of 30-day all-cause mortality and severe morbidity.
- The FOCUS randomized, controlled trial (n = 2016) [47] examined a transfusion trigger of 100 g/L versus 80 g/L in patients with either a history of, or risk factors for, cardiovascular disease following hip-fracture surgery and found no difference in the combined outcome of death or inability to walk 10 feet at 60 days (46.1% versus 48.1% respectively, odds ratio 0.92, 95% confidence interval 0.73–1.16).

Septic shock

The evidence to support RBC transfusion in anemic septic shock patients is also conflicting, with mixed results demonstrating benefit only in the presence of pre-existing microcirculation derangements [33].

- The landmark early goal-directed therapy in severe sepsis trial by Rivers *et al.* [48] incorporated a hematocrit target of 30 g/L (or approximate Hb 100 g/L) as part of an early resuscitation strategy, which demonstrated a significant survival benefit. However, RBC transfusion was only one facet of a bundle of therapies included in the algorithm making benefit attributable to transfusion alone impossible to discern.
- The most recent Surviving Sepsis Guidelines (2012) [49] endorses a restrictive transfusion strategy (trigger of Hb <70 g/L, targeting Hb 70–90 g/L) in the absence of "extenuating circumstances" amongst severely septic patients in whom hypoperfusion has been resolved.
- The role of RBC transfusion may be better understood upon completion of the TRISS trial (Transfusion Requirements in Septic Shock Trial) (NCT01485315). This study, with a planned enrollment of 1000 patients, aims to compare the effect of a restrictive (transfusion trigger Hb <70 g/L) versus liberal (trigger Hb <90 g/L) on 90 day all-cause mortality amongst septic shock patients.

Neuro-critical care

Those suffering from acute neurological stresses, including ischemic stroke, subarachnoid hemorrhage (SAH) and traumatic brain injury are thought to be particularly susceptible to secondary ischemia from altered/decreased tissue oxygen delivery and/or uptake and utilization. Preclinical studies have demonstrated the biologic plausibility of oxygen delivery optimization in the brain. However, numerous observational data in human subjects across brain injury etiologies have again demonstrated conflicting benefit of RBC transfusion.

- In the small subgroup analysis of neurologic patients (n = 67) in the TRICC trial [50], the authors were unable to demonstrate benefit in the liberal transfusion group, but conversely did not demonstrate harm in the restrictive group. The very small numbers make this difficult to interpret.
- The only existing RCT is a small study of aneurysmal SAH patients (n = 44) [51] in which patients were randomized to either a restrictive transfusion trigger (Hb 100 g/L) or a liberal trigger (Hb 115 g/L). However, this study was underpowered to evaluate any clinically meaningful outcome.
- A recent systematic review of comparative studies of RBC transfusion in the neuro-critically ill [52] found only six studies in the literature, and concluded that insufficient evidence existed to support or refute a restrictive transfusion trigger in this population. Among the studies included, in which high risk of bias existed, as well as a lack of assessment of long-term outcomes, no benefit in mortality or length of hospital stay was demonstrated in the lower transfusion trigger groups.

A practical approach to RBC transfusion

Recommendations by the ASA Task Force on Blood Component Therapy [53] state, and remain valid today, that transfusion is:

- "rarely required above an Hb of 100 g/L,"
- "almost always indicated when Hb is <60 g/L."

Current evidence supports a restrictive strategy (Hb ≤70 g/L) for transfusion in most ICU settings. More definitive data is still required for certain specific patient populations, including patients with cardiovascular diseases and acute neurologic injuries. Until such time, a higher transfusion trigger (Hb 80-90 g/L) is clinically acceptable in the context of critical illness.

References

1. De Benoist B, McLean E, Egil I, Cogswell M. *Worldwide Prevalence of Anaemia 1993-2005*. WHO 2008.

2. Hébert PC, Tinmouth A, Corwin H. Anemia and red cell transfusion in critically ill patients. *Crit Care Med* 2003; 31(12) : S672-7.

3. Vincent JL, Baron J-F, Reinhart K *et al.* Anemia and blood transfusion in critically ill patients. *J Am Med Assoc* 2002; 288 : 1499-507.

4. Walsh TS, Lee RJ, Maciver CR *et al.* Anemia during and at discharge from intensive care: the impact of restrictive blood transfusion practice. *Intensive Care Med* 2006; 32 : 100-9.

5. Corwin HL, Gettinger A, Pearl RG *et al.* The CRIT Study: Anemia and blood transfusion in the critically ill–current clinical practice in the United States. *Crit Care Med* 2004; 32 : 39-52.

6. Nguyen B, Bota D, Melot C, Vincent J-L. Time course of hemoglobin concentrations in nonbleeding intensive care unit patients. *Crit Care Med* 2003; 31 : 406-10.

7. Von Ahsen N, Muller C, Serke S *et al.* Important role of non-diagnostic blood loss and blunted erythropoietic response in the anaemia of medical intensive care patients. *Crit Care Med* 1999; 27 : 2630-9.

8. Bloos F, Reinhart K. Venous oximetry. *Intensive Care Med* 2005; 31 : 911-13.

9. Madjdpour C, Spahn DR. Allogeneic red blood cell transfusion: physiology of

oxygen transport. *Best Pract Res Clin Anaesthesiol* 2007; 21 : 163–71.

10. Hébert PC, Hu LQ, Biro GP. Review of physiologic mechanisms in response to anemia. *Can Med Assoc J* 1997; 156 (Supplement) : S27–40.

11. Creteur J, Neves AP, Vincent J-L. Near-infrared spectroscopy technique to evaluate the effects of red blood cell transfusion on tissue oxygenation. *Crit Care* 2009; 13 Suppl 5 : S11.

12. Suttner S, Piper SN, Kumle B *et al.* The influence of allogeneic red blood cell transfusion compared with 100% oxygen ventilation on systemic oxygen transport and skeletal muscle oxygen tension after cardiac surgery: retracted. *Anesth Analg* 2004; 99 : 2–11.

13. Hébert PC, McDonald BJ, Tinmouth A. Clinical consequences of anemia and red cell transfusion in the critically ill. *Crit Care Clin* 2004; 20 : 225–35.

14. Carson JL, Duff A, Poses R *et al.* Effect of anaemia and cardiovascular disease on surgical mortality and morbidity. *Lancet* 1996; 348 : 1055–9.

15. Carson JL, Noveck H, Berlin J, Gould S. Mortality and morbidity in patients with very low postoperative Hb levels who decline blood transfusion. *Transfusion* 2002; 42 : 812–8.

16. Wu WC, Rathore SS, Wang Y *et al.* Blood transfusion in elderly patients with acute myocardial infarction. *N Engl J Med* 2001; 345 : 1230–6.

17. Ronco C, Bowry S, Tetta C. Dialysis Patients and Cardiovascular Problems: Can Technology Help Solve the Complex Equation ? *Blood Purif* 2006; 24 : 39–45.

18. Van Iperen CE, Gaillard CA, Kraaijenhagen RJ *et al.* Response of erythropoiesis and iron metabolism to recombinant human erythropoietin in intensive care unit patients. *Crit Care Med* 2000; 28 : 2773–8.

19. Zarychanski R, Turgeon AF, McIntyre L, Fergusson DA. Erythropoietin-receptor agonists in critically ill patients: a meta-analysis of randomized controlled trials. *CMAJ* 2007; 177 : 725–34.

20. Hébert P, Wells G, Martin C *et al.* Variation in red cell transfusion practice in the intensive care unit: a multicentre cohort study. *Crit Care* 1999; 3 : 57–63.

21. Dietrich KA, Conrad SA, Hebert CA *et al.* Cardiovascular and metabolic response to red blood cell transfusion in critically ill volume-resuscitated nonsurgical patients. *Crit Care Med* 1990; 18 : 940–4.

22. Casutt M, Seifert B, Pasch T *et al.* Factors influencing the individual effects of blood transfusions on oxygen delivery and oxygen consumption. *Crit Care Med* 1999; 27 : 2194–200.

23. Conrad SA, Dietrich KA, Hebert CA, Romero MD. Effect of red cell transfusion on oxygen consumption following fluid resuscitation in septic shock. *Circ Shock* 1990; 31 : 419–29.

24. Lorente JA, Landín L, De Pablo R *et al.* Effects of blood transfusion on oxygen transport variables in severe sepsis. *Crit Care Med* 1993; 21 : 1312–8.

25. Marik PE, Sibbald WJ. Effect of stored-blood transfusion on oxygen delivery in patients with sepsis. *JAMA* 1993; 269 : 3024–9.

26. Steffes CP, Bender JS, Levison MA. Blood transfusion and oxygen consumption in surgical sepsis. *Crit Care Med* 1991; 19 : 512–7.

27. Raghavan M, Marik PE. Anemia, allogenic blood transfusion, and immunomodulation in the critically ill. *Chest* 2005; 127 : 295–307.

28. Gilliss BM, Looney MR, Gropper MA. Reducing noninfectious risks of blood transfusion. *Anesthesiology* 2011; 115 : 635–49.

29. Zallen G, Moore EE, Ciesla DJ *et al.* Stored red blood cells selectively activate human neutrophils to release IL-8 and secretory PLA2. *Shock* 2000; 13 : 29–33.

30. Toy P, Gajic O, Bacchetti P *et al.* Transfusion-related acute lung injury: incidence and risk factors. *Blood* 2012; 119 : 1757–67.

31. Lin Y, Saw C-L, Hannach B, Goldman M. Transfusion-related acute lung injury

prevention measures and their impact at Canadian Blood Services. *Transfusion* 2012; 52 : 567–74.

32. Landers DF, Hill GE, Wong KC, Fox IJ. Blood transfusion-induced immunomodulation. *Anesth Analg* 1996; 82 : 187–204.

33. McIntyre L, Tinmouth AT, Fergusson DA. Blood component transfusion in critically ill patients. *Curr Opin Crit Care* 2013; 19 : 326–33.

34. Tinmouth A, Fergusson D, Yee IC, Hébert PC. Clinical consequences of red cell storage in the critically ill. *Transfusion* 2006; 46 : 2014–27.

35. Purdy FR, Tweeddale MG, Merrick PM. Association of mortality with age of blood transfused in septic ICU patients. *Can J Anaesth* 1997; 44 : 1256–61.

36. Vamvakas EC, Carven JH. Transfusion and postoperative pneumonia in coronary artery bypass graft surgery: effect of the length of storage of transfused red cells. *Transfusion* 1999; 39 : 701–10.

37. Vamvakas EC, Carven JH. Length of storage of transfused red cells and postoperative morbidity in patients undergoing coronary artery bypass graft surgery. *Transfusion* 2000; 40 : 101–9.

38. Zallen G, Offner PJ, Moore EE et al. Age of transfused blood is an independent risk factor for postinjury multiple organ failure. *Am J Surg* 1999; 178 : 570–2.

39. Hébert PC, Wells G, Blajchman MA et al. A multicenter, randomized, controlled clinical trial of transfusion requirements in critical care. Transfusion Requirements in Critical Care Investigators, Canadian Critical Care Trials Group. *N Engl J Med* 1999; 340 : 409–17.

40. Marik PE, Corwin HL. Efficacy of red blood cell transfusion in the critically ill: a systematic review of the literature. *Crit Care Med* 2008; 36 : 2667–74.

41. Carson JL, Carless PA, Hébert PC. Transfusion thresholds and other strategies for guiding allogeneic red blood cell transfusion. *Cochrane database Syst Rev* 2012; 4(5) : CD002042.

42. Rao S V, Jollis JG, Harrington RA et al. Relationship of blood transfusion and clinical outcomes in patients with acute coronary syndromes. *J Am Med Assoc* 2004; 292 : 1555–62.

43. Hébert PC, Yetisir E, Martin C et al. Is a low transfusion threshold safe in critically ill patients with cardiovascular diseases? *Crit Care Med* 2001; 29 : 227–34.

44. Carson JL, Brooks MM, Abbott JD et al. Liberal versus restrictive transfusion thresholds for patients with symptomatic coronary artery disease. *Am Heart J* 2013; 165 : 964–71.

45. Spiess BD, Ley C, Body SC et al. Hematocrit value on intensive care unit entry influences the frequency of Q-wave myocardial infarction after coronary artery bypass grafting. The Institutions of the Multicenter Study of Perioperative Ischemia (McSPI) Research Group. *J Thorac Cardiovasc Surg* 1998; 116 : 460–7.

46. Hajjar LA, Vincent J-L, Galas FRBG et al. Transfusion requirements after cardiac surgery: the TRACS randomized controlled trial. *J Am Med Assoc* 2010; 304 : 1559–67.

47. Carson JL, Terrin ML, Noveck H et al. Liberal or restrictive transfusion in high-risk patients after hip surgery. *N Engl J Med* 2011; 365 : 2453–62.

48. Rivers E, Nguyen B, Havstad SA. Early Goal-Directed Therapy in the Treatment of Severe Sepsis and Septic Sho et al. *N Engl J Med* 2001; 345 : 1368–77.

49. Dellinger RP, Levy MM, Rhodes A et al. Surviving sepsis campaign: international guidelines for management of severe sepsis and septic shock: 2012. *Crit Care Med* 2013; 41 : 580–637.

50. Mcintyre LA, Fergusson DA, Hutchison JS et al. Effect of a liberal versus restrictive transfusion strategy on mortality in patients with moderate to severe head injury. *Neurocrit Care* 2006; 5 : 4–9.

51. Naidech AM, Shaibani A, Garg RK et al. Prospective, randomized trial

of higher goal hemoglobin after subarachnoid hemorrhage. *Neurocrit Care* 2010; 13 : 313–20.

52. Desjardins P, Turgeon AF, Tremblay MH *et al*. Hemoglobin levels and transfusions in neurocritically ill patients: a systematic review of comparative studies. *Crit Care* 2012; 16(2) : R54.

53. American Society of Anesthesiologists Task Force on Blood Component Therapy Practice guidelines for blood component therapy. *Anesthesiology* 1996; 84 : 732–47.

Coagulation problems in the critically ill

Alejandro Lazo-Langner

Coagulation disorders are a very common finding in critically ill patients. They include abnormalities in platelets, coagulation factors and the fibrinolytic system, and in general they are due to three mechanisms: impaired production or synthesis, peripheral destruction, consumption, sequestration or accelerated loss, and dysfunction.

This chapter will review the epidemiology of coagulation abnormalities in the ICU, the general mechanisms of coagulopathy, the differential diagnosis of specific abnormalities, and the general principles of management of these patients.

Epidemiology of coagulation abnormalities in critically ill patients

Abnormalities in platelet count

- Thrombocytopenia (defined as a platelet count $<150\ 000 \times 10^9$/L) is present in one-third to one-half of all patients admitted to an ICU for a medical condition [1].
- Platelet counts $<100\ 000 \times 10^9$/L can be found in up to one-quarter of patients, whereas counts $<50\ 000 \times 10^9$/L are present in about 15% of patients.
- The incidence of thrombocytopenia is higher in surgical and trauma patients: about 40% of them have platelet counts $<100\ 000 \times 10^9$/L.
- Platelet counts $<50\ 000 \times 10^9$/L are associated with a four- to fivefold higher bleeding risk and about 90% of critically ill patients with intracranial bleeding have a platelet count $<100\ 000 \times 10^9$/L.
- Thrombocytopenia has been found to be an independent predictor of mortality in numerous studies [2,3].
- Persistent thrombocytopenia for more than 4 days or a drop in the platelet count >50% during an ICU stay is related to a four- to sixfold increase in mortality [4].

Abnormalities in global coagulation assays

- Global coagulation assays (prothrombin time, PT, or activated partial thromboplastin time, aPTT) are found to be prolonged in 14–28% of ICU patients.
- Prolongation of coagulation assays as reflected by a PT or aPTT ratio greater than 1.5 (i.e. the ratio of the patient's coagulation time compared to a control) predicts excessive bleeding.
- Prolonged PT or aPTT are independent predictors of mortality in trauma patients.

Handbook of ICU Therapy, third edition, ed. John Fuller, Jeff Granton and Ian McConachie. Published by Cambridge University Press. © Cambridge University Press 2015.

Other coagulation abnormalities

- Elevated D-dimer and fibrin degradation products (FDPs) can be found in intensive care patients (42%), trauma patients (80%) and patients with sepsis (99%).
- Low fibrinogen levels are frequently found in ICU patients and are related to increased mortality [5].
- Low levels of the natural anticoagulants antithrombin and protein C are found in approximately half of trauma patients and up to 90% of patients with sepsis [6].
- Evidence of hyperfibrinolysis can be found in 57% of trauma patients and is also a predictor of mortality [7].

Mechanisms of coagulopathy

The coagulation system is a highly phylogenetically preserved system and has a fundamental role for survival. In addition to its pivotal function of maintaining the integrity of the vascular bed it has a number of additional functions that are increasingly recognized. These nonhemostatic functions explain the frequent and profound disruption of the coagulation system observed in critically ill patients.

Coagulation system and inflammation

- Natural anticoagulant pathways, in particular the protein C system, play a central role in the regulation of inflammation.
- Deficiency in the protein C system is associated with a general dysregulation of the coagulation system in sepsis.
- Binding of activated protein C to the endothelial protein C receptor (EPCR) potentiates its anticoagulant and anti-inflammatory effects.
- In sepsis, the presence of proteolytic enzymes such as neutrophil elastase results in degradation of the inactive protein C with subsequent deficiency.
- Additionally, EPCR is downregulated in sepsis, which may negatively affect the protein C system.
- Proinflammatory cytokines such as TNF-α and IL-1 downregulate the expression of thrombomodulin, the endothelial target of thrombin, resulting in a lower activation of inactive protein C.
- Additionally, a relative protein S (the cofactor of protein C) deficiency can result from an increase in the complement component C4bBP from acute phase reaction, because C4bBP forms a complex with protein S [2,3,8].
- All of these alterations result in a prothrombotic state.

Coagulation system and immunity

- There is increasing evidence of the role of the hemostatic system in immunity.
- In the presence of a thrombus (either arterial or venous) monocytes and neutrophils are swiftly recruited to the vessel wall and the nascent clot.
- Platelets interact with neutrophils in response to bacterial products and trigger the release of neutrophil extracellular traps or NETs, which are constituted by neutrophil intracellular components and have important antibacterial functions, but are also potent activators of the coagulation system.

- Coagulation factors such as thrombin and activated factor X, as well as platelets, are capable of regulating the effector functions of immune cells.
- Under normal circumstances the activation of coagulation by immune cells serves a role in the response to pathogens by exerting direct antimicrobial effects and limiting bacterial spreading.
- However, the concurrent activation of coagulation and inflammation might induce a vicious loop resulting in excessive activation of immune cells and pathological thrombus formation [9].

Coagulation system and vascular homeostasis

- The coagulation system interacts with the renin–angiotensin system at multiple levels. These interactions could result in bidirectional alterations of both systems, potentially leading to a prothrombotic state or altering the vessel tone. Examples where these interactions might be relevant are sepsis and hypertensive emergencies.
- The Prekallikrein–Kallikrein–high-molecular-weight kininogen (PK-K-HMWK) system, also known as the contact pathway, can stimulate the coagulation system through activation of coagulation factor XII.
- Angiotensinase C (PRCP) converts PK to K. This reaction also generates bradykinin (a vasodilator peptide) from kininogen.
- Under conditions of sepsis or exposure to artificial surfaces (e.g. extracorporeal circuits) factor-XII-dependent coagulation activation can be observed.
- PRCP also degrades angiotensin II to angiotensin, resulting in vasodilatation.
- The angiotensin-converting enzyme (ACE) degrades bradykinin and converts angiotensin I to angiotensin II, resulting in enhanced vasoconstriction and inhibition of the fibrinolytic system [10,11].
- Bradykinin (1–5) – a degradation product of bradykinin – inhibits thrombin-induced platelet aggregation [10].
- Stimulation of AT2 receptors enhances bradykinin formation.
- Angiotensins I, II and III induce expression of tissue factor by stimulating the AT1 receptor. This overexpression of tissue factor results in a thrombogenic endothelium.

Coagulation system and tissue remodeling

- The fibrinolytic system has been found to play an important role in tissue and vascular remodeling, mainly through activation of matrix metalloproteinases and their regulators. These enzymes are involved in the degradation of extracellular matrix components and are crucial in many processes, including angiogenesis and wound healing.
- Plasmin and plasminogen activators can regulate the activation of growth factors and are involved in tissue proliferation.
- Plasminogen activator inhibitor-type1 (PAI-1), the main regulator of plasmin generation, is involved in cell adhesion and migration and has an active role in carcinogenesis.
- Alterations in the fibrinolytic system have been associated with venous, but mainly arterial, thrombosis and atherogenesis [12,13].

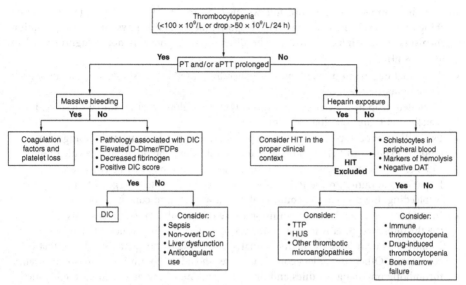

Figure 7.1 Diagnostic algorithm for coagulation abnormalities in critically ill patients. (Adapted and modified from [2]). Abbreviations: aPTT activated partial thromboplastin time; DAT direct antiglobulin test; DIC disseminated intravascular coagulation; FDPs fibrin(ogen) degradation products; HIT heparin-induced thrombocytopenia; HUS hemolytic uremic syndrome; PT prothrombin time; TTP thrombotic thrombocytopenic purpura.

Coagulation abnormalities in critically ill patients

Identifying the coagulation abnormalities developing in critical patients might be not straightforward. Characteristics to be considered in the differential approach include timing, severity, underlying disorders, drug exposure and other clinical or laboratory findings. These might help to determine the mechanism of coagulopathy. A simplified diagnostic algorithm is shown in Figure 7.1.

Thrombocytopenia

In critically ill patients thrombocytopenia is usually multifactorial and related to illness severity. Its magnitude correlates with the length of ICU stays and also with mortality. It is important to recognize the underlying cause in order to establish an effective management plan.

- The major mechanisms of thrombocytopenia include hemodilution, increased consumption, increased destruction, decreased production and sequestration.
- The major causes of thrombocytopenia and their relative incidences include sepsis (52%), disseminated intravascular coagulation (25%), massive blood loss (8%), thrombotic microangiopathy (1%), heparin-induced thrombocytopenia (1%), immune thrombocytopenia (1%) and drug-induced thrombocytopenia (10%) [4].

Diagnostic approach to thrombocytopenia in critically ill patients

When evaluating a patient with thrombocytopenia in the ICU, clinicians must consider the time of onset of the thrombocytopenia, the nadir platelet count and the dynamic course of the platelet count. In general, after an initial drop in the platelet count (for example, after cardiac surgery) an increase follows, usually around 3 or 4 days later, frequently reaching higher levels than baseline. This response indicates that physiologic compensation mechanisms remain intact. However, the differential diagnosis is not straightforward in many cases [4].

- A gradual decline in platelet count is generally caused by consumptive coagulopathy or bone marrow failure.
- A sudden drop in platelet count, especially if it develops after an initial increase, is usually due to immunologic causes.
- Pseudothrombocytopenia, an *in vitro* phenomenon due to platelet clumping when blood is exposed to EDTA anticoagulant in test tubes, should always be ruled out.
- In all cases, the underlying medical or surgical conditions must be considered. In patients admitted to the ICU with thrombocytopenia after surgery, trauma or bleeding, the drop in the count is almost always due to consumption.
- In medical patients, the most common cause of thrombocytopenia is sepsis, and the thrombocytopenia is usually moderate ($50–100 \times 10^9$/L). When the platelet count is less than 50×10^9/L, disseminated intravascular coagulation (DIC) must be considered. Other, much less common causes include autoimmune thrombocytopenia, thrombotic microangiopathies and drugs. In patients living or traveling to endemic areas, malaria should be considered.
- If thrombocytopenia is associated with a thrombotic complication, the diagnostic considerations must include antiphospholipid antibodies syndrome and heparin-induced thrombocytopenia in patients with recent heparin exposure.
- Heparin-induced thrombocytopenia (HIT) should be considered in patients with recent exposure to heparin, if the thrombocytopenia develops between days 5 and 10–14 after an initial heparin exposure, is associated with a thrombotic complication or skin necrosis, the nadir is between 20 and 100×10^9/L, and there is no alternative explanation [14].
- In patients with severe thrombocytopenia ($<20 \times 10^9$/L) the most common cause is sepsis, but marrow infiltrative conditions such as acute leukemia, myelodysplastic syndromes or myelopthisis should be considered, in particular if other cell lines are affected.
- A gradual decrease in platelet count may indicate multiorgan failure and the development of consumptive coagulopathy – DIC.
- DIC frequently presents with other coagulation abnormalities in addition to the thrombocytopenia, such as prolonged coagulation times, decreased levels of coagulation factors, and increased FDPs [2–4].

Prolonged coagulation times

Critically ill patients frequently develop prolongation of global coagulation times (PT and aPTT). Although these tests are a practical way of measuring one or multiple coagulation factors, they might not reflect the hemostatic function *in vivo*.

- In general, PT or aPTT will be prolonged if coagulation factors drop below 50% of normal. However, there is great variation depending on reagents or instruments used.

- The International Normalized Ratio (INR) is a ratio of the PT in a patient compared to a control that is normalized in reference to an international standard. Although it has greatly increased its use to evaluate global coagulation in an attempt to allow better standardization, it has only been validated for monitoring anticoagulant therapy with vitamin K antagonists such as warfarin or acenocoumarol.
- Deficiencies in coagulation factors are usually due to consumption, impaired synthesis or massive loss. A less common cause is the presence of inhibitors (acquired hemophilia, acquired von Willebrand's disease, lupus anticoagulants) [2,3].

Diagnostic approach to prolonged coagulation times in critically ill patients

- Causes of isolated PT (or INR) prolongation include factor VII deficiency, mild vitamin K deficiency, mild liver insufficiency and use of vitamin K antagonists.
- Causes of isolated aPTT prolongation include factors VIII, IX or XI deficiency, use of unfractionated heparin (or low-molecular-weight heparin overdose), acquired inhibitors (most frequently against factor VIII), factor XII or PK deficiencies and hemophilia A (factor VIII deficiency) or B (factor IX deficiency).
- Causes of concurrent prolongation of PT and aPTT include factors X, V, II or fibrinogen deficiencies, severe vitamin K deficiency, use of vitamin K antagonists, liver failure, massive loss and consumption (DIC).

Disseminated intravascular coagulation (DIC)

This is a frequent complication in critically ill patients caused by systemic intravascular activation of the hemostatic system resulting in the formation of microvascular thrombi, which can in turn contribute to worsening organ dysfunction.

- Proinflammatory cytokines released by mononuclear and endothelial cells during a severe inflammatory response result in thrombin generation mediated by the tissue factor–factor VIIa pathway. This activation concurrently with a decrease in the function of the anticoagulant antithrombin and protein C systems, and an inhibition of the fibrinolytic system mediated by high levels of PAI-1, result in progressive activation and consumption of platelets and coagulation factors, leading to intravascular fibrin deposition and microvascular thrombi. In serious cases the thrombocytopenia and the depletion of coagulation factors might lead to major bleeding.
- DIC frequently presents with several coagulation abnormalities including thrombocytopenia, and prolonged coagulation times as a result of a decrease in coagulation factors. It also results in increased FDPs.
- A diagnosis of DIC depends on the presence of a combination of coagulation abnormalities in the appropriate setting; however, some scoring systems have been developed with high diagnostic sensitivity and specificity.
- The International Society on Thrombosis and Haemostasis scoring system includes risk assessment, major laboratory criteria (platelet count, PT, FDPs) and specific criteria (thrombin, protein C, thrombin–antithrombin complexes) [15].
- The Japanese Association for Acute Medicine DIC score includes platelet count, PT, FDPs and evidence of systemic inflammatory response [16].
- DIC score is an independent predictor of mortality [17].

Other coagulation abnormalities

Routine coagulation tests such as PT, aPTT and platelet count do not account for all possible defects potentially leading to bleeding complications. Special tests are needed to confirm such conditions and involvement of the hematology service is necessary in the assessment and management of these abnormalities.

Platelet function defects

- Platelet function defects are frequently present in critically ill patients.
- Platelet function can be abnormal as a result of systemic conditions, in particular uremia and severe liver failure.
- Several drugs can affect platelet function and lead to hemorrhagic complications, including aspirin, thienopyridines, nonsteroidal anti-inflammatory drugs, hirudins (e.g lepirudin and bivalirudin) and abciximab.
- In cardiac patients, exposure of blood to extracorporeal circuits can induce severe platelet dysfunction.
- No routine laboratory tests can identify platelet dysfunction. The use of bleeding time has been abandoned due to its notorious unreliability. Other tests such as platelet aggregometry and closure time (PFA100 analyzer) can help to better identify these defects, but they are not widely available and their interpretation is not straightforward [2].

Hyperfibrinolysis (primary)

- This condition is manifested by a marked activation of the fibrinolytic system and it can lead to serious hemorrhagic problems.
- It is relatively rare and it can be observed typically in patients with acute promyelocytic leukemia and prostate cancer.
- Patients exposed to extracorporeal circuits can also present this condition as a result of plasminogen release from the endothelium.
- Treatment with thrombolytic agents, typically for ischemic cardiac or cerebral events, results in an induced hyperfibrinolytic state.
- Patients present with high levels of D-dimer or FDPs and low levels of fibrinogen, plasminogen, or α-2 antiplasmin or FDPs, Other tests such as euglobulin lysis time can help to identify this condition [2].

Principles of management of patients with coagulation abnormalities

The cornerstone of the management of critically ill patients with coagulation abnormalities is the proper and timely management of the underlying condition. However, supportive measures are frequently needed. Adequate transfusional support with packed red blood cells is important. Recent evidence confirms that erythrocytes play an active role in supporting thrombin generation [18]. Improvement of hematocrit has been shown to improve hemostasis *in vitro* [19] and some studies suggest it might also decrease mortality in some groups of patients [20]. Correction of metabolic abnormalities such as acidosis, hypothermia and hypocalcemia should also be pursued, since all of these will have a negative impact on the hemostatic function [21]. Maintaining adequate tissue perfusion is also fundamental, and consideration should be given to the use of permissive hypotension, which has been found to reduce coagulopathy in trauma patients [22].

Platelet abnormalities

- In general, patients with a platelet count of less than 10×10^9/L should be managed with prophylactic platelet transfusions which have been shown to decrease, albeit not eliminate, major bleeding events [23].
- Patients with higher platelet counts (20–50 $\times 10^9$/L) should also receive platelet transfusions in the presence of bleeding. In patients with platelet dysfunction and major bleeding, platelet transfusions can be indicated, even in the case of normal platelet counts.
- Platelet transfusions are more effective in cases of thrombocytopenia due to increased consumption or impaired production. In cases of conditions leading to increased platelet destruction (such as immune thrombocytopenia) they are usually not helpful and are reserved only for cases of critical bleeding. In such cases other treatments, such as intravenous immunoglobulin, steroids, immunosuppressive agents or thrombopoietin mimetics might be necessary.
- In cases of suspected or confirmed heparin-induced thrombocytopenia, cessation of heparin and use of alternative anticoagulants such as lepirudin, argatroban or fondaparinux should be instituted. Platelet transfusions are usually contraindicated since they might aggravate the condition and should be reserved for cases with critical bleeding. Warfarin initiation should be postponed until normalization of platelet count [14].

Coagulation factor deficiencies

- In cases of coagulation factor deficiencies, they can be replenished by using fresh frozen plasma, or coagulation factor concentrates. Plasma is usually reserved for patients with bleeding events; however, a risk of volume overload exists if large amounts are required.
- Use of coagulation factor concentrates can be considered in cases of single factor deficiencies.
- Prothrombin complex concentrates are indicated for the rapid reversal of warfarin-associated coagulopathy. Their use outside this context (e.g. for replenishing a global coagulation factor deficiency) should be considered off-label and it cannot be routinely recommended. Consideration should be given only in extreme cases. Additionally, these agents do not replenish all coagulation factors and hemostatic defects might persist.
- Use of fibrinogen concentrates or cryoprecipitates should be considered in patients with critically low levels of fibrinogen, in particular in patients with active bleeding or at high risk, such as patients with acute promyelocytic leukemia.
- Recombinant activated factor VII (rFVIIa) is approved for the treatment of bleeding in hemophiliac patients with inhibitors. A great deal of anecdotal evidence exists suggesting improved hemostatic function in bleeding patients after using this agent. A meta-analysis suggested that the use of rFVIIa reduces blood transfusion and it may reduce mortality, but increases the risk of arterial thrombosis [24]. However, a well-designed randomized, controlled trial failed to show improvement in mortality or relevant clinical outcomes in patients with intracranial hemorrhage, in spite of a

reduction of hematoma growth [25]. Therefore, the use of this agent is not recommended routinely and it should only be considered in cases of life-threatening events as a last resource.

- 1-Deamino-8-D-arginine vasopressin (DDAVP) induces release of von Willebrand factor from endothelial cells, resulting in a significant increase of this factor and its associated factor VIII, with a subsequent hemostatic response. Its main use is in the treatment of patients with certain types of von Willebrand's disease and mild hemophilia A, but it has been used with success to treat patients with platelet dysfunction secondary to uremia.

- Antifibrinolytic agents such as ε-aminocaproic acid or tranexamic acid can be used to reduce blood loss and transfusion requirements. The use of tranexamic acid has been shown to reduce mortality in bleeding trauma patients and it seems to be safe [26,27].

Conclusions

Coagulation abnormalities are frequent in critically ill patients. Treatment of the underlying condition is fundamental in the management of these abnormalities. Early identification and intervention of these complications is essential to improve clinical outcomes. The use of supportive measures is paramount and prohemostatic agents should be considered with caution, depending on the underlying mechanism of coagulopathy. A multidisciplinary approach is necessary to improve the outcomes in these patients.

References

1. Vanderschueren S, De Weerdt A, Malbrain M et al. Thrombocytopenia and prognosis in intensive care. Crit Care Med 2000; 28 : 1871–6.

2. Levi M, Opal SM. Coagulation abnormalities in critically ill patients. Crit Care 2006; 10 : 222.

3. Levi M, Schultz M. Coagulopathy and platelet disorders in critically ill patients. Minerva Anestesiol 2010; 76 : 851–9.

4. Greinacher A, Selleng K. Thrombocytopenia in the intensive care unit patient. Hematology Am Soc Hematol Educ Program 2010; 2010 : 135–43.

5. Inaba K, Karamanos E, Lustenberger T et al. Impact of fibrinogen levels on outcomes after acute injury in patients requiring a massive transfusion. J Am Coll Surg 2013; 216 : 290–7.

6. Bernard GR, Vincent JL, Laterre PF et al. Efficacy and safety of recombinant human activated protein C for severe sepsis. N Engl J Med 2001; 344 : 699–709.

7. Raza I, Davenport R, Rourke C et al. The incidence and magnitude of fibrinolytic activation in trauma patients. J Thromb Haemost 2013; 11 : 307–14.

8. Della VP, Pavani G, D'Angelo A. The protein C pathway and sepsis. Thromb Res 2012; 129 : 296–300.

9. Engelmann B, Massberg S. Thrombosis as an intravascular effector of innate immunity. Nat Rev Immunol 2013; 13 : 34–45.

10. Dielis AW, Smid M, Spronk HM et al. The prothrombotic paradox of hypertension: role of the renin-angiotensin and kallikrein-kinin systems. Hypertension 2005; 46 : 1236–42.

11. Hagedorn M. PRCP: a key to blood vessel homeostasis. Blood 2011; 117 : 3705–6.

12. Meltzer ME, Doggen CJ, de Groot PG et al. The impact of the fibrinolytic system on the risk of venous and arterial thrombosis. Semin Thromb Hemost 2009; 35 : 468–77.

13. Zorio E, Gilabert-Estelles J, Espana F et al. Fibrinolysis: the key to new pathogenetic mechanisms. Curr Med Chem 2008; 15 : 923–9.

14. Arepally GM, Ortel TL. Heparin-induced thrombocytopenia. *Annu Rev Med* 2010; 61 : 77–90.

15. Taylor FB, Jr., Toh CH, Hoots WK *et al.* Towards definition, clinical and laboratory criteria, and a scoring system for disseminated intravascular coagulation. *Thromb Haemost* 2001; 86 : 1327–30.

16. Singh RK, Baronia AK, Sahoo JN *et al.* Prospective comparison of new Japanese Association for Acute Medicine (JAAM) DIC and International Society of Thrombosis and Hemostasis (ISTH) DIC score in critically ill septic patients. *Thromb Res* 2012; 129 : e119–e125.

17. Dhainaut JF, Yan SB, Joyce DE *et al.* Treatment effects of drotrecogin alfa (activated) in patients with severe sepsis with or without overt disseminated intravascular coagulation. *J Thromb Haemost* 2004; 2 : 1924–33.

18. Whelihan MF, Zachary V, Orfeo T, Mann KG. Prothrombin activation in blood coagulation: the erythrocyte contribution to thrombin generation. *Blood* 2012; 120 : 3837–45.

19. Eugster M, Reinhart WH. The influence of the haematocrit on primary haemostasis in vitro. *Thromb Haemost* 2005; 94 : 1213–8.

20. Sheth KN, Gilson AJ, Chang Y *et al.* Packed red blood cell transfusion and decreased mortality in intracerebral hemorrhage. *Neurosurgery* 2011; 68 : 1286–92.

21. Spahn DR, Bouillon B, Cerny V *et al.* Management of bleeding and coagulopathy following major trauma: an updated European guideline. *Crit Care* 2013 19; 17 : R76.

22. Morrison CA, Carrick MM, Norman MA *et al.* Hypotensive resuscitation strategy reduces transfusion requirements and severe postoperative coagulopathy in trauma patients with hemorrhagic shock: preliminary results of a randomized controlled trial. *J Trauma* 2011; 70 : 652–63.

23. Stanworth SJ, Estcourt LJ, Powter G *et al.* A no-prophylaxis platelet-transfusion strategy for hematologic cancers. *N Engl J Med* 2013; 368 : 1771–80.

24. Hsia CC, Chin-Yee IH, McAlister VC. Use of recombinant activated factor VII in patients without hemophilia: a meta-analysis of randomized control trials. *Ann Surg* 2008; 248 : 61–8.

25. Mayer SA, Brun NC, Begtrup K *et al.* Efficacy and safety of recombinant activated factor VII for acute intracerebral hemorrhage. *N Engl J Med* 2008 15; 358 : 2127–37.

26. Roberts I, Perel P, Prieto-Merino D *et al.* Effect of tranexamic acid on mortality in patients with traumatic bleeding: prespecified analysis of data from randomised controlled trial. *BMJ* 2012; 345 : e5839.

27. Shakur H, Roberts I, Bautista R *et al.* Effects of tranexamic acid on death, vascular occlusive events, and blood transfusion in trauma patients with significant haemorrhage (CRASH-2): a randomised, placebo-controlled trial. *Lancet* 2010 3; 376 : 23–32.

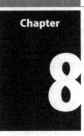

Airway management in critically ill patients

Titus C Yeung and Donald EG Griesdale

Introduction

In contrast to the elective perioperative setting, intubations of critically ill patients are high-risk procedures, with up to a third of patients experiencing a severe, life-threatening complication [1–4]. The reasons for this are multiple:

- Patients often have limited physiologic reserves [5] and there may be limited time for optimization.
- There is an increased risk of both difficult laryngoscopy and difficult intubation when compared to the operating room [1–3].
- Intubations may be performed by individuals with varying expertise [1, 5].

Airway assessment and documentation

- Most intubations in the critically ill are urgent rather than emergent. This allows time to perform a quick, but focused assessment of the airway.
- The acronym "LEMON" evaluation tool is used to assess the potential difficulty of an airway [6] and has been validated in patients presenting to the emergency department (see Figure 8.1).
- Predictors of difficult mask ventilation and difficult intubation are listed in Table 8.1.
- Nonreassuring physical exam features have a low to moderate sensitivity (20–62%) and a moderate to fair specificity (82–97%) [7], thus the clinician must always be prepared for the unanticipated difficult airway. Documentation of airway management following intubation is essential. Important features to document include: Cormack–Lehane glottis view, number of intubation attempts, primary method and adjunct used to secure the airway, and complications (if any).
- A difficult airway occurs when an individual trained in airway management experiences difficulty with either mask ventilation, intubation, or both (adapted from the American Society of Anesthesiologists) [8].
- An airway management algorithm is presented in Figure 8.2.

Based on the perceived difficulty, there are two basic approaches to intubating a patient:

1. "Rapid sequence induction and intubation (RSII)" with abolition of spontaneous ventilation, or
2. "Awake" technique with maintenance of spontaneous ventilation.

Handbook of ICU Therapy, third edition, ed. John Fuller, Jeff Granton and Ian McConachie. Published by Cambridge University Press. © Cambridge University Press 2015.

L   Look externally
Look at the patient externally for characteristics that are known to cause difficult laryngoscopy, intubation or ventilation.

E   Evaluate the 3-3-2 rule
In order to allow alignment of the pharyngeal, laryngeal and oral axes and therefore simple intubation, the following relationships should be observed. The distance between the patient's incisor teeth should be at least 3 finger breadths (1), the distance between the hyoid bone and the chin should be at least 3 finger breadths (3), and the distance between the thyroid notch and the floor of the mouth should be at least 2 finger breadths (2).

1 - Inter incisor distance in fingers.
2 - Hyoid mental distance in fingers.
3 - Thyroid to floor of mouth in
     fingers.

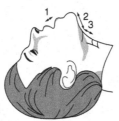

M   Mallampati
The hypopharynx should be visualized adequately. This has been done traditionally by assessing the Mallampati classification. The patient is sat upright, told to open the mouth fully and protrude the tongue as far as possible. The examiner then looks into the mouth with a light torch to assess the degree of hypopharynx visible. In the case of a supine patient, Mallampati score can be estimated by getting the patient to open the mouth fully and protrude the tongue and a laryngoscopy light can be shone into the hypopharynx from above.

| Class I: soft palate, uvula, fauces, pillars visible | Class II: soft palate, uvula, fauces visible | Class III: soft palate, base of uvula visible | Class IV: hard palate only visible |

O   Obstruction?
Any condition that can cause obstruction of the airway will make laryngoscopy and ventilation difficult. Such conditions are epiglottis, peritonsillar abscesses and trauma.

N   Neck mobility
This is a vital requirement for successful intubation. It can be assessed easily by getting the patient to place their chin down onto their chest and then to extend their neck so they are looking towards the ceiling. Patients in hard collar neck immobilization obviously have no neck movement are therefore harder to intubate.

Figure 8.1 The LEMON airway assessment method. (Reproduced from [6] with permission from BMJ Publishing Group Ltd.)

Optimization

- There is often time for patient optimization prior to intubation to help minimize the risks during the procedure.
- Using an intubation checklist can help minimize the risk of complications [9,10].

Table 8.1 History and physical exam features predictive of difficult mask ventilation and difficult endotracheal intubation

Mask ventilation	Intubation
Snoring or obstructive sleep apnea	History of difficult intubation
Beard	Interincisor distance < three fingers
Mallampati iii or iv	Mallampati iii or iv
Age ≥55	Decreased neck range of motion
Limited jaw protrusion	Prominent overbite
Thyromental distance < three fingers	Thyromental distance < three fingers
Body mass index ≥30	
Lack of teeth	
Thick/obese neck anatomy	

Adapted from [8,38–40].

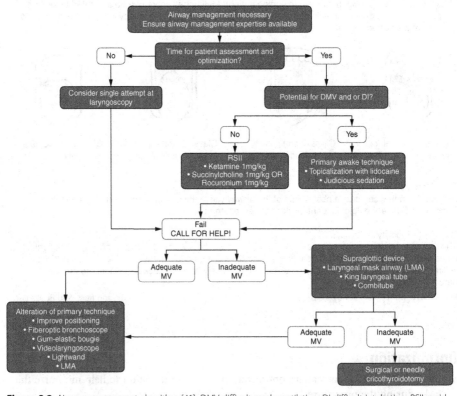

Figure 8.2 Airway management algorithm [41]. DMV difficult mask ventilation; DI difficult intubation; RSII rapid sequence induction and intubation; MV mask ventilation.

- If the patient is suspected to have a full stomach and at high risk of aspiration, a naso-gastric tube may be passed to evacuate stomach contents.
- Proper positioning of the patient in the sniffing position facilitates glottis exposure [11].
- Patients should be preoxygenated with a fractional inspiratory concentration of oxygen (FiO_2) of 1.0 or by using noninvasive positive-pressure ventilation (NIPPV) [12].
- However, critically ill patients may be minimally responsive to preoxygenation [2] and severe hypoxemia (O_2 saturation <80%) is common in the intubation of critically ill patients [13,14].
- Hypotension is common during the intubation period. Adequate intravenous (IV) access is essential prior to intubation. Appropriate volume loading with IV fluids and immediate availability of vasopressors can help minimize the hemodynamic instability during this time.

Rapid sequence induction and intubation (RSII)

- Critically ill patients should be assumed to have a full stomach and therefore at risk of vomiting and aspiration during intubation. The period of highest risk of aspiration is between the administration of sedatives and time of cuff inflation after successful intubation. This risk is further increased if the patient is bag-mask ventilated with insufflation of air in the stomach.
- RSII helps mitigate these risks by administering a predetermined dose of induction and paralytic medications to minimize the time at risk.
- While giving predetermined doses of induction and paralytic minimizes this time of vomiting risk, it may lead to relative anesthetic over- or underdosing.

In critically ill patients with hemodynamic instability, the dose of induction agents can be reduced. This will minimize the hemodynamic side effects of the drugs.

- Ketamine (1–2 mg/kg IV) is an ideal induction agent for intubation of critically ill patients with sepsis due to its stable hemodynamic profile [15].
- Etomidate (0.3 mg/kg IV) also possesses a stable hemodynamic profile, but causes adrenal insufficiency that corrects by 48 hours [16], which may lead to increased mortality in patients with sepsis [17], leading to concerns with its use in this patient population [18,19].
- Propofol (1–2 mg/kg IV) is also used as an induction agent. However, given its peripheral vasodilatory and negative inotropic properties, its use should be limited in critically ill patients.

Neuromuscular blockade agents should only be used by a physician who is experienced with intubation when a difficult airway is not anticipated. Otherwise, an awake or spontaneous breathing mode should be employed. Neuromuscular blockade agents include depolarizing agents (succinylcholine) and nondepolarizing agents (e.g. rocuronium).

- Succinylcholine (1–1.5 mg/kg IV) potentially provides better intubating conditions compared to rocuronium (1 mg/kg). [20,21].
- However, succinylcholine is contraindicated in patients with a history of malignant hyperthermia, hyperkalemia, significant burns or muscle injury, stroke, spinal-cord injury and neuromuscular diseases such as Duchenne's muscular dystrophy.

Controversies in RSII

- Traditionally, bag-mask ventilation (BMV) was not used in RSII to avoid the risk of aspiration with insufflation of the stomach. However, in patients with hypoxemia, the risk of aspiration should be balanced by the risk of prolonged hypoxemia. In this situation, gentle mask ventilation with an oral airway may be used to maintain oxygenation.
- Cricoid pressure during RSII to occlude the upper esophageal sphincter after paralysis has also been described. This was thought to minimize the amount of passive regurgitation of stomach contents and subsequent aspiration. However, cricoid pressure is not proven to protect against aspiration and may worsen glottic view, impair BMV, increase the risk of aspiration by inducing vomiting and retching [22], and potentially even cause esophageal trauma if the patient retches against a closed glottis. A reasonable approach may be to apply cricoid pressure, but minimize or remove it if it impairs intubation or BMV.

Awake intubation

- The primary goal of an "awake" intubation is to maintain spontaneous ventilation.
- While the fiberoptic bronchoscope is the most common approach used in the operating room, achieving an awake intubation can be used with any modality, as long as spontaneous ventilation is maintained.

Crucial steps in the procedure include:

- Good patient communication, as cooperation greatly facilitates this procedure.
- Adequate topicalization of the airway with local anesthesia. This can be achieved via nebulization, atomization or direct application of 2% lidocaine, or a combination of these techniques. Care should be taken to remain under the recommended total dose of 5 mg/kg.
- Judicious sedation – while some sedation may be necessary for the procedure, critically ill patients will be extremely sensitive to any sedative medication. Therefore, if any sedation is required, judicious doses should be used (i.e. midazolam 0.5 mg IV or ketamine 0.3 mg/kg IV at a time). Dexmedetomidine, a centrally acting selective α-2 agonist, is increasingly being used for sedation during awake intubation [23].
- Establish a backup plan – since this is an anticipated difficult airway, a backup plan is essential. This may include involving other expertise (i.e. anesthesia or surgical colleagues) as well as having other adjunct tools and possibly a surgical airway setup prepared.

Adjunct devices

- Many airway devices have been developed in addition to direct laryngoscopy to provide an alternative or rescue option for intubation.
- Each device and technology has its own advantages and disadvantages and may work well in certain situations while failing in others. It is important to recognize the limitations of each device in order to maximize its benefit.
- Gum-elastic bougie is a 60 cm endotracheal tube introducer whose tip is at a 35° angle. It is useful in situations with poor glottis visualization (e.g. Cormack–Lehane grade III

or IV) or a small glottis aperture (e.g. pharyngeal swelling or mass). It is placed under direct visualization using a laryngoscope and confirmation of placement is obtained by feeling the tip making contact with the tracheal rings as it is introduced into the trachea and until a definitive endpoint is met (mainstem bronchus). An endotracheal tube (ETT) is then placed over the bougie and advanced into the trachea. If the esophagus is accidentally intubated, neither the tracheal rings nor a definitive endpoint will be felt. Visualizing with a laryngoscope as the ETT is passed over the bougie will help facilitate a smoother intubation.

- Video laryngoscopes are indirect, rigid, fiberoptic laryngoscopes with a camera mounted at the end of the blade. There are a variety of devices with varying blade angles and sizes [24]. Examples include: Glidescope® videolaryngosope, McGrath® Video Laryngoscope and the Pentax Airway Scope®. While video laryngoscopes may obtain a view of the glottis easily, advancing the tube through the glottis may be challenging [25]. The view afforded by video laryngoscopes will be obscured by secretions or blood.
- Fiberoptic intubating bronchoscopy is a technique generally used in patients with a difficult airway in an awake fashion. The oropharynx is well topicalized with local anesthetic and judicious amounts of sedation are given to facilitate intubation. With an endotracheal tube loaded onto the fiberoptic bronchoscope, the scope is then passed gently through the glottis and into the trachea. After further topicalization, the patient is asked to take a deep breath and the endotracheal tube is then gently advanced through the glottis and into the trachea. Endotracheal placement of the tube is then confirmed prior to withdrawal of the scope.
- Laryngeal mask airway (LMA) is a supraglottic device that provides a conduit for ventilation. In the emergent situation, it is a valuable rescue device for a failed airway [26]. There are many different insertion techniques described. Generally, the cuff is deflated and well lubricated and advanced along the hard palate until it reaches the supraglottic area. The insertion may be facilitated by providing a jaw-lift procedure and/ or by inserting the LMA upside down until it reaches the posterior oropharynx and then flipped into position. Furthermore, the LMA may act as a conduit for intubation. The Fastrach® LMA has an accompanying Fastrach endotracheal tube, which can be inserted through the LMA into the glottis. Alternatively, other techniques are described using a fiberoptic bronchoscope.

Failed or unanticipated difficult airway

- A failed airway is a life-threatening emergency that mandates an immediate call for help.
- The clinician must always be prepared for an unanticipated difficult airway because of the poor discriminative ability of the physical exam.
- Furthermore, a severely hypoxic patient with poor physiologic reserve may not allow for adequate time to preoxygenate and intubate.
- If the patient cannot be intubated, then immediate mask ventilation should be performed using oral or nasopharyngeal airways with a two-person technique if required.
- If mask ventilation is not adequate, then a supraglottic airway device (e.g. laryngeal mask airway or King LT) should be immediately inserted. If adequate ventilation ensues, a plan can be formulated for definitive airway control.

- If a "cannot intubate, cannot ventilate" situation develops despite a supraglottic airway device, then a surgical airway should be considered to establish definitive control of the airway.

Surgical airway

- The indication for a surgical airway is a "cannot intubate, cannot ventilate" patient.
- Unless a practitioner has previous surgical airway experience, a cricothyroidotomy is the easiest surgical procedure to obtain airway control.
- Both an open surgical approach and a percutaneous approach (using commercially developed kits and Seldinger technique) are described.
- Relative contraindications to a surgical airway include distorted neck anatomy, pre-existing infection and/or coagulopathy.

Post-intubation management

- The post-intubation period is very high risk for complications, including esophageal intubation and hemodynamic compromise.
- Confirmation of endotracheal tube placement is paramount given the high morbidity of unrecognized esophageal intubations. Waveform capnography is the most reliable method [27] and is a Class I recommendation in certain guidelines [28]. We believe waveform capnography should be used to confirm endotracheal placement [11].
- Once intubated, the minimum volume of air should be used to fill the endotracheal tube cuff to minimize the risk of post-extubation stridor [29].
- Post-intubation hypotension can occur from a variety of causes, including sedation for intubation, positive-pressure ventilation or hypovolemia. Intravascular fluids and vasopressors should be readily available to maintain end-organ perfusion. Avoiding agitation by giving short-term sedation will allow for easier resuscitation.
- Once the patient's hemodynamics are stabilized, a recruitment maneuver (CPAP 40 cmH_2O for 30 s) has been shown to improve short-term oxygenation [30].
- A portable chest X-ray should be obtained to confirm placement and look for potential complications (e.g. pneumothorax, aspiration).

Reducing complications in intubation

- Intubation is a complex interaction between patient-, environmental- and practitioner-related factors [26].
- Multiple attempts at intubation are associated with severe complications around the time of intubation [1,31,32].
- Experience in airway management is crucial to reduce the number of intubation attempts [33].
- Familiarity with more than one technique is important for intubation success [34].
- High-fidelity simulation is gaining more popularity in training and allows for experience in airway management in respiratory arrest scenarios [35–37]. While it remains unclear whether this skill and experience translates into improved success in real-life airway management, it may still be a valuable education tool, particularly in less experienced trainees.

- Development and use of an intubation checklist for use in critically ill patients is associated with fewer life-threatening complications, even in the hands of experienced providers [11].

The Fourth National Audit Project of the Royal College of Anesthesists and Difficult Airway Society (NAP4)

- In 2011, the Fourth National Audit Project of the Royal College of Anaesthetists and Difficult Airway Society studied airway complications outside of the operating room, specifically the ICU and emergency department [10].
- A high proportion of complications occurred after hours with less experienced staff performing airway procedures.
- A high rate of complications involved obese patients and these were associated with worse outcomes. Failed intubations and problems with tracheostomies were common.
- The absence of capnography contributed to the failure to recognize esophageal intubations.
- Factors that contributed or caused complications included communication, education and training, equipment and resources, patient risk factors and judgment.

Recommendations to minimize complications in the ICU include:
- Use of capnography to confirm endotracheal placement
- Adequate expertise and staff to provide airway support
- Use of an intubation checklist to improve communication, prepare the patient, equipment and team and identify a backup plan
- Acknowledging the difficult airway and potential for significant morbidity of obese patients.

Conclusion

Airway management including intubation can be a challenge in critically ill patients. It is important to recognize that there are multiple factors that will influence the process of intubation, including patient anatomic variables, hemodynamic variables, the urgency of intubation and practitioner experience. Developing a standardized approach and a well thought-out backup plan to recognize and manage any potential difficult situation will help minimize the risk to the patient.

References

1. Griesdale DEG, Bosma TL et al. Complications of endotracheal intubation in the critically ill. *Intensive Care Med* 2008; 34 :1835–42.

2. Jaber S, Amraoui J, Lefrant JY et al. Clinical practice and risk factors for immediate complications of endotracheal intubation in the intensive care unit: a prospective, multiple-center study. *Crit Care Med* 2006; 34 : 2355–61.

3. Schwartz DE, Matthay MA, Cohen NH. Death and other complications of emergency airway management in critically ill adults. A prospective investigation of 297 tracheal intubations. *Anesthesiology* 1995; 82 : 367–76.

4. Simpson GD, Ross MJ, McKeown DW, Ray DC. Tracheal intubation in the critically ill: a multi-centre national study of practice and complications. *Br J Anaesth* 2012; 108 : 792–9.

5. Hirsch-Allen AJ, Ayas N, Mountain S et al. Influence of residency training on multiple attempts at endotracheal intubation. *Can J Anesth* 2010; 57 : 823–9.

6. Reed MJ, Dunn MJ, McKeown DW. Can an airway assessment score predict difficulty at intubation in the emergency department? *Emerg Med J* 2005; 22 : 99–102.

7. Shiga T, Wajima Z, Inoue T, Sakamoto, A. Predicting difficult intubation in apparently normal patients: a meta-analysis of bedside screening test performance. *Anesthesiology* 2005;103 : 429–37.

8. Apfelbaum JL, Hagberg CA, Caplan RA et al. Practice guidelines for management of the difficult airway: an updated report by the American Society of Anesthesiologists Task Force on Management of the Difficult Airway. *Anesthesiology* 2013; 118 : 251–70.

9. Jaber S, Jung B, Corne P et al. An intervention to decrease complications related to endotracheal intubation in the intensive care unit: a prospective, multiple-center study. *Intensive Care Med* 2010; 36 : 248–55.

10. Cook T, Woodall N, Harper J, Benger J. Fourth National Audit Project. Major complications of airway management in the UK: results of the Fourth National Audit Project of the Royal College of Anaesthetists and the Difficult Airway Society. Part 2: intensive care and emergency departments. *Br J Anaesth* 2011; 106 : 632–42.

11. Benumof JL. Management of the difficult adult airway. With special emphasis on awake tracheal intubation. *Anesthesiology* 1991; 75 : 1087–110.

12. Baillard C, Baillard C, Fosse JP et al. Noninvasive ventilation improves preoxygenation before intubation of hypoxic patients. *Am J Respir Crit Care Med* 2006; 174 : 171–7.

13. Cheney FW, Posner KL, Lee LA et al. Trends in anesthesia-related death and brain damage: a closed claims analysis. *Anesthesiology* 2006; 105 : 1081–6.

14. Mort TC. Preoxygenation in critically ill patients requiring emergency tracheal intubation. *Crit Care Med* 2005; 33 : 2672–5.

15. Jabre P, Combes X, Lapostolle F et al. Etomidate versus ketamine for rapid sequence intubation in acutely ill patients: a multicentre randomised controlled trial. *Lancet* 2009; 374 : 293–300.

16. Vinclair M, Broux C, Faure P et al. Duration of adrenal inhibition following a single dose of etomidate in critically ill patients. *Intensive Care Med* 2008; 34 : 714–9.

17. Finfer S. Corticosteroids in septic shock. *N Engl J Med* 2008; 358 : 188–90.

18. Griesdale DE. Etomidate for intubation of patients who have sepsis or septic shock – where do we go from here ? *Crit Care* 2012; 16 : 189.

19. Annane D. ICU physicians should abandon the use of etomidate! *Intensive Care Med* 2005; 31 : 325–6.

20. Sluga M, Ummenhofer W, Studer W et al. Rocuronium versus succinylcholine for rapid sequence induction of anesthesia and endotracheal intubation: a prospective, randomized trial in emergent cases. *Anesthesia and Analgesia* 2005; 101 : 1356–61.

21. Perry JJ, Lee JS, Sillberg VA, Wells GA. Rocuronium versus succinylcholine for rapid sequence induction intubation. *Cochrane Database Syst Rev* 2008 Apr 16; (2) : CD002788.

22. El-Orbany M, Connolly LA. Rapid sequence induction and intubation: current controversy. *Anesth Analg* 2010; 110 : 1318–25.

23. Cattano D, Lam NC, Ferrario L, et al. Dexmedetomidine versus remifentanil for sedation during awake fiberoptic intubation. *Anesthesiol Res Pract*; 2012 : 753107.

24. Levitan RM, Heitz JW, Sweeney M, Cooper RM. The complexities of tracheal intubation with direct laryngoscopy and alternative intubation devices. *Ann Emerg Med* 2011; 57 : 240–7.

25. Griesdale DEG, Liu D, McKinney J, Choi PT. Glidescope(®) video-laryngoscopy versus direct laryngoscopy for endotracheal intubation: a systematic review and meta-analysis. *Can J Anesth* 2012; 59 : 41–52.

26. American Society of Anesthesiologists. Practice guidelines for management of the difficult airway: an updated report by the American Society of Anesthesiologists Task Force on Management of the Difficult Airway. *Anesthesiology* 2003; 98 :1269–77.

27. Grmec, S. Comparison of three different methods to confirm tracheal tube placement in emergency intubation. *Intensive Care Med* 2002; 28 : 701–4.

28. Neumar RW, Otto CW, Link MS *et al.* Part 8: adult advanced cardiovascular life support: 2010 American Heart Association Guidelines for Cardiopulmonary Resuscitation and Emergency Cardiovascular Care. *Circulation* 2010; 122 : S729–67.

29. Jaber S, Chanques G, Matecki S *et al.* Post-extubation stridor in intensive care unit patients. Risk factors evaluation and importance of the cuff-leak test. *Intensive Care Med* 2003; 29 : 69–74.

30. Constantin JM, Futier E, Cherprenet AL *et al.* A recruitment maneuver increases oxygenation after intubation of hypoxemic intensive care unit patients: a randomized controlled study. *Crit Care* 2010; 14 : R76.

31. Sakles JC, Chiu S, Mosier J, Walker C and Stolz U. The importance of first pass success when performing orotracheal intubation in the emergency department. *Acad Emerg Med* 2013; 20, 71–8.

32. Hasegawa K, Shigemitsu K, Hagiwara Y *et al.* Association between repeated intubation attempts and adverse events in emergency departments: an analysis of a multicenter prospective observational study. *Ann Emerg Med* 2012; 60 : 749–54.

33. Hirsch-Allen AJ, Ayas N, Mountain S *et al.* Association between year of residency training and multiple attempts at endotracheal intubation. *Can J Anaesth* 2010; 57 : 823–9.

34. Aziz MF, Healy D, Kheterpal S *et al.* Routine clinical practice effectiveness of the Glidescope in difficult airway management: an analysis of 2,004 Glidescope intubations, complications, and failures from two institutions. *Anesthesiology* 2011; 114 : 34–41.

35. Kory PD, Eisen LA, Adachi M *et al.* Initial airway management skills of senior residents: simulation training compared with traditional training. *Chest* 2007; 132 : 1927–31.

36. Mayo PH, Hackney JE, Mueck JT *et al.* Achieving house staff competence in emergency airway management: results of a teaching program using a computerized patient simulator. *Crit Care Med* 2004; 32 : 2422–7.

37. Rosenthal ME, Adachi M, Ribaudo V *et al.* Achieving housestaff competence in emergency airway management using scenario based simulation training: comparison of attending vs housestaff trainers. *Chest* 2006; 129 : 1453–8.

38. Kheterpal S, Han R, Tremper KK *et al.* Incidence and predictors of difficult and impossible mask ventilation. *Anesthesiology* 2006; 105 : 885–91.

39. Karkouti K, Rose DK, Wigglesworth D, Cohen MM. Predicting difficult intubation: A multivariable analysis. *Can J Anesth* 2000; 47 : 730–739.

40. El-Orbany M, Woehlck HJ. Difficult mask ventilation. *Anesth Analg* 2009; 109 : 1870–1880.

41. Griesdale DE, Henderson WR, Green RS. Airway management in critically ill patients. *Lung* 2011; 189 : 181–92.

Noninvasive mechanical ventilation

Mark Soth and Thomas Piraino

Noninvasive positive-pressure ventilation (NIPPV) is very similar to invasive ventilation in that it supports improved gas exchange and decreased respiratory muscle work.

- NIPPV refers to a bilevel mode that has not only CPAP (continuous positive airway pressure), which is referred to as EPAP (endpositive airway pressure), but also when a patient triggers a breath, the machine increases pressure to the inspiratory positive airway pressure (IPAP).
- The ΔP between the IPAP and EPAP is analogous to pressure support (PS) of conventional ventilation.
- CPAP or EPAP are analogous to positive end-expiratory pressure (PEEP) during invasive ventilation.

Although CPAP and NIPPV are different, for ease of reference both will be referred to as NIPPV in this text, except where the difference is important.

The main difference of NIPPV from invasive ventilation is that it uses a mask or helmet interface rather than an endotracheal tube.

- This offers the advantages of being readily taken on and off to facilitate weaning, maintaining some ability to communicate, and avoids the complications of sedation and ventilator-associated pneumonia.
- The main disadvantages of NIPPV are no direct protection of the airway, no deep suctioning below the vocal cords, limited ability to apply high pressures and development of intolerance to the mask over time.

Hence, the ideal NIPPV candidate:

- Protects their airway
- Has strong cough and minimal secretions
- Tolerates the interface well
- Has a quickly reversible condition or is able to breathe comfortably for periods off NIPPV.

Noninvasive positive-pressure ventilation is not advisable in patients with poor airway protection, copious secretions, recent esophageal surgery, severe active cardiac ischemia or with facial burns or trauma.

Handbook of ICU Therapy, third edition, ed. John Fuller, Jeff Granton and Ian McConachie. Published by Cambridge University Press. © Cambridge University Press 2015.

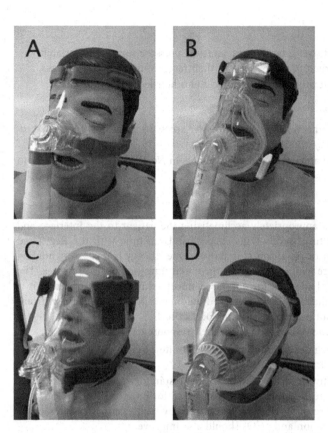

Figure 9.1 NIPPV interfaces.

Choosing an interface

The main interface options are a nasal mask (Figure 9.1A), full-face mask (Figure 9.1B) or total face mask (Figure 9.1C,D). There is also a helmet available in some jurisdictions, but not in North America (not shown).

Nasal mask

Pros: Comfortable and nonclaustrophobic. Patient can talk easily.

Cons: Difficult to maintain pressures if a high amount needed or in mouth-breathers, which makes it a poor choice in acute respiratory failure.

Full-face mask

Pros: Able to obtain higher pressures and covers both nose and mouth.

Cons: Various models have contraptions to relieve pressure, but patients can develop pressure sores, particularly over the nose. May have leaks from facial hair or variability in patient's chin, nose and cheek structure.

Total face mask

Pros: Spreads pressure out over a larger area, so fewer pressure sores. Less variability between patients' facial structure on the edge of their face, so may have fewer leaks.
Cons: Some patients find it more claustrophobic and others less than a full mask.

Helmet

Pros: Nothing strapped to the patient's face, so easier access to mouth. Not strapped to the patients face in case they vomit.
Cons: A more complicated apparatus and not available in North America. Less access to the upper chest and neck.

Initiating NIPPV

Successful NIPPV hinges on appropriately acclimatizing the patient to the interface and titrating the pressures to optimal levels. This entails hands-on time with the Registered Nurse, Respiratory Therapist or physician at initiation. One strategy is to start by holding the mask on the patient's face while talking with them and titrating up the pressures. The mask is then strapped on and adjusted for optimal comfort, while minimizing leaks. It is important to note that the machine will detect and automatically adjust for a significant amount of leaking, so it is not necessary to have a perfect seal.

The patient needs to be monitored closely for their response to NIPPV.

- At our institution, this includes continuous cardiac monitor, oxygen saturation monitor and a moderate- to high-intensity staffing area.
- The most sensitive objective measure to watch is the respiratory rate, which should decrease as the work of breathing decreases. Also watch for improvement in heart rate and the patient's level of respiratory distress suggested by their respiratory accessory muscle use. Oxygen saturation and pCO_2 should also improve.
- These improvements should occur within the first 30 to 60 minutes of initiating NIPPV.
- If they are not, then you need to consider making adjustments, whether the patient's underlying condition is likely to rapidly improve in the near future (e.g. diuresis for heart failure), or whether the patient is failing NIPPV and needs to be intubated.

Selecting and adjusting CPAP pressure

Continuous positive airway pressure is physiologically similar to PEEP. It has the benefits of decreasing cardiac preload and afterload. It also increases recruitment of alveoli with higher opening and closing pressures, resulting in more surface area for gas exchange and improved oxygenation. Hence, CPAP can be titrated for both its respiratory and cardiovascular effects.

- Generally in congestive heart failure, CPAP of at least 8–10 cm H_2O is used and often higher.
- Patients with chronic obstructive pulmonary disease (COPD) also benefit from PEEP in the above range, due to the effect of splinting open of smaller airways allowing relief of gas trapping – similar to what patients accomplish on their own with pursed lip breathing.

One key point to remember about CPAP and NIPPV is that without an endotracheal tube, the patient needs a patent airway for the machine to sense and deliver breaths.

- In patients with obstructive sleep apnea (OSA), it is essential to set the CPAP or EPAP at a level above what is needed to prevent obstruction.

- Insufficient CPAP or EPAP in OSA may manifest as nontriggering of the IPAP, thoracic paradoxical breathing or worsening gas exchange – particularly when sleeping.

Selecting and adjusting the IPAP pressure

The IPAP level in NIPPV is the maximum pressure that the machine delivers when a respiratory effort is detected. The difference between IPAP and EPAP, referred to as ΔP, is like pressure support of conventional ventilation. A higher ΔP helps augment respiratory muscular effort, augmenting tidal volumes to improve CO_2 elimination, while decreasing the "work of breathing." It is important to remember that unlike increasing PEEP in the PS/CPAP mode of invasive ventilation, when increasing EPAP, one must also increase IPAP by the same amount or the ΔP will decrease.

- The level of IPAP required is very patient specific. It is important to acclimatize the patient to the pressures, but also be cautious not to use insufficient pressure.
- Generally, IPAPs in the 15–20 cm H_2O range are used and titrated to the patients response, as described in the "Initiating NIPPV" section.
- Pressures in the mid to high 20s are also used at times, but can be limited due to mask leak or patient tolerance.

NIPPV for acute exacerbation of COPD

The largest amount of supportive evidence for the use of NIPPV (particularly bilevel) is in the management of COPD exacerbation. Complications arising from dynamic hyperinflation in this population lead to excessive elastic and resistive forces that increase respiratory muscle workload and ultimately lead to respiratory failure. Intubation and invasive mechanical ventilation become difficult because of the complicated lung mechanics associated with COPD.

- The use of NIPPV in these patients results in lower failure rates compared to standard medical therapy, lower requirement for intubation, lower mortality and decreased length of stay in hospital [1,2].
- The level of applied EPAP helps to splint open airways at risk of collapsing, and the delivered pressure (IPAP) assists with the increased respiratory muscle workload.

NIPPV for acute cardiogenic pulmonary edema

The use of NIPPV for acute cardiogenic pulmonary edema (ACPE) is aimed at treating the respiratory complications related to the presence of pulmonary edema.

- The use of CPAP alone may increase the functional residual capacity, reduce atelectasis, improve respiratory system compliance, reduce right-to-left intrapulmonary shunting and improve cardiac output.
- However, because there is often an associated increased respiratory workload with ACPE, the use of bilevel NIPPV may be more appropriate for the patient to reduce the amount of respiratory distress.
- Meta-analysis of randomized trials of over 3000 patients supports either CPAP or NIPPV for the treatment of ACPE to decrease intubation and mortality [3].
- However, the studies comparing CPAP to bilevel tended to use CPAP in the 10 cm H_2O range compared to EPAP in the bilevel arms in the 5 cm H_2O range. Since PEEP and its equivalents are important to the physiology of ACPE, this

difference may make the bilevel results appear less optimal. Given that, when using bilevel, we use EPAP in the 10 cm H_2O range.

- The patient presentation and response to therapy should therefore influence the choice of mode and pressures used.

There is controversy when NIPPV is considered in the setting of myocardial ischemia. With modern ultrasensitive troponin assays to detect myocardial distress and damage, it is common for there to be some component of ischemia. NIPPV has not been shown to cause myocardial infarction [3].

- If patients do not have an excellent and rapid response to NIPPV, then NIPPV may increase the myocardial demand compared to fully sedating and intubating the patients.
- Conversely, intubation may be associated with its own hemodynamic swings and complications.
- Judgment and expertise is needed, but NIPPV can be considered for those with predominantly ACPE, a mild troponin rise and unconcerning ECG.
- Those with higher-risk features of cardiac ischemia biochemically or on ECG should have a low threshold for intubation to offload myocardial demand and facilitate cardiac catheterization, if appropriate.

NIPPV for pneumonia

Since pneumonia significant enough to cause respiratory failure is often accompanied by increased pulmonary secretions and often takes several days for significant improvement, it is not an ideal condition for NIPPV and there is a high failure rate. There is very little evidence in this area.

- One RCT has been done in COPD patients presenting with pneumonia and showed a decrease in intubation [4].
- In non-COPD patients, one small RCT of NIPPV for severe respiratory failure showed decreased intubation and mortality in the subgroup with pneumonia [5].
- Given the paucity of evidence, there is no strong recommendation for or against use of NIPPV in pneumonia.

It should also be noted that the patients with pneumonia in the studies quoted did not have ARDS or multiorgan failure and NIPPV is likely not appropriate in these settings.

NIPPV for ARDS

Acute respiratory distress syndrome (ARDS) is not a good candidate disease for NIPPV, since it is slow to resolve and patients have very severe pulmonary dysfunction, and the literature has been discouraging.

- While CPAP and NIPPV have been shown to improve gas exchange, they do not reduce the eventual need for intubation or mortality [6].
- Patients with ARDS are also prone to the effects of stress placed on the lungs by positive-pressure ventilation and a controlled ventilatory approach targeting small lung volumes is more appropriate.

NIPPV for immunocompromised patients

There is evidence demonstrating that noninvasive ventilation decreases the risk of ventilator-associated pneumonia. This may be of particular importance in patients with underlying immunosuppression.

- A prospective, randomized controlled trial of noninvasive ventilation compared with standard oxygen therapy for immunosuppressed patients in acute respiratory failure found a significant reduction in the need for intubation, and a significant improvement in survival to hospital discharge [7].
- After separating the results into subgroups it appears that the benefit of NIPPV in these patents is specific to immunosuppression secondary to hematologic cancer and neutropenia.
- However, with the small study size of 52 patients, strong conclusions cannot be drawn.

The potential for improved outcomes for immunosuppressed patients may be limited by the severity of the underlying condition and whether or not the respiratory failure is an isolated and treatable cause.

NIPPV as an adjunct to weaning

The use of NIPPV to facilitate extubation and to prevent extubation failure has been studied in critical care patients.

- For patients with acute-on-chronic respiratory failure NIPPV was successful at allowing early extubation, resulting in decreased time required for invasive mechanical ventilatory support despite failing a spontaneous breathing trial (SBT), without an increase in extubation failure [8].
- The reduction in extubation failure, and a reduction in mortality, has been demonstrated in patients with chronic respiratory disorders who successfully passed a spontaneous breathing trial, but had an increase in hypercapnia after the SBT [9].
- A recent randomized controlled trial found that the use of NIPPV post-extubation in patients intubated for acute respiratory failure significantly reduced extubation failure within 48 hours. This was significant after the exclusion of COPD patients. The absolute risk reduction was 33.9% with a number needed to treat (NNT) of 3 for avoiding reintubation [10].
- Meta-analysis of 11 trials with 623 patients suggests a mortality benefit (odds ratio 0.39), particularly in the subpopulation of patients with COPD [11].

Small studies tend to overestimate treatment effects, but even accounting for that, systematic use of NIPPV as a strategy to facilitate extubation, prevent extubation failure and even reduce mortality in patients with underlying chronic respiratory disease appears beneficial.

It is important to distinguish proactive NIPPV use as a weaning adjunct from NIPPV use for unplanned extubation failure.

- One large randomized trial of NIPPV for extubated patients who developed respiratory failure was stopped early due to increased mortality compared to the usual strategy of reintubating these patients promptly [12].

- The NIPPV arm of this study had an average use of 12 hours of NIPPV prior to reintubation with the main reason for reintubation being lack of improvement compared to reintubation within an average of 2 hours in the standard care arm.

If one does consider a trial of NIPPV as rescue for a failed extubation, then the patient must have an excellent rapid response to NIPPV with a low threshold for reintubation. Furthermore, this is best in patients with a rapidly treatable cause for the extubation failure, such as fluid overload rather than more slow-to-resolve conditions like pneumonia or ARDS.

References

1. Ram FS, Picot J, Lightowler J, Wedzicha JA. Non-invasive positive pressure ventilation for treatment of respiratory failure due to exacerbations of chronic obstructive pulmonary disease. *Cochrane Database Syst Rev* 2004; (3) : CD004104.

2. Chandra D, Stamm JA, Taylor B *et al.* Outcomes of noninvasive ventilation for acute exacerbations of chronic obstructive pulmonary disease in the United States, 1998–2008. *Am J Respir Crit Care Med* 2012; 185 : 152–9.

3. Mariani, J, Macchia, A, Belsiti, C *et al.* Noninvasive ventilation in acute cardiogenic pulmonary edema: a meta-analysis of randomized controlled trials. *J Cardiac Fail* 2011; 17 : 850–9.

4. Confalonieri, M, Potena, A, Carbone, G *et al.* Acute respiratory failure in patients with severe community-acquired pneumonia: a prospective randomized evaluation of noninvasive ventilation. *Am J Respir Crit Care Med* 1999; 160 : 1585–91.

5. Ferrer, M, Esquinas, A, Leon, M *et al.* Noninvasive ventilation in severe hypoxemic respiratory failure a randomized clinical trial. *Am J Resp Crit Care Med* 2003;168 : 1438–44.

6. Delclaux C, L'Her E, Alberti C, Mancebo J *et al.* Treatment of acute hypoxemic nonhypercapnic respiratory insufficiency with continuous positive airway pressure delivered by a face mask: a randomized controlled trial. *JAMA* 2000; 284 : 2361–7.

7. Hilbert, G, Gruson, D, Vargas F *et al.* Noninvasive ventilation in immunosuppressed patients with pulmonary infiltrates, fever, and acute respiratory failure. *N Engl J Med* 2001; 344 : 481–7.

8. Girault C, Daudenthun I, Chevron V *et al.* Noninvasive ventilation as a systematic extubation and weaning technique in acute-on-chronic respiratory failure: a prospective, randomized controlled study. *Am J Respir Crit Care Med* 1999; 160 : 86–92.

9. Ferrer M, Sellarés J, Valencia M *et al.* with chronic respiratory disorders: randomised controlled trial. *Lancet* 2009; 374 : 1082–8.

10. Ornico SR, Lobo SM, Sanches HS *et al.* Noninvasive ventilation immediately after extubation improves weaning outcome after acute respiratory failure: a randomized controlled trial. *Crit Care* 2013; 17 (2) : R39.

11. Zhu F, Liu Z, Long X *et al.* Effect of noninvasive positive pressure ventilation on weaning success in patients receiving invasive mechanical ventilation: a meta-analysis. *Chin Med J* 2013; 126 : 1337–43.

12. Esteban A, Frutos-Vivar F, Ferguson ND *et al.* Noninvasive positive-pressure ventilation for respiratory failure after extubation. *N Engl J Med* 2004; 350 : 2452–60.

Nutrition

Ilya Kagan and Pierre Singer

Introduction

Simple starvation in nonstressed subjects is associated with glycolysis and protein break-down to provide amino acids and glucose through gluconeogenesis. The body adapts to protein-sparing metabolism. In stress, such as trauma, surgery or severe sepsis, these adaptations are reduced secondary to:

- Increased proinflammatory mediators production like IL-1 and TNF-α
- Increased production of cortisol, catecholamines and growth hormone
- Activation of coagulation and fibrinolysis
- Activation of lipid mediators
- Insulin resistance
- Accelerated proteolysis and increased release of glutamine.

The critically ill patient is very sensitive to variations in the intake of nutrients. Excess substrate administration:

- Increases oxidative stress, inducing reactive oxygen species and stimulating inflammatory pathways
- May disturb liver function tests and the CO_2 load on the respiratory system may increase the duration of ventilator support [1].

In contrast, hypocaloric regimens can decrease oxidative stress, but multiple observational studies have shown that nutritional support resulting in an energy deficit is associated with an increase in morbidity and mortality [2,3].

- However, in a large observational study, the lowest mortality was associated with administration of 80% of the calorie intake [4].
- Others [5] found that a cumulative negative energy balance of more than 10 000 kcal was associated with the poorest outcome.

  Several physiological processes are associated with increasing severity of illness:

- Obligatory glucose production via gluconeogenesis (with muscle breakdown supplying amino acids).
- Preferential use of fat in sepsis.

Handbook of ICU Therapy, third edition, ed. John Fuller, Jeff Granton and Ian McConachie. Published by Cambridge University Press. © Cambridge University Press 2015.

- Muscle loss and proteinolysis associated with negative nitrogen balance. This destruction of the muscles is mainly related to autocannibalism of the muscle [6]. Prolonged immobilization increases this muscle loss [7].

Reasons for feeding the critically ill patient

- Enteral nutrition may prevent gut mucosal atrophy.
- Glucose administration reduces protein breakdown.
- Adequate administration of protein (1.5 g/kg/day is the optimal dose) reduces negative nitrogen balance and its complications [8–10] such as tissue breakdown (ICU patients lose 1% of lean body mass per day – mainly muscle).
- Adequate administration of calories (progressively increasing to 25 kcal/kg/day or to a target defined by indirect calorimetry) improves the protein synthesis rate and decreases the negative energy balance, improving morbidity and mortality [11,12].

Nutritional status

Nutritional status prior to critical illness is important:

- Severely malnourished patients with BMI below 18.5 kg/m^2 are associated with increased mortality as well as increased morbidity.
- Severely morbid obesity (BMI >40 kg/m^2) is also associated with increased mortality [13].
- Nutritional risk screening [14] identifies any critically ill patient as being at nutritional risk and therefore a candidate for formal nutritional assessment and therapy.
- Frequently, the loss of muscle mass and muscle function (sarcopenia) is obvious, but in others cases is masked by obesity or edema. Elderly patients are more at risk.

Assessment of nutritional status

Over- and undernutrition, as well as micronutrient disturbances are frequent in the ICU. The height and the ideal weight should be compared with the actual weight if available. A history of loss of appetite, weight, decrease in function and in strength are important. However, no measurement (anthropometric or from the laboratory) accurately defines nutritional disturbancies.

- Indirect calorimetry can evaluate resting energy expenditure [15].
- A hand-grip dynamometer is useful for determining muscle strength and may reflect lean body mass.
- Abdominal computerized tomography, if performed, can evaluate precisely abdominal fat mass and lean body mass [16].
- Bioelectrical impedance, which quantitatively measures lean body mass, as well as fat mass and extracellular water may be helpful in stable patients without water shifts.

Early or late feeding

- Immediately after acute illness, autophagy [17] provides the body with nutrients for the early stages after injury. Prolonged starvation is deleterious and therefore nutritional support should be started. A debate exists regarding the optimal timing of beginning nutrition.
- Stabilization of hemodynamic status should first be obtained (although there is no increase in hemodynamic instability with early enteral nutrition) [18].

- Enteral nutrition (EN) should be attempted within 24–48 hours if there are no contraindications. If not, there is a rapid onset of gut mucosal atrophy and one loses the beneficial effects of enteral feeding on metabolism and hormonal gut production of incretins (which stimulate insulin secretion and suppress glucagon secretion) [19].
- Some authors do not recommend early parenteral nutrition (PN) because, in some studies, it has led to increased morbidity (such as infection rate and length of ventilation) [20]. Others recommend administering supplemental PN only after 3 days delay in nutrition, or if 60% of the calorie target is not reached – they describe a decrease in infection rate and duration of ventilator support [21]. Finally, a large randomized trial in patients with relative contraindications to early enteral nutrition compared standard care, including enteral feeding when possible, to early PN. They did not find any difference in mortality or length of stay between the two groups, but the PN group had a shorter duration of invasive ventilation [22].
- Thus, PN should be started in a patient who is severely malnourished or with a nonfunctioning GI tract.

Nutritional composition

Energy and protein requirements

- Predictive equations are inaccurate in critical illness. Measured energy expenditure compared to most of the predictive equations show unacceptable errors and a very low accuracy [23] in the predictive equations. Indirect calorimetry is the gold standard to assess resting energy expenditure. Limitations exist such as patients with high FiO_2, chest drainage, hemodynamic or ventilatory instability. The European Society of Enteral and Parenteral Nutrition (ESPEN) guidelines recommend [11] the administration of energy as close as possible to the measured energy expenditure obtained by indirect calorimetry, in order to decrease negative energy balance.
- In the absence of indirect calorimetry, resting energy expenditures vary usually from 22 to 24 kcal/kg/day, according to Kreymann et al. [24]. Thus, in the absence of indirect calorimetry, ICU patients should probably receive 25 kcal/kg/day. However, a tight calorie-control study based on regular energy expenditure measurements demonstrated that the tight calorie-control group had a higher energy and protein intake compared to a group receiving 25 kcal/kg/day. There was a trend towards improved hospital mortality in the tight calorie-control group (25). All patients receiving less than their targeted enteral feeding after 2 days should be considered for supplementary PN.
- Protein losses can be measured, but in practice 1–1.5 g/kg/day are required (11). Protein requirement increases during hypocaloric feeding and in patients with acute renal failure on continuous renal replacement therapy. Receiving adequate protein intake may be more important than achieving the target energy requirement in order to maintain nitrogen balance.

Composition of nonprotein calories

There should be a balanced ratio between carbohydrates and lipids in the prescription of the nonprotein calories.

- Carbohydrate (CHO) intake is essential in the critically ill patient, providing a unique substrate to the brain, the white and red blood cells, and surgical or traumatic wounds.

The upper limit of glucose utilization is 5 mg/kg/min and this limit should not be exceeded. Excessive CHO will increase the risks of hyperglycemia and infection, liver-function test disturbances and respiratory compromise in patients with limited respiratory reserves due to an overproduction of CO_2 [26].

- Lipids are preferentially metabolized in sepsis. They are taken up by the reticulo-endothelial system and are integrated in the membranes of the cells modifying prostaglandin metabolism and cell membrane composition. Soy-bean-based lipids may increase the inflammatory process and other markers of oxidative stress and other lipids are being evaluated for use in parenteral nutrition (27). It is controversial, but the American Society of Parenteral and Enteral Nutrition recommend no lipid be administered in parenteral nutrition formulations in the first week of parenteral nutrition (28). The use of fish-oil-based lipids is discussed below.

Note: If propofol is infused for sedation one must remember that this is dissolved in a fat emulsion equivalent to 10% intralipid.

Other nutritional requirements

- Water (25 to 30 mL/kg/day) and standard electrolytes need to be supplied. Magnesium and phosphate supplements may be required, mainly if refeeding syndrome is suspected. In this case, close monitoring of the electrolytes is mandatory.
- Vitamins, supplied in the form of a commercial multivitamin preparation, should be administered every day [29,30]. In the long term, vitamins B12, K and folate supplements may be required.
- Antioxidants such as selenium have been administered in some countries and may be associated with a better outcome, e.g. in sepsis [31]. However, selenium requirements vary according to different countries and systemic administration should be cautious and ideally after verification of the blood level.
- Trace element supplements are also mandatory, especially in patients who are subject to large losses, such as patients with burns, fistulas, open abdomen therapies and continuous renal replacement therapy. Double daily doses are required in these circumstances [32].

Oral feeding

Inadequate oral energy intake in the first 7 days following extubation has been described [33]. According to the ESPEN Nutrition Day Audit, slightly more than 25% of the ICU patients are being fed orally at any time [34]. The key goal is to identify patients who exhibit increased respiratory risk before beginning oral alimentation. Gastrointestinal dysmotility disorders are frequent, secondary to administered sedative and other medications or disease pathophysiology. Specific dietary recommendations should be made after a satisfactory simple bedside swallowing assessment administered by a trained provider. Then, specific diet can be prescribed.

Enteral nutrition

- EN is strongly recommended in preference to PN wherever possible.
- Without stimulation the gastrointestinal mucosa rapidly atrophies.
- Bowel sounds are not a sign of small-bowel normal peristalsis, but are from gastric or colonic origin.

- There seems no advantage to measuring gastric residual volume in terms of achieving calorie target or prevention of ventilator-associated pneumonia [35]. However, a tube positioned in the duodenum or the jejunum has the advantage of enabling successful administration of more calories [36].
- Prokinetic drugs (metoclopramide and erythromycin) are useful in improving gut motility and absorption [11].
- EN is beneficial to gut enterocytes, enteroendocrine cells, Paneth cells and the Goblet cells, and may reduce bacterial and toxin translocation through the gut wall.
- Enteral feeding reduces GI bleeding from stress ulcers.
- EN decreases infective complications in surgical patients [37].
- Many commercial preparations include fibers, fish oil and γ-linolenic acid, antioxidants, arginine, glutamine, leucine, branched-chain amino acids, pre- and probiotics. All are approximately 1 kcal/mL, but dense calorie formulas are helpful in anuric patients in whom fluid restriction is important.
- EN is cheaper than PN and with less metabolic and infectious complications.
- No need for "starter" diluted feeds. If problems occur, start at a lower rate rather than diluting the feed.
- Continuous pump feeding is better than intermittent bolus feeding – less risk of aspiration.
- Fine bore tubes are difficult to aspirate from, block easily and have few advantages in the critically ill patient.

Complications of enteral nutrition

- Malposition of tubes – always check with chest X-ray, mainly for duodenal tubes.
- Aspiration – watch for large residual volumes. Half sitting position is the best preventive measure for aspiration.
- Diarrhea – very common. Check for antibiotics and other medications as causes of diarrhea. *Clostridium difficile* infection must always be excluded. In the absence of these causes treat symptomatically rather than automatically stopping the feed. Fiber may be important.
- Infection/contamination – feeds are excellent bacteria growth media.
- Blockage of tubes – flush all medications with water or pancreatic enzymes.
- Constipation – often due to inadequate H_2O intake or possibly lack of fiber.
- Multiple studies have shown that nutritional goals/volumes of enteral feed are often unmet on many days in many patients in ICU.

Parenteral nutrition

- Discussed recently in the literature especially regarding the timing of starting PN (early versus late) [20–22].
- Should be prescribed in gastrointestinal failure such as ileus, severe diarrhea, malabsorption, short-bowel syndrome or high-output fistula.
- Supplemental PN may be given if EN is not reaching the targeted goal [11].
- More expensive.
- More metabolic problems such as hyperglycemia, hypertriglyceridemia, electrolyte disturbances.
- Requires dedicated central venous access (with all its complications).

- Incidence of infectious complications related to the care of the site rather than the type of site (e.g. tunneled versus nontunneled).
- Refeeding syndrome [38] may occur if full calorie nutrition is abruptly introduced after a period of starvation. This causes hormonal changes, chiefly increases in insulin and decreases in glucagon release, resulting in fluid and electrolyte shifts. Hypophosphatemia, hypokalemia and hypomagnesemia are the most common electrolyte changes seen. Hypophosphatemia may cause respiratory failure due to respiratory muscle weakness [39]. Although commonest with PN, this can also occur when EN is instituted.
- The use of PN supplied by the manufacturer as a multichamber bag (activated and mixed prior to administration) was found in a large, retrospective database to be associated with significantly fewer bloodstream infections when compared with traditional solutions compounded in hospital pharmacies [40].

Hyperglycemia

- Frequent in ICU patients and may be related more to increased production from gluconeogenesis rather than decreased utilization (unless septic).
- When starting IV insulin to control glucose, ensure a constant glucose intake.
- High glucose levels are associated with higher rate of septic complications, while tight control using insulin is associated with a high rate of hypoglycemia [41].
- Less evidence is available to support very tight glucose control (80 to 110 mg/dL) with recent recommendations supporting higher targets of 100 to 150 mg/dL up to even 180 mg/dL, according to some scientific societies. However, no consensus has been reached. This is further discussed in the chapter on endocrine problems.

Note: Convert mg/dL to mmol/L by multiplying value by 0.0555.

Nutrition in acute respiratory failure

As for any malnourished patient, the ventilated patient suffering from malnutrition should be fed progressively to avoid refeeding syndrome. The calorie target should be obtained using indirect calorimetry to avoid overfeeding, which will increase VCO_2 production [26], and hyperglycemia and underfeeding, which will increase lean body mass wasting. Enough protein should be administered. In ALI and ARDS adequate amounts of eicosapentaenoic acid and γ-linolenic acid have been demonstrated to improve oxygenation, and morbidity and mortality [42,43]. The bolus administration of the same nutrients even in larger amounts has not shown the same effects [44].

Novel nutritional substrates

We should distinguish between substitution of nutrients that are lacking, supplementation of nutrients administered in excess of normal requirements and pharmaco nutrition (the use of specific nutrients in addition to regular nutrition for specific purposes [1]). However, many of these nutrients have been supplied in combination preparations limiting our ability to identify the direct effect of a specific nutrient.

Fish oil

- Omega (Ω) classification relates to the double bond nearest the last carbon of the chain of a fatty acid.

- Ω-3 fatty acids are essential for the body and are found in small quantities in normal diets.
- Ω-3 can be added to enteral or parenteral nutritional products.
- Ω-3 fatty acids are able to be incorporated in the cell membrane and to change its function. Fluidity is increased, cell signaling processes are modified and lipid mediators are influenced. The Ω-6 fatty acid arachidonic acid yields highly inflammatory prostaglandins and leukotrienes, whereas Ω-3 fatty acids favor production of less inflammatory prostaglandins [45].
- Patients with ALI and ARDS may benefit from enteral nutrition enriched in Ω-3 fatty acids, together with γ-linoleic acid, improving oxygenation as well as reducing duration of ventilation and length of stay [42,43].
- IV administration of Ω-3 fatty acids as a supplement in PN improves liver-function-test disturbances and has been shown to decrease infection rate and length of stay of surgical patients staying in the ICU without improving overall survival [46].

Glutamine

- Classified as a semi-essential amino acid that can be synthesized *de novo* in health, but is a conditionally essential amino acid in catabolic and stress states.
- Glutamine levels are usually decreased in critical illness. Humans have 24–48 hours of glutamine stores to maintain glutamine levels after injury [47].
- Large amounts of glutamine are released from the muscle in response to stress.
- Glutamine is a fuel for rapidly dividing cells, such as intestinal mucosa, lymphocytes and macrophages, is a precursor for synthesis of nucleic acids and preserves glutathione and antioxidant capacity.
- Glutamine has been previously recommended to be administered as a supplementation in ICU patients receiving total PN [11] at the dose of 0.3 to 0.5 g/kg/day.
- Enteral glutamine has been found to improve morbidity in multiple trauma and burns patients [48].
- A recent large, prospective randomized study (REDOXS study) [48] found the supplemental administration of glutamine in severely ill patients to increase mortality in patients with multiple organ failure. Current guidelines still support the administration of glutamine in ICU patients but these guidelines may need to be revised [49].

Arginine

- A nonessential amino acid thought to be important for wound healing, collagen deposition and immune function.
- A precursor of nitric oxide potentially increasing vasodilatation.
- Specific supplementation is no longer recommended in the ICU during acute illness since it potentially may increase mortality in sepsis [50].

Fiber, pro- and prebiotics

- Fiber added to enteral nutrition may reduce the incidence of diarrhea [51], but this is still considered controversial. Fermentation of soluble fiber by gut bacteria is an important source of short-chain fatty acid substrates for colonocytes.

- A recent meta-analysis suggests that the administration of probiotics (beneficial live bacteria) to critically ill patients does not significantly reduce mortality, but does reduce the incidence of VAP and ICU length of stay [52]. However, caution should be exercised before considering the use of probiotics owing to an increase in mortality in patients with pancreatitis given probiotics [53].
- Prebiotics (oligofructose, galacto-oligosaccharides and lactulose which stimulate the normal gut bacterial flora) can be administered alone or with probiotics. They may reduce systemic inflammation, improve the immunological status of the intestinal mucosa and help prevent infections. However, large studies are required to give definitive recommendations [54].

Summary

Nutritional support in critically ill patients requires:

- Recognition of nutritional status of the patient
- Accurate target of energy and protein requirement
- Appropriate choice of nutrients
- Avoidance of under- and overfeeding.
- Appropriate choice of route of nutrients
- Appropriate metabolic monitoring.

References

1. Singer P, Hiesmayr M, Biolo G et al. Pragmatic approach to nutrition in the ICU. Clin Nutr 2013; 33 : 246–51.

2. Villet S, Chiolero RL, Bollmann MD et al. Negative impact of hypocaloric feeding and energy balance on clinical outcome in ICU patients. Clin Nutr 2005; 24 : 502–9.

3. Dvir D, Cohen J, Singer P. Computerized energy balance and complications in critically ill patients: an observational study. Clin Nutr 2006; 25 : 37–44.

4. Kutsogiannis L, Alberda C, Gramlich L, et al. Early use of supplemental parenteral nutrition in critically ill patients: results of an international multicenter observational study. Crit Care Med 2011; 39 : 2691–9.

5. Bartlett RH, Allyn PA, Medley T. Nutritional therapy based on positive caloric balance in burn patients. Arch Surg 1977; 112 : 974–80.

6. Biolo G, Bosutti A, Iscra F et al. Contribution of the ubiquitin-proteasome pathway to overall muscle proteolysis in hypercatabolic patients. Metabolism 2000; 49 : 689–91.

7. Biolo G, Ciocchi B, Stulle M et al. Calorie restriction accelerates the catabolism of lean body mass during 2 wk of bed rest. Am J Clin Nutr 2007; 86 : 366–72.

8. Wolfe RR, Goodenough RD, Burke JF et al. Response of protein and urea kinetics in burn patients to different levels of protein intake. Ann Surg 1983; 197 : 163–71.

9. Ishibashi N, Plank LD, Sando K et al. Optimal protein requirements during the first 2 weeks after the onset of critical illness. Crit Care Med 1998; 26 : 1529–35.

10. Hoffer LJ. Protein and energy provision in critical illness. Am J Clin Nutr 2003; 78 : 906–11.

11. Singer P, Berger MM, Van den Berghe G et al. ESPEN Guidelines on Parenteral Nutrition: Intensive care. Clin Nutr 2009; 33 : 387–400.

12. MJ Allingstrup MJ, N Esmailzadeh N, A Wilkens Knudsen et al. Provision of protein and energy in relation to measured requirements in intensive care patients. Clin Nutr 2012; 31 : 462–8.

13. Tremblay A, Bandi V. Impact of body mass index on outcomes following critical care. Chest 2003; 123 : 1202–7.

14. Kondrup J, Rasmussen HH, Hamberg O et al. Nutritional risk screening (NRS 2002): a new method based on analysis of controlled clinical trials. Clin Nutr 2002; 22 : 321.

15. Lev S, Cohen J, Singer P. Indirect calorimetry measurements in the ventilated critically ill patient: facts and controversies – the heat is on. Crit Care Clin 2010; 26:1–9.

16. Chan T. Computerized method for automatic evaluation of lean body mass from PET/CT: comparison with predictive equations. J Nucl Med 2012; 53 : 130–7.

17. Choi AMK, Ryter SW, Levine B Autophagy in human health and disease. N Eng J Med 2013; 368 : 651–62

18. Khalid I, Doshi P, DiGiovine B. Early enteral nutrition and outcomes of critically ill patients treated with vasopressors and mechanical ventilation. Am J Crit Care 2010 : 19 : 261–8.

19. Singer P, Pichard C, Heideggeret CP et al. Considering energy deficit in the intensive care unit. Curr Opin Clin Nutr Metab Care 2010; 13:170–6.

20. Casaer MP, Mesotten D, Hermans G et al. Early versus late parenteral nutrition in critically ill patients. N Eng J Med 2011; 37:601–9.

21. Heidegger CP, Berger MM, Graf S et al. Optimization of energy provision with supplemental parenteral nutrition (SPN) improves the clinical outcome of critically ill patients : a randomized controlled trial. Lancet. 2013; 381 : 385–93.

22. Doig GS, Simpson F, Sweetman EA et al. Early parenteral nutrition in critically ill patients with short-term relative contraindications to early enteral nutrition: a randomized controlled trial. JAMA 2013; 309 :2130–8.

23. Reid C. Frequency of under and overfeeding in mechanically ventilated ICU patients: causes and possible consequences. J Hum Nutr Diet 2006; 19 : 13–22.

24. Kreymann G, DeLegge MH, Luft G et al. The ratio of energy expenditure to nitrogen loss in diverse patient groups: a systematic review. Clin Nutr 2012; 31: 168–75.

25. Singer P, Anbar R, Cohen J et al. The Tight Calorie Control Study (TICACOS): a prospective, randomized, controlled study of nutritional support in critically ill patients. Intensive Care Med 2009; 37: 601–9.

26. Herve P, Simmonneau G, Girard P et al. Hypercapnic acidosis induced by nutrition in mechanically ventilated patients: glucose versus fat. Crit Care Med 1985 : 13:537–40.

27. Siqueira J, Smiley D, Newton C et al. Substitution of standard soybean oil with olive oil-based lipid emulsion in parenteral nutrition: comparison of vascular, metabolic, and inflammatory effects. J Clin Endocrinol Metab 2011; 96 : 3207–16.

28. McClave SA, Martindale RG, Vanek VW et al. Guidelines for the Provision and Assessment of Nutrition Support Therapy in the Adult Critically Ill Patient: Society of Critical Care Medicine (SCCM) and American Society for Parenteral and Enteral Nutrition (A.S.P.E.N.). JPEN 2009; 33: 277–316.

29. Manzanares W, Hardy G. Thiamine supplementation in the critically ill. Curr Opin Clin Nutr Metab Care 2011; 14 : 610–7.

30. Higgins DM, Wischmeyer PE, Queensland KM et al. Relationship of vitamin D deficiency to clinical outcomes in critically ill patients. JPEN 2012; 36 : 713–20.

31. Alhazzani W, Jacobi J, Sindi A et al. The effect of selenium therapy on mortality in patients with sepsis syndrome: a systematic review and meta-analysis of randomized controlled trials. Crit Care Med 2013; 41 : 1555–64.

32. Berger M, Shenkin A, Revelly J et al. Copper, selenium, zinc and thiamine balances during continuous venovenous hemodiafiltration in critically ill patients. Am J Clin Nutr 2004; 80 : 410–16.

33. Peterson SJ, Tsai AA, Scala CM et al. Adequacy of oral intake in critically ill patients 1 week after extubation. J Am Diet Assoc 2010; 110 : 427–33.

34. Alvárez-Falcón A, Ruiz-Santana S. Oral feeding. World Rev Nutr Diet 2013; 105 : 43–9.

35. Reignier J, Mercier E, Le Gouge A et al. Clinical Research in Intensive Care and

Sepsis (CRICS) Group. Effect of not monitoring residual gastric volume on risk of ventilator-associated pneumonia in adults receiving mechanical ventilation and early enteral feeding: a randomized controlled trial. *JAMA* 2013; 309 : 249–56.

36. Zhang Z, Xu X, Ding J et al. Comparison of postpyloric tube feeding and gastric tube feeding in intensive care unit patients: a meta-analysis. *Nutr Clin Pract* 2013; 28 : 371–80.

37. Moore FA, Feliciano DV, Andrassy RJ et al. Early enteral feeding, compared with parenteral, reduces postoperative septic complications. The results of a meta-analysis. *Ann Surg* 1992; 216: 172–83.

38. Byrnes MC, Stangenes J. Refeeding in the ICU: an adult and pediatric problem. *Current Opinion in Clinical Nutrition and Metabolic Care* 2011; 14 : 186–92.

39. Patel U, Sriram K. Acute respiratory failure due to refeeding syndrome and hypophosphatemia induced by hypocaloric enteral nutrition. *Nutrition* 2009; 25 : 364–7.

40. Pontes-Arruda A, Zaloga G, Wischmeyer P et al. Is there a difference in bloodstream infections in critically ill patients associated with ready-to-use versus compounded parenteral nutrition? *Clin Nutr* 2012; 31 : 728–34.

41. Finfer S, Wernerman J, Preiser JC et al. Clinical review: consensus recommendations on measurement of blood glucose and reporting glycemic control in critically ill adults. *Crit Care* 2013; 17 : 229.

42. Gadek JE, DeMichele SJ, Karlstad MD et al. Enteral Nutrition in ARDS Study Group: effect of enteral feeding with eicosapentaenoic acid, gamma-linolenic acid, and antioxidants in patients with acute respiratory distress syndrome. *Crit Care Med* 1999; 27:1409–20.

43. Singer P, Theilla M, Fisher H. Benefit of an enteral diet enriched with eicosapentaenoic acid and gamma-linolenic acid in ventilated patients with acute lung injury. *Crit Care Med* 2006; 34 : 1033–8.

44. Stapleton RD, Martin TR, Weiss NS et al. A phase II randomized placebo-controlled trial of omega-3 fatty acids for the treatment of acute lung injury. *Crit Care Med* 2011; 39 : 1655–62.

45. Singer P, Shapiro H, Theilla M et al. Anti-inflammatory properties of omega-3 fatty acids in critical illness: novel mechanisms and an integrative perspective. *Intensive Care Med* 2008; 34 : 1580–9.

46. Pradelli L, Mayer K, Muscaritoli M et al. n-3 fatty acid-enriched parenteral nutrition regimens in elective surgical and ICU patients: a meta-analysis. *Crit Care* 2012; 16 : R184.

47. Askanazi J, Carpentier YA, Michelsen CB. Muscle and plasma amino acids following injury: influence of intercurrent infection. *Ann Surg* 1980; 192: 78–82.

48. Heyland D, Muscedere J, Wischmeyer PE et al. Canadian Critical Care Trials Group. A randomized trial of glutamine and antioxidants in critically ill patients. *N Engl J Med* 2013; 368 : 1489–97.

49. Preiser JC, Berré PJ, Van Gossum A et al. Metabolic effects of arginine addition to the enteral feeding of critically ill patients. *JPEN* 2001; 25 : 182–7.

50. Kalil AC, Danner RL. L-Arginine supplementation in sepsis: beneficial or harmful? *Curr Opin Crit Care* 2006; 12 : 303–8.

51. Spapen H, Diltoer M, Van Malderen C et al. Soluble fiber reduces the incidence of diarrhea in septic patients receiving total enteral nutrition: a prospective, double-blind, randomized, and controlled trial. *Clin Nutr.* 2001; 20 : 301–5.

52. Barraud D, Bollaert PE, Gibot S. Impact of the administration of probiotics on mortality in critically ill adult patients: a meta-analysis of randomized controlled trials. *Chest* 2013; 143 : 646–55.

53. Morrow LE, Gogineni V, Malesker MA. Synbiotics and probiotics in the critically ill after the PROPATRIA trial. *Curr Opin Clin Nutr Metab Care* 2012; 15 : 147–50.

54. Manzanares W, Hardy G. The role of prebiotics and synbiotics in critically ill patients. *Curr Opin Clin Nutr Metab Care* 2008; 11 : 782–9.

Electrolyte and metabolic acid–base problems

Harneet Kaur, Julio P Zavala Georffino, Daniel Castro Pereira, Bhupesh Khadka, Joseph Dreier and Clay A Block

Metabolic acidosis

Definition

Metabolic acidosis [1] can be defined as a low arterial blood pH in conjunction with low serum bicarbonate concentration caused either by increased acid generation/decreased acid secretion or loss of bicarbonate.

Approach to metabolic acidosis

- Calculation of anion gap/serum AG (anion gap) = measured cations – measured anions
- Serum AG = Na – (Cl + HCO₃)
- Normal AG is 12 ± 2. Since much of the unmeasured anion is albumin, AG must be adjusted in patients with hypoalbuminemia – decrease AG by 2.5 mEq/L for every 1 g/dL reduction in the serum albumin concentration.

Causes

Different causes and classification of metabolic acidosis are outlined below:

Anion gap	Nonanion gap
Lactic acidosis	Toluene ingestion
Diabetic ketoacidosis	Diarrhea or other intestinal losses
Starvation-induced ketoacidosis	Chronic kidney disease and tubular dysfunction
Ingestions like methanol, ethylene glycol, aspirin (salicylates), toluene, diethylene glycol, propylene glycol	Type 1 (distal) renal tubular acidosis (RTA)
Chronic kidney disease (uremia)	Type 2 (proximal) RTA
D-lactic acidosis	Type 4 RTA (hypoaldosteronism)
Pyroglutamic acid (5-oxoproline)	

Handbook of ICU Therapy, third edition, ed. John Fuller, Jeff Granton and Ian McConachie. Published by Cambridge University Press. © Cambridge University Press 2015.

Anion gap metabolic acidosis

- **MUD PILES.** Acronym representing methanol, uremia, diabetes, paraldehyde, iron (and isoniazid), lactate, ethylene glycol and salicylate (and starvation).
- **GOLDMARK.** This acronym represents glycols (ethylene and propylene), oxoproline, L-lactate, D-lactate, methanol, aspirin, renal failure and ketoacidosis.
- **Ethylene glycol/methanol poisoning.** Associated with severe AG metabolic acidosis. Ethylene glycol is a component of antifreeze and solvents. If left untreated, can lead to cardiopulmonary symptoms and renal failure often accompanied by abundant calcium oxalate crystals in the urine. Along with AG, osmolar gap (measured osmolality – calculated osmolality) is also elevated. Therapy includes supportive treatment, and it is crucial to reduce the metabolism of the parent compound, as well as to accelerate the removal of metabolites from the body. Fomepizole inhibits alcohol dehydrogenase and prevents formation of toxic metabolites. Hemodialysis should also be used for quick removal of parent compound and metabolites.
- **Salicylate toxicity.** If taken in toxic concentrations can lead to increased lactic acid production. Also causes respiratory alkalosis by stimulating the respiratory center. Treatment includes conservative management and alkalinization of blood and urine. Alkalemia causes ionization of salicylic acid, which leads to decreased accumulation of drug in CNS and also favors increased excretion in urine since it is poorly reabsorbed in the tubules. If serum level >80 mg/dL, hemodialysis should be done to quickly remove the drug.
- **5-oxoprolinemia/pyroglutamic academia.** Presents with elevated AG and should be considered where the high AG is not explained by other culprits in GOLDMARK. Pyroglutamic acidemia is generally a rare inherited disorder presenting in infancy because of deficiency of either glutathione synthetase or 5-oxoprolinase. It has also been described in adults as an acquired form. This usually occurs in association with acetaminophen (Tylenol), flucloxacillin and vigabatrin, particularly in severe sepsis, liver or renal failure. This is due to reversible inhibition of glutathione synthetase. Diagnosed by urine organic acid screen, which identifies puroglutamic aciduria. Therapy includes cessation of known culprit and use of N-acetylcysteine (replenishes glutathione stores).

Nonanion-gap MA

Renal and extrarenal causes

To differentiate between renal and extrarenal causes one can measure the urine ammonia excretion, but this is often not readily available. We can indirectly measure it by the urine anion gap.

$$UAG = (Urine\ Na + urine\ K) - Urine\ Cl$$

Negative UAG is seen in extrarenal causes and positive UAG is indicative of renal (renal tubular acidosis or RTA) etiology.

RTA is classified below :

	Proximal RTA type II	Distal RTA type IV	Classic distal RTA type I
Defect	Reabsorption of HCO_3	Decreased aldosterone secretion or effect (H^+ and K^+ excretion)	H^+ excretion
Urine pH	Variable	<5.5	>5.5
Plasma potassium	Decreased	Increased	Decreased
Diseases	Fanconi syndrome Systemic lupus erythematosus Multiple myeloma/ amyloid Tenofovir Acetazolomide and topiramate Aminoglycoside Heavy metals Vitamin D deficiency	Hypoaldosteronism Renal disease, most often diabetic nephropathy Nonsteroidal anti-inflammatory drugs Calcineurin inhibitors ACE inhibitors and angiotensin II receptor blockers Heparin Primary adrenal insufficiency	Sjögren's syndrome Systemic lupus erythematosus Rheumatoid arthritis Ifosfamide Amphotericin B Lithium carbonate Hyperparathyroidism Vitamin D intoxication Sarcoidosis Obstructive uropathy Idiopathic

Acid–base analysis

- First step is to determine whether patient is acidemic or alkalemic, based on arterial pH.
- Next step: determine whether it is a primary respiratory or metabolic disorder by measuring arterial PCO_2 and serum bicarbonate level.
- If respiratory problem is present, assess if acute or chronic by comparing pH and $PaCO_2$.
- If a metabolic acidosis is present, determine whether it is anion gap or nonanion gap.
- In metabolic disturbances, determine whether the respiratory system is adequately compensating. (Winter's formula: Expected $PCO_2 = 1.5 \times$ serum bicarbonate $+8 \pm 2$). This is then compared to the actual PCO_2 to assess the degree of respiratory compensation of metabolic acidosis. (In addition, a PCO_2 less than calculated suggests primary respiratory alkalosis, while if greater it suggests primary respiratory acidosis.)
- If an anion-gap acidosis exists, determine the presence of any concomitant metabolic disturbances by using the $\Delta AG/\Delta HCO_3$ ratio.

ΔAG = measured AG – normal AG

ΔHCO_3 = normal bicarbonate – measured bicarbonate

Ratio between 1 and 2: pure high AG metabolic acidosis. Ratio >2: mixed acid–base disorder.

Treatment

- The treatment of metabolic acidosis can vary markedly with the underlying disorder.
- In severe metabolic acidosis, assuming that respiratory function is normal, a pH of 7.20 would be reasonable to target and usually requires raising the serum bicarbonate to 10 to 12 mEq/L. The deficit can be calculated by the formula:

$$HCO_3 \text{ deficit} = HCO_3 \text{ space} \times HCO_3 \text{ deficit per liter}$$
$$= 0.5 \times \text{lean body weight} \times (24 - HCO_3)$$

- Sodium bicarbonate can be given as oral tablets, powder, as a hypertonic bicarbonate bolus or isotonic sodium bicarbonate. For patients with volume depletion, administration of three ampules of bicarbonate (each contains 50 mEq of sodium bicarbonate) in 1 L of dextrose 5% in water (D5W) solution will help with both volume expansion and alkalinization.
- Replace 50% of deficit in the first 24 hours and determine future dosage based on response to therapy and target bicarbonate.
- Renal replacement therapy is employed for refractory severe metabolic acidosis.

Metabolic alkalosis

Definition

Metabolic alkalosis [2–4] is defined as a rise in the plasma bicarbonate concentration, either by adding bicarbonate to the plasma or by failure to excrete the excess bicarbonate in the urine, pH >7.45.

Pathophysiology

Generation of metabolic alkalosis:

- Elevation in plasma HCO_3 concentration is induced by H^+ loss from the GI tract (vomiting) or in the urine (diuretics). H^+ is derived from the intracellular dissociation of H_2CO_3:

$$CO_2 + H_2O \longleftrightarrow H_2CO_3 \longleftrightarrow H^+ + HCO_3^-$$

- Metabolic alkalosis is also produced by the administration of HCO_3 by H^+ movement into the cells and K^+/Cl^- depletion. A transcellular H^+ shift typically occurs with hypokalemia. Chloride depletion alkalosis occurs when the fluid that is lost contains Cl^- but no bicarbonate. The severity of this process is generally limited by buffering of the excess extracellular HCO_3^- by cell and bone buffers.

Causes of chloride-responsive metabolic alkalosis:

- Vomiting, nasogastric suction
- Thiazides
- Metolazone
- Loop diuretics
- Chronic hypercapnia
- Diarrhea
- Villous adenoma of colon.

Causes of chloride-resistant metabolic alkalosis:

- Mineralocorticoid excess (hyperaldosteronism, Cushing's syndrome, ACTH-secreting tumor, renin-secreting tumor)
- Syndrome of apparent mineralocorticoid excess
- Bartter syndrome, Gitelman's syndrome
- Decreased effective circulating volume in the setting of heart failure/cirrhosis
- Renal failure
- Hypokalemia.

Metabolic alkalosis associated with alkali administration:

- Sodium bicarbonate
- Lactate in Ringer's solution
- Parenteral nutrition – acetate, glutamate
- Citrate (blood products, plasma exchange)
- Milk alkali syndrome
- Dialysis.

Clinical features

Mild to moderate metabolic alkalosis is asymptomatic. Hyocalcemia and hypokalemia can develop, which cause cardiac arrhythmias, especially in patients with ischemic heart disease. If serum HCO_3 level is >50 mmol/L, patients can develop seizures, delirium and tetany.

Investigations

- Elevated serum bicarbonate >30 mmol/L and hypokalemia is diagnostic
- Checking the blood gas may help, but is not required to make a diagnosis
- If the etiology is not clear, then mixed disorder should always be suspected and blood gas is warranted
- Urine chloride concentration :
  - Less than 25 mEq/L – Vomiting, diarrhea, post-hypercapnia, cystic fibrosis, low chloride intake
  - Urine chloride greater than 40 mEq/L – Primary mineralocorticoid excess, diuretics, alkali load, Bartter/Gitelmen syndrome and severe hypokalemia
  - The urine chloride concentration may not be useful in patients who are unable to maximally conserve Cl^- due to tubular defects as occurs with renal failure or severe hypokalemia (<2.0 mEq/L).

Treatment

Chloride-responsive alkalosis

- The increase in bicarbonate resorption can be counteracted by administration of normal saline or by volume expansion. Increased distal chloride delivery will increase the bicarbonate secretion in the collecting tubule. Effect can be monitored by increases in the urine pH (>7).

Chloride-resistant alkalosis

- Typically seen in edematous states (heart failure, cirrhosis, nephrotic syndrome) following diuretic therapy
- Treatment includes discontinuing diuretics, trial of acetazolamide, dialysis
- Acetazolamide is a carbonic anhydrase inhibitor that increases the excretion of bicarbonate and potassium. Need to monitor for hypokalemia and treat if present. Dose – 250 mg to 375mg once or twice daily. Effect can be monitored by increase in urine pH (>7). It can sometimes cause increase in PCO_2 levels, which is clinically insignificant.

Disorders of sodium and water balance

Overview

- Disorders of sodium and water balance [5–9] are present in 28.7% of patients admitted to ICU. Hyponatremia occurs in 12–13% and hypernatremia in 12–17% of critically ill patients, both associated with higher mortality compared with patients with normal sodium levels.
- In a steady state, the ingestion of water and sodium must match their excretion. Almost all sodium filtrated by the glomeruli is reabsorbed in the tubules, so sodium problems are related almost exclusively to problems of water balance.

Key hormones

Antidiuretic hormone (ADH) via opening of water channels in collecting ducts, regulates sodium concentration. The stimuli for secretion of ADH are:

- Increased plasma osmolality: normal osmolality is between 280–285 mOsm/kg (osmotic secretion).
- Arterial "underfilling" (nonosmotic secretion) due to decreased cardiac output, vasodilation or both.
- *Aldosterone*, the primary hormone that regulates total body sodium and volume via reabsorption of sodium *in exchange* for potassium and/or H^+ in collecting ducts. The stimuli for secretion are hypovolemia and hyperkalemia.

Hyponatremia

Definition

Hyponatremia is defined as plasma Na^+ <135 mmol/L

Pathophysiology

- In hyponatremia the main pathophysiologic disorder is water retention leading to an excess of water relative to sodium, which is due to increased ADH in almost all hyponatremic states.
- ADH secretion may be "appropriate" in response to the stimuli described above.
- ADH secretion may be "inappropriate," when it is activated in the absence of the stimuli described previously. (The most common disorder is syndrome of inappropriate ADH, SIADH.)

- In a few cases, ADH secretion may be appropriately suppressed and other mechanisms may explain hyponatremia:
  - The normal kidney capacity to excrete electrolyte free water is 15–20 L per 24 hours (~10% of GFR). Patients with primary polydipsia usually overcome the kidney capacity to excrete water, drinking more than this and producing hyponatremia.
  - The maximal urinary dilutional capacity is 50 mOsm/kg. Thus a person with diminished solute intake (100 mOsm/day) that drinks 3 L/day, is able to excrete 2 L/day and will retain water every day and have hyponatremia (beer-drinkers not eating or tea and toast diet).
  - Loop diuretics are more potent than thiazide diuretics, but the latter are more likely to produce hyponatremia.
  - Reset osmostat is a phenomenon in which the set point for plasma osmolality is reduced; therefore ADH secretion and thirst are stimulated at this lower level to maintain plasma [Na$^+$] there. This disorder can be seen during pregnancy and in patients with severe malnutrition.

Causes/classification

- Normo-osmolar hyponatremia – laboratory abnormality in which an excess of plasma proteins or lipids increase the nonaqueous portion of the plasma sample, which leads to a false report of low serum sodium concentration.
- Hyperosmolar hyponatremia – an osmotically active solute accumulates in extracellular fluid, leading to water shifts and diluting the sodium content. Hyperglycemia is the most common etiology. There is a fall in plasma sodium concentration of 1.6–2.4 mmol/L for every 5.54 mmol/L rise in plasma glucose. Other etiologies are mannitol, sorbitol and glycine.
- Hypo-osmolar hyponatremia – "true" hyponatremia can be also further subdivided (see Figure 11.1.)

Hypovolemic hyponatremia

- Renal losses: diuretic excess, mineralocorticoid deficiency, salt losing nephritis, osmotic diuresis, bicarbonaturia, ketonuria
- Extra renal losses: vomiting, diarrhea, "third space" burns, pancreatitis.

Euvolemic hyponatremia

- Glucocorticoid deficiency, hypothyroidism, psychiatric disorders (primary polydipsia), tea and toast diet, beer potomania, reset osmostat, SIADH, exercise-associated hyponatremia, reset osmostat.
- SIADH: emotional or physical stress, pain, nausea, tumors, CNS disorders, pulmonary diseases, drugs (nicotine, chlorpropamide, tolbutamide, clofibrate, cyclophosphamide, morphine, barbiturates, carbamazepine, NSAIDs, acetaminophen, antipsychotics, antidepressants, omeprazole, ACE inhibitors, MDMA).

Hypervolemic hyponatremia

- Heart failure, cirrhosis, nephrotic syndrome, renal failure.

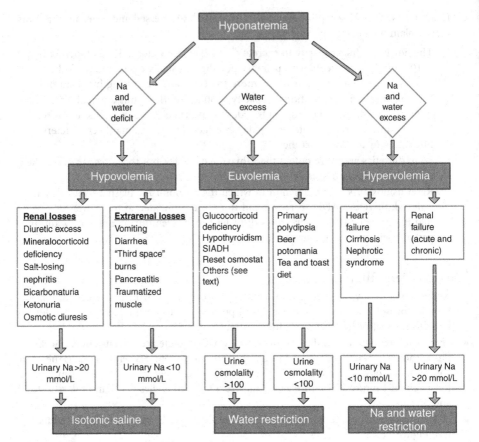

Figure 11.1 Causes and work-up of hypo-osmolar hyponatremia.

Clinical presentation

- Symptomatic hyponatremia: osmotic intracellular water shift leading to cerebral edema. Initially patients may complain of malaise, nausea, headache and progress to severe neurological manifestations like confusion and lethargy that may lead to stupor, seizures and coma, when serum sodium concentration falls below 115–120 mmol/L.
- Asymptomatic hyponatremia: generally slower/more insidious onset.

Management

Work-up

- Plasma osmolality: "true" hyponatremia should be hypo-osmolar and therefore should have low plasma osmolality (<280 mOsm/kg). Useful to differentiate from hyperosmolar and hypo-osmolar causes.
- Evaluate volume status. A careful physical exam and history of present illness will help to establish the differential diagnosis of hyponatremia, including presence of signs/

symptoms of volume depletion (hypotension, tachycardia, orthostatic, etc.) and fluid overload (edema, shortness of breath, orthopnea, PND, JVP, crackles, etc.)

- Urine osmolality: normal response to hyponatremia should be dilute urine (urine osmolality <100 mOsm/L). Nondilute urine indicates the presence of ADH. Dilute urine also may be found in disorders like primary polydipsia and low solute intake states like tea and toast diet and beer potomania (described above).
- Urinary Na^+. Helps in the bedside assessment of effective circulating volume and to differentiate between renal and extrarenal losses of sodium (see Figure 11.1).
- Other tests: TSH, cortisol levels.

Treatment

Acute hyponatremia (rapid development of hyponatremia in 48 hours)

Acute symptomatic hyponatremia may be a very serious clinical situation and needs treatment regardless of etiology. Treatment of choice is infusion of 3% NaCl, also known as hypertonic saline, which contains 513 mmol/L of Na. The rate of infusion can be determined by estimation of the change in serum sodium using 1 L of hypertonic saline over 24 hours using the Adrogue–Madias formula :

Change in Na = [(Na in infused fluid + K in infused fluid) – serum Na]/ [TBW + 1]

TBW: Total body water (weight × 0.5 if female, × 0.6 if male)

As an example, a 66 kg female presents with serum Na of 105 mmol/L and with stupor. Using the formula, the change in Na^+ will be 12 mmol if given 1 L of hypertonic saline

$$Change\ in\ Na = [(513 + 0) - 105]/[(66 \times 0.5) + 1]$$
$$= 408/[33 + 1]$$
$$= 12$$

Therefore, 100 mL of hypertonic saline will increase serum Na^+ by 1.2 mmol. As the patient is symptomatic, an initial infusion of 100–200 mL/h would be appropriate, without exceeding a correction of >10 mmol/L in 24 hours. In this patient no more than 900 mL of hypertonic saline should be use in the first 24 hours and serum sodium levels should be monitored every 4 hours in order to make appropriate adjustments.

Chronic hyponatremia (development of hyponatremia in >48 hours)

A slow process of adaptation in the brain (exclusion of osmolytes like phosphocreatine, myoinositol and amino acids) will decrease intracellular osmolality and avoid cerebral edema. Therefore rapid correction of chronic hyponatremia may lead to osmotic demyelination. Different strategies, depending on the etiology, can be used to excrete the excess of water.

- Fluid restriction is primary treatment for SIADH. It is important to note that the daily fluid intake should be restricted to less than 24 hour urine output and insensible losses, to be effective.
- Loop diuretics enhance excretion of water by interfering with the concentration gradient necessary to reabsorb water in the distal nephron. Can be used in cases of hypervolemia.

- Demeclocycline (600–1200 mg/day), a tetracycline antibiotic that causes nephrogenic DI and resistance to ADH should be considered only if other measures have failed, because of potential side effects, including nephrotoxicity, which is reversible.
- Vasopressin antagonists (tolvaptan) are effective in euvolemic and hypervolemic hyponatremia. They are approved for short-term treatment of hyponatremia, but their long-term effect and impact in clinical outcomes is still unknown.

Hypernatremia

Definition

Hypernatremia is defined as plasma $[Na^+]$ >145 mmol/L and reflects cellular dehydration.

Pathophysiology

Increases in plasma osmolality are sensed by hypothalamic cells, which stimulate thirst and also the release of ADH. The development of hypernatremia involves increased water losses in the setting of inadequate intake and, very rarely, excessive sodium intake.

- Inadequate intake → primary hypodipsia (hypothalamic or osmo-receptor dysfunction, advanced age), decreased access to water (post-operative, intubated, handicapped patients and with mental impairment like delirium or dementia).
- Increased renal water loss → osmotic diuresis, diabetes insipidus (DI), loop diuretics, post-acute kidney injury (AKI), post-obstructive diuresis.
- Increased extrarenal water loss → gastrointestinal losses, skin losses, increased insensible losses (skin, respiratory tract).
- Increased salt intake → excessive Na administration (saline or bicarbonate), hyperalimentation, salt ingestion, mineralocorticoid excess.

Clinical presentation

- May be related to cellular dehydration because of loss of intracellular water. Initially patients may present with general/nonspecific symptoms like anorexia, nausea, vomiting that may progress to more prominent neurological symptoms like altered mental status, irritability, focal neurological deficits and if acute and severe, coma and seizures. Other symptoms include polyuria and polydipsia as presenting symptoms of DI.
- Clinical signs of volume status will help in the initial assessment and work-up.

Causes/classification

Hypovolemic hypernatremia

Decreased total body water and decreased total body sodium:

- Renal losses: osmotic diuresis (glucose, mannitol, urea, high-protein feeds), loop diuretics, post-AKI diuresis, post-obstructive diuresis.
- Extrarenal losses: gastrointestinal (vomiting, diarrhea, NG suctioning, entero-cutaneous fistula), skin (sweating, burns).

Euvolemic hypernatremia

Decreased total body water and normal total body sodium:

- Renal losses: diabetes insipidus (DI):

    ADH dependent → central DI (trauma, neurosurgery, brain tumors, infiltrative disorders, hypoxic encephalopathy, bleeding, infection, aneurysm), hereditary (X-linked recessive), gestational DI.

    Acquired nephrogenic DI → hypercalcemia, hypokalemia, drug-induced (lithium, demeclocycline, amphotericin B, foscarnet), chronic kidney disease, malnutrition.

- Extrarenal losses: increased insensible losses (skin, respiratory tract, fever).

Hypervolemic hypernatremia

Increased total body sodium and decreased or normal total body water:

- Excessive sodium administration: saline or bicarbonate
- Hyperalimentation (total parenteral nutrition)
- Mineralocorticoid excess.

Management
Work-up (see Figure 11.2)

- Assess volume status (vital signs, orthostatic change, jugular venous pressure (JVP), skin turgor, peripheral edema).
- Evaluate urine osmolality, plasma osmolality, urinary Na^+, urinary output (UOP)

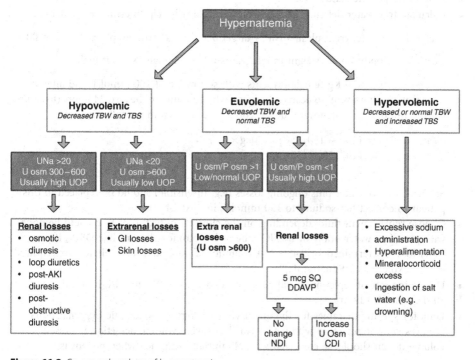

Figure 11.2 Causes and work up of hypernatremia.

- In hypovolemic hypernatremia, high UOP, urinary Na^+ >20 mmol/L and urine osmolality 300–600 mOsm/kg will correlate with renal losses of free water (see above), whereas low UOP, urinary Na^+ <20 and elevated urine osmolality >600 mOsm/kg will correlate with GI and skin losses.
- In euvolemic hypernatremia, patients with low UOP and elevated urine osmolality (>600 mOsm/kg, Uosm/Posm >1) correlate with extra renal losses, whereas patients with high urinary output and low urine osmolality (<300 mOsm/kg, Uosm/Posm <1) will correlate with diabetes insipidus.
- To determine central versus nephrogenic DI, subcutaneous vasopressin/ 1-deamino-8-D-arginine vasopressin (DDAVP) administration will help the differentiation. No change in urine osmolality after administration of exogenous vasopressin, 5 µg subcutaneously (SQ) will be diagnostic of nephrogenic DI. It is important to remember that central and nephrogenic DI may also be partial and will present with relatively normal UOP and urine osmolality between 300 and 600 mOsm/kg.
- Hypervolemic hypernatremia may be determined by physical examination and careful clinical history.

Treatment

The goals of treatment in hypernatremia are to decrease ongoing water losses and replace the free-water deficit. The following approach is suggested:

- Determine volume status
- Calculate free-water deficit. The following formula will help to estimate the deficit:

Water deficit = (current plasma Na^+ – target plasma Na^+)/(target plasma Na^+) × TBW

TBW: Total body water (weight in kilograms × 0.5 if female, × 0.6 if male)

As an example, a 70 Kg female presents with serum Na of 160 mmol/L and altered mental status. If we want to decrease serum Na by 10 mmol in the next 24 hours (to serum Na 150 mmol/L), the free-water deficit could be calculated in the following way:

$$\text{Water deficit} = (160 - 150/150) \times (70\text{kg} \times 0.5)$$
$$= (10/150) \times (35)$$
$$= 2.5 \text{ L}$$

So, 2.5 L of free water plus ongoing losses (e.g. insensible) should be replaced in this patient to correct her sodium to 150 mmol/L in next 24 hours.

- Choose replacement fluid: depending on the clinical context, repletion could be done with pure free water orally or by NG tube or hypotonic solutions like D5W, if pure water loss is determined, or 0.45% NaCl solution if water and salt repletion are required (in hypovolemic hypernatremia).
- Determine rate of repletion: usually recommended to be 0.5 mmol/L/h or a decrease of 10–12 mmol/24 hours.
- Look for specific therapies for the underlying etiology: hypovolemic hypernatremia requires volume repletion with 0.45% NaCl. If severe volume depletion is present, volume deficit should be corrected with NS initially and then when patient is

hemodynamically stable, correct free-water deficit. In central DI, administration of DDAVP (vasopressin analog) is the therapy of choice. In nephrogenic DI a, thiazide diuretic will induce mild volume depletion and decrease distal delivery of salt and water, reducing free-water excretion.

Disorders of potassium [10–13]
Hypokalemia
Overview

- Most common electrolyte abnormality in hospitalized patients
- It is usually defined as a serum potassium of less than 3.5 mmol/L
- Given the fact that untreated hypokalemia is associated with high morbidity and mortality, it is critical to recognise and treat these disorders promptly.

Pathophysiology

- Potassium is the most abundant cation in the body. It is predominantly restricted to the intracellular space, such that only 2% is located extracellularly and the remaining 98% is in the intracellular compartment. The ratio of intracellular to extracellular potassium (Ki/Ke) is the major determinant of resting membrane potential, and is regulated primarily by the sodium-potassium ATPase pump located on the plasma membrane of most cells.
- The daily intake of potassium in the western diet is between 80 and 120 mmol. The kidney is the major route of potassium excretion, accounting for 90% of potassium loss daily. The remaining 10% is excreted through the gastrointestinal tract.
- Potassium is also regulated on a short-term basis by transcellular shift.
- Symptoms include fatigue, weakness, leg cramps, constipation and rhabdomyolysis, and ascending paralysis and respiratory difficulties in severe cases. The rate of potassium change determines symptom severity.
- Cardiac dysrhythmias may also be the only presenting symptom.

Causes
Increased loss

- Renal losses: diuretics are the most common cause of hypokalemia, with loop diuretics inhibiting the NaK2Cl channel and thiazide diuretics blocking the NaCl cotransporter, resulting in increased distal delivery of sodium and thus secretion of potassium via a favorable electrochemical gradient.
- GI losses: diarrhea, villous adenoma, VIPoma.

Transcellular shift
Drugs:

- β-2 sympathomimetic (albuterol)
- Phosphodiesterase inhibitors (i.e. theophylline and caffeine)
- Exogenous insulin
- Calcium-channel blockers
- Antipsychotic drugs – risperidone, quetiapine (rarely)

Elevated extracellular pH:
- Respiratory and metabolic alkalosis
- Hypokalemic periodic paralysis

Decreased intake:
- Inadequate dietary intake is an unusual cause of hypokalemia, given a patient would need to consume less than 1 gram (25 mmol) per day.

Miscellaneous:
- Hypomagnesemia
- Genetic syndromes – Liddle's, Bartter, Gitelman's syndromes
- Amphotericin B.

Clinical features
- Often asymptomatic with mild hypokalemia (serum potassium of 3.0–3.5 mmol/L)
- Generalized weakness/ascending paralysis can occur with serum potassium of <2.5 mmol/L
- Impairment of respiratory function can occur with serum potassium <2.0 mmol/L
- In patients with cardiac ischemia, heart failure or left ventricular hypertrophy, even mild-to-moderate hypokalemia increases the likelihood of cardiac arrhythmias
- Rhabdomyolysis/muscle tenderness
- Chronic hypokalemia has been observed to cause hypertension and chronic kidney disease.

Diagnosis
- ECG – U-waves, T-wave flattening or ST segment changes.
- Check urine potassium secretion (either 24 hour urine collection or spot urine potassium/creatinine ratio); 24 hour urine potassium >30 mmol/day or spot urine potassium/creatinine ratio of >13 represents inappropriate renal losses.
- Assessment of acid–base status, e.g. for distal and proximal renal tubular acidosis or metabolic alkalosis.
- Measurement of the renin, aldosterone and cortisol concentrations under appropriate conditions like hypertension, metabolic alkalosis to rule out hyperaldosteronism and mineralocorticoid excess.
- Diuretic and/or laxative abuse often mimics these rare syndromes ruled out by urinary test for diuretics panel and stool test for phenolphthalein.

Treatment
- Potassium replacement can be given orally or IV, depending upon severity of hypokalemia; IV is usually reserved for severe hypokalemia (<2.7 mmol/L). The rate of IV replacement should not exceed 20 mmol/h and cardiac rhythm should be monitored. Oral preparations; KCl, K phosphate, K bicarbonate.
- Care should be taken to avoid too rapid administration or overcorrection.

- Treat underlying hypomagnesemia if present.
- There is no simple formula for calculating the amount needed in patients in whom potassium loss is continuing. Typically, 40 to 100 mmol of supplemental potassium chloride is needed each day to maintain serum potassium concentrations near or within the normal range in patients receiving diuretics.
- A good rule of thumb is 10 mEq of potassium will raise the serum potassium by 0.1 mmol/L for potassium >3 mmol/L. For potassium <3 mmol/L, total body deficit may be large.
- In resistant hypokalemia, potassium-sparing diuretic therapy may be a viable option, depending on the clinical circumstance.

Hyperkalemia
Overview
- Hyperkalemia is the most common potentially life-threatening electrolyte disorder. Renal excretion is extremely efficient, and large amounts of potassium can be eliminated within a few hours.
- Toxic effects are mainly due to skeletal and cardiac muscle depolarization. Neuromuscular effects of hyperkalemia are influenced by many other factors, including sodium and calcium. Any cause of decreased delivery of sodium to the distal tubule will impair potassium excretion and result in elevated plasma levels. Lysis of cells and transcellular shift in the setting of acidemia will increase serum potassium.

Causes
- Acute or chronic renal insufficiency
- Drugs: angiotensin-converting enzyme inhibitors (ACEI) or angiotensin receptor blockers (ARB), trimethoprim, spironolactone, succinylcholine, digitalis toxicity, heparin, penicillin G, β-blockers.
- Tumor lysis syndrome
- Pseudohyperkalemia (mechanical trauma during venipuncture, repeated fist clenching during blood draw can lead to efflux of potassium out of muscle cells)
- Metabolic acidosis
- Rhabdomyolysis
- Pseudohypoaldosteronism type 1 and type 2 (Gordon's syndrome)
- Insulin deficiency, hyperglycemia
- High-volume blood transfusions
- Iatrogenic – by excessive administration of oral or IV potassium.

Clinical features
- Muscle weakness, flaccid paralysis, ascending paralysis especially with serum potassium levels >7 mEq/L
- Electrocardiograms typically pick up potassium toxicity prior to onset of symptoms

- Cardiac toxicity is dependent on both the absolute serum potassium level and the rate of rise in the level
- Arrhythmias and heart blocks
- Bradycardia (rare) – poorly responsive to atropine or cardiac pacing
- Ventricular tachycardia (more common with hypokalemia)
- Ventricular fibrillation (poorly responsive to cardioversion when potassium remains elevated)
- Asystole
- Pulseless electrical activity.

Diagnosis

- Suspected from the clinical context and confirmed in the laboratory
- Pseudohyperkalemia should be ruled out in anyone without any clinical suggestion of hyperkalemia
- Physical findings are usually absent or nonspecific, although hyperactive reflexes and, in rare cases, flaccid paralysis may occur. Cardiac toxicity is the most dangerous feature of hyperkalemia. Clinically, the most prominent manifestations are found on the electrocardiogram
- ECG findings chronologically in descending order of frequency: peaked T-waves, prolonged PR interval, loss of P-wave, widened QRS, merging of QRS and T-wave to form a sine wave pattern
- Check renal function, CK levels, electrolytes, ABG for metabolic acidosis, renin/ aldosterone if underlying endocrinopathy is suspected.

Treatment

Stabilize cardiac membrane

- Calcium salts – decrease cardiac membrane excitability. Intended for life-threatening ECG changes, but also used when peaked T-waves are seen. Effective within minutes of administration, but action is limited to 30–60 min.
- Given as IV calcium gluconate 1000 mg or calcium chloride 500–1000 mg over few minutes with cardiac monitoring. Dose can be repeated in 5 min if ECG changes persist.

Potassium shift into cells

- Insulin therapy: causes influx of potassium by stimulating the activity of the Na-K-ATPase pump in skeletal muscle
- Regular insulin 10 units administered IV (reduces potassium 0.65–1 mmol/L). Dextrose 50 g IV is coadministered with insulin to prevent hypoglycemia (should not be given without insulin as may worsen hyperkalemia via solvent drag)
- β-agonist therapy: activate Na-K ATPase pumps through β-2 receptor stimulation in a manner that is additive to the effect of insulin. Albuterol can be given as 10 to 20 mg in 4 mL of saline by nebulization over 10 minutes or as 0.5 mg by intravenous infusion. Side effects include tachycardia and potentiation of angina symptoms

- Sodium bicarbonate: can shift potassium from the extracellular to the intracellular space by increasing blood pH. Only beneficial with concomitant metabolic acidosis. Usually given as isotonic solution with 150 mEq of sodium bicarbonate in one liter of D5W over 2–4 hours.

Removal of potassium

- Hemodialysis (HD): employed for refractory hyperkalemia. Most effective and reliable way to remove potassium from the body via diffusion over a transmembrane gradient. HD can remove up to 25–40 mmol per hour. On average 1 mmol/L can be removed in the first hour and 1 mmol/L over the next 2 hours, since the concentration gradient declines with treatment.
- Cation exchange resins work by exchanging calcium or sodium for potassium. Available as sodium polystyrene sulfonate, which can be given orally (15–30 g, 3–4 times/day). When a more rapid effect is desired, the resin can be given as a retention enema; 50 g of resin is suspended in a mixture of 50 mL. Side effects – intestinal necrosis in patients with ileus or obstruction.
- Diuretics: loop/thiazide diuretics are theoretically effective, but efficacy is not proven. Should be used with caution to avoid volume depletion.

Disorders of calcium [14–17]
Overview
- Total body calcium is 1000 g to 1300g – extracellular space contains only 0.1%, the rest is localized in bone. Only 50% is ionized (active), 40% bound to albumin and 10% bound to anions.
- Total calcium reflects levels of free calcium if plasma levels of protein, pH and anions are normal. Adjusted calcium for hypoalbuminemia = measured Ca (mg/dL) + (0.8 × [4 – albumin (gm/dL)]). Acidemia decreases Ca binding to protein, increasing ionized calcium as a fraction of total calcium. Each 0.1 unit decrease in pH increases ionized Ca by 0.05 mmol/L. Each 0.1 increase in pH decreases ionized Ca by 0.14 mg/dL. Therefore, ionized Ca measurement is recommended in the ICU, especially during renal replacement therapy.
- Ionized calcium <0.8 mmol/L or >1.4 mmol/L is independently associated with intensive care unit and hospital mortality.

Hypocalcemia
Definition
Ca concentration <2.1 mmol/L or ionized Ca <1.16 mmol/L. Frequent in hospitalized patients, affecting up to 88% in the ICU – associated with severity of illness not a specific illness per se.

Pathophysiology in the critically ill
- Precipitation into tissues
- Complex formation with lactate-containing fluids and citrate from blood products or anticoagulation during renal replacement therapy

- Decreased renal suppression of the parathyroid gland by hypo- or hypermagnesemia
- Resuscitation-induced hemodilution in trauma patients
- Spurious hypocalcemia with use of gadolinium during MRI as it interferes with colorimetric-based calcium assays, but ionized calcium assays remain unaffected.

Causes

- Vitamin D deficiency
- Hypoparathyroidism
- Pseudohypoparathyroidism
- Tissue consumption of calcium (pancreatitis, hungry bone syndrome, rhabdomyolysis, tumor lysis)
- Drugs (foscarnet, biphosphonates).

Clinical manifestations

- Difficult to assess if on sedatives or neuromuscular blockade
- Neuromuscular irritability: perioral numbness, tetany, bronchial spasm, Trousseau's and Chvostek's signs
- Trousseau's sign: carpopedal spasm induced by inflation of a blood pressure cuff to 20 mmHg above systolic blood pressure for 3 minutes
- Chvostek's sign: tapping the facial nerve anterior to earlobe, positive if twitching of the lip. It is neither sensitive nor specific
- Psychiatric manifestations
- Papilledema
- Cardiovascular: congestive heart failure and QTc prolongation.

Management

- IV calcium if symptomatic or Ca concentration of <1.75 mmol/L or ionized Ca <0.8 mmol/L: 1 to 2 g followed by 0.3 to 1.0 mg/kg/h of elemental calcium
- PO calcium if asymptomatic, up to 2000 mg daily
- Hypomagnesemia and hyperphosphatemia should be corrected concomitantly
- Phosphate and bicarbonate should not be infused with Ca (precipitation)
- Calcium gluconate 10% (10 mL vial) contains 93 mg of elemental calcium
- Calcium chloride 10% (10 mL vial) contains 270 mg of elemental calcium (painful, vein sclerosing)
- Calcium carbonate 1250 mg contains 500 mg of elemental calcium.

Hypercalcemia
Definition

Mild (2.6–2.9 mmol/L)
Moderate (3.0–3.4 mmol/L)
Severe ($\geq$ 3.5 mmol/L)

Causes

- Endocrine: hyperparathyroidism (most common in ambulatory setting), familial hypocalciuric hypercalcemia (FHHC), hyper- and hypothyroidism, adrenal insufficiency, pheochromocytoma, VIPoma.
- Malignancy (most common in inpatient setting): bone metastasis, parathormone (PTH), PTHrp (parathyroid-related peptide), calcitriol or 1-25(OH)2D (the hormonally active form of vitamin D)
- Granulomatous disease: sarcoidosis, tuberculosis (TB), fungal
- Exogenous agents: milk alkali, lithium, thiazides
- Miscellaneous: immobilization, post-renal failure with rhabdomyolysis, disseminated CMV.

Clinical manifestations

- Symptoms are related more to rate of rise of serum calcium and volume depletion than absolute serum calcium
- Gastrointestinal: nausea, vomiting, constipation, pain
- Neuromuscular: change in mental status, lethargy, weakness
- Renal: polyuria and volume depletion
- Cardiovascular: hypertension, short QT interval, can trigger digitalis toxicity.

Diagnosis (investigations)

- If PTH high: hyperparathyroidism or FHHC
- If PTH low: check PTHrp, 25(OH)2 vitamin D and 1-25(OH)2 vitamin D.

Further workup/diagnostic features are listed below:

Diagnosis	PTH	Ca	P	25-OHD3	1-25-(OH)2D3
pHPT	H	H	L/N	N	H
FHHC	N/H	N (H)	N (L)	N	N (L)
Thyrotoxicosis	L	L	N/L	N	N/L
PTHrp	L (H)	L	L/N	N	L
Lymphoma and Hodgkin's	L	L	N/H	N	H
Metastatic bone disease	L	L	N/H	N	L
Immobilization	L	L	N/L	N	L
Post-acute renal failure with rhabdomyolysis	L	N/L	N/H	L	H
Granulomatous disease	L	L	N/L	N	HH
Milk alkali syndrome	L	L	N/L		
Vitamin D intoxication	L	L	N/H	HH	N/L/H

pHPT = primary hyperparathyroidism. H, high; L, low; N, normal.

Treatment

Treatment options are outlined below:

Intervention	Dosage	Indication
Intravenous saline	200–500 mL/h	Universal
Furosemide	20–40 mg IV	Fluid overload only, not to be used routinely
Oral phosphorus	Neutraphos 250 mg PO QID	If hypophosphatemia
Pamidronate	60–90 mg IV over 2 h	Universal (in preference in HHM)
Alternative to pamidronate is zoledronate	4 mg IV over 15 min	Universal (in preference in HHM)
Glucocorticoids	Prednisone 60 mg PO	Vitamin D intoxication, sarcoidosis (rarely HHM)
Mithramycin	25 µg/kg over 4–6 h	In preference in HHM, parathyroid carcinoma
Calcitonin	4–8 IU/kg SQ or IM q 12 h	Universal (adjuvant drug)
Gallium nitrate	100–200 mg/m^2 of BSA IV over 24-h period for 5 days	In preference in HHM
Hemodialysis	Ca2$^+$ -free dialysate. Use with extreme caution as death has been reported. Reduced calcium in dialysate is preferable	Hypercalcemic crisis and renal insufficiency

HHM = humoral hypercalcemia of malignancy.

Disorders of magnesium [18–19]

Overview

- Average-sized adult: total body magnesium (Mg) 21–25 g (15 mmol/kg) i.e. 1750–2000 mEq or 875–1000 mmol
- 67% in bone, 31% intracellular and 1–2% extracellular
- Plasma distribution: 70% free and filtered by kidneys, the rest mostly bound to albumin (not filtered)
- Normal range: 1.7–2.3 mg/dL or 0.71–0.96 mmol/L (1 mmol/L = 2.4 mg/dL = 2 mEq/L)
- Average US dietary intake per person: 300 mg/day (30–40% absorbed in jejunum and ileum, the rest excreted in stool; reabsorbed up to 80% if severe Mg deficiency)
- Dietary sources: green vegetables, meat, fish and milk/milk products.

Pathophysiology

- Unlike other electrolytes, Mg is at least 50% reabsorbed by cortical thick ascending loop of Henle (TAL) – mainly passive transport via potential difference created by sodium-potassium-two chloride (Na-K-2Cl) channel
- 40% or less reabsorbed by proximal convoluted tubule (PCT)
- 10% or less reabsorbed by distal convoluted tubule (DCT) and collecting duct
- Roughly 3500 mg/d is filtered and almost all (99%) is reabsorbed while rest is excreted in urine. During magnesium deficiency, kidneys will reduce excretion to <10 mg/d to conserve Mg but this may take up to 3–5 days to occur physiologically.

Factors affecting renal reabsorption of Mg:

- PCT: proportional to sodium transport, which is influenced by extracellular volume (ECV) status
- TAL: ECV status by influencing luminal flow rate; plasma Mg concentration (increased plasma concentration, decreases reabsorption); hyperparathyroidism (increases reabsorption); hypercalcemia (decreases reabsorption); metabolic acidosis, hyperthyroidism, alcohol (decreases reabsorption).

Hypomagnesemia
Definition
Less than 1.7 mg/dL or 0.71 mmol/L (corrected for hypoalbuminemia).

Causes
Impaired intestinal absorption
- Starvation/decreased dietary intake/inadequate Mg in TPN (most common scenario is in ICU patients with dietary limitation and use of loop diuretics)
- Malabsorption/steatorrhea/diarrhea
- Surgical bowel resection
- Alcohol from decreased dietary Mg and also direct tubular dysfunction leading to increased excretion.

Increased renal excretion
- ECV expansion
- Osmotic diuretics (hyperglycemia in uncontrolled DM, ketoacidosis-DKA)
- Loop diuretics by inhibiting Na-K-2Cl channel
- Drugs (cisplatin, aminoglycoside, cyclosporine, amphotericin B, tacrolimus, pentamidine, cetuximab, foscarnet, proton-pump inhibitors)
- Post-obstructive diuresis or diuretic phase of ATN
- Congenital (Bartter syndrome).

Miscellaneous
- Hungry bone syndrome
- Acute pancreatitis
- Hypercalcemia

- Chronic metabolic acidosis
- Citrate-rich fluid replacement post-liver transplant.

Clinical features

- Hypomagnesemia leads to hypocalcemia (decreased PTH release and action) and hypokalemia (increased renin/aldosterone and tubular secretion)
- Symptoms include apathy, nausea, seizures, Chvostek's and Trousseau's sign; arrhythmias (QRS widening, QT prolongation, torsades, VF, increased risk of digoxin toxicity); hyper-reflexia (deep tendon reflexes), tetany.

Diagnosis

- Fractional excretion of

$$Mg = \frac{(U\ mg \times plasma\ Cr)}{UCr \times (Plasma\ Mg \times 0.7)} \times 100\%$$

- >2% or 24-hour urine Mg >10–30 mg means inappropriate renal magnesium wasting; less than these numbers indicate kidney is appropriately conserving magnesium in the setting of hypomagnesemia.

Treatment

Severe magnesium deficiency i.e. Mg 0.5 mmol/L

- 1–1.5 mEq/kg IV in first 24 hours at divided doses and close monitoring of plasma level
- Then, 0.5–1 mEq/kg IV daily until level normalizes. (Monitor for hypotension, deep tendon reflexes, facial flushing or feeling of warmth while giving IV Mg)
- Magnesium sulfate is commonly used to supplement magnesium intravenously. It is available as 10%, 25% and 50% solutions (commonly used is 50%); 1 g of 50% magnesium sulfate gives 8 mEq elemental magnesium; 1–2 g can be given within 5–10 min in emergent situation.

Less severe magnesium deficiency

- Oral supplements with 30–60 mEq/d in 3–4 divided doses. Magnesium oxide 400 mg tablet contains 20 mEq elemental Mg while magnesium chloride 535 mg tablet (long acting) contains 5.3 mEq of elemental Mg (diarrhea less compared to magnesium oxide)
- Amiloride or potassium-sparing diuretics for hypomagnesemia caused by loop diuretics or other drugs listed above under cause section.

Note: reduce the magnesium supplements to 50% if GFR <30 mL/min and monitor level closely. Replace magnesium before Ca or K supplements in order for body to retain supplemented K or Ca.

Hypermagnesemia

Definition

Mg >2.3 mg/dL or 0.96 mmol/L.

Causes

Increased magnesium load

- IV Mg, e.g. treatment of preeclampsia or eclampsia
- Oral agents, e.g. elemental preparations/antacids/laxatives and enemas/Epsom salts.

Renal insufficiency

- Usually when GFR falls <30 mL/min
- Usually after an increased Mg load the level normalizes within 8 hours if normal renal function present.

Clinical features

- When Mg levels between 4–5 mg/dL or 1.6–2 mmol/L: lethargy, confusion, nausea, mild hypotension; decreased deep tendon reflexes; increased PR, QRS complex and QT interval
- Mg >10 mg/dL: respiratory depression, coma, bradycardia and heart block; hypotension – moderate to severe; muscle weakness; cardiac arrest when >15–20 mg/dL.

Treatment

- Asymptomatic/mild: observation – no treatment
- Symptomatic or level >10 mg/dL:
    - Emergent – IV calcium gluconate (elemental calcium 15 mg/kg over 4 hours)
    - Less urgent – ECV expansion and loop diuretics (if normal renal function, otherwise hemodialysis).

Disorders of phosphorus [20–23]

Overview

- Incidence of hypophosphatemia varies between 0.2% and 2.2% for all admitted patients, but has been reported as high as 21.5% or even higher in selected patient series.
- Intensive care unit (ICU) patients are at increased risk of hypophosphatemia due to the presence of multiple causal factors including volume expansion, diuretics, metabolic acidosis, respiratory alkalosis, refeeding syndrome and others.
- It mainly occurs within the first 3 days of admission, in particular in patients with preserved renal function.

Pathophysiology

- Phosphorus is an essential mineral that is usually found in nature combined with oxygen as phosphate. In a healthy 70-kg adult, the total body phosphorus content is around 700 g (23 000 mmol); 80% is present in the skeleton as crystalline hydroxyapatite, 9% in the skeletal muscle, 10.9% in the viscera and 0.1% in the extracellular fluid.

- The total plasma concentration of phosphorus is 3.9 mmol/L. This plasma concentration is determined by the dietary intake, intestinal absorption, renal tubular reabsorption and shifts between the intracellular and extracellular spaces.
- The average diet provides 800–1500 mg (20–40 mmol) of phosphorus daily; 70% of the phosphate is absorbed in the gut, mainly in the duodenum and jejunum, stimulated through 1,25-dihydroxyvitamin D3 and with passive diffusion of phosphate ions.
- Under steady-state conditions, the kidney is the most important regulator of the serum phosphate level, ensuring that urinary phosphate output is equivalent to the net phosphate absorption from the intestine.
- Phosphate acts as a buffer for the maintenance of plasma and urinary pH 1–5.
- Phosphate is a component of 2,3-diphosphoglycerate in the supply of oxygen to the tissue and it is the source of adenosine triphosphates, the body's main reservoir of energy for several physiological processes. Thus, hypophosphatemia can lead to tissue hypoxia and disruption of cellular function.

Hypophosphatemia
Definition
Serum phosphate level <2.5 mg/dL (0.8 mmol/L).

Causes
- Decreased intestinal absorption
    . Severe dietary phosphate restriction
    . Phosphate binding antacids
    . Vitamin D deficiency/resistance
    . Secretory diarrhea
    . Steatorrhea
    . Vomiting.
- Internal redistribution (most frequent)
    . Recovery from malnutrition
    . Recovery from diabetic ketoacidosis
    . Respiratory alkalosis (e.g. sepsis, anxiety, mechanical ventilation, heat stroke, salicylate overdose, hepatic coma, gout, alcohol withdrawal)
    . Hormonal and other agents (e.g. insulin, glucagon, epinephrine, dopamine, β-2 agonists, steroids, xanthine derivatives)
    . Rapid cell proliferation/uptake (e.g. hungry bone syndrome, acute leukemia, Burkitt's lymphoma).
- Increased urinary excretion
    . Hyperparathyroidism
    . Disorders of vitamin D metabolism (e.g. vitamin D deficiency, X-linked hypophosphatemic rickets).
    . Renal tubular defects (e.g. Fanconi syndrome, chronic alcoholism)
    . Diuretics

- . Metabolic acidosis
- . Glucocorticoid/mineralocorticoid therapy.
- Volume expansion
- Parathyroid hormone-related protein
- Kidney transplantation
- Extracorporeal loss with continuous renal replacement therapy.

Clinical manifestations

Appear when the serum phosphate level is <2 mg/dL.

- Musculoskeletal – weakness, myalgias, rhabdomyolysis, osteopenia, osteomalacia
- Cardiovascular – congestive heart failure, arrhythmias
- Pulmonary – respiratory failure, failure of weaning from ventilator
- Neurologic – coma, seizures, encephalopathy, parasthesias
- Hematologic – hemolysis, leukocyte dysfunction, platelet dysfunction.

Treatment

- An important side effect of oral phosphate supplementation is diarrhea. For patients with overt symptoms and for those who cannot take milk or tablets, intravenous infusion of phosphate can be administered.
- There are weight-based regimens, giving 0.08 mmol/kg (2.5 mg/kg) or 0.16 mmol/kg (5 mg/kg) over 6 hours, depending on the severity of the expected phosphate deficit.
- Close monitoring of serum phosphate level and other ions is crucial.
- The faster replacement therapy takes place, the more likely that side effects will occur.
- Side effects of intravenous phosphate repletion are hypocalcemia, metastatic calcification, hyperkalemia associated with potassium-containing supplements, volume excess, hypernatremia, metabolic acidosis and hyperphosphatemia.

Hyperphosphatemia
Definition

Serum phosphorus >4.5 mg/dL (1.45 mmol/L).

Causes

- Tumor lysis syndrome
- Rhabdomyolysis
- Exogenous phosphate load (after the ingestion of sodium-phosphate laxatives and as bowel preparation for colonoscopy)
- Acute or chronic kidney disease
- Increased tubular reabsorption of phosphate
- Vitamin D toxicity
- Bisphosphonates
- Hypoparathyroidism
- Acromegaly
- Familial tumoral calcinosis.

Clinical features

- Severe hyperphosphatemia can cause life-threatening hypocalcemia
- Hyperparathyroidism in chronic kidney disease patients
- Acute kidney injury secondary to acute phosphate nephropathy.

Treatment

- Phosphate restriction and phosphate binders (sevelamer, Ca carbonate, Ca acetate)
- Hemodialysis/hemofiltration for resistant hyperphosphatemia.

References

1. Gabow PA. Disorders associated with an altered anion gap acidosis. *Kidney Int* 1985; 27 : 472–83.

2. Galla JH, Luke RG. Pathophysiology of metabolic alkalosis. *Hosp Pract (Off Ed)* 1987; 22 : 123–30, 139–41, 145–6.

3. Webster NR, Kulkarni V. Metabolic alkalosis in the critically ill. *Crit Rev Clin Lab Sci* 1999; 36 : 497–510.

4. Pahari DK, Kazmi W, Raman G, Biswas S. Diagnosis and management of metabolic alkalosis. *J Indian Med Assoc* 2006; 104 : 630–4, 636.

5. Schrier RW. Decreased effective blood volume in edematous disorders: what does this mean ? *J Am Soc Nephrol* 2007; 18 : 2028–31.

6. Schrier RW, Bansal S. Diagnosis and management of hyponatremia in acute illness. *Curr Opin Crit Care* 2008; 14 : 627–34.

7. Adrogue HJ, Madias NE. Hyponatremia. *N Eng J Med* 2000; 342 : 1581–89.

8. Adrogue HJ, Madias NE. Hypernatremia *N Engl J Med* 2000; 342 : 1493.

9. Palevsky PM, Bhagrath R, Greenberg A. Hypernatremia in hospitalized patients. *Ann Intern Med* 1996; 124 : 197–203.

10. Gennari FJ. Hypokalemia. *N Engl J Med* 1998; 339 : 451–8.

11. Levinsky. Management of Emergencies: Hyperkalemia. *N Engl J Med* 1966; 274 : 1076–7.

12. Fisch C. Relation of electrolyte disturbances to cardiac arrhythmia. *Circulation* 1973; 47 : 408–19.

13. Sedlacek M, Schoolwerth AC, Remillard BD. Electrolyte Disturbances in the Intensive Care Unit. *Semin Dial* 2006; 19 : 496–501.

14. Zivin JR, Gooley T, Zager RA, Ryan MJ. Hypocalcemia: a pervasive metabolic abnormality in the critically ill. *Am J Kidney Dis* 2001; 37 : 689–98.

15. McCurdy MT, Shanholtz CB. Oncologic emergencies. *Crit Care Med* 2012; 40 : 2212–22.

16. R. Ziegler. Hypercalcemic crisis. *J Am Soc Nephrol* 2001; 12 : S3–9.

17. Egi M, Kim I, Nichol A, *et al.* Ionized calcium concentration and outcome in critical illness. *Crit Care Med* 2011; 39 : 314–21.

18. Assadi F. Hypomagnesemia: an evidence-based approach to clinical cases. *Iran J Kidney Dis* 2010; 4 : 13–9.

19. Sedlacek M, Schoolwerth AC, Remillard BD. Critical care issues for the nephrologist: electrolyte disturbances in the intensive care unit. *Seminars in dialysis* 2006; 19 : 496–501.

20. Stoff JS. Phosphate homeostasis and hypophosphatemia. *Am J Med* 1982;72 : 489–95.

21. Marik PE, Bedigian MK. Refeeding hypophosphatemia in critically ill patients in an intensive care unit: a prospective study. *Arch Surg* 1996; 131 : 1043–7.

22. Arrambide K, Toto RD. Tumor lysis syndrome. *Semin Nephrol* 1993; 13 : 273.

23. Fournier A, Morinière P, Ben Hamida F *et al.* Use of alkaline calcium salts as phosphate binder in uremic patients. *Kidney Int Suppl* 1992; 38 : S50.

Chapter 2

Principles of IPPV and care of the ventilated patient

Mohit Bhutani and Ian McConachie

Mechanical ventilation, especially intermittent positive-pressure ventilation (IPPV) is the mainstay of modern intensive care practice and of fundamental importance to intensive care unit (ICU) therapy.

Care of the ventilated patient
General issues

- Airway. Access via cuffed tracheal tube or tracheostomy. Secure the tube. Do not overinflate the tracheal cuff. Cuff pressure should be regularly measured, even in tubes with a high-volume/low-pressure cuff. Tracheostomy site should be maintained.
- Maintain appropriate emergency airway and other equipment and drugs – either at the bedside or within easy reach.
- Change circuits, tubing etc. according to local infection control guidelines.
- Provide adequate humidification and clearance of secretions. The absence of humidification will encourage heat loss and dehydration of the upper respiratory tract. This can cause upper airway epithelial damage, and difficulties with clearance of dry secretions. Conversely, excess heat and/or humidification can cause problems.
- Routine nursing care, including care of the unconscious patient.
- Appropriate mouth care and hygiene.
- Monitor appropriately. In view of the unpredictable and complex effects of IPPV on the cardiopulmonary system, be prepared to monitor the central vascular pressures and cardiac output (CO). An arterial line is mandatory to facilitate blood gas sampling for all but the shortest periods of ventilation.
- Nasogastric (NG tube) or feeding tube to relieve gastric distension and permit administration of medications and nutrition.
- Ensure patient comfort as far as possible – see chapter on sedation and analgesia.
- Ensure adequate nutrition and hydration – see chapter on nutritional support.

Specific issues
Deep-vein thrombosis prophylaxis

Deep-vein thrombosis (DVT) prophylaxis is a requirement among patients requiring mechanical ventilation in the ICU setting. Pharmacological prophylaxis is most common,

Handbook of ICU Therapy, third edition, ed. John Fuller, Jeff Granton and Ian McConachie. Published by Cambridge University Press. © Cambridge University Press 2015.

but mechanical devices may also be effective and preferred where the risk of bleeding is high. Low-molecular-weight heparins (LMWH) are thought to be associated with less bleeding (and less heparin-induced thrombocytopenia) than standard unfractionated heparin (UH); however, trials comparing these two agents have not reliably shown this [1].

Updated guidelines for DVT prophylaxis in critically ill patients have recently been published [1]. Current recommendations include the following:

- No need for routine ultrasound screening for DVT in critically ill patients.
- Recommendation for the use of LMWH or UH for the prevention of DVT.
- If the patient is actively bleeding or at increased risk for bleeding, the use of intermittent pneumatic compression devices or graduated compression stockings is recommended until the bleeding risk is reduced. Thereafter, when clinically safe to do so, LMWH or UH is preferred.

Pressure area care

The reported incidence of pressure ulcers (PU) in the ICU ranges from 1–64% [2]. This wide range is due to variability in both the patient populations studied and definitions used in these studies. There are several risk factors for the development of PUs in the ICU [2,3]:

- Perfusion and oxygenation problems
- High acute physiology and chronic health evaluation II (APACHE II) score
- Skin maceration due to incontinence or poor wound healing
- Anemia
- Increased length of stay.

The usefulness of the commonly used Waterlow pressure sore risk (PSR) scale in the ICU has been established [3]. In that study, when a patient had a PSR score >25 on admission, the risk of developing a pressure sore was significantly increased.

Eye care

Eye problems, especially microbial keratitis, can have devastating effects on vision in survivors from ICU. The incidence and prevalence is unknown. Pseudomonas is commonly the reported infecting organism.

- In a small study [4], 60% of ventilated patients receiving sedation for more than 48 h had developed corneal erosion when assessed using the ocular slit lamp, especially in those patients who were unable to close their eyes. Protective eyelid taping was effective in preventing and treating the corneal erosion.

The use of an algorithm has been proposed [5] to reduce the incidence of these problems:

- Lids closed: no specific treatment
- Conjunctiva exposed: use of 4-hourly lubricants
- Cornea exposed: use of tape over eyes + 4-hourly lubricants
- Prone position: use of tape over eyes + 4-hourly lubricants.

One must not forget to administer chronic eye medications to ventilated patients, especially medication for glaucoma. It is important to be aware that other medications may affect intraocular pressures.

- For example, the use of dopamine is associated with increased intraocular pressures in critically ill patients [6]. This may not be a problem in normal patients, but may represent a significant risk in patients with glaucoma.

Daily assessment and management planning

The ventilated patient should receive a full clinical examination each day with special focus on the cardiopulmonary system. In addition, a suggested structured program for assessment and management planning is presented in Table 12.1.

Table 12.1 Daily management plan/checklist.

Is the diagnosis accurate?
If not, what investigations are necessary?

Are the treatments correct?
 Right dose?
 Right duration?
 Adjustment for renal or hepatic dysfunction?
 Secure from allergy or toxicity?

Consider the supportive therapy:
 Is there a need for inotropic or vasopressor support? If so, are they on appropriate dose of drug?
 Stress ulcer prophylaxis?
 DVT prophylaxis?

Consider the hemodynamics:
 Adequate organ perfusion?
 Adequate filling?
 Appropriate hematocrit?
 Adequate monitoring?
 Signs of myocardial or other ischemia?

Consider the ventilation:
 What is the FiO_2?
 Is the tidal volume (TV) appropriate for patient support and lung protection?
 Is the positive end-expiratory pressure (PEEP) adequate?
 Are recruitment maneuvers necessary?
 Appropriate mode?
 Can they wean? If not, why not?

Consider the lungs:
 Are secretions present? Changing?
 Does the airway resistance or lung compliance need to be measured?
 Appropriate humidification?
 Are they head up?

Can they be mobilized to a chair? If not, why not?

Is sedation appropriate? What is depth? Is it stopped daily?

Are you communicating appropriately with the patient, even if sedated?
Do relatives need information or counselling?

Are nursing issues addressed, such as pressure area, eye care and oral care and given as appropriate?

Check parameters of liver and renal function. Is renal support required?

Is the gut working? Gut protection prescribed? Prokinetics? Enteral nutrition? Diarrhea or constipation?

Adequate caloric intake? Adequate nutrition?

What bacteriological evidence is there of need for antibiotics?
What specimens have been sent? When? Need repeating?
Is the white cell count rising/falling? Temperature?

Is there adequate vascular access? How old are the lines? Any evidence for line sepsis?
Is there need to change circuits, IV tubing etc?
Are tubes, lines etc. secure?

Have you checked for focal neurological signs?

Have specialist referrals been done?

The contributions of Dr D Kelly, Blackpool Victoria Hospital, Blackpool, UK to this plan/checklist are acknowledged.

Airway management

The choice is between oral tracheal tubes, nasal tracheal tubes and tracheostomy tubes. Each has its advantages, disadvantages and complications. Table 12.2 outlines the advantages and disadvantages of oral and nasal tracheal tubes.

General problems with any of these airway interventions include:

- Bypassing upper airway defenses against infection
- Loss of natural humidification of inspired gases
- Less effective cough
- Potential for long-term damage to airway
- Increased work of breathing due to increased airway resistance.

Overall, most would agree that oral tracheal tubes are preferred to nasal tracheal tubes for most situations in the adult ICU and that nasal tubes in modern ICUs are of largely historical interest only.

The role of chest X-rays

All new admissions to ICU will need a chest X-ray (CXR), even if only as a baseline. In the past it was considered important to perform daily CXRs on ventilated patients. This practice has been questioned, both as to its usefulness in clinical decision-making and its impact on ICU outcomes:

- Studies show us that clinical examination can effectively predict the need for radiography [7].
- Studies examining the value of routine daily CXR found that this practice was not associated with a reduction in ICU or hospital length of stay or mortality [8]. Further, a meta-analysis of clinical trials examining the use of selective imaging in the ICU supports these conclusions [9].

Thus CXRs should be performed largely on the basis of clinical change in the patient's condition. In particular, regular CXRs performed on patients who are rapidly improving seems pointless.

Table 12.2 Oral and nasal tracheal tubes

Oral tubes	
Advantages	Usually smooth nontraumatic insertion Easy suction of secretions Familiarity
Disadvantages	Patient discomfort/sedation requirements Obstruction by bite Problems with oral hygiene and mouth care Tracheal damage if cuff overinflated (reduced by low-pressure cuffs) Occasionally difficult to secure (e.g. patients with beards) Dental trauma on insertion Molding at body temperature and movement within the oropharynx
Nasal tubes	
Advantages	Better comfort (i.e. less sedation requirements) Easy fixation Less oropharyngeal movement
Disadvantages	Sinusitis as occult source of sepsis False passages created during insertion Bacteremia on insertion Nasal erosions Epistaxis on insertion Difficult for suction Tracheal damage, as for above Longer than oral tubes, slightly increased work of breathing

Exceptions to the above include CXRs following central-line insertion or following intubation; that is, those circumstances where clinical assessment of placement position may be unreliable. In addition, many would still argue for occasional "screening" CXRs to be performed in long-stay ventilated patients, but this is not a validated practice.

Principles of ventilatory support

- IPPV should only be used where there is a reasonable chance of survival.
- It should not be used as the last therapeutic act in a dying patient, purely because it is available. Patients who are clearly dying should be allowed to do so without a period of inappropriate therapy on a ventilator.

The prime indication for IPPV outside of the operating theatre is respiratory failure, but modern ICU practice recognizes the value of early ventilation as part of organ support in other critically ill patients, especially in the presence of shock or cardiac failure.

Indications

Indications for IPPV include:

- Post-operative management: for patients that are unable to be safely extubated following the surgical procedure, either due to an underlying condition, the nature of the surgery or complications of the surgery. Examples include patients with morbid obesity, post-operative hypothermia, pre-existing lung disease, cardiac surgery and gross abdominal distension.

- Diseases causing airway obstruction:

  Central: tumor, laryngeal edema, tracheal stenosis
  Peripheral: status asthmaticus, acute exacerbation of COPD (AECOPD)

- Diseases causing hypoventilation:

  Central: stroke, intracerebral hemorrhage, drug overdose
  Peripheral: neuromuscular weakness (e.g. amyotrophic lateral sclerosis, Guillan–Barré syndrome)

- Chest wall disease (ex. kyphoscoliosis)
- Alveolar respiratory disease: pneumonia (ex. community or hospital acquired, aspiration), hemorrhage syndromes, alveolar proteinosis, acute respiratory distress syndrome (ARDS)
- Cardiovascular disease: cardiac arrest, severe shock of any etiology, congestive heart failure (CHF)
- Other: to provide organ support prior to organ donation, trauma, pneumothorax, pulmonary embolism
- The difficult decision is often not whether to ventilate a patient but more often *when* to ventilate a patient (apart from acute emergencies, e.g. cardiac arrest). This is difficult to be precise about and although clinical parameters exist to help guide in the decision, ultimately the decision to provide IPPV should take into account the entire clinical situation.

Some clinical parameters that may assist in the decision include:

- Level of consciousness, inability to clear secretions, trauma
- RR >35/min
- Vital capacity <10 mL/kg
- Maximal inspiratory pressure (MIP) less than –25 cm H_2O
- Rising $PaCO_2$ on arterial blood gas, despite interventions
- Refractory hypoxemia.

Often trends in physical and physiological variables are more useful than absolute values [10].

In acknowledging this, one must not forget that hypercarbia usually develops relatively slowly, whereas acute hypoxia can be lethal within minutes. It is better to intubate early rather than too late!

Contraindications to IPPV

There are no true contraindications to IPPV. However, the decision to withhold IPPV in patients with respiratory failure is a clinical decision that is routinely made. This decision can be difficult to make and requires the judgment of experienced practitioners.

- Ideally, the family and other healthcare professionals involved in caring for the patient should be part of the decision to provide or withhold IPPV.
- The patient's wishes should be paramount, but unfortunately when the situation arises, the patient is often unable to become rationally involved due to their illness.

- This highlights a need to establish the patient's desires for the level of supportive care on admission to hospital if possible. This would include referring to any advanced directives or living wills that the patient may have already completed, in addition to discussing the topic with the patient (or their designated legal advocate).

The development and widespread use of noninvasive positive-pressure ventilation (NIPPV), such as CPAP or bilevel ventilation, has greatly reduced the need for IPPV for many common conditions, such as COPD and CHF exacerbations. There are well-established indications and contraindications for NIPPV [11,12]:

- Indications: AECOPD, CHF, hypoxemic respiratory failure, post-extubation respiratory failure
- Contraindications: cardiac arrest, inability to protect the airway, decreased level of consciousness, patient at increased risk of aspiration, facial trauma/surgery, noncooperative patient.

A failed trial of noninvasive support does not necessarily mean that IPPV is inappropriate. However, just because a patient is considered suitable for a trial of noninvasive support does not automatically mandate invasive ventilation if it fails.

Physiological effects of IPPV
Cardiovascular effects
The two main physiological effects of IPPV are:

1. Lung volumes are increased, often significantly compared to spontaneous ventilation:
   - Large TVs cause a rise in pulmonary vascular resistance (PVR). This may lead to acute pulmonary hypertension and right ventricular (RV) compromise. This is due to the overinflated alveoli causing compression of the alveolar blood vessels. (Conversely, shallow breathing, e.g. during weaning, can also increase PVR, partly by collapsing alveoli, causing a fall in diameter of extra-alveolar pulmonary blood vessels and partly by development of hypoxic pulmonary vasoconstriction.)
   - Hyperinflation can occasionally "squeeze" the heart in the cardiac fossa causing falls in cardiac output (CO) analogous with cardiac tamponade. This is occasionally seen in status asthmaticus or severe AECOPD.
2. Intrathoracic pressure (ITP) is increased at all points in the respiratory cycle, compared to the "negative" pressures generated during spontaneous ventilation:
   - The heart operates as a "pressure chamber within a pressure chamber" (as described by Pinsky from Pittsburgh) and it is therefore not surprising that changes in ITP affect cardiac function.
   - Thus changes in ITP are transmitted to the cardiac chambers during ventilation.
   - Inspiration during IPPV increases ITP and therefore increases right atrial (RA) pressure relative to atmospheric pressure, leading to a decreased gradient for venous return, reduced RV filling and reduced RV stroke volume [13]. In addition, the increased ITP decreases the gradient across the left ventricle (LV), resulting in decreased LV afterload. The decreased venous return and LV afterload tends to reduce intrathoracic blood volume.

- Conversely, with decreased ITP, as occurs with spontaneous breathing during inspiration, the opposite is achieved; for example, decreased RA pressure, increased gradient for venous return, increased RV stroke volume, increased LV transmural pressure and increased LV afterload. The combined effect is to increase intrathoracic blood volume.
- The decreased venous return and therefore decreased CO with IPPV is the major hemodynamic effect of ventilation in most patients. As it relates to ITP, the decreased CO is worse if the ventilator is set to provide either a high TV (high-peak ITP) or a prolonged inspiratory time (high-mean ITP). PEEP also exacerbates the fall in venous return.
- Venous return and CO can be restored by either fluid infusion or sympathetic drugs, both of which restore the gradient for venous return, despite further increases in RA pressure.

Thus, increased ITP reduces venous return (pre-load), but also reduces afterload on the heart due to effects on transmural pressure.

- Which of these effects predominates depends on several factors, for example presence of hypovolemia and, most importantly, the state of the heart.
- Any beneficial effect on afterload in the normal heart is limited by the fall in venous return.
- In the failing heart the CO is relatively insensitive to changes in pre-load (flat part of the Starling curve), but exquisitely sensitive to small reductions in afterload. Thus, in heart failure, there may be beneficial effects on CO from increases in ITP with ventilation. In addition it will be crucial in the failing heart to avoid large falls in ITP, as may occur during labored spontaneous breathing, as this can dramatically increase both pre-load and afterload, producing pulmonary edema.

With high ITP, RV afterload usually increases due to increasing PVR and development of acute pulmonary hypertension. Thus, high thoracic pressures can reduce LV filling due to RV distension, pushing the septum to the left to reduce LV chamber size (known as interventricular independence). This effect of excessive high thoracic pressure can counteract the beneficial effects on LV afterload.

Thus the cardiovascular consequences of IPPV are complex and vary in differing disease states.

Respiratory effects

- IPPV causes a potential increase in ventilation and perfusion (V/Q) mismatch due to preferential ventilation of the nondependent, poorly perfused lung regions. Positive end-expiratory pressure in general will improve oxygenation by recruitment of poorly ventilated lung regions [14].
- In the supine position, functional residual capacity (FRC) will be reduced, due in part to upward displacement of the abdominal contents. This contributes to an increase in microatelectasis, and an increase in physiologic shunt. This can be mitigated by increasing mean airway pressure through the utilization of PEEP.
- Decreased pulmonary perfusion if CO falls with IPPV causes an increase in alveolar dead space.
- Surfactant secretion is also reduced by prolonged IPPV.

In addition, both respiratory muscle and diaphragmatic weakness can develop in patients receiving IPPV. The mechanism is presumed to be due to the more general complication of critical illness polyneuropathy, a well-described complication of the critically ill.

Other systemic consequences of IPPV

- GI: increased risk of stress ulcers, decreased splanchnic circulation [15]
- Renal: renal dysfunction [16]
- CNS: the inhibition of venous drainage from the head may also result in an increase in the intracranial pressure (ICP).

Beneficial effects

There is a considerable reduction in the work of breathing and improved gas exchange with the use of IPPV. This is achieved by:

- Improvement in alveolar expansion, particularly where there is lobar collapse, often secondary to progressive hypoventilation and exhaustion
- Recruitment of collapsed lung units, thereby reducing physiologic shunt
- Oxygenation usually, but not always, does increase
- Secretions are easily removed by suction or bronchoscopy
- It is often only with IPPV support that adequate analgesia can be given to some patients (e.g. with multiple injuries).

Limitations of IPPV

- IPPV does not reverse any intrinsic lung problem
- The ventilator should be viewed as *adjunctive* rather than primary support
- From the moment a patient is connected to the ventilator, the goal should be to remove them from it as soon as it is safe to do so
- The results of ventilation are best when it is given as pure temporary support of a patient with a relatively healthy lung (e.g. drug overdose, hypothermia, post-operative patient)
- For patients with existing pulmonary and cardiac disorders, the aim is to support respiration, while allowing time for other measures to be effective (e.g. antibiotics, diuretics, steroids etc.)
- The results are worst when IPPV is instituted in conditions for which there is *no* specific therapy for the underlying problem (e.g. ARDS).

Goals of ventilatory support

The overall goals of IPPV are to reduce the work of breathing. This is achieved by the following:

- *Maintain adequate oxygenation*: the two main determinants of arterial oxygenation are the inspired oxygen concentration and the mean airway pressure. This was first observed in neonates undergoing IPPV, but was later observed in adult patients with ARDS [17]. Arguably, all other manipulations known to increase oxygenation, for example, increased TV, PEEP, inverse ratio ventilation exert their beneficial effect secondary to an increase in mean airway pressure. However, not all methods of increasing airway pressure may be of equal benefit to the patient (e.g. a minimum level of PEEP may be crucial).

- *Maintain adequate ventilation*: IPPV should be used to help normalize the $PaCO_2$ to maintain a normal pH. However, conditions do exist, where permissive hypercapnea is accepted in order to prevent complications of IPPV, such as barotrauma.
- Achieve patient/ventilator synchrony by use of more flexible modes and/or by use of sedation.
- Minimize complications of IPPV: both respiratory and cardiac.

Initial ventilator settings

The following are guidelines for initial ventilator settings in patients requiring IPPV. The mode of ventilation, the patient's clinical circumstances and evolving needs will impact these parameters.

- **Set inspired oxygen concentration**: Initially 100% is sensible if there is doubt regarding the adequacy of oxygenation. This may avoid the patient suffering a period of ongoing hypoxia. One could use the pulse oximeter or arterial blood gas (ABG) analysis to titrate the FiO_2.
- **Adjust the FiO_2 to the lowest percentage required to meet oxygenation goals**: Typically, a minimum goal would be to achieve an arterial PO_2 of at least 60 mm Hg and/or saturations of 90%. Patients with ARDS may tolerate a lower PaO_2 ("permissive hypoxemia") so as to limit the dangers from excessive TVs or airway pressures [18,19,20].
- **Set tidal volume (TV)**: a TV of 6–8 mL/kg predicted body weight is a reasonable initial setting. Current research supports TVs at the lower end of this scale to avoid complications of IPPV (see below).
- **Set respiratory rate (RR)**: an initial RR of 10–14 breaths/min will suffice. Lower rates may be appropriate in certain circumstances (status asthmaticus or ARDS). As with TV, this will need to be adjusted to the clinical scenario.
- **Set PEEP**: almost without exception patients benefit from at least 5 cm PEEP if only to limit the required inspired oxygen concentration and prevent "low-level barotrauma" (see below). The full recruitment effect may not be seen for several hours.
- **Set I:E ratio**: usual inspiratory:expiratory (I:E) ratio is 1:2. (Patients with ARDS are discussed elsewhere, but they may need this to be adjusted, including using a reverse I:E ratio.) Care should be taken if the patient is at risk of air trapping.
- Usual inspiratory flow rate of approximately 50–100 L/min.
- It is considered desirable to set the ventilator, as soon as possible, to allow the patient to maintain spontaneous respiratory efforts in order to limit respiratory muscle wasting and shorten the duration of ventilatory support [21].
- Set volume and pressure alarms.
- Set reasonable trigger sensitivity (either flow or pressure triggered) so as to be able to initiate spontaneous breaths if appropriate. The trigger should not be too sensitive, as this may result in dysynchrony.

All must be adjusted according to clinical response and frequent assessment. Lung-protective strategies are discussed more fully in the chapters on modes of ventilation and ARDS.

Ventilator-induced lung injury (VILI)

The acute lung injury due to mechanical ventilation is termed VILI. Part of this relates to airway pressures – barotrauma.

Barotrauma

- Barotrauma strictly refers to any complication of ventilation related to thoracic pressures and could therefore include the cardiac effects, but most limit barotrauma to pneumothorax, pneumomediastinum, subcutaneous emphysema and the rare occurrence of systemic air embolus.
- The mechanism of barotrauma is probably related to alveolar and bronchiolar distension leading to eventual airway disruption and interstitial gas formation. It is generally accepted that high levels of PEEP, endobronchial intubation and underlying lung disease, especially acute lung injury, increase the incidence of barotraumas [10,22,23]. Many now recommend that plateau airway pressures be maintained, where possible, below 35 cm H_2O [10,24].
- It has become accepted in recent years that "low-level barotrauma" can occur. Here, in the absence of PEEP, repetitive opening and closure of alveoli cause damage from shearing forces [25].

Volume trauma or volutrauma

- It is now believed that in many acute lung disorders, especially ARDS, the disease process is heterogenous; that is, there are small, relatively normal areas of lung in conjunction with areas of diseased lung (known as the "baby lung" concept). If sufficiently high TVs are used to recruit the diseased areas, then the normal areas will be overdistended and damaged. Thus conventional IPPV may contribute to further parenchymal lung damage.
- The term "volutrauma" itself was coined to emphasize the role of excessive inflation volumes in secondary lung damage. Confusion arose because most early animal studies of barotrauma raised the airway pressure by increasing TV. A very elegant study examined pressure and volume truly independently for the first time (using a veterinary "iron lung" to generate volume without increasing pressure and thoraco-abdominal binding to increase thoracic pressures without altering TV). The authors clearly showed that histological lung damage only occurred in the high-volume group [26].
- High TVs in critically ill patients cause the release of inflammatory mediators into the circulation. A study of patients with acute lung injury demonstrated that low PEEP/ high TV mechanical ventilation was associated with cytokine release into the circulation within 1 h [27]. This could be avoided by application of a lung-protective strategy of high PEEP/low TV.

Ventilator care bundles

In recent years there has been much interest in ventilator care bundles. This approach to consistent, evidence-based management comprises the bundling together of various aspects of care, each individually known or believed to improve patient care. It is hoped that by attention to detail, use of protocols and daily checklists to improve compliance with the individual care aspects, improvements in overall care and outcome will be achieved. Much of the focus on ventilator bundles of care is aimed at reducing infectious complications of ventilation. For example, if various interventions believed to reduce the incidence of ventilator-associated pneumonia (VAP) are implemented together, this should result in reductions in the incidence of such VAP. However, despite widespread introduction and use of these bundles, RCT evidence for improvements in outcome and reductions in VAP is sparse [28].

- Commonly known bundles include the FAST HUG bundle [29] and the Institute for Health Improvement ventilator bundle [30].
- The FAST HUG bundle includes feeding, analgesia, sedation, thromboembolic prophylaxis, head-of-bed elevation, stress ulcer prevention and glucose control.
- The IHI ventilator bundle includes: elevation of the head of the bed to 45°, daily sedation hold and assessment of readiness to extubate, daily oral chlorhexidine rinses, proton-pump inhibitors or H_2 receptor antagonists, anticoagulants or compression devices.

Many clinicians have little problem with the concept of bundles, despite the lack of prospective data supporting the bundle (as opposed to studies on individual aspects of the bundle in isolation), but are concerned that more appropriate interventions may not be included in the bundle or that different parts of the bundle, in time, may be less well supported in the literature (e.g. normalization of glucose in the critically ill patient).

Other common bundles of relevance to the critically ill patient are the sepsis bundles from the Surviving Sepsis Campaign and bundles related to care of vascular catheters.

References

1. Guyatt GH, Akl E, Crowther M et al. Executive summary: Antithrombotic Therapy and Prevention of Thrombosis, 9th edn: American College of Chest Physicians Evidence-Based Clinical Practice Guidelines. Chest 2012; 141 (Suppl) : 7–47S.

2. Theaker C, Mannan M, Ives N, Soni N. Risk factors for pressure sores in the critically ill. Anaesthesia 2000; 55 : 221–4.

3. Weststrate JT, Hop WC, Aalbers AG et al. The clinical relevance of the waterlow pressure sore risk scale in the ICU. Intens Care Med 1998; 24 : 815–20.

4. Imanaka H, Taenaka N, Nakamura J, Aoyama K et al. Ocular surface disorders in the critically ill. Anesth Analg 1997; 85 : 343–6.

5. Suresh P, Mercieca F, Morton A, Tullo AB. Eye care for the critically ill. Intens Care Med 2000; 26 : 162–6.

6. Brath PC, MacGregor DA, Ford JG, Prielipp RC. Dopamine and intraocular pressure in critically ill patients. Anesthesiology 2000; 93 : 1398–400.

7. Krivopal M, Shlobin OA, Schwartzstein RM. Utility of daily routine portable chest radiographs in mechanically ventilated patients in the medical ICU. Chest 2003; 123 : 1607–14.

8. Bhagwanjee S, Muckart DJ. Routine daily chest radiography is not indicated for ventilated patients in a surgical ICU. Intens Care Med 1996; 22 : 1335–8.

9. Oba Y, Zaza T. Abandoning daily routine chest radiography in the intensive care unit: meta-analysis. Radiology 2010;255 : 386–95.

10. Slutsky AS. Mechanical Ventilation. American College of Chest Physicians Consensus Conference. Chest 1993; 104 :1833–59.

11. International Consensus Conference in Intensive Care Medicine: noninvasive positive pressure ventilation in acute respiratory failure. Am J Respir Crit Care Med 2001; 163 : 283–91.

12. Celikel T, Sungur M Ceyhan B, Karakurt S. Comparison of noninvasive positive pressure ventilation with standard medical

therapy in hypercapnic acute respiratory failure. *Chest* 1998; 114 : 1636.

13. Qvist J, Pontoppidan H, Wilson RS *et al.* Hemodynamic responses to mechanical ventilation with PEEP: the effect of hypervolemia. *Anesthesiology* 1975; 42 : 45–55.

14. Ralph DD, Robertson HT, Weaver LJ. Distribution of ventilation and perfusion during positive end-expiratory pressure in the adult respiratory distress syndrome. *Am Rev Resp Dis* 1985; 131 : 54–60.

15. De Backer D. The effects of positive end-expiratory pressure on the splanchnic circulation. *Intensive Care Med* 2000; 26 : 361–3.

16. Uchino S, Kellum JA, Bellomo R *et al.* Acute renal failure in critically ill patients: a multinational, multicenter study. *JAMA* 2005; 294 : 813–8.

17. Marini JJ, Ravenscraft SA. Mean airway pressure: physiologic determinants and clinical importance – Part 2: Clinical implications. *Crit Care Med* 1992; 20 : 1604–16.

18. Bugge JF. Pressure limited ventilation with permissive hypoxia and nitric oxide in the treatment of adult respiratory distress syndrome. *Eur J Anaesthesiol* 1999; 16 : 799–802.

19. The Acute Respiratory Distress Syndrome Network. Ventilation with lower tidal volumes as compared with traditional tidal volumes for acute lung injury and the acute respiratory distress syndrome. *N Engl J Med* 2000; 342 : 1301.

20. Chiumello D, Pelosi P, Calvi E *et al.* Different modes of assisted ventilation in patients with acute respiratory failure. *Eur Respir J* 2002; 20 : 925–33.

21. Putensen C, Zech S, Wrigge H *et al.* Long-term effects of spontaneous breathing during ventilatory support in patients with

acute lung injury. *Am J Respir Crit Care Med* 2001; 164 : 43–9.

22. Gammon RB, Shin MS, Groves RH Jr *et al.* Clinical risk factors for pulmonary barotrauma: a multivariate analysis. *Am J Respir Crit Care Med* 1995; 152 : 1235–40.

23. Schnap LM, Chin DP, Szaflarski N, Matthay MA. Frequency and importance of barotrauma in 100 patients with acute lung injury. *Crit Care Med* 1995; 23 : 272–8.

24. Boussarsar M, Thierry G, Jaber S *et al.* Relationship between ventilatory settings and barotrauma in the acute respiratory distress syndrome. *Intensive Care Med* 2002; 28 : 406–13.

25. Muncedere JG, Mullen JBM, Gan AS, Slutsky AS. Tidal ventilation at low airway pressures can augment lung injury. *Am J Resp Crit Care Med* 1994; 149 : 1327–34.

26. Dreyfuss D, Soler G, Basset G, Saumon G. High inflation pressure pulmonary oedema – respiratory effects of high airway pressure, high tidal volume, and positive endexpiratory pressure. *Am Rev Respir Dis* 1988; 137 : 1159–64.

27. Stuber F, Wrigge H, Schroeder S *et al.* Kinetic and reversibility of mechanical ventilation-associated pulmonary and systemic inflammatory response in patients with acute lung injury. *Intens Care Med* 2002; 28 : 834–41.

28. O'Grady N, Murray PR, Ames N. Preventing ventilator-associated pneumonia: does the evidence support the practice? *JAMA* 2012; 307 : 2534–9.

29. Vincent JL. Give your patient a fast hug (at least) once a day. *Crit Care Med* 2005; 33 : 1225–9.

30. Marwick C, Davey P. Care bundles: the holy grail of infectious risk management in hospital? *Curr Opin Infect Dis* 2009; 22 : 364–9.

13 Modes of ventilation and ventilator strategies

Tania Ligori

Mechanical ventilation is in many cases the cornerstone of supportive care for respiratory failure. It has the potential to improve gas exchange, as well as decrease work of breathing.

That said, mechanical ventilation is not an entirely benign therapy and the clinician is tasked with attempting to deliver the benefits of positive-pressure ventilation while minimizing the potential for lung injury and hemodynamic instability.

This chapter will review the characteristics of common modes of invasive mechanical ventilation and discuss strategies and evidence for lung-protective ventilation. The use of noninvasive ventilatory techniques is covered elsewhere.

Modes of mechanical ventilation

- In general, a mode of ventilation can be broadly classified by the amount of work the ventilator performs relative to the patient during inspiration.
- In controlled modes, the ventilator is responsible for initiating and delivering each breath and assumes the entire work of breathing.
- Assist or support modes allow the patient to initiate a breath, but partially offset the work of breathing.
- More specifically, a ventilator mode can be defined by the features of the inspiratory breath delivered, regardless of the degree of support.
- These defining variables include the trigger, the limit (or target) and the cycle [1].

Inspiratory breath characteristics

Trigger

The trigger describes the variable that initiates a breath. A ventilator-triggered breath is initiated after a set time has elapsed, reflecting the set respiratory rate. A patient-triggered breath occurs when the patient makes an inspiratory effort sufficient to cause a change in either flow or pressure in the ventilator circuit.

Limit/target

This is the pressure, volume or flow target during inspiration.

Handbook of ICU Therapy, third edition, ed. John Fuller, Jeff Granton and Ian McConachie. Published by Cambridge University Press. © Cambridge University Press 2015.

Cycle

This is the variable that ends the inspiratory phase and signals the start of passive expiratory gas flow. The cycle variable can be time, tidal volume or a decrease in flow to a prespecified percentage of the peak inspiratory flow.

Controlled modes of ventilation

Volume control ventilation (VCV)

Volume control ventilation is volume-limited and time-cycled. A predetermined tidal volume is delivered at a set respiratory rate. In this mode, an inspiratory flow profile must be specified and is usually a property of the ventilator. Flow is most commonly delivered as a square (constant) waveform, but it can also be decelerating or sinusoidal. Peak inspiratory flow or inspiratory time must also be selected by the clinician and determines the duration of inspiration. The ventilator will then deliver each breath with the same flow-time profile, thus generating the same tidal volume. Thus, at a given respiratory rate, in the absence of system leaks, minute ventilation is guaranteed. Airway pressure, however, will vary depending on the mechanics (resistance and compliance) of the respiratory system [2].

Pressure control ventilation (PCV)

Pressure control ventilation is pressure-limited and time-cycled. One must set a desired pressure limit, respiratory rate and inspiratory time (or I:E ratio) on the ventilator. Gas flows quickly from the ventilator until the target pressure in the respiratory system is achieved. At that point, flow decelerates to maintain a constant pressure profile for the duration of the inspiratory time. In this case, tidal volume is the dependent variable and will change based on the mechanics of the respiratory system [3].

High-frequency oscillatory ventilation (HFOV)

The use of HFOV was first described in the neonatal population. In HFOV, a constant distending pressure (or mean airway pressure, MAP) is generated, maintaining lung inflation. The MAP is usually higher than that generated with conventional modes of ventilation. Unlike other modes of ventilation, both inspiration and expiration are active processes and are controlled by the ventilator piston. Tidal volumes are generated by pressure oscillations around the MAP baseline at a frequency between 3 and 10 Hz (180–600 breaths per minute). These rapid oscillations result in very small tidal volumes, consistent with a lung-protective strategy [4]. Unfortunately, HFOV has not been shown to improve mortality in ARDS (see below).

Assisted modes of ventilation

Assist control ventilation (ACV)

Assist control ventilation can be either volume- or pressure-limited. Essentially, the ventilator is set just as in PCV or VCV. The difference, however, is that the patient may trigger the ventilator for any and/or every breath. Each breath, whether triggered or not, will be delivered according to the same clinician-set parameters. If the patient does not trigger the ventilator (i.e. is paralyzed or heavily sedated), a minimum number of breaths are guaranteed and this mode becomes indistinguishable from PCV or VCV.

Pressure support ventilation (PSV)

Pressure support ventilation is pressure-limited and flow-cycled. Every breath is patient-triggered and thus the patient determines the respiratory rate. During inspiration, patient effort signals the ventilator to increase gas flow until the airway pressure reaches the preset pressure support level. For any given value of pressure support, tidal volume is determined by patient effort, as well as the mechanics of the respiratory system. When inspiratory flow decreases below a threshold value, usually a certain percentage of peak inspiratory flow, the ventilator cycles to expiration. This decrement in flow is taken to reflect inspiratory muscle relaxation and the end of inspiration.

Airway pressure release ventilation (APRV)

Airway pressure release ventilation is a time-cycled mode that alternates between two levels of airway pressure, a high pressure (P_{high}) and a low pressure (P_{low}). Most of the time is spent at P_{high}, in order to keep alveoli recruited, with brief cycling to P_{low} (usually less than 1 s duration) in order to allow ventilation. The patient is allowed or in fact is meant to breath throughout the respiratory cycle. Spontaneous breathing has the advantage of improving ventilation of dependent alveoli, requiring less sedation and potentially preserving diaphragm function [4,5].

Proportional assist ventilation (PAV)

Proportional assist ventilation is a patient-triggered mode of ventilation. It is unique in that it is not pressure-, volume- or flow-limited. With PAV, the clinician sets the *proportion* of work that will be provided by the ventilator with each breath. By calculating the resistance and elastance of the respiratory system, the ventilator determines the amount of flow and volume assistance required to deliver each breath, according to the proportion of work it has been set to give. The remainder of the work is left to the patient. For example, a PAV setting of 50% means that the ventilator will provide 50% of the work required for inspiration. In essence, the ventilator amplifies the patient's inspiratory effort. By adapting to changing lung mechanics and patient demand, this mode is felt by some clinicians to improve patient–ventilator synchrony, that is, matching between the patient's spontaneous respiratory efforts and the ventilator's gas delivery [6].

Neurally adjusted ventilatory assist (NAVA)

Neurally adjusted ventilatory assist is an assisted mode of ventilation that attempts to improve patient–ventilator synchrony. With NAVA, the electrical activity of the diaphragm is measured continuously using electromyography (EMG) electrodes near the distal end of a specialized esophageal probe. The electrical activity is used to signal gas flow, which begins as soon as the diaphragm is stimulated by the phrenic nerve. As the diaphragm relaxes in expiration, gas flow subsides. Similar to PAV, the ventilator provides assistance in proportion to patient effort. In this case, the pressure delivered is proportional to the measured electrical activity of the diaphragm. The clinician sets the degree of support, that is the pressure to be delivered per unit of EMG activity measured. Currently, the use of NAVA is predominantly limited to investigational settings [6,7].

Positive end-expiratory pressure (PEEP)

Positive end-expiratory pressure is the pressure above atmospheric pressure that is maintained in the respiratory system throughout the entire respiratory cycle. It is not, as the name would suggest, only present at end-expiration. It is synonymous with CPAP (continuous positive airway pressure) but, by convention, is the term applied to patients receiving invasive mechanical ventilation.

From a pulmonary perspective, using PEEP can maintain alveolar recruitment [8]. This can have several potential benefits, including:

- Improved oxygenation by reducing atelectasis and intrapulmonary shunting
- Decreased lung injury by minimizing cyclic alveolar collapse
- Increased functional residual capacity
- Improved lung compliance.

As alveoli become overdistended, however, gas exchange can be compromised by one or more possible mechanisms:

- Barotrauma (i.e. pneumothorax)
- Compression of the blood vessels around the distended alveoli, which can:
  i. Increase physiological dead space
  ii. Divert blood to other poorly ventilated regions (if present) thereby increasing the shunt fraction
  iii. Increase pulmonary vascular resistance, thereby decreasing pulmonary blood flow.

The increased intrathoracic pressure generated by PEEP may produce hemodynamic effects as well [9]:

- Right ventricular pre-load and left ventricular afterload usually decrease
- Pulmonary vascular resistance may either increase or decrease, depending in part on the PEEP-induced changes in lung volume [10]
- Pulmonary vascular resistance in turn contributes to right ventricular afterload and right ventricular output
- The net effect of these changes influences left ventricular stroke volume and ultimately cardiac output.

Ventilatory strategies

Although mechanical ventilation can be life-saving, it has the potential to cause lung injury via several proposed mechanisms. These are:

- Barotrauma – exposure to high transpulmonary pressures
- Volutrauma – overdistension due to high tidal volumes
- Atelectrauma – repetitive opening and closing of alveoli
- Biotrauma – release of inflammatory mediators from distention of the lungs that can have injurious effects on nonpulmonary organs.

Together, these mechanisms constitute what is termed "ventilator-induced lung injury" or VILI [11]. A lung-protective strategy aims to minimize VILI. Practically, this involves:

- Limiting lung stress and strain (i.e. limiting tidal volume and plateau pressure/transpulmonary pressure)
- Applying positive end-expiratory pressure (PEEP) at a level sufficient to keep the lung recruited and prevent atelectrauma [12].

Low tidal volume ventilation

The concept of lung-protective ventilation (LPV) evolved from the study of patients with acute lung injury (ALI) and acute respiratory distress syndrome (ARDS).

- In the past, ventilation strategies aimed at maximizing gas exchange in ALI/ARDS would sometimes include the use of tidal volumes as high as 10–15 ml/kg.
- It was later recognized, however, that ARDS is a heterogeneous disease in the lung. Some areas of the lung become fluid-filled, consolidated and difficult to expand, while other areas remain quite normal.
- Effectively, the overall amount of lung that can be ventilated is reduced, giving rise to the concept of the "baby lung" – a smaller effective lung volume available for gas exchange [13].
- Ventilating the "baby lung" with high tidal volumes can result in regional overdistension of normal lung units and cause injury.
- Thus, lung-protective ventilation involves ventilating with smaller tidal volumes, 4–6 mL/kg, and minimizing plateau pressures (a surrogate of end-inspiratory transpulmonary pressure).

In 2000, the ARDSNet group published the largest multicentered randomized controlled trial examining the effect of low tidal volume ventilation on mortality in ARDS [14].

- In this study, the control (conventional) arm was ventilated with an initial tidal volume of 12 mL/kg predicted body weight to achieve a plateau pressure ≤50 cm H_2O while the experimental (lung-protective) arm was ventilated with a tidal volume of 6 mL/kg and plateau pressure ≤30 cm H_2O.
- The study was stopped early, after an interim analysis showed a 22% relative risk reduction in mortality with the protective lung-ventilation strategy. There was also a greater number of ventilator-free days in the group treated with lower tidal volumes.

Adopting a ventilation strategy using low tidal volumes may result in hypercapnia.

- Tolerating a higher $PaCO_2$ in an attempt to minimize lung injury is termed *permissive hypercapnia.*
- Hypercapnia (and the accompanying respiratory acidosis that may occur in the absence of buffering) is generally well tolerated [15].
- There is some thought that hypercapnia may actually be protective in acute lung injury, but the current evidence is insufficient to advocate for the use of permissive hypercapnia as a therapy in its own right [16].

The benefits of low tidal volume ventilation in patients without ALI/ARDS remain unclear [17].

Positive end-expiratory pressure

The optimal level of PEEP to use as part of a lung-protective strategy in ALI/ARDS has not been conclusively established. Three major randomized, controlled trials in the last decade have compared the use of higher versus lower PEEP strategies in combination with low tidal volume ventilation [18–20].

- The ALVEOLI and LOVS studies titrated PEEP values using a table of predetermined PEEP/FiO_2 combinations based on the oxygenation status of the patient.

- The Express trial adjusted PEEP on the basis of pulmonary mechanics. Patients in the high PEEP group had PEEP set to reach a plateau pressure of 28–30 cm H_2O compared to the minimal distension group in which a PEEP of 5–9 cm H_2O was maintained.
- Each of these studies failed to demonstrate a significant mortality benefit between groups. In the LOVS and Express trials, however, the higher PEEP groups required less rescue interventions for refractory hypoxemia.
- A meta-analysis of all three trials confirmed these findings [21]. Examining the data from all 2299 patients, there was no statistically significant difference in overall hospital mortality between the higher and lower PEEP groups. In the group of patients with ARDS (PaO_2/FiO_2 ratio <200) at baseline, however, those in the higher PEEP group were more likely to survive to hospital discharge. The group with ALI (but not ARDS) did not experience benefit with higher PEEP.
- Perhaps then it is the patients with more severe disease that benefit from higher end-expiratory pressure. In fact, using CT scanning, Gattinoni *et al.* showed that patients with more severe disease were those that had more recruitable lung on imaging and were also more likely to respond to the application of external PEEP [13].

A novel method for adjusting PEEP by calculating transpulmonary pressures (TPP) was described in a small pilot study by Talmor *et al.* in 2008 [22]. Transpulmonary pressure, the effective alveolar distending pressure, is calculated as airway pressure minus pleural pressure. Esophageal pressure can be used as a surrogate for pleural pressure although there has been some criticism of this practice in ARDS patients. By monitoring transpulmonary pressures, the authors of this study propose that it is possible to adjust PEEP to prevent repetitive alveolar collapse (maintain positive end-expiratory TPP) and lung overdistention (limit end-inspiratory TPP). They hypothesized that PEEP guided by esophageal pressure monitoring would lead to improved oxygenation compared to a strategy of titrating PEEP based on the ARDSNet trial protocol. This study did in fact find improved oxygenation and respiratory system compliance in the esophageal pressure group up to 72 hours following randomization. Mortality at 28 days was also better, but the study was not powered for this outcome. Further study is necessary to draw any clear conclusions with regards to the use of this technique, but the idea of tailoring PEEP to the individual patient is very interesting.

High-frequency oscillatory ventilation (HFOV)

The concept of lung-protective ventilation also renewed interest in the use of HFOV in adult ARDS. By delivering tidal volumes that are smaller than dead-space, and preventing cyclic alveolar collapse by maintaining a high end-expiratory distending pressure, HFOV would seem like the ideal ventilator mode in ARDS.

Early studies suggested potential benefit to the use of HFOV in ARDS, but the studies were small and the control groups received ventilation that would generally be considered injurious by today's standards [23–26].

Two larger trials aimed to resolve this issue by randomizing patients with new-onset ARDS to receive either HFOV or a strategy using lung-protective ventilation [27,28].

- There was no mortality benefit to HFOV at 30 days in the OSCAR trial.
- In the OSCILLATE trial, the goal was to randomize 1200 patients. After 548 patients were enrolled, the trial was stopped early for safety concerns. There was an increase in in-hospital mortality in the HFOV group (relative risk for death 1.33 (95% confidence interval, 1.09–1.64; $p = 0.005$)).

Therefore, the evidence does not support early institution of HFOV in ARDS at this time. Whether this holds true for HFOV as a rescue mode of ventilation in ARDS is not currently known.

References

1. Gould T, de Beer JMA. Principles of artificial ventilation. *Anaesth Intensive Care Med* 2007; 8 : 91–101.

2. Koh SO. Mode of mechanical ventilation: volume controlled mode. *Crit Care Clin* 2007; 23 : 161–67.

3. Nichols D, Haranath S. Pressure control ventilation. *Crit Care Clin* 2007; 23 : 183–99.

4. Fan E, Stewart T. New modalities of mechanical ventilation: high-frequency oscillatory ventilation and airway pressure release ventilation. *Clin Chest Med* 2006; 27 : 615–25.

5. Modrykamien A, Chatburn R, Ashton R. Airway pressure release ventilation: an alternative mode of mechanical ventilation in acute respiratory distress syndrome. *Cleve Clin J Med* 2011; 78 : 101–10.

6. Kacmarek RM. Proportional assist ventilation and neutrally adjusted ventilation ventilatory assist. *Respir Care* 2011; 56 : 140–8.

7. Terzi N, Piquilloud L, Roze H *et al*. Clinical review: update on neurally adjusted ventilatory assist – resport of a round-table conference. *Crit Care* 2012; 16 : 225.

8. Acosta P, Santisbon E, Varon J. The use of positive end-expiratory pressure in mechanical ventilation. *Crit Care Clin* 2007; 23 : 251–61.

9. Luce JM. The cardiovascular effects of mechanical ventilation and positive end-expiratory pressure. *J Am Med Assoc* 1984; 252 : 807–11.

10. West JB. *Respiratory Physiology: The Essentials*. Baltimore: Lippincott Williams & Wilkins; 2008.

11. Dreyfuss D, Saumon G. Ventilator-induced lung injury: lessons from experimental studies. *Am J Respir Crit Care Med* 1998; 157 : 294–323.

12. Gattinoni L, Carlesso E, Brazzi L, Caironi P. Postive end-expiratory pressure. *Curr Opin Crit Care* 2010; 16 : 39–44.

13. Gattinoni L, Caironi P, Cressoni M *et al*. Lung recruitment in patients with the acute respiratory distress syndrome. *N Engl J Med* 2006; 354 : 1775–86.

14. The Acute Respiratory Distress Syndrome Network. Ventilation with lower tidal volumes as compared with traditional tidal volumes for acute lung injury and the acute respiratory distress syndrome. *New Engl J Med* 2000; 342 : 1301–8.

15. Laffey JG, O'Croinin D, McLoughlin P, Kavanagh BP. Permissive hypercapnia – role in protective lung ventilatory strategies. *Intensive Care Med* 2004; 30 : 347–56.

16. Ismaiel NM, Henzler D. Effects of hypercapnia and hypercapnic acidosis on attenuation of ventilator-associated lung injury. *Minerva Anestesiol* 2011; 77 : 723–33.

17. Lipes J, Bohmehrani A, Lellouche F. Low tidal volume ventilation in patients without acute respiratory distress syndrome: a paradigm shift in mechanical ventilation. *Crit Care Res Pract* 2012 : 416862.

18. The National Heart, Lung, and Blood Institute ARDS Clinical Trials Network. Higher versus lower positive end-expiratory pressures in patients with the acute respiratory distress syndrome. *N Engl J Med* 2004; 351 : 327–36.

19. Meade MO, Cook DJ, Guyatt GH *et al*. Ventilation strategy using low tidal volumes, recruitment maneuvers, and high positive end-expiratory pressure for acute lung injury and acute respiratory distress

syndrome; a randomized controlled trial. *J Am Med Assoc* 2008; 299 : 637–45.

20. Mercat M, Richard JM, Vielle B, *et al.* Positive end-expiratory pressure setting in adults with acute lung injury and acute respiratory distress syndrome: a randomized controlled trial. *J Am Med Assoc* 2008; 299 : 646–55.

21. Briel M, Meade M, Mercat M *et al.* Higher vs lower positive end-expiratory pressure in patients with acute lung injury and acute respiratory distress syndrome: systematic review and meta-analysis. *J Am Med Assoc* 2010; 303 : 865–73.

22. Talmor D, Sarge T, Malhotra A *et al.* Mechanical ventilation guided by esophageal pressure in acute lung injury. *N Engl J Med* 2008; 259 : 2095–104.

23. Fort P, Farmer C, Westerman J *et al.* High-frequency oscillatory ventilation for adult respiratory distress syndrome: a pilot study. *Crit Care Med* 1997; 25 : 937–47.

24. Derdak S, Mehta S, Stewart TE *et al.* High-frequency oscillatory ventilation for acute respiratory distress syndrome in adults: a randomized, controlled trial. *Am J Respir Crit Care Med* 2002; 166 : 801–8.

25. Papzian L, Gainnier M, Marin V *et al.* Comparison of prone positioning and high-frequency oscillatory ventilation in patients with acute respiratory distress syndrome. *Crit Care Med* 2005; 33 : 2162–71.

26. Bollen CW, van Well GTJ, Sherry T *et al.* High frequency oscillatory ventilation compared with conventional mechanical ventilation in adult respiratory distress syndrome: a randomized controlled trial. *Crit Care* 2005; 9(4) : R430–9.

27. Young D, Lamb SE, Shah S *et al.* High-frequency oscillation for acute respiratory distress syndrome. *N Engl J Med* 2013; 368 : 806–13.

28. Ferguson ND, Cook DJ, Guyatt GH *et al.* High-frequency oscillation in early acute respiratory distress syndrome. *N Engl J Med* 2013; 368 : 795–805.

Discontinuing mechanical ventilation

Ron Butler

The key points of this chapter are as follows :

- Instituting mechanical ventilation for acute respiratory failure is life-saving. For most patients, the point that they transition to recovery from their acute respiratory failure and are ready to have ventilation discontinued is easily missed.
- Prolonging ventilation unnecessarily is associated with additional morbidity for the patient.
- Discontinuing ventilation when patients are not ready is associated with additional morbidity for the patient.
- Systematically looking for readiness to discontinue ventilation and standardizing the process with protocols decreases the time spent on a ventilator and reduces the risk of requiring reintubation.
- Utilizing nurse and respiratory-therapist-led protocols for weaning standardizes the approach to patients and generally results in patients having ventilation discontinued earlier.
- Sedation can have a tremendous impact on the duration of ventilation. Systematically reassessing the need and dose of sedation can shorten time on the ventilator.
- Noninvasive ventilation can be utilized as part of the strategy for discontinuing ventilation. The evidence supporting its use is strongest in patients with chronic obstructive lung disease. In this setting it can be used as a weaning strategy.
- Noninvasive ventilation as a rescue strategy for those that develop respiratory failure following extubation is not well supported by the literature and should be used cautiously.
- Tracheostomy is most useful in the patients that have prolonged weaning from the ventilator. A strategy of early tracheostomy is not supported by the literature.

Introduction

Weaning has been the term that has been associated with discontinuing mechanical ventilation for decades. By definition this means to remove from a source of dependence and yet for most patients their first attempt at discontinuing mechanical ventilation is successful. A classification system for weaning patients from mechanical ventilation was published in 2007 [1]:

1. Simple: proceed from the initiation of weaning to successful extubation on the first attempt without difficulty.
2. Difficult: patients who fail initial weaning and require up to three spontaneous breathing trials (SBT), or as long as 7 days from the initial SBT to achieve successful weaning.

Handbook of ICU Therapy, third edition, ed. John Fuller, Jeff Granton and Ian McConachie. Published by Cambridge University Press. © Cambridge University Press 2015.

3. Prolonged: patients who fail at least three weaning attempts or require more than 7 days of weaning after the first spontaneous breathing trial.

The proportion of patients' weaning from mechanical ventilation in a cohort study of medical surgical ICUs in Vienna in each category were: 59% simple, 26% difficult, 14% prolonged [2].

- The key factor for patients in the simple category is ensuring that clinicians are systematically looking at patients for their readiness to discontinue ventilation.
- Patients in the prolonged category represent a relatively small proportion of the critical care population in a mixed medical surgical ICU, but they consume a considerably greater proportion of total ventilator days and require much time and effort in order to discontinue ventilation.
- They are often weak and deconditioned having had prolonged ICU stays, often with multiple comorbidities, and most of them would meet the definition of chronically critically ill (see chapter on Chronic critical illness).
- Strategies to discontinue ventilation in this group include: careful attention to nutritional support, active involvement of physiotherapy to improve strength and endurance, attention to sleep and treatment of delirium, and optimization of underlying comorbidities.
- The term weaning is most apt for this group as it is a slow and gradual process.

Most of the literature around weaning has been developed studying the patients that are in the simple and difficult categories.

Discontinuing ventilation versus extubation

For most critically ill patients the time that they are ready to have ventilation discontinued coincides with their readiness to extubate and within the literature, studies that have defined the approach have often linked the two together. Nevertheless it is important to distinguish the criteria for each separately, as there are times where a patient may not require ventilation and yet not be ready for extubation.

Readiness to discontinue ventilation

1. Reversal (complete or partial) of process that necessitated ventilation
2. Ability to sustain oxygenation without mechanical support
3. Ability to perform the work of breathing.

Readiness for extubation

1. Ability to maintain and protect airway
2. Ability to cough and clear secretions.

Predictors

The ability to discern when patients are ready to discontinue ventilation has been a long-standing goal of clinicians. The dilemma is that maintaining patients on a ventilator longer than required risks morbidity, wastes resources and delays patient recovery, but extubating

Table 14.1 Threshold values for successful weaning

Parameter	Threshold values for successful weaning
Vital Capacity	More than 10–15 mL/kg
Minute ventilation	Less than 10–15 L/min
Negative inspiratory pressure	More negative than –20 to – 30 cm H_2O
Respiratory rate[*]	Less than 30–38 breaths per minute
Tidal volume[*]	More than 4–6 mL/kg
Frequency/tidal volume (f/V_T)[*]	Less than 60–105

[*] measured during brief period of unsupported breathing

patients when they are not ready similarly risks major morbidity or mortality, wastes resources and delays patient recovery [3,4].

- Determining whether a patient can be oxygenated adequately without mechanical support is relatively simple.
- However, knowing when sufficient reversal of the process that put the patient on the ventilator has occurred or whether a patient can adequately perform the work of breathing is more difficult.

A number of variables have been studied as predictors for the success of weaning and extubation.

- A sample of some of these predictors and the range of the threshold values that were studied are shown in Table 14.1.
- In a comprehensive review of these predictors, published in 2001 [5], it was noted that none of the predictors were particularly powerful at predicting success and failure.
- Some of the threshold values produced predictors that had good sensitivity, but poor specificity. A test that is simple to perform that when negative rules out successful weaning can be used as a useful screening test.
- The rapid shallow breathing index (f/V_T) with a threshold value of 105 has a 92% sensitivity and has been incorporated into many weaning protocols in this fashion. Patients with an f/V_T greater than 105 are very unlikely to be successfully weaned; anyone with a value less than that should be further evaluated with a spontaneous breathing trial.

Spontaneous breathing trials

The landmark study by Ely *et al.* [3] demonstrated the importance of systematically screening patients for readiness for discontinuing mechanical ventilation and then progressing patients to an SBT. The daily screening criteria from the trial are listed in Table 14.2.

When patients satisfy all the criteria on the daily screen, an SBT is initiated. SBTs are typically performed on T-piece, CPAP or pressure support of 5 to 8 cm H_2O for 30 minutes to 2 hours [3,6]. Patients are monitored for tolerance using both objective and subjective criteria. Criteria to discontinue a spontaneous breathing trial are outlined in Table 14.3.

Table 14.2 Daily screening criteria

Daily screening criteria
PaO$_2$/FiO$_2$ >200, PEEP ≤5 cm H$_2$O
Adequate cough during suctioning
f/V$_T$ ≤105
No infusion of sedatives or vasopressors

Table 14.3 Criteria to discontinue spontaneous breathing trial

Criteria to discontinue spontaneous breathing trial
Respiratory rate greater than 35 for 5 minutes or longer
SaO$_2$ <90%
Heart rate >140 or sustained changes in heart rate >20% from baseline
Systolic BP >180 or <90 mmHg
Increased anxiety or diaphoresis

Patients that successfully complete a spontaneous breathing trial need to be evaluated for extubation readiness. When this protocol is followed in patients in mixed medical surgical ICUs, the reported reintubation rate at 48 hours ranges from 3–19% [1]. Patients that are unable to complete the spontaneous breathing trial are placed back on restful ventilatory support and re-evaluated at least daily for further spontaneous breathing trials. Evaluation of the possible reasons for failure allows clinicians to attempt to improve the probability of success with the next SBT.

SBTs versus other weaning techniques

Traditionally there have been three approaches to discontinuing ventilation:

1. Spontaneous breathing trial. This traditionally means going from full ventilatory support to trying the patient off the ventilator. Originally done utilizing a T-piece, which is simply an oxygen source connected to the endotracheal tube, it is now also performed on CPAP or with a low level of pressure support.
2. Synchronized intermittent mandatory ventilation (SIMV) wean. This utilized the SIMV mode and involved a stepwise reduction in the ventilator rate allowing the patient to assume a greater proportion of the work of breathing. Traditionally when the ventilator rate was reduced to four breaths per minute and if the patient tolerated this level of support they were considered weaned.
3. Pressure support wean. Pressure support was set to provide ventilatory support and then gradually decreased in a stepwise fashion allowing the patient to assume a greater proportion of the work of breathing. When the patient tolerated pressure support from 5–8 cm H$_2$O they were considered weaned.

Two studies conducted in the 1990s addressed which approach was best in a population that was considered difficult to wean by virtue of the fact that they had failed an initial SBT in order to be enrolled in the study [7,8].

- One study found that SBTs were most effective, while the other found pressure support to be superior. In both studies, the SIMV technique was the least effective.
- An international observational study published in 2011 [9] demonstrated that SBTs were being used in over 80% of patients who were considered simple to wean, but the majority of patients in the difficult and prolonged weaning category had gradual reduction of support as the method of weaning. The majority of those patients had reduction of pressure. This is perhaps not surprising, as the evidence for the SBT is best established for the simple to wean category and many of the patients requiring prolonged weaning represented the weaning failures in the clinical trials that established the SBT as the accepted standard.

Protocols

Protocols are decision support tools that provide explicit directions and have been effectively utilized for discontinuing ventilation. Most protocols address screening for readiness for discontinuing ventilation, the conduct of SBTs and finally evaluation for extubation for those passing the SBT. A number of studies have looked at the use of protocols for discontinuing ventilation.

- Although not all of the studies have had positive results, a recent meta-analysis of the trials [10] demonstrated a 25% reduction in the duration of mechanical ventilation when discontinuing ventilation was protocolized.

The impact of sedation

Critically ill patients often require sedation early in their critical illness to help stabilize them and increase their tolerance to mechanical ventilation. However, unless there is a systematic approach to re-evaluating both the need for sedation and the dose required to achieve the sedative goal, patients can receive more sedation than they require and this prolongs their ventilation.

- In the study by Kress [11], a strategy of daily awakening shortened the time on a ventilator by over 2 days and ICU stay by 3 days. Furthermore, far fewer patients in the intervention group received investigations for delayed awakening.
- In a randomized trial that combined both daily awakening and spontaneous breathing trials there was shorter duration of ventilation, ICU length of stay and lower mortality in the intervention group [12].

Early mobilization

Patients ventilated for acute respiratory failure are often sedated and immobile for days, attached to a ventilator.

- Patients managed in this fashion quickly lose muscle mass and become deconditioned. There is also evidence that full mechanical ventilation can induce diaphragm dysfunction in a very short time [13].
- Recent evidence supports that even critically ill ventilated patients can often begin to be safely mobilized early in their critical illness. Benefits include increased exercise capacity, improved functional status at hospital discharge and reduced time on the ventilator [14].

Use of noninvasive ventilation in weaning

Noninvasive ventilation (NIV) has been advocated as a weaning strategy.

- A systematic review of noninvasive ventilation as a weaning strategy in patients invasively ventilated for respiratory failure of any etiology identified five studies, with a total of 171 patients [15]. These studies weaned patients using either a strategy of early extubation followed by immediate application of NIV, or continued invasive ventilatory weaning.
- The review found there was a reduction in mortality, ventilator-associated pneumonia, length of stay and a nonsignificant reduction in the proportion of weaning failures.
- However, several of the studies included in the review were either exclusively or predominantly COPD patients, a population where the indication and benefit for NIV is well established [16].
- This strategy appears promising; however, whether it applies more broadly beyond the COPD population needs further study.

The use of noninvasive ventilation as a technique to avoid reintubation following post-extubation respiratory failure has not been as successful. There have been two randomized trials that have examined this [17,18].

- In both cases the application of noninvasive ventilation once respiratory distress started in the post-extubation period did not reduce the need for reintubation.
- In the larger multicenter study, the use of noninvasive ventilation did delay the time to reintubation by almost 10 hours; however, the mortality rate in the group randomized to noninvasive ventilation was significantly higher than the group randomized to standard therapy [18].

Weaning failures

Defining weaning failure has become more complicated now that NIV may be used as a weaning technique, transitioning patients from full invasive support to noninvasive ventilatory support. Weaning failure includes failure of one or more SBTs, as well as reintubation and/or resumption of ventilatory support within 48 hours following extubation. There are many causes of weaning failure, and in the case of patients in the prolonged weaning category often there are multiple issues contributing to the weaning failure.

A systematic approach to try and identify the cause(s) of failure allows the clinician to try and optimize the patient for the next attempt at weaning. In the case of patients in the prolonged weaning category, addressing these issues may take days to weeks. Between weaning attempts, patients should be provided sufficient support on the ventilator so that they can rest and recover.

Causes of weaning failure:

- Severe/prolonged critical illness
- Pre-existing comorbid conditions, e.g. COPD, chronic renal failure, congestive heart failure
- Neurologic: excess sedation, delirium, critical illness polyneuropathy
- Respiratory: increased work of breathing: reduced compliance (bronchospasm, edematous lungs, reduced chest wall compliance from obesity), increased metabolic rate, increased dead space, imposed work of breathing from endotracheal tube or tracheostomy tube, inappropriate ventilator settings.

Table 14.4 Reasons for reintubation

Reasons for reintubation (some patients will have more than one)
Upper airway obstruction
Hypoxemia
Respiratory acidosis
Signs of increased respiratory work
Cardiac failure
Atelectasis
Decreased consciousness

- Reduced respiratory muscle capacity: generalized weakness, deconditioning, diaphragmatic paralysis, myopathy
- Cardiac: unrecognized coronary ischemia, diastolic dysfunction, valvular disease
- Malnutrition: prolonged negative nitrogen balance and protein depletion
- Metabolic: electrolyte disturbances
- Psychologic: anxiety, depression.

Extubation failures

The causes of failure from an RCT on SBTs are shown in Table 14.4 [6].

Not all extubation failures are the same:

- Patients that required reintubation from upper airway obstruction had a mortality rate of 11%, compared to 36% for those that required reintubation from any of the other causes. The 11% mortality compared favorably with the mortality rate of those patients that were successfully extubated and never required reintubation (12.5%) [6].
- Extubation failures can be classified as early (minutes to few hours) or late (hours to 2 days). Failures associated with upper airway obstruction usually occur early.

The role and timing of tracheostomy in weaning

Tracheostomy is often performed in ICU patients for prolonged respiratory support or weaning. The introduction of bedside percutaneous techniques for placement has largely replaced the need to go to the operating room for this procedure. The perceived benefits to tracheostomy include: a more secure airway, easier transition on and off ventilation during weaning, easier communication for the patient, increased comfort, easier mouth care, earlier mobilization and decreased work of breathing. However tracheostomy is not without risks, which include: bleeding, wound infection, tracheal stenosis and occasionally death.

Traditionally, tracheostomy was considered after 10–14 days of ventilation. More recently the role of early tracheostomy has been explored.

- A systematic review in 2008 analyzed seven studies of early versus late tracheostomy and did not demonstrate any benefit to early tracheostomy in terms of short- or long-term mortality, ventilator-associated pneumonia or duration of mechanical ventilation [19].

- A recent large multicenter randomized controlled trial of early (less than 4 days of ventilation) or late (after 10 days) tracheostomy did not demonstrate any benefits in short- or long-term mortality or ICU length of stay. Where 92% of patients in the early group received a tracheostomy, only 45% of the late group required a tracheostomy [20].

In patients who require tracheostomy for prolonged weaning, the approach of progressive lengthening of trach-mask trials appears more effective for weaning than continued reduction of pressure support and then ventilator discontinuation [21].

Decannulation

When the patient's condition improves and they are tolerating significant periods off the ventilator, consideration may be given to downsizing the tracheostomy tube. There are now tracheostomy tubes with low profile cuffs that can be utilized throughout the weaning process and maintained in place until the patient is ready to be decannulated.

- With a smaller tube in place corking the tracheostomy may be better tolerated, allowing speech and evaluation of swallowing.
- When ventilation has been successfully discontinued and the patient no longer needs the tracheostomy for secretion clearance, the patient can be decannulated.
- An intermediate step of exchanging the cuffed tracheostomy tube for an uncuffed tube is not always necessary.

The stoma should be covered by a dry, occlusive dressing and allowed to heal spontaneously. Note that decannulation results in an increase in dead space, which can increase the WOB by more than 30% [22].

References

1. Boles JM, Bion J, Connors A, et al. Weaning from mechanical ventilation. Eur Respir J 2007; 29 : 1033–56.

2. Funk G-C, Anders S, Breyer M-K., et al. Incidence and outcome of weaning from mechanical ventilation according to new categories Eur Respir J 2010; 35 : 88–94.

3. Ely EW, Baker AM, Dunagan DP et al. Effect on the duration of mechanical ventilation of identifying patients capable of breathing spontaneously. N Engl J Med 1996;335 : 1864–9.

4. Frutos-Vivar F, Esteban A, Apezteguia C et al. Outcome of reintubated patients after scheduled extubation. J Crit Care 2011; 26 : 502–9.

5. Meade M, Guyatt G, Cook D et al. Predicting success in weaning from mechanical ventilation. Chest 2001; 120 : 400S–4S

6. Esteban A, Alía I, Tobin MJ, et al. Effect of spontaneous breathing trial duration on outcome of attempts to discontinue mechanical ventilation. Am J Respir Crit Care Med 1999; 159 : 512–18.

7. Brochard L, Rauss A, Benito S et al. Comparison of three methods of gradual withdrawal from ventilatory support during weaning from mechanical ventilation. Am J Respir Crit Care Med 1994; 150 : 896–903.

8. Esteban A, Frutos F, Tobin MJ et al. A comparison of four methods of weaning patients from mechanical ventilation. New Engl J Med 1995 332 : 345–50.

9. Penuelas O, Frutos-Vivar F, Fernandez C et al. Characteristics and outcomes of ventilated patients according to time to liberation from mechanical ventilation. Am J Respir Crit Care Med 2011; 184 : 430–7.

10. Blackwood B, Alderdice F, Burns K, Cardwell C. Use of weaning protocols for reducing duration of mechanical ventilation in critically ill adult patients: Cochrane systematic review and meta-analysis. BMJ 2011; 342: c7237.

11. Kress JP, Pohlman AS, O'Connor MF, Hall JB. Daily interruption of sedative infusions in critically ill patients undergoing mechanical ventilation. *N Engl J Med* 2000; 342 : 1471–7.

12. Girard TD, Kress JP, Fuchs BD, *et al.* Efficacy and safety of a paired sedation and ventilator weaning protocol for mechanically ventilated patients in intensive care (Awakening and Breathing Controlled trial): a randomised controlled trial. *Lancet* 2008; 371 : 126–34.

13. Schweickert WD, Pohlman MC, Pohlman AS *et al.* Early physical and occupational therapy in mechanically ventilated, critically ill patients: a randomised controlled trial. *Lancet* 2009; 373 : 1874–82.

14. Levine S, Nguyen T, Taylor N *et al.* Rapid disuse atrophy of diaphragm fibers in mechanically ventilated humans. *N Engl J Med* 2008; 358 : 1327–35.

15. Burns KEA, Adhikari NKJ, Meade MO. Noninvasive positive pressure ventilation as a weaning strategy for intubated adults with respiratory failure. *Can J Anaesth* 2006; 53 : 305–15.

16. Ram FS, Picot J, Lightowler J, Wedzicha JA. Non-invasive positive pressure ventilation for treatment of respiratory failure due to exacerbations of chronic obstructive pulmonary disease. *Cochrane Database Syst Rev* 2004; (1) : CD004104.

17. Keenan SP, Powers C, McCormack DG, Block G. Noninvasive positive-pressure ventilation for postextubation respiratory distress: a randomized controlled trial. *JAMA* 2002; 287 : 3238–44.

18. Esteban A, Frutos-Vivar F, Ferguson ND, Arabi Y, *et al.* Noninvasive positive-pressure ventilation for respiratory failure after extubation. *N Engl J Med* 2004; 350 : 2452–60

19. Wang F, Wu Y, Bo L, *et al.* The timing of tracheotomy in critically ill patients undergoing mechanical ventilation: a systematic review and meta-analysis of randomized controlled trials. *Chest* 2011; 140 : 1456–65.

20. Young D, Harrison DA, Cuthbertson BH *et al.* Effect of early vs late tracheostomy placement on survival in patients receiving mechanical ventilation the TracMan randomized trial. *JAMA.* 2013; 309 : 2121–9

21. Jubran A, Grant BJB, Duffner LA, *et al.* Effect of pressure support vs unassisted breathing through a tracheostomy collar on weaning duration in patients requiring prolonged mechanical ventilation. *JAMA* 2013; 309 : 671–7

22. Chadda K, Louis B, Benaissa L *et al.* Physiological effects of decannulation in tracheostomised patients. *Intens Care Med* 2002; 28 : 1761–7.

Chapter 15

Vasoactive drugs

Daniel H Ovakim

Many critically ill patients require cardiovascular support and, in addition to appropriate fluid resuscitation, vasoactive drugs are vital tools in achieving hemodynamic resuscitation targets aimed at:

- Improving oxygen delivery through optimizing cardiac output, organ blood flow and organ perfusion pressure.
- Augmenting catecholamine action, either directly by interacting with receptors found throughout the cardiovascular system or by inhibiting catecholamine metabolism.

In general:

- Vasopressors increase blood pressure, whereas inotropes increase cardiac output.
- Inodilators increase cardiac output, but cause peripheral vasodilation, which can lower blood pressure.
- Mixed agents, such as dopamine and epinephrine, increase both cardiac output and blood pressure.

Role of fluids:

- Intravascular volume repletion is crucial prior to initiation of vasopressors.
- Vasopressors are often ineffective and can result in an increased risk of adverse effects when used in the setting of inadequate intravascular volume.
- Whenever possible, vasopressors should be initiated only when fluid resuscitation fails to restore adequate pressure.

Structure of the autonomic nervous system

The autonomic nervous system is composed of the sympathetic and parasympathetic nervous systems.

- Sympathetic nervous system: comprised of the thoracolumbar outflow, characterized by short pre-ganglionic fibers and long post-ganglionic fibers.
- Parasympathetic nervous system: made up of the craniosacral outflow with long pre-ganglionic fibers and short post-ganglionic fibers that are typically located in close proximity to the target organ.

Handbook of ICU Therapy, third edition, ed. John Fuller, Jeff Granton and Ian McConachie. Published by Cambridge University Press. © Cambridge University Press 2015.

Neurotransmitters

- Acetylcholine is the primary mediator of both the sympathetic (pre-ganglionic) and parasympathetic (pre- and post-ganglionic) nervous systems.
- Sympathetic post-ganglionic neurons release norepinephrine, with the exception of sweat glands, where the primary neurotransmitter is acetylcholine.
- Epinephrine (adrenaline) is produced in the adrenal medulla, the central nervous system and the para-aortic bodies.

Receptor physiology

Adrenoreceptors

Adrenergic receptors (adrenoreceptors) are an integral part of the sympathetic nervous system. They are responsive to the endogenous catecholamines norepinephrine (noradrenaline) and epinephrine.

There are two main classes of adrenergic receptors, α and β, which have several subtypes.

Alpha receptors

- α_1 receptors are found primarily in blood vessels. Activation of these receptors leads to contraction of vascular smooth muscle resulting in vasoconstriction.
- α_2 receptors are located on the presynaptic nerve terminals, and mediate feedback inhibition of post-synaptic norepinephrine release by inhibiting pre-synaptic release of acetylcholine.
- Activation of post-synaptic peripheral α_2 receptors can result in vasoconstriction.

Beta receptors

- β_1 receptors are located in the heart and intestinal smooth muscle. Stimulation of these receptors results in positive inotropy and chronotropy. Other actions include stimulation of renin release from the juxtaglomerular apparatus of the kidney.
- β_2 receptors are found in bronchial, uterine, intestinal and vascular smooth muscle, and stimulation results in muscle relaxation, leading to bronchodilatation, relaxation of intestinal smooth muscle and vasodilation.
- The normal heart contains both β_1 and β_2 receptors at a ratio of 3:1. This ratio can be altered (3:2) in severe heart failure due to downregulation of β_1 receptors.

Receptor activity

The effects at adrenoreceptors are mediated via second messenger systems involving G-proteins, coupled to either adenylate cyclase (β receptors) or phospholipase C (α_1 receptors). The end result is phosphorylation of intracellular proteins that propagate and amplify the response to stimulation.

Agonism versus antagonism

- An agonist is any agent that either directly or indirectly stimulates a particular adrenoreceptor, thereby eliciting a pharmacologic response.
- An antagonist may occupy its target receptor, however does not elicit a response.

Dopaminergic receptors

There are two subtypes of dopaminergic receptors – D_1 and D_2. Both are present in the central nervous system (CNS) and at peripheral sites:

- D_1 receptors are found in vascular and mesenteric smooth muscle – stimulation leads to relaxation and subsequent vasodilation.
- Stimulation of dopaminergic receptors found in the renal and splanchnic beds results in increased renal and splanchnic blood flow, leading to diuresis and natriuresis.

Catecholamine metabolism

Catecholamine synthesis occurs in blood plasma via four enzymes [1].

1. Tyrosine hydroxylase converts tyrosine to DOPA (dihydroxyphenylalanine), which is the rate-limiting step in catecholamine synthesis. Sympathetic stimulation accelerates this process, whereas excess catecholamine inhibits it.
2. DOPA decarboxylase coverts DOPA to dopamine.
3. Dopamine-β-hydroxylase converts dopamine to norepinephrine.
4. Phenylethanolamine N-methyltransferase converts norepinephrine to epinephrine.

Once released, catecholamines are subject to reuptake into the post-synaptic neuron or they are metabolized by monoamine oxygenase (MAO) or catechol-O-methyltransferase (COM-T).

Vasopressors

The primary effects of vasopressors are to increase systemic vascular resistance (SVR) and mean arterial pressure (MAP). They also promote vasoconstriction in capacitance vessels, increasing venous return and cardiac output.

- Recent data also suggest that vasopressors may have a role in cardiogenic shock by improving coronary perfusion pressure [2].
- They can also be considered in hypovolemic or obstructive shock as a bridge to treating the underlying cause.

Details on the dosing and clinical effects of these agents are summarized in Table 15.1.

Norepinephrine

Endogenous norepinephrine (NE) is stored in neuronal vesicles [1].

- NE is predominantly used for its potent effect at α_1 receptors, leading to vasoconstriction and an increase in MAP.
- It also has activity at β_1 receptors, though less so than epinephrine, leading to a neutral effect on cardiac output, stroke volume and cardiac filling pressure.
- Reflex bradycardia in response to carotid baroreceptor stimulation overcomes the chronotropic effects of this agent.
- NE has a wide dose range, reflecting downregulation of α receptors with prolonged use
- NE is recommended as the first-line vasopressor in septic shock following an initial fluid challenge [3].

Table 15.1 Dosing, duration of action, receptor activity and clinical effect of vasoactive drugs

Vasoactive medication/ dosing	Dose	Duration of action (min)	Relative receptor activity				Hemodynamic effects			
			α_1	Dop	β_1	β_2	CO	HR	SVR	MAP
Vasopressors										
Norepinephrine (µg/min)	2–40	1–2	4+	−	2+	−	↔/↑	↔/↑	↑↑↑	↑↑↑
Vasopressin (units/min)	0.03	20[a]	-	−	−	−	↔/↑	↔	↑↑↑	↑↑↑
Phenylephrine (µg/min)	100–180	15–20	3+	−	−	−	↔/↑	↔/↓	↑↑	↑↑
Inotropic agents (inodilators)										
Dobutamine (µg/kg/min)	2–20	2–4	−/+	−	3+	+	↑↑↑	↑↑	↓↓	↔/↓
Milrinone (µg/kg/min); 50 µg/kg bolus	0.25–0.75	150[a b]	−	−	2+	+	↑↑↑	↑	↓↓	↓
Isoproterenol (µg/min)	2–10	10–15	-	-	3+	3+	↑↑	↑↑	↓	↓
Mixed agents										
Epinephrine (µg/min)	2–20	3–5	1+	−	4+	4+	↑↑↑	↑↑↑	↓	↔
Dopamine (µg/kg/min)	1–4	2–10	−	2+	−	−	↑	↑	↓	↔
	3–10		−/+	2+	2+	−	↑↑	↑↑	↑	↑
	10–20		2+	2+	3+	-	↔	↑↑	↑↑	↑↑
Hypotensive agents										
Nitroglycerin (µg/min)	2.5–50	1–4[a]	-	-	-	-	-	-	↓	↓
Nitroprusside (µg/kg/min)	0.3–2	1–10	-	-	-	-	-	-	↓	↓
Esmolol (mg/kg/min); 1.5 mg/kg load	0.15–0.3	9[a]	-	-	↓	-	↓	↓	↔/↓	↔/↓

[a] half-life
[b] prolonged in renal failure
1+–4+: relative potency of individual agents at named receptor, 4+ being the most potent, − = no activity at that receptor
CO: cardiac output
HR: heart rate
SVR: systemic vascular resistance
MAP: mean arterial pressure
↑: relative effect on individual physiologic parameter, ↑ representing mild increase, ↑↑↑ major increase, ↔ neutral or no effect, ↓ decrease.

- A recent study comparing norepinephrine to dopamine showed improved mortality when used as the initial vasopressor agent in cardiogenic shock [2].

Phenylephrine

Phenylephrine is a synthetic potent α_1 agonist, with almost no activity on β receptors. It is used primarily to correct vasodilation in volume-replete patients unresponsive to norepinephrine.

- Due to its potent vasoconstricting effects, phenylephrine can lead to a profound reflex bradycardia, as well as reduction in cardiac output.
- It may have a role in treating vasoplegia related to spinal shock or following cardio-pulmonary bypass, as well as in correcting tachyarrhythmia-related hypotension.

Ephedrine

- Ephedrine acts primarily on α- and β-adrenergic receptors, but with less potency. It also acts indirectly by facilitating release of endogenous norepinephrine.
- Ephedrine is primarily used in the setting of post-anesthesia-induced hypotension.

Vasopressin

Vasopressin is a naturally occurring compound synthesized in the hypothalamus and released from the posterior pituitary gland. It has both vasopressor and antidiuretic activity, mediated via vasopressin receptors (V_1 and V_2).

- V_2 receptors are located in the renal-collecting tubules and stimulation promotes water reabsorption.
- V_1 receptors are expressed in vascular smooth muscle and are responsible for vasoconstriction.
- It has been demonstrated that in early septic shock, the level of circulating vasopressin rises; however, during prolonged shock this level falls. It has been estimated that this relative deficiency is seen in a third of patients and may contribute to refractory hypotension [4].

The use of vasopressin should therefore be viewed in terms of replacing a relative deficiency, rather than exogenous administration.

- A low-dose vasopressin infusion may confer some benefit in these patients and allow withdrawal or reduction of catecholamines [5,6].
- The Vasopressin And Septic Shock Trial (VASST) demonstrated that a low-dose infusion of vasopressin (0.03 units/min) reduced mortality in patients with less severe septic shock (defined as requiring less than 15 µg/min norepinephrine on study enrollment), and confirmed that patients could be weaned off of norepinephrine earlier [7].
- Vasopressin should not be regarded as a titratable agent, rather, should be used at a fixed dose (0.02–0.04 units/min).

Complications of vasopressors

Moderate to high doses of vasopressors can have several adverse effects, including:

- Tachycardia in patients that are inadequately volume resuscitated.
- Coronary artery constriction precipitating ischemia and infarction.

- Increased afterload leading to myocardial dysfunction, decreased stroke volume and cardiac output
- Limb ischemia and necrosis
- Impairment of splanchnic blood flow, leading to ulceration, ileus, malabsorption and bowel infarction [8,9].

However, several recent findings may mitigate these concerns:

- In severe sepsis the use of norepinephrine improves splanchnic blood flow, oxygen delivery and oxygen uptake [9].
- In the normal mammalian circulation, norepinephrine infusion has been shown to improve renal and coronary blood flow [10].
- The addition of norepinephrine to patients unresponsive to dobutamine has been shown to increase cardiac output [11].

Inotropic agents (inodilators)

Inotropes are used to improve myocardial contractility, resulting in increased cardiac output (Table 15.1).

Dobutamine

Dobutamine is a synthetic catecholamine and potent β_1 agonist and weak β_2 agonist. It is a mixture of two isomers that are structurally similar to epinephrine.

- The D-isomer is a potent β_1 and β_2 agonist; however, it also has α_1 antagonist effect.
- The L-isomer has primarily β_1 activity, though it possesses some α_1 agonist activity.

The primary effect of dobutamine is via β_1 receptor agonism, leading to increased cardiac output by augmenting contractility and stroke volume, which may in part be due to improved ventricular compliance [11,12]. Stimulation of $\beta2$ receptors leads to peripheral vasodilation.

- The dose-dependent increase in cardiac output with dobutamine is often accompanied by a proportional decrease in SVR, resulting in lowering of blood pressure. Adverse effects on blood pressure are more likely in patients with inadequate intravascular volume.
- Dobutamine increases cardiac workload and myocardial O_2 consumption, which can stress an already stressed myocardium [13].Through increased cardiac output, dobutamine may exert a beneficial effect on renal function [14].
- Dobutamine can result in dose-limiting tachyarrhythmias and ventricular ectopy.
- Dobutamine is a first-line agent in the management of cardiogenic shock, and myocardial dysfunction in the setting of septic shock.
- As a single agent, it is best reserved for patients without severe hypotension.
- In hypotensive patients, dobutamine can be used in combination with a vasopressor, such as norepinephrine, which may improve coronary perfusion pressure [2,15].

Milrinone

Milrinone is a synthetic phosphodiesterase-3 inhibitor, which acts to increase intracellular cAMP, producing inotropy independent of the β adrenergic receptor.

- Milrinone also enhances ventricular relaxation (lusitropy), which may lead to improved coronary perfusion.
- Milrinone has no reported effect on myocardial O_2 consumption [13].
- Milrinone also increases cAMP in vascular smooth muscle, promoting vasodilation, which can lead to hypotension, more so in patients with inadequate intravascular volume [13].
- Milrinone has a significantly longer half-life compared to catecholamines, which is further prolonged in the setting of renal dysfunction.
- Milrinone is used primarily in cardiogenic shock, particularly when other agents, and conservative measures (diuresis, nitrates) have failed.
- Prolonged use of milrinone requires caution, as an earlier study demonstrated an increase in hypotension and a nonsignificant increase in mortality in patients receiving more than 48 h of milrinone, a finding that may be worse in patients with ischemic cardiomyopathy [16].
- Other phospodiesterase inhibitors have been used in Europe, e.g. enoximone. Its effects are similar to those of milrinone.

Isoproterenol

Isoproterenol (Isuprel) is primarily an inotropic and chronotropic agent.

- Similar to dobutamine, it acts upon β_1 and β_2 adrenergic receptors; however, unlike dobutamine it has a stronger chronotropic effect and higher affinity for β_2 receptors, leading to pronounced hypotension.
- It is primarily used in patients with hypotension related to bradycardia.

Mixed agents

Mixed agents possess characteristics of both vasopressors and inotropes. The major agents in this class include epinephrine and dopamine (Table 15.1).

Epinephrine

Epinephrine is the major endogenous sympathomimetic agent. It is synthesized, stored and released from the chromaffin cells of the adrenal medulla.

It is active at all adrenoreceptors and infusion results in an increase in cardiac output and blood pressure with an accompanying tachycardia.

The use of epinephrine as a single agent is attractive; however, there are potential serious side effects associated with its use:

- It has potent dysrhythmogenic effects.
- It increases cardiac workload, which may result in myocardial ischemia.
- Though the use of epinephrine has been shown to reduce splanchnic blood flow [8,17], there is no clinical evidence that the use of epinephrine results in adverse clinical outcomes [15,18,19].
- Administration of epinephrine may lead to lactic acidosis in patients with severe sepsis, which may result from reduction in hepatic blood flow or direct stimulation of skeletal muscle β2 adrenergic receptors [20].
- Metabolic disturbances such as hyperglycemia and hypokalemia can occur.

In the most recent iteration of the surviving sepsis guidelines, epinephrine is recommended as a second-line agent for the treatment of sepsis-induced hypotension unresponsive to fluid resuscitation and norepinephrine [3].

Epinephrine remains the agent of choice in the cardiac arrest situation and in the treatment of anaphylaxis.

Dopamine

Dopamine acts at α, β and dopaminergic receptors, with the specific receptor activity varying depending on dose.

- Traditional teaching is that at low doses (<5μg/kg/min) dopaminergic effects predominate, leading to improved renal blood flow. The β and α effects, seen at concentrations of 5–10 μg/kg/min and >10 μg/kg/min, respectively, allow the drug to be used as an inotrope and a vasopressor.
- Individual variation does not often allow for prediction of effects at a given dose. In addition, the clearance of dopamine is reduced in critically ill patients, further diminishing the precision of targeting a particular dose to effect [21] and only serves to increase the risk of adverse effects.
- A recent trial comparing dopamine to norepinephrine in patients with shock demonstrated an increase in the number of adverse events for patients that received dopamine. In the subset of patients with cardiogenic shock, dopamine was associated with a significant increase in mortality [2].
- Two recent meta-analyses examining the use of dopamine in septic shock demonstrated that the use of dopamine was associated with an increased risk of mortality and higher risk of cardiac arrhythmia when compared to norepinephrine [22,23].

Based on this information, there is almost no justification to use dopamine in a critically ill patient population [24]. However, dopamine continues to be in widespread use, with many perceiving it as relatively safe [25].

Adverse effects of dopamine

- Use at moderate to high doses is often complicated by tachycardia and tachyarrhythmias.
- There is evidence to suggest harmful effects of dopamine on neuro-endocrine function, with infusions inhibiting prolactin, growth hormone and thyroid-stimulating hormone release [26].
- Dopamine has immunosuppressive effects though the inhibition of T-cell proliferation [27].
- Dopamine may also reduce gastric mucosal perfusion in septic patients [28].

"Renal-dose" dopamine

Historically, low (renal)-dose dopamine was used for the prevention and treatment of acute renal failure.

- Although both diuresis and natriuresis can be demonstrated following dopamine administration, the increase in urinary flow likely results from improved renal blood flow secondary to an increased cardiac output.

- Despite the often firm belief in the concept of "renal-dose dopamine," there is substantial evidence against this claim [29–31].

Dopexamine

Dopexamine is a relatively new drug with primarily β_2 agonist activity. It is a synthetic analog of dopamine and also demonstrates agonism at dopaminergic receptors.

- Dopexamine has primarily been tested in clinical trials of perioperative optimization, thus there is limited evidence to support its use as an alternative to currently available agents [32–34].
- A recent animal study has suggested that dopexamine may exert an anti-inflammatory effect and confer protection against endotoxemia-related multiorgan failure, independent of any hemodynamic alteration [35].
- The suggested mechanism for such an effect is the different effect of adrenoceptor stimulation on the inflammatory response, β_1 stimulation being proinflammatory, while β_2 and α_1 stimulation are anti-inflammatory [36]. This adds a whole new dimension to a debate on choice of inotropic drug! Studies showing significant effects on clinical outcome are, however, lacking.

Hypotensive agents

There are several clinical situations in which a patient will require acute lowering of their blood pressure:

- Obstetrical patient with severe gestational hypertension (pre-eclampsia).
- Malignant hypertension/hypertensive emergency.
- Intracranial hemorrhage requiring precise blood pressure control.

Therapy is directed at rapidly lowering blood pressure to minimize end-organ damage. Commonly used agents are detailed below.

Directly acting vasodilators

Nitroglycerin (NTG)

Predominantly causes venodilation resulting in reduced preload (Table 15.1). Useful in patients with myocardial ischemia and ventricular failure. Given by intravenous (IV) infusion.

Hydralazine

Direct arteriodilator. Can be given orally or administered IV as a bolus (10–20 mg every 1–2 hours) or infusion. Mainstay in the treatment of pregnancy-induced hypertension, though applicable to many clinical scenarios.

Sodium nitroprusside

Arterio- and venodilator that acts by stabilizing smooth-muscle membrane. Infusion leads to compensatory tachycardia, as well as worsening of V/Q mismatch due to intrapulmonary shunting, resulting in oxygen desaturation.
Caution with prolonged use re: cyanide toxicity.

Adrenergic receptor antagonists

Labetalol

Acts at α_1 and β receptors, the latter predominating, especially on intravenous administration. Easily titratable; useful in obstetric hypertensive emergencies.

Esmolol

Rapidly acting, selective β_1 blocker. Its extremely short life (9 minutes) makes it eminently suitable for IV infusion.

Phentolamine

Competitive α blocker used in the treatment of hypertension associated with pheochromocytoma.

Summary and general points

- Inotropic agents increase cardiac output.
- MAP will usually increase as a secondary effect.
- Choice of vasoactive drug depends on the goals of therapy.
- Match the mechanism of action of a drug with the desired therapeutic goal.
- Consider the agent (or combination of agents) that best addresses the abnormality that needs to be corrected.
- Choice of agent depends on the pharmacology of the agents, and effect on α and β receptors.
- When titrating vasopressor doses, the commonly suggested target MAP is 65 mmHg, though a higher target can be used in patients with baseline hypertension.
- Regardless of the initial agent chosen, the dose should be titrated to effect (blood pressure or marker of end-organ perfusion). Additional agents can be added if the initial agent fails to reach target.
- Drug responsiveness diminishes over time, requiring constant dose titration and adjustment.
- Prolonged exposure (>72 h) to inotropic agents leads to a downregulation of β_1 receptors, necessitating dose titration, which does necessarily indicate deterioration in the patient's condition.
- With the exception of vasopressin and milrinone, vasoactive drugs are rapidly acting with a short half-life (Table 15.1), making them easily titratable and weanable, depending on attainment of desired endpoints.
- Whenever possible, drugs with α adrenergic affects should be only given into a central vein, as extravasation can lead to tissue necrosis.
- Appropriate monitoring should be in place prior to the commencement of any infusions.
- Patients on high doses of single or multiple agents may be significantly sensitive to even brief interruptions of the infusion. Starting a new infusion shortly before the near-empty syringe or bag runs out can minimize this risk.

References

1. Wesfall TC, Westfall DP. Neurotransmission. The autonomic and somatic motor nervous sytems. In: Brunton LL, Lazo, JS, Parker KL, editors. *Goodman and Gilman's The Pharmacological Basis of Therapeutics*, 11th edn. New York: McGraw-Hill; 2006 : 137–77.

2. De Backer D, Biston P, Devriendt J et al. Comparison of dopamine and norepinephrine in the treatment of shock. *N Engl J Med* 2010; 362 : 779–89.

3. Dellinger RP, Levy MM, Rhodes A et al. Surviving Sepsis Campaign: International guidelines for management of severe sepsis and septic shock: 2012. *Crit Care Med* 2013; 41 : 580–637.

4. Sharshar T, Blanchard A, Paillard M et al. Circulating vasopressin levels in septic shock. *Crit Care Med* 2003; 31 : 1752–8.

5. Malay MB, Ashton Jr RC, Landry DW, Townsend RN. Low-dose vasopressin in the treatment of vasodilatory septic shock. *J Trauma* 1999; 47 : 699–703.

6. Patel BM, Chittock DR, Russell JA, Walley KR. Beneficial effects of short term vasopressin infusion during severe septic shock. *Anaesthesiology* 2002; 96 : 576–82.

7. Russell JA, Walley KR, Singer J et al. Vasopressin versus norepinephrine infusion in patients with septic shock. *N Engl J Med* 2008; 358 : 877–87.

8. De Backer D, Creteur J, Silva E, Vincent J-L. Effects of dopamine, norepinephrine, and epinephrine on the splanchnic circulation in septic shock: Which is best? *Crit Care Med* 2003; 31 : 1659–7.

9. Meier-Hellmann A, Specht M, Hannemann L et al. Splanchnic flow is greater in septic shock treated with norepinephrine than in severe sepsis. *Int Care Med* 1996; 22 : 1354–9.

10. Di Giantomasso D, May CN, Bellomo R. Norepinephrine and vital organ blood flow. *Int Care Med* 2002; 28: 1804–9.

11. Martin C, Viviand X, Arnaud S et al. Effects of norepinephrine plus dobutamine or norepinephrine alone on left ventricular performance of septic shock patients. *Crit Care Med* 1999; 7 : 1708–13.

12. Pawha R, Anel R, Alahdad MT et al. Cardiovascular response to dobutamine in septic shock. *Crit Care Med* 1999; 27 : A136.

13. Bayram M, De Luca L, Massie B, Gheorghiade M. Reassessment of dobutamine, dopamine, and milrinone in the management of acute heart failure syndromes. *Am J Cardiol* 2005; 96 (Suppl) : 47–58.

14. Duke DJ, Briedis JH, Weaver RA. Renal support in critically ill patients: low-dose dopamine or low-dose dobutamine? *Crit Care Med* 1994; 22 : 1893–4.

15. Annane D, Vignon P, Renault A et al. Norepinephrine plus dobutamine versus epinephrine alone for management of septic shock: a randomized trial. *Lancet* 2007; 370 : 676–84.

16. Cuffe MS, Califf RM, Adams KF Jr et al. Short-term intravenous milrinone for acute exacerbation of chronic heart failure. A randomized controlled trial. *JAMA* 2002; 287 : 1541–47.

17. Meier-Hellman A, Reinhart K, Bredle DL et al. Epinephrine impairs splanchnic perfusion in septic shock. *Crit Care Med* 1997; 25 : 399–404.

18. Myburg JA, Higgins A, Jovanovska A et al. A comparison of epinephrine and norepinephrine in critically ill patients. *Int Care Med* 2008; 34 : 2226–34.

19. Seguin P, Bellissant E, Le Tulzo Y et al. Effects of epinephrine compared with the combination of dobutamine and norepinephrine on gastric perfusion in septic shock. *Clin Pharmacol Ther* 2002; 71 : 381–8.

20. Day NP, Phu NH, Bethell DP et al. The effects of dopamine and adrenaline infusions on acid–base balance and systemic haemodynamics in severe infections. *Lancet* 1996; 348 : 219–223.

21. Juste RN, Moran L, Hooper J, Soni N. Dopamine clearance in critically ill patients. *Int Care Med* 1998; 24 : 1217–20.

22. De Backer D, Aldecoa C, Njimi H, Vincent JL. Dopamine versus norepinephrine in the treatment of septic shock: a meta-analysis. *Crit Care Med* 2012; 40 : 725–30.

23. Vasu TS, Cavallazzi R, Hirani A *et al.* Norepinephrine or dopamine for septic shock: a systematic review of randomized controlled trials. *J Intensive Care Med* 2012; 27 : 172–8.

24. Holmes CL, Walley KR. Bad medicine: low-dose dopamine in the ICU. *Chest* 2003; 123 : 1266–75.

25. Sakr Y, Reinhart K, Vincent JL *et al.* Does dopamine administration in shock influence outcome? Results of the Sepsis Occurrence in Acutely Ill Patients (SOAP) Study. *Crit Care Med* 2006; 34 : 589–97.

26. Van den Berghe G, de Zegher F. Anterior pituitary function during critical illness and dopamine treatment. *Crit Care Med* 1996; 24 : 1580–90.

27. Devins SS, Miller A, Herndon BL *et al.* Effects of dopamine on T-lymphocyte proliferative responses and serum prolactin concentrations in critically ill patients. *Crit Care Med* 1992; 20 : 1644–9.

28. Neviere R, Mathieu D, Chagnon JL *et al.* The contrasting effects of dobutamine and dopamine on gastric mucosal perfusion in septic patients. *Am J Resp and Crit Care Med* 1996; 154 : 1684–8.

29. Bellomo R, Chapman M, Finfer S *et al.* Low dose dopamine in patients with early renal dysfunction: a placebo-controlled randomised trial. Australian and New Zealand Intensive Care Society (ANZICS) Clinical Trials Group. *Lancet* 2000; 356 : 2139–43.

30. Kellum JA, Decker JM. Use of dopamine in acute renal failure: a meta-analysis. *Crit Care Med* 2001; 29 : 1526–31.

31. Marik PE. Low-dose dopamine: a systematic review. *Int Care Med* 2002; 28 : 877–3.

32. Wilson J, Woods I, Fawcett J *et al.* Reducing the risk of major elective surgery: a randomised controlled trial of preoperative optimisation of oxygen delivery. *Br Med J* 1999; 318 : 1099–103.

33. Takala J, Meier-Hellmann A, Eddleston J *et al.* Effect of dopexamine on outcome after major abdominal surgery: a prospective randomized, controlled multicenter study. *Crit Care Med* 2000; 28 : 3417–23.

34. Stone MD, Wilson RJT, Cross J, Williams BT. Effect of adding dopexamine to intraoperative volume expansion in patients undergoing major elective surgery. *Br J Anaesth* 2003; 91 : 619–24

35. Bangash MN, Patel NSA, Benetti E *et al.* Dopexamine can attenuate the inflammatory response and protect against organ injury in the absence of significant effects on hemodynamics or regional microvascular flow. *Crit Care* 2013; 17 : R57–67.

36. Uusaro A, Russell JA. Could anti-inflammatory actions of catecholamines explain the possible beneficial effects of supranormal oxygen delivery in critically ill surgical patients ? *Intensive Care Med* 2000; 26 : 299–304.

Chapter

16

Optimizing antimicrobial therapy in the ICU

Stephen Y Liang and Anand Kumar

Introduction

- Infections are common among intensive care unit (ICU) patients. On any given day, up to 70% of ICU patients receive antimicrobials for treatment of or prophylaxis against infection [1].
- Appropriate and timely administration of antimicrobial therapy in the ICU reduces morbidity and mortality in patients with serious infections, particularly when complicated by severe sepsis or septic shock [2,3].
- In view of growing antimicrobial resistance worldwide, with fewer and fewer novel agents in development, optimal use of existing antimicrobials is imperative in critically ill patients.

Approach to infection in the critically ill patient

- The decision to initiate antimicrobial therapy should rest upon a reasonable clinical suspicion for infection, buttressed by a thorough diagnostic evaluation.
- The respiratory tract, abdomen, bloodstream and genitourinary system are the most common sites of infection in patients admitted to the ICU [1]. Soft-tissue infections are also common, but are frequently missed in the early stages.
- In patients that have undergone invasive procedures or prolonged hospitalization, healthcare-associated infections (e.g. central-line-associated bloodstream infection, ventilator-associated pneumonia, catheter-associated urinary tract infection, surgical-site infection, decubitus ulcers and *Clostridium difficile* infection) must also be considered.
- Fever is a common presentation of infection, although it may be blunted or absent in the elderly, the immunocompromised, burn victims and patients receiving renal replacement therapy. It is important to remember that thromboembolic disease (e.g. deep-vein thrombosis, pulmonary embolus), medications, transfusion-related reactions, adrenal insufficiency, certain malignancies and a host of other noninfectious processes may also manifest as fever in the ICU.
- An initial laboratory investigation should include a complete blood count with differential, metabolic panel, liver function test, coagulation studies and urinalysis. HIV testing is recommended in high-risk populations.
- Whenever possible, microbiological cultures from probable sites of infection (e.g. blood, urine, sputum, wound) should be obtained before initiating antimicrobials to maximize yield and guide therapy. Depending on clinical suspicion, invasive procedures such as

Handbook of ICU Therapy, third edition, ed. John Fuller, Jeff Granton and Ian McConachie. Published by Cambridge University Press. © Cambridge University Press 2015.

lumbar puncture, thoracentesis or paracentesis should be performed to secure cultures and rule out infection. However, antimicrobial therapy should never be delayed in an unstable patient to obtain cultures. This is particularly true for suspected meningitis, rapidly progressive necrotizing infections and septic shock.

- If a central-line-associated bloodstream infection (CLABSI) is suspected, at least one blood culture should be drawn through the infected catheter and one culture from a peripheral site. The offending catheter should be removed and the catheter tip sent for culture in the setting of sepsis, septic thrombophlebitis or tunnel infection.
- If ventilator-associated pneumonia (VAP) is suspected, bronchoscopy with broncheoalveolar lavage may be considered to more accurately culture the lower respiratory tract.
- If a catheter-associated urinary tract infection (CAUTI) is suspected, urinalysis and urine culture should be obtained from the sampling port of the catheter and not from the collection bag. An infected urinary catheter should be removed immediately.

- *Clostridium difficile* infection should always be on the differential of any ICU patient presenting with diarrhea, ileus or toxic megacolon, particularly in the setting of leukocytosis and recent antibiotic exposure. A stool specimen should be sent for *C. difficile* toxin by immunoassay or polymerase chain reaction.
- Effective source control (i.e. drainage of infected fluid collections, debridement of infected or necrotic tissue, removal of infected hardware, catheters or other medical devices) is crucial to ensuring the success of antimicrobial therapy.

Principles of antimicrobial therapy

The optimization of antimicrobial therapy in the ICU can be challenging. While *in vitro* antimicrobial susceptibilities of an infecting microorganism may serve as a logical starting point for selecting appropriate therapy, hemodynamic instability, immunocompromised states, and frequent multiorgan dysfunction resulting in altered drug metabolism and clearance *in vivo* often conspire to complicate the situation. Inadequate antimicrobial therapy not only fosters resistance, but also increases morbidity and mortality risk.

A rational approach to antimicrobial therapy in critical illness should encompass the following aspects:

- Appropriate spectrum of coverage
- Pharmacokinetics and pharmacodynamics
- Adequate dosing to sustain activity
- Drug toxicity
- Early administration
- Periodic reassessment of effect.

Multidisciplinary involvement of critical care pharmacists and infectious disease specialists can further enhance antimicrobial prescribing in ICU and improve patient outcomes [4,5].

Determining the spectrum of coverage

The appropriate spectrum of antimicrobial coverage should be determined in the context of risk of major adverse consequences in case of error. Broader coverage is mandated in life-threatening infections such as septic shock, where inappropriate therapy substantially increases the risk of death [6]. Empiric antimicrobial coverage is often necessary in the ICU, given that a causative pathogen is seldom known at the time of presentation.

- Initial antibiotic selection should be guided by a determination of community-acquired versus healthcare-associated infection, with an added emphasis in the latter on coverage of multidrug-resistant organisms (e.g. methicillin-resistant *Staphylococcus aureus*, vancomycin-resistant enterococcus, multidrug-resistant Gram-negative bacilli).
- Chronic comorbid diseases (e.g. diabetes mellitus, chronic kidney disease, chronic obstructive pulmonary disease) and immunocompromised states (e.g. human immunodeficiency virus infection, malignancy, solid organ or bone marrow transplantation, chronic corticosteroid use) may also factor into empiric coverage of specific organisms (e.g. *Pseudomonas aeruginosa*), as well as multidrug-resistant organisms associated with frequent healthcare exposure.

In general, critical illness warrants broad-spectrum coverage of Gram-positive and Gram-negative organisms, with one or more antibiotics to maximize the likelihood of treating the causative microorganism on initial presentation (Table 16.1).

- Empiric Gram-positive coverage (including methicillin-resistant *S. aureus*) is often achieved using vancomycin. Alternative agents may include daptomycin (if the infection is nonpulmonary), linezolid or ceftaroline.
- If *P. aeruginosa* infection is not suspected, empiric Gram-negative coverage may consist of a third-generation cephalosporin (ceftriaxone, cefotaxime), β-lactam/β-lactamase inhibitor (e.g. piperacillin-tazobactam) or carbapenem (e.g. meropenem, imipenem).
- If *P. aeruginosa* infection is suspected, an antipseudomonal cephalosporin (cefepime, ceftazidime), β-lactam/β-lactamase inhibitor (e.g. piperacillin-tazobactam), carbapenem (meropenem, imipenem), monobactam (aztreonam), fluoroquinolone (ciprofloxacin), or aminoglycoside (e.g. gentamicin) is appropriate.

In certain high-risk populations, antifungal coverage may be indicated (Table 16.2).

- Risk factors for candidemia include central venous catheters, total parenteral nutrition, hemodialysis, prior broad-spectrum antibiotics, gastrointestinal procedures and immunocompromised states, including neutropenia [7,8].
- Initial antifungal therapy with an echinocandin (micafungin, caspofungin, anidulafungin) provides broad coverage of *Candida albicans* and non-*albicans* species in critical illness [9]. Alternatives may include a lipid formulation of amphotericin B or voriconazole.

Combination empiric therapy using antibiotics with different mechanisms of action is associated with decreased mortality in severe sepsis and septic shock [6,10–13], likely attributable to an extended spectrum of coverage, as well as synergistic effects, at least in some circumstances (e.g. septic shock).

- Empiric double coverage of *Pseudomonas aeruginosa* and other Gram-negative infections remains controversial and should be reserved for patients with neutropenia or serious infection (pneumonia, meningitis, endocarditis, bacteremia) at high risk for multidrug-resistant organisms [14]. Septic shock is another emerging situation where data suggests that targeted combination therapy can improve outcome [11,12].

Table 16.1 Common antibiotics used in critical care

Antibiotic/dose	Spectrum	Lipophilicity	PK/PD	Toxicity	Dosing considerations
Piperacillin/tazobactam 3.375 g IV q6 hrs 4.5 g IV q6 hrs (P. aeruginosa)	Streptococci, MSSA, ampicillin-sensitive enterococcus, Gram-negatives (including P. aeruginosa at higher dose), anaerobes	Hydrophilic	T > MIC	Interstitial nephritis, ↓Hgb, ↓WBC, ↓platelets	Adjust dose based on CrCl
Ampicillin/sulbactam 1.5–3.0 g IV q6 hrs	Streptococci, MSSA, Gram-negatives (excluding P. aeruginosa), anaerobes	Hydrophilic	T > MIC	Interstitial nephritis, ↓Hgb, ↓WBC, ↓platelets	Adjust dose based on CrCl
Ceftriaxone 1–2 g IV q12–24 hrs	Streptococci, MSSA, Gram-negatives (excluding P. aeruginosa)	Hydrophilic	T > MIC	↑AST and ALT, ↑bilirubin, biliary sludging, ↓Hgb, ↓WBC	No dose adjustment necessary in renal or hepatic impairment
Cefepime 1–2 g IV q8 hrs	Streptococci, MSSA, Gram-negatives (including P. aeruginosa)	Hydrophilic	T > MIC	Seizure, encephalopathy (elderly, renal impairment), ↑AST and ALT, ↓Hgb, ↓WBC	Adjust dose based on CrCl
Ceftaroline 600 mg IV q12 hrs	Streptococci, MSSA, MRSA, Gram-negatives (excluding P. aeruginosa)	Hydrophilic	T > MIC	↑AST and ALT, ↓Hgb, ↓WBC	Adjust dose based on CrCl
Meropenem 500 mg IV q6 hrs or 1 g IV q8 hrs	Streptococci, MSSA, Gram-negatives (including P. aeruginosa and ESBL-producing organisms), anaerobes	Hydrophilic	T > MIC	Seizure, ↑AST and ALT, ↓Hgb, ↓WBC	Adjust dose based on CrCl
Vancomycin [23] 15 mg/kg IV q12 hrs (starting dose)	Streptococci, MSSA, MRSA, enterococci (excluding VRE)	Hydrophilic	AUC/MIC	Nephrotoxicity, ototoxicity, red man syndrome, ↓WBC, ↓platelets	Adjust dose based on CrCl Check trough prior to 3rd or 4th dose (goal: 15–20 µg/mL for serious infections)

Drug/Dose	Coverage	Property	PK/PD	Adverse effects	Dose adjustment
Linezolid 600 mg PO/IV q12 hrs	Streptococci, MSSA, MRSA, enterococci (including VRE)	Lipophilic	T > MIC AUC/MIC	↓WBC, ↓platelets, serotonin syndrome (if pt on an SSRI or MAOI)	No dose adjustment necessary in renal or hepatic impairment
Daptomycin 4–6 mg/kg IV q24 hrs	Streptococci, MSSA, MRSA, enterococci (including VRE)	Hydrophilic	C_{max}/MIC	↑CPK, rhabdomyolysis, eosinophilic pneumonia	Adjust dose based on CrCl
Tigecycline 100 mg IV loading dose, then 50 mg IV q12 hrs	Streptococci, MSSA, MRSA, enterococci (including VRE), Gram-negatives (excluding *P. aeruginosa*), anaerobes	Lipophilic	AUC/MIC	Nausea, vomiting, acute pancreatitis	Adjust dose based on hepatic function; no dose adjustment necessary in renal impairment
Ciprofloxacin 400 mg IV q12 hrs 400 mg IV q8 hrs (*P. aeruginosa*)	Gram-negatives (including *P. aeruginosa* with q8 hr dosing)	Lipophilic	C_{max}/MIC AUC/MIC	Seizure, QT prolongation, tendon rupture, multiple drug interactions (including warfarin), avoid in myasthenia gravis	Adjust dose based on CrCl
Gentamicin/ tobramycin [34,35] *Traditional dose:* 2 mg/kg IV q12 hrs *Extended-interval dose:* 5 mg/kg IV q24 hrs	Gram-negatives (including *P. aeruginosa*), enterococci (when combined with penicillin or vancomycin for synergy)	Hydrophilic	C_{max}/MIC	Nephrotoxicity, ototoxicity	Adjust dose based on CrCl *Traditional dose:* check peak (goal: 8–10 µg/mL in serious infection) and trough (goal: <1 µg/mL) with 3rd or 4th dose *Extended-interval dose:* check drug concentration 6–14 hours after 1st dose and adjust dosing interval using nomogram [34]

ESBL: extended-spectrum β-lactamase; MAOI: monoamine oxidase inhibitor; MRSA: methicillin-resistant *Staphylococcus aureus*; MSSA: methicillin-sensitive *Staphylococcus aureus*; SSRI: selective serotonin reuptake inhibitor; VRE: vancomycin-resistant enterococcus.

Table 16.2 Common antifungals used in critical care

Antibiotic/dose	Spectrum[a]	Lipophilicity	PK/PD	Toxicity	Dosing considerations
Micafungin[b] 100 mg IV q24 hrs	Candida albicans, non-albicans Candida spp (C. glabrata, C. krusei, C. parapsilosis, C. tropicalis), Aspergillus spp	Water-soluble, lipophilic	C_{max}/MIC AUC/MIC	↑AST and ALT	No dose adjustment necessary in renal or hepatic impairment
Voriconazole 6 mg/kg IV q12 hrs × 2 loading doses, then 4 mg/kg IV q12 hrs or 200–300 mg PO q12 hrs	Most Candida spp, Aspergillus spp, Fusarium spp, Scedosporium apiospermum	Lipophilic	AUC/MIC	Visual disturbances, ↑AST and ALT, pancreatitis, QT prolongation, multiple drug interactions	Avoid IV if CrCl <50 mL/min (PO route preferred); adjust dose based on hepatic function
Fluconazole 800 mg IV loading dose, then 400 mg IV q24 hrs	C. albicans, non-albicans Candida spp (C. parapsilosis, C. tropicalis)	Weakly lipophilic	AUC/MIC	↑AST and ALT, QT prolongation, multiple drug interactions	Adjust dose based on CrCl
Liposomal amphotericin B 3–5 mg/kg IV q24 hrs	Most Candida spp, Aspergillus spp, Fusarium spp, Zygomycetes (e.g. Mucor)	Lipophilic	C_{max}/MIC AUC/MIC	Nephrotoxicity, infusion-related reactions, ↓K^+, ↓Mg^{2+}	No dose adjustment necessary in renal or hepatic impairment

[a] Antifungal susceptibilities should always be confirmed by in vitro assessment of mean inhibitory concentration.
[b] Other echinocandins, depending on institutional availability, include caspofungin and anidulafungin. While the dosing of these agents differs, spectrum, lipophilicity, PK/PD, toxicity, and dosing considerations are similar to that of micafungin.

When available, institutional antibiograms can help shape empiric therapy by providing local antimicrobial susceptibility patterns of commonly encountered microorganisms.

When a pathogen is identified, the spectrum of antimicrobial therapy should be narrowed, based on susceptibility testing and clinical response.

Understanding pharmacokinetics and pharmacodynamics

Pharmacokinetics (PK) is the study of how absorption, distribution and clearance (e.g. metabolism, excretion) of an administered antimicrobial affects drug concentrations in the host over time.

Absorption from the gastrointestinal tract in a critically ill patient is often poor due to diminished gut perfusion, bowel edema or ileus. Therefore, intravenous drug administration is favored in the ICU to achieve consistent and therapeutic drug levels.

Antimicrobial penetration of tissues can differ from organ to organ, leading to variable *distribution* that may be further impaired in critical illness.

- Adequate drug concentrations are often readily attained in highly vascular structures such as the lung, pleura, peritoneum and synovial joints.
- The blood–brain barrier can present a significant obstacle to achieving adequate drug levels in the central nervous system. High plasma drug concentrations are often necessary to ensure adequate levels in the cerebrospinal fluid.
- Penetration into avascular targets, including abscesses and necrotic tissue, is generally poor and requires surgical drainage or debridement. Likewise, vascular insufficiency may also present a challenge to adequate drug delivery to infected tissues.
- Impaired tissue perfusion secondary to severe sepsis and septic shock may also result in lower drug concentrations in target tissues.

Distribution of antimicrobials is further influenced by patient size, fat composition and tissue edema.

- Apparent *volume of distribution* (V_d) is defined as the total amount of drug administered (D) divided by the plasma drug concentration (C), and describes the relative theoretical distribution of a drug within body compartments.
- Interstitial third-spacing secondary to increased capillary permeability in sepsis coupled with aggressive fluid resuscitation can increase the V_d for hydrophilic antimicrobials (e.g. β-lactams, carbapenems, glycopeptides, linezolid, aminoglycosides), leading to lower tissue and plasma drug concentrations [15]. The same is seen in other conditions associated with increased interstitial volume, including cirrhosis, renal failure, congestive heart failure and trauma.
- Hypoalbuminemia may increase the V_d for highly protein-bound antimicrobials (e.g. ceftriaxone, ertapenem), leading to lower tissue and plasma concentrations in the setting of increased interstitial volume.
- Lipophilic antimicrobials (e.g. fluoroquinolones, macrolides, clindamycin, tigecycline) possess a high V_d at baseline and are less affected by increased interstitial volume.

Clearance is defined as the volume of blood cleared of drug per unit time. It represents the elimination of a drug through glomerular filtration and/or hepatic metabolism.

- Many critically ill patients develop acute kidney injury, which can lead to impaired drug clearance and high plasma drug concentrations.

- Renal clearance of antimicrobials may also be augmented in sepsis due to increased cardiac output and renal blood flow, leading to lower plasma drug concentrations. Higher or more frequent antimicrobial dosing may be necessary.
- Acute liver injury in sepsis may result in impaired hepatic metabolism and clearance of certain antimicrobials, requiring dose adjustment.

Pharmacodynamics (PD) is the study of how drug concentrations impact the host, and more importantly, the infecting microorganism.

The minimum inhibitory concentration (MIC) is the lowest concentration of an antimicrobial necessary to inhibit bacterial growth *in vitro*. It is a measure of pathogen response to a static concentration of antimicrobial, as opposed to the variable concentrations achieved in clinical practice with intermittent dosing.

- A microorganism is considered susceptible to an antimicrobial if the MIC is 1/16 to 1/4 of the peak achievable serum concentration (or urine concentration if the pathogen is urinary).
- A susceptible MIC can be misleading, particularly if antimicrobial concentrations at target sites (e.g. cerebrospinal fluid, biliary tract, pancreas, prostate, avascular tissues) fail to equilibrate well with serum. Treatment failure despite a satisfactory MIC may also occur if an antimicrobial is highly protein bound and sufficient tissue levels cannot be achieved, as only unbound drug is pharmacologically active.
- Conversely, an antimicrobial with a nonsusceptible or intermediately susceptible MIC may be highly effective if well concentrated at the target site (e.g. aminoglycosides in urosepsis) or if the drug is known to have a post-antibiotic effect (e.g. aminoglycosides, fluoroquinolones), resulting in substantial bacterial killing or inhibition, despite subtherapeutic concentrations.
- The MIC should never be used as the sole determinant in selecting an antimicrobial.

Antimicrobial effects can be described in terms of their ability to inhibit (bacteriostatic) or kill (bactericidal) an infecting microorganism *in vitro*.

- A bactericidal drug has a minimum bactericidal concentration (MBC) that is only 2 to 4 times the MIC.
- A bacteriostatic drug has an MBC that is greater than 16 times the MIC.
- An alternate definition for cidality requires a minimum of 3 log killing in 24 hours with any value less than that indicative of static activity.
- Historically, bactericidal drugs have been favored in the treatment of endocarditis, meningitis, osteomyelitis and bacterial infections in neutropenic patients, although many bacteriostatic agents have been used with success [16]. Cidal drugs are favored in septic shock, wherever possible.

Establishing and maintaining antimicrobial activity through appropriate dosing

Antimicrobial therapy should begin at maximum recommended dosing in the setting of life-threatening infection [17,18]. This is often higher than the usual dose (e.g. 1.5 g of vancomycin or 750 mg of levofloxacin). The initial loading dose should be further guided by an assessment of the V_d.

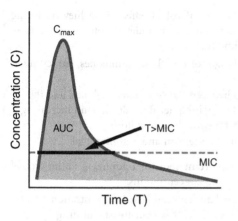

Figure 16.1 Pharmacokinetic/pharmacodynamics indices commonly used in optimizing antimicrobial therapy.

- Increased capillary permeability in sepsis can increase the V_d of hydrophilic antimicrobials, necessitating a larger loading dose to attain optimal serum concentrations and saturate body compartments. Subsequent maintenance doses and frequency of administration should be adjusted based on daily reassessment of clearance.
- Renal function should be determined by estimation of the creatinine clearance (CrCl) rather than following serum creatinine alone. Calculations of creatinine clearance are typically based on static values. In acute renal failure, such calculations will normally overestimate creatinine clearance and, conversely, they will underestimate creatinine clearance during renal recovery. In the absence of diuretic therapy, urine output may also provide a marker for real-time renal clearance.

Antimicrobial efficacy can be maximized through dosing strategies based on PK/PD indices (Figure 16.1). Most antimicrobial effects fall into one of the following categories:

Time-dependent: optimal antimicrobial effect occurs during the time (T) in which the drug concentration exceeds the MIC for a given dosing interval (T > MIC).

- Examples: β-lactams (penicillins, cephalosporins, carbapenems), linezolid, clindamycin
- Effect is optimized by increasing T > MIC through more frequent dosing, or in some cases, prolonged or continuous intravenous infusion [19]. The latter two remain controversial.
- T >4 × MIC for ≥60% or T >90% MIC of the dosing interval is recommended with intermittent dosing. With continuous infusion, T > MIC is typically 100% for most pathogens [20,21].

Concentration-dependent: optimal antimicrobial effect occurs at the peak concentration (C_{max}) reached after administration of the drug.

- Examples: aminoglycosides, fluoroquinolones, metronidazole, daptomycin
- Effect is optimized by increasing the ratio between C_{max} and the MIC (C_{max}/MIC) through higher drug dosing for a given dosing interval. The prolonged post-antibiotic effect (PAE) of many of these drugs allows for less frequent (extended interval) dosing, particularly in the case of aminoglycosides.
- C_{max}/MIC ratio ≥ 10–12 is preferable when treating Gram-negative infections with aminoglycosides [22].

Time- and concentration-dependent: optimal antimicrobial effect is achieved during T > MIC and when C_{max} is high. Both parameters define an index of total drug exposure known as the area under the concentration-time curve (AUC).

- Examples: vancomycin [23], linezolid, aminoglycosides, fluoroquinolones, tetracyclines, tigecycline, azithromycin
- Effect is optimized by increasing the ratio between the AUC over 24 hours and the MIC (AUC_{0-24}/MIC) by increasing C_{max} through higher drug dosing and increasing T > MIC through frequent dosing and therapeutic drug monitoring.
- Effective AUC_{0-24}/MIC ratios vary with microorganism and antimicrobial.

Therapeutic drug monitoring (TDM) is an important tool for optimizing antimicrobial dosing through direct measurement of serum drug concentrations.

- Antimicrobials appropriate for TDM ideally have an established concentration effect and/or concentration–toxicity relationship, significant patient-to-patient drug concentration variability, and a low therapeutic index (where the difference between therapeutic and toxic doses is small).
- TDM is routinely employed to guide aminoglycoside and glycopeptide (e.g. vancomycin) dosing. While β-lactams are subject to marked PK variability in the critically ill, TDM for these agents is not routinely available in many clinical settings.

Special populations

Obese patients (defined as having a body mass index $\geq$30) can present with significant variations in V_d and clearance [24].

- Many antimicrobials exhibit an increased V_d in obese patients, often requiring specific weight-based dosing regimens, depending on whether the antimicrobial is hydrophilic or lipophilic.
- While baseline renal clearance may be higher in obese patients, comorbid diseases (e.g. diabetes mellitus, hypertension) contributing to renal insufficiency are also common and may require dose reduction to avoid toxicity.

Burn patients may develop increased capillary permeability and hypoalbuminemia leading to interstitial edema and increased V_d, followed by a hyperdynamic state marked by increased cardiac output and renal clearance [25]. While higher and more frequent dosing of antimicrobials is usually necessary, TDM is warranted to ensure effective drug concentrations.

Renal replacement therapy (RRT), including continuous renal replacement therapy (CRRT) and sustained low-efficiency dialysis (SLED), is often employed to manage acute renal failure in the ICU. Therapeutic drug concentrations may be problematic to achieve due to enhanced removal. Individualized dosing regimens based on trough monitoring are recommended [26–28].

Extracorporeal membrane oxygenation (ECMO) can complicate antimicrobial therapy through drug sequestration within the circuit and hemodilution leading to increased V_d [29]. Antimicrobial dosing recommendations continue to evolve with increasing use of ECMO in the ICU.

Minimizing drug toxicity

- Adverse effects, drug–drug interactions and toxicity profiles should factor prominently into the selection of an antimicrobial.
- Where possible, attempts should be made to prevent further exacerbation of underlying renal or hepatic insufficiency, either from comorbid disease or acute organ dysfunction in the setting of critical illness.

Administering timely antimicrobial therapy

- Rapid administration (<1 hour) of effective intravenous antimicrobial therapy is recommended in the setting of severe sepsis, with or without septic shock [3].
- Initiation of antimicrobial therapy within the first hour of hypotension related to septic shock has been associated with a 79.9% survival rate [2]. With each ensuing hour of delay, survival is reduced by 7.6%, resulting in a survival rate of 42% at 6 hours.
- Delayed antimicrobial therapy also adversely impacts outcomes in patients with bacteremia, fungemia, pneumonia, meningitis and other serious infections [30].

Reassessing for effect

- Antimicrobial therapy should be continuously re-examined in the ICU to assess for efficacy, toxicity and appropriateness.
- As the patient clinically improves, de-escalation, or narrowing, of empiric antimicrobial coverage is strongly recommended, especially if a causative microorganism and its susceptibilities have been established. Clinical response alone, however, is sufficient to support judicious de-escalation even in culture-negative situations.
- The goals of de-escalation are to reduce selective pressure on bacteria, prevent antimicrobial resistance and minimize drug toxicity.
- While further research is needed, antimicrobial de-escalation has not been shown to harm patients, at least in healthcare-associated pneumonia, and may reduce antimicrobial costs [31].
- Final duration of antimicrobial therapy should be guided by clinical improvement and limited to the shortest effective course wherever possible.

Clinical deterioration or failure to improve on an antimicrobial regimen is frequent grounds for changing or adding antimicrobials. However, it is also important to identify potential causes for antimicrobial failure.

- Gaps in empiric coverage may allow microorganisms not originally isolated in bacterial culture to persist. Additional consideration should be given to investigating mycobacteria, fungi and viral etiologies through specialized cultures and other diagnostics.
- Inadequate optimization of PK and PD parameters may result in suboptimal serum and tissue antimicrobial concentrations, despite demonstrated *in vitro* susceptibility.
- Abscesses, foreign bodies (including medical devices), and poorly perfused tissues present barriers to antimicrobial penetration. Additional source control may be necessary.

- Noninfectious processes (e.g. rheumatologic disease, occult malignancy, drug fever) are unlikely to improve with antimicrobial therapy.
- If an infection has not been identified, either immediate discontinuation or commitment to a shortened course of empiric therapy should be strongly considered and has been associated with lower costs and antimicrobial resistance without increased mortality risk or length of stay [32,33].

Summary

- Antimicrobials play an integral part in the management of infectious diseases in the ICU.
- Optimal use of antimicrobials can be achieved through methodical selection and administration of the right drug, at the right dose, at the right time.
- A dynamic approach emphasizing daily reassessment of the appropriateness and necessity of antimicrobial therapy in the ICU is the key to preventing antimicrobial overutilization and future drug resistance.

References

1. Vincent JL, Rello J, Marshall J et al. International study of the prevalence and outcomes of infection in intensive care units. *JAMA* 2009; 302 : 2323–9.

2. Kumar A, Roberts D, Wood KE et al. Duration of hypotension before initiation of effective antimicrobial therapy is the critical determinant of survival in human septic shock. *Crit Care Med* 2006; 34 : 1589–96.

3. Dellinger RP, Levy MM, Rhodes A et al. Surviving sepsis campaign: international guidelines for management of severe sepsis and septic shock: 2012. *Crit Care Med* 2013; 41 : 580–637.

4. MacLaren R, Bond CA, Martin SJ, Fike D. Clinical and economic outcomes of involving pharmacists in the direct care of critically ill patients with infections. *Crit Care Med* 2008; 36 : 3184–9.

5. Raineri E, Pan A, Mondello P et al. Role of the infectious diseases specialist consultant on the appropriateness of antimicrobial therapy prescription in an intensive care unit. *Am J Infect Control* 2008; 36 : 283–90.

6. Kumar A, Ellis P, Arabi Y et al. Initiation of inappropriate antimicrobial therapy results in a fivefold reduction of survival in human septic shock. *Chest* 2009; 136 : 1237–48.

7. Chow JK, Golan Y, Ruthazer R et al. Risk factors for albicans and non-albicans candidemia in the intensive care unit. *Crit Care Med* 2008; 36 : 1993–8.

8. Hachem R, Hanna H, Kontoyiannis D et al. The changing epidemiology of invasive candidiasis: Candida glabrata and Candida krusei as the leading causes of candidemia in hematologic malignancy. *Cancer* 2008; 112 : 2493–9.

9. Pappas PG, Kauffman CA, Andes D et al. Clinical practice guidelines for the management of candidiasis: 2009 update by the Infectious Diseases Society of America. *Clin Infect Dis* 2009; 48 : 503–35.

10. Micek ST, Welch EC, Khan J et al. Empiric combination antibiotic therapy is associated with improved outcome against sepsis due to Gram-negative bacteria: a retrospective analysis. *Antimicrob Agents Chemother* 2010; 54 : 1742–8.

11. Kumar A, Safdar N, Kethireddy S, Chateau D. A survival benefit of combination antibiotic therapy for serious infections associated with sepsis and septic shock is contingent only on the risk of death: a meta-analytic/meta-regression study. *Crit Care Med* 2010; 38 : 1651–64.

12. Kumar A, Zarychanski R, Light B et al. Early combination antibiotic therapy yields improved survival compared with monotherapy in septic shock: a propensity-matched analysis. *Crit Care Med* 2010; 38 : 1773–85.

13. Díaz-Martín A, Martínez-González ML, Ferrer R et al. Antibiotic prescription patterns in the empiric therapy of severe sepsis: combination of antimicrobials with different mechanisms of action reduces mortality. Crit Care 2012;16; R223.

14. Paul M, Benuri-Silbiger I, Soares-Weiser K, Leibovici L. Beta lactam monotherapy versus beta lactam-aminoglycoside combination therapy for sepsis in immunocompetent patients: systematic review and meta-analysis of randomised trials. BMJ 2004; 328 : 668.

15. Rea RS, Capitano B, Bies R et al. Suboptimal aminoglycoside dosing in critically ill patients. Ther Drug Monit 2008; 30 : 674–81.

16. Pankey GA, Sabath LD. Clinical relevance of bacteriostatic versus bactericidal mechanisms of action in the treatment of Gram-positive bacterial infections. Clin Infect Dis 2004; 38 : 864–70.

17. Roberts JA, Lipman J. Pharmacokinetic issues for antibiotics in the critically ill patient. Crit Care Med 2009; 37 : 840–51.

18. Roberts JA, Joynt GM, Choi GY et al. How to optimise antimicrobial prescriptions in the Intensive Care Unit: principles of individualised dosing using pharmacokinetics and pharmacodynamics. Int J Antimicrob Agents 2012; 39 : 187–92.

19. Roberts JA, Webb S, Paterson D et al. A systematic review on clinical benefits of continuous administration of beta-lactam antibiotics. Crit Care Med 2009; 37 : 2071–8.

20. McKinnon PS, Paladino JA, Schentag JJ. Evaluation of area under the inhibitory curve (AUIC) and time above the minimum inhibitory concentration (T>MIC) as predictors of outcome for cefepime and ceftazidime in serious bacterial infections. Int J Antimicrob Agents 2008; 31 : 345–51.

21. Sinnollareddy MG, Roberts MS, Lipman J, Roberts JA. beta-lactam pharmacokinetics and pharmacodynamics in critically ill patients and strategies for dose optimization: a structured review. Clin Exp Pharmacol Physiol 2012; 39 : 489–96.

22. Moore RD, Lietman PS, Smith CR. Clinical response to aminoglycoside therapy: importance of the ratio of peak concentration to minimal inhibitory concentration. J Infect Dis 1987; 155 : 93–9.

23. Zelenitsky S, Rubinstein E, Ariano R et al. Vancomycin pharmacodynamics and survival in patients with methicillin-resistant Staphylococcus aureus-associated septic shock. Int J Antimicrob Agents 2013; 41 : 255–60.

24. Janson B, Thursky K. Dosing of antibiotics in obesity. Curr Opin Infect Dis 2012; 25 : 634–49.

25. Blanchet B, Jullien V, Vinsonneau C, Tod M. Influence of burns on pharmacokinetics and pharmacodynamics of drugs used in the care of burn patients. Clin Pharmacokinet 2008; 47 : 635–54.

26. Roberts DM, Roberts JA, Roberts MS et al. Variability of antibiotic concentrations in critically ill patients receiving continuous renal replacement therapy: a multicentre pharmacokinetic study. Crit Care Med 2012; 40 : 1523–8.

27. Choi G, Gomersall CD, Tian Q et al. Principles of antibacterial dosing in continuous renal replacement therapy. Crit Care Med 2009; 37 : 2268–82.

28. Bogard KN, Peterson NT, Plumb TJ et al. Antibiotic dosing during sustained low-efficiency dialysis: special considerations in adult critically ill patients. Crit Care Med 2011; 39 : 560–70.

29. Shekar K, Fraser JF, Smith MT, Roberts JA. Pharmacokinetic changes in patients receiving extracorporeal membrane oxygenation. J Crit Care 2012; 27:741 e9–18.

30. Funk DJ, Kumar A. Antimicrobial therapy for life-threatening infections: speed is life. Crit Care Clin 2011; 27 : 53–76.

31. Masterton RG. Antibiotic de-escalation. Crit Care Clin 2011; 27 : 149–62.

32. Singh N, Rogers P, Atwood CW et al. Short-course empiric antibiotic therapy for patients with pulmonary infiltrates in the intensive care unit. A proposed solution for

indiscriminate antibiotic prescription. *Am J Respir Crit Care Med* 2000; 162 : 505–11.

33. Schlueter M, James C, Dominguez A *et al.* Practice patterns for antibiotic de-escalation in culture-negative healthcare-associated pneumonia. *Infection* 2010; 38 : 357–62.

34. Bailey TC, Little JR, Littenberg B *et al.* A meta-analysis of extended-interval dosing versus multiple daily dosing of aminoglycosides. *Clin Infect Dis* 1997; 24 : 786–95.

35. Craig WA. Optimizing aminoglycoside use. *Crit Care Clin* 2011; 27 : 107–21.

Chapter

Sedation, analgesia and neuromuscular blockade

17

Brian Pollard

Introduction

The origins of the specialty of intensive care are closely allied with the specialty of anesthesia and it is therefore not surprising that the ICU patient originally received very deep sedation bordering on general anesthesia, often with the use of a muscle relaxant [1]. Invasive procedures and routine procedures all tend to be easier in a completely unconscious patient rather than one who is only lightly sedated. This is not a valid reason to provide deep sedation and during the last 30 years, there has been a wider appreciation of the negative effects of continuous deep sedation and muscular relaxation. The patient in the modern ICU tends therefore to be sedated for the initial period and then allowed to be run at a level of sedation that is just enough to provide anxiolysis and compliance with management. Newer drugs have facilitated the process because the level of sedation can be changed rapidly.

Sedation

In the modern ICU the degree of sedation is tailored to the needs of each individual patient and kept as low as possible. Every patient is different, but the principal indications for sedation can be summarized as follows.

Control of stress and anxiety

The ICU is a frightening and alien environment for a patient to encounter. Not only that, but patients find themselves subjected to a significant number of unknown, invasive and possibly painful procedures. Some degree of sedation is therefore necessary, at least for the initial period and intermittently thereafter during a patient's stay on the ICU.

Control of intracranial pressure

In a patient with a raised intracranial pressure, any straining or attempting to breathe out of synchrony with the ventilator may cause spikes in the ICP. Sedation will help to prevent these.

Control of seizures and spasms

Appropriate choice of sedation will help to reduce the frequency and severity of seizures and spasms, and may form a very useful contribution to the management of epilepsy, tetanus and other related conditions.

Handbook of ICU Therapy, third edition, ed. John Fuller, Jeff Granton and Ian McConachie. Published by Cambridge University Press. © Cambridge University Press 2015.

Safe transport

Transporting a patient between departments or hospitals is a potentially hazardous activity. Increasing the level of sedation reduces the risk and provides a calm patient for the transfer.

Compliance with procedures

A routine part of management of a critically ill patient involves simple nursing procedures, as well as more complex and invasive ones. A sedated patient will be more compliant with these procedures and any stress will be reduced.

Facilitate/tolerate controlled ventilation

The early ICU ventilators were modifications of those used in the operating room. Modern modes of ventilatory support that synchronize with the patient's own respiratory pattern have made it easier for the lightly sedated patient to comply with ventilatory support [2,3]. In addition the development of techniques of percutaneous tracheostomy has also helped.

Promote a more natural sleep pattern

Patients in the ICU rarely have a normal sleep cycle [4]. They experience reduced rapid eye movement and slow wave sleep. Sleep deprivation will accentuate confusion and increase the likelihood of delirium. It is probably impossible to provide a natural sleep pattern within the 24-hour environment that is the ICU, but any attempt to promote this will be beneficial.

Agitation and delirium

Agitation is common in the ICU patient and may make patients uncooperative, difficult to monitor and problematic to treat. Delirium and agitation can also pose risks to both patients and staff. Sedation will reduce these issues in the short term, but conversely it is thought that a period of sedation may of itself contribute to the development of delirium and confusion in the post-ICU period.

Reduction of metabolic and hormonal response to critical illness

Appropriately managed sedation will contribute to a decrease in the work of breathing as well as myocardial oxygen demand. There is also a reduction in the extent of the metabolic and hormonal response to critical illness.

Sedative agents

A sedative agent for use on the ICU should provide a calm, relaxed patient who is pain and stress free and will comply with all aspects of management. One agent will not provide everything and it is common to use two or more agents together. A sedative and analgesic combination is common and in some cases the analgesic contributes to the sedation. Sedative agents should ideally have the following properties:

- Short half-life (easy to control)
- Suitable for infusion administration
- Cheap

- Water soluble
- No adverse effects (short term or long term)
- No venous irritation
- No cardiovascular or respiratory depression
- Minimal potential for dependence.

Midazolam: a short-acting benzodiazepine, it may be administered by bolus (1–2 mg), but more commonly is given by infusion (1–5 mg/h). Although relatively short acting, it has the potential to accumulate, especially in patients with impaired hepatic or renal function [5]. Midazolam is also extensively protein bound, leading to a potential increase in depth of sedation and prolongation of action in patients with low albumin.

Propofol: a short-acting general anesthetic agent, propofol is administered by infusion (1–5 mg/kg/h) although can also be given by bolus to provide rapid effect. It has less hangover than other agents and will significantly shorten weaning from the ventilator [6]. Although relatively expensive, it is cost effective in terms of shorter weaning times after a prolonged infusion [7]. A bolus dose may exhibit a short-lived cardiodepressant effect.

Clonidine: this centrally acting α_2 agonist is effective in producing background sedation and helping to control agitation, delirium and anxiety. It also attenuates sympathetic responses to stress [8, 9] and has an opioid-sparing effect, allowing a decrease in the quantity of opioids required to achieve a given level of analgesia. The usual dose is 50–250 μg IV

Dexmedetomidine: another α_2 agonist with similar effects to clonidine. It also exhibits analgesic effects, together with the capacity to attenuate the cardiovascular stress responses [10]. Its popularity is increasing [11].

Isoflurane and desflurane: these inhalational anesthetic agents are effective sedatives at appropriate inhaled concentrations. They are not routinely used for long-term ICU sedation on the grounds of cost and the requirement for specialized ventilators fitted with vaporizers and efficient scavenging systems.

Other agents: temazepam is not routinely used for ICU sedation, but is sometimes used as a hypnotic in an effort to restore a "normal" sleep cycle. Diazepam has a long half-life and possesses pharmacologically active metabolites. It is unsuitable for routine use in the ICU patient, but may have a place for occasional use in the nonventilated patient suffering from severe acute anxiety. Haloperidol is a major tranquilizer and finds occasional use in the ICU patient to help to control agitation. Etomidate usage is associated with adrenal suppression and it should not be used by infusion in the ICU.

Analgesia

It is common for an ICU patient to experience pain at some time during their period of ICU care [12, 13]. Post-operative surgical patients have painful wounds and necessary procedures such as vascular cannulation, wound dressing, tracheal intubation, endobronchial suctioning and physiotherapy may cause pain. Poor pain control may lead to agitation and exacerbate anxiety.

Analgesic agents

An analgesic agent should provide pain relief without any other adverse effects. The ideal analgesic would have properties similar to those for the ideal sedative agent, above.

Tolerance to opioid infusions is common in the ICU patient. Dependence may also develop and typical narcotic withdrawal reactions may be seen and may be difficult to manage. A useful side effect of the opioid family is to suppress respiratory drive and the cough reflex, and thus help to reduce attempts to breathe out of phase with controlled ventilation.

Morphine: morphine can be given by bolus (5–10mg) or infusion (1–5 mg/h) and is probably the commonest opioid analgesic in the ICU. It is cheap and has analgesic, anxiolytic and sedative actions with minimal cardiovascular depression. It does possess pharmacologically active metabolites that may accumulate in patients with renal insufficiency [14].

Fentanyl: fentanyl (bolus 50–100μg or infusion 1–5 μg/kg/h) is a popular analgesic with excellent cardiovascular stability. It may accumulate following long-term administration.

Alfentanil: alfentanil (5 mg bolus then infusion 2–5 mg/h) is less popular and not available in some countries. It is predictably short-acting after brief administration but a long-term infusion may lead to prolongation of effect.

Remifentanil: remifentanil (infusion 1–10 μg/kg/h) has a rapid onset of action (<60 s), a predictable metabolic profile and a relatively constant short half-life of 2–3 min. It is unaffected by renal failure [15]. It can be used for long periods without the risk of accumulation.

Paracetamol (acetaminophen): a useful analgesic agent that has a morphine-sparing effect. It may be used for its weak analgesic properties, as well as for its antipyretic effect. It is not usually adequate when used alone.

Other analgesics: the nonsteroidal anti-inflammatory drugs tend not to be routinely used in ICU patients because of their multiple pharmacological effects and side effects, but may have a role on occasions. Tramadol may also find an occasional use.

Regional blockade: many regional techniques may be used in the ICU patient [16]. Epidural, intrapleural and transversus abdominis plane (TAP) blocks are often used and lend themselves to continuous infusions of local analgesic agents, especially following thoracic, abdominal and pelvic injury or surgery. Local infiltration prior to vascular cannulation should always be considered, even in the sedated patient.

Management of sedation and analgesia

The goal is to provide a patient who:

- is pain-free
- is clear, calm and cooperative during the day
- has sufficient restful sleep at night
- can be rapidly weaned from ventilatory support when ready
- is at as light a level of sedation as possible while maintaining comfort.

These goals are difficult to achieve because the ideal drug or drug combination does not exist. Every patient is different and the same patient may behave differently at different times. Drug accumulation is common in the critically ill (many have impaired renal or hepatic function) and tolerance to the agents used develops. Increased levels of sedation and/or analgesia are often needed during invasive procedures, but returning the infusion rate to preprocedure levels may be less easy. In the past there has been a tendency to oversedate ICU patients to make them easier to manage and this temptation must be resisted. There does nevertheless remain a group of patients who do need deep sedation and adequate sedation must not be withheld in these patients.

Excessively deep sedation may result in:

- Cardiovascular depression
- Respiratory depression
- Depressed immune function
- Suppression of cough reflex
- Prolonged weaning (with increased risk of opportunist infection)
- Difficulty in neurological assessment
- Gastrointestinal stasis
- Increased risk of pressure sore development
- Increased risk of venous thromboembolism
- Physical and/or psychological drug dependence leading to withdrawal complications
- Increased risk of drug interactions
- Increased costs (drug costs and those due to increased length of stay).

The sedation of a critically ill patient is one of the most important aspects of their management. Every patient is unique and the choice (and dose) of agents must be matched to the patient and individually titrated to a definable endpoint. This will differ between patients and also in the same patient at different times.

Opioids provide excellent analgesia, but cannot be relied upon to provide adequate sedation if given alone. The coadministration of a sedative agent (commonly midazolam or propofol) is necessary. Remember that the drugs will tend to potentiate each other's sedative activity and individual titration is mandatory.

Monitoring the level of sedation is important to ensure that individual patient goals are met. Every ICU should have written guidelines or protocols describing optimum sedation practice for all classes of patient.

A regular (daily in many cases) sedation "hold" is recommended [17]. In this technique, all sedation infusions are stopped completely and the patient constantly observed. This allows staff to assess conscious level and minimize the risk of undetected drug accumulation. The infusions are then recommenced when necessary, but possibly at a new reduced rate. Where accumulation is occurring the interrupted infusion(s) may not need recommencing for several hours, allowing clearance of excess sedative agent and potentially shortening time to wean from ventilatory support. Remember that a sedation hold may be inadvisable for some patients, for example those with significant ischemic heart disease.

Tolerance to sedatives and analgesic drugs may develop. It is more common in patients on long-term infusions than those sedated for a short time and results in a progressive increase in the amount of drug required to produce a given effect [18,19].

Drug dependence may occur in the ICU patient and withdrawal of the causative agent can be challenging. Sudden cessation or too rapid weaning may precipitate an acute withdrawal reaction [20]. This can be manifest in a number of ways, which include tachycardia, hypertension, fever, tachypnea, mydriasis, agitation, delirium, seizures, opioid craving, cramps, muscle pains and dysesthesia [21]. Some of these may be particularly difficult to see in the ventilated patient. A gradual reduction in sedative and opioid infusion rates and/or supplementation with drugs such as methadone or diazepam may help decrease the incidence of withdrawal phenomena.

The establishment of balanced sedation and analgesia, and its subsequent smooth withdrawal, may be further complicated as a result of a patient's pre-existing habituation to recreational substances, e.g. alcohol, nicotine and street drugs. Consideration of appropriate replacement therapy for habituated patients whilst in intensive care has been suggested, although it remains a subject of debate.

Measuring sedation

In order to achieve the best level of sedation for each patient, a method of measuring it is useful. Both subjective and objective methods exist, the former being more commonly used because the latter remain to be fully evaluated in the ICU patient. Many ICUs have their own individualized scoring systems developed as a modification of an existing system. Visual analog scales are very limited in the ICU, but some units use them as one component of their scoring system.

Subjective techniques

- The Ramsay system is popular [22]. It scores comfort, sedation, anxiety and agitation on a six-point scale and has been shown to have good reliability. The six individual response descriptors are not mutually exclusive, which may produce some difficulties in interpretation [23, 24].
- The Richmond Agitation–Sedation Scale (RASS) [25] scores patients on a 10-point scale from unrouseable to combative. It has more specific descriptors than the Ramsey scale and has been claimed to provide more accurate assessments.

Objective techniques

- Continuous electro-encephalography (EEG) should represent the gold standard because it is measuring the effect of the drugs on the target organ, the brain. Unfortunately it is impractical for routine use because it requires a trained specialist technician to record and interpret it. In addition, each drug has its own EEG pattern and there are significant variations between individual patients.
- Bispectral index (BIS) has been extensively researched for the measurement of depth of anesthesia in the operating room. Logic would suggest that, as the drugs used for ICU sedation are the same as those used in general anesthesia, then BIS may have a role in the ICU patient. The inbuilt BIS algorithms have been developed for the anesthetized patient and whereas BIS shows an effect with sedation, the significant variability between patients and drugs remains a problem [26–28].
- Auditory evoked potentials (AEP) have been developed as a tool for assessing depth of anesthesia. There is insufficient research in the ICU patient to be able to determine whether they have a role in ICU sedation [29].
- Electrical impedance tomography (EIT) examines the changes in impedance within the brain on the injection of a very small alternating current. It is in its infancy, but if its potential can be harnessed then it might provide a viable window on the brain and allow us to develop a real objective sedation monitor [30].

Muscular relaxation

In the 1980s, neuromuscular blockade formed a vital part of the management of a patient on the ICU. The principal reason would seem to be a belief that in order to secure effective controlled ventilation, muscular paralysis was required. The ICU ventilators at the time were modifications of those used in the operating room and tended to control the breathing whatever the patient did. Muscle relaxation was therefore advantageous in many patients. The development of modern ICU ventilators has helped to drive the move away from muscular relaxation, as well as a realization that paralysis is unnecessary most of the time and the possible adverse effects of long-term paralysis. In the modern ICU muscle relaxants are given for specific short-term indications and not as a routine.

Indications for the use of a muscle relaxant include:

- Tracheal intubation. Suxamethonium (succinylcholine) (1–1.5 mg/kg) is the usual agent of choice, but any of the other agents may be used if circumstances permit.
- To optimize ventilation. There are circumstances where neuromuscular blockade is advantageous for optimum management of ventilation. In severe acute asthma, peak inflation pressures are less when a relaxant is used. In patients with critical oxygenation and/or poor lung compliance (especially with inverse ratio, prone or high-frequency ventilation) then a muscle relaxant will often improve oxygenation.
- Raised intracranial pressure. Coughing and breathing out of phase with the ventilator may produce sudden potentially damaging surges in intracranial pressure. These are usually attenuated by muscular relaxation.
- Transport. Safe transport of the critically ill ventilated patient is often facilitated by the use of a muscle relaxant.
- Airway procedures. Tracheostomy and bronchoscopy are usually safer when the patient is paralyzed.
- Control of muscle spasms. In some situations, e.g. tetanus or rabies, painful and potentially damaging muscle spasms may occur. These are abolished or attenuated by using a muscle relaxant. Epileptic seizures would of course be abolished by the use of a muscle relaxant, but this is not recommended because the seizure activity would not be suppressed by the relaxant, only the external manifestations.

Neuromuscular blockade can result in several undesirable problems in the ICU patient. Awareness is possible if concomitant sedation is inadequate. Critical care myopathy/ neuropathy may be accentuated, particularly if a steroid-based relaxant is used. Disuse atrophy has been reported, which may delay weaning from ventilation and subsequent rehabilitation. Active coughing is prevented, which will impair the ability to clear secretions from the airway.

Neuromuscular blocking agents

Suxamethonium (succinylcholine)

This depolarizing relaxant only finds a place in rapid onset, short-duration situations, in particular tracheal intubation. A dose of 1.5mg/kg has an onset within 60 seconds and a duration of 3–5 minutes. It must be given with caution (or ideally avoided) in cases of raised potassium, muscular denervation, spinal-cord injury, raised intracranial pressure, burns and malignant hyperpyrexia susceptibility.

Atracurium

This is an ideal muscle relaxant for use by infusion (0.5–1 mg/kg/h). It has no active metabolites and its metabolism (and therefore half-life) is independent of all organ systems. It has excellent cardiovascular stability, although some histamine release has been reported following a bolus dose. Some patients demonstrate tolerance to its effects, necessitating an escalation in infusion rate to maintain a constant block.

Cis-atracurium

This is the main active isomer in atracurium (the racemate). The only differences are less tendency to histamine release and increased cost. Infusion rate is 50–200 μg/kg/h.

Vecuronium

This intermediate-duration muscle relaxant is also suitable for continuous infusion administration (50–200 μg/kg/h). It has an active metabolite, which may accumulate in cases of hepatic or renal dysfunction, although in practice this is rarely a problem. Long-term use has been reported to possibly be associated with the condition of steroid-induced myopathy.

Rocuronium

The properties of rocuronium are very similar to vecuronium, but it has no active metabolite. The onset of action is more rapid when given in a bolus dose. By infusion the dose is 300–600 μg/kg/h.

Pancuronium

This steroid relaxant is still available in some countries. It has a long duration of action and a slow onset. It is not suitable for infusion administration. Bolus dose is 0.1 mg/kg. It may produce a tachycardia following a bolus dose.

Monitoring neuromuscular blockade

All patients receiving a muscle relaxant should have their level of neuromuscular blockade regularly checked. The recommended technique is to use a peripheral nerve stimulator. Any accessible nerve/muscle combination may be used, but the commonest nerves to use are the ulnar nerve, common peroneal nerve and facial nerve. The train-of-four technique is recommended. A level of block where one or two "twitches" are present out of the four is the most appropriate level to aim for most of the time. Deeper levels of block may, very occasionally, be necessary. Reversal of a neuromuscular block is routine in the operating room, but rarely required in the ICU.

References

1. Murdoch S, Cohen A. Intensive care sedation: a review of current British practice. *Intens Care Med* 2000; 26 : 922–8.

2. Hilbert G, Clouzeau B, Nam Bui H, Vargas F. Sedation during noninvasive ventilation. *Minerva Anesteziol* 2012; 78 : 842–46.

3. Karir V, Hough CL, Daniel S *et al.* Sedation practices in a cohort of critically ill patients receiving prolonged mechanical ventilation. *Minerva Anestiziol* 2012; 78 : 801–9.

4. Aurell J, Elmquist D. Sleep in the surgical intensive care unit: continuous poly-graphic recording of nine patients

receiving postoperative care. *Br Med J* 1985; 290 : 1029–32.

5. Shelly MP, Mendel L, Park GR. Failure of critically ill patients to metabolise midazolam. *Anaesthesia* 1987; 42 : 619–26.

6. Roekarts PMHJ, Huygen FJPM, DeLange S. Infusion of propofol versus midazolam for sedation in the intensive care unit following coronary artery bypass surgery. *J Cardiothorac Vasc Anesth* 1993; 7 : 142–7.

7. Barrientos-Vega R, Mar-Sanchez-Soria M, Morales-Gracia C *et al.* Prolonged sedation of critically ill patients with midazolam or propofol: impact on weaning and cost. *Crit Care Med* 1997; 25 : 33–40.

8. Kulkarni SK, Parale MP, Kulkarni GK. Clonidine in alcohol withdrawal: a clinical report. *Methods Find Exp Clin Pharmacol* 1987; 9 : 697–8.

9. Cushman PJ, Sowers JR. Alcohol withdrawal syndrome: clinical and hormonal responses to α-2 adrenergic treatment. *Alcoholism* 1989; 13 : 361–4.

10. Venn RM, Grounds RM. Comparison between dexmedetomidine and propofol for sedation in the intensive care unit: patient and clinician perceptions. *Br J Anaesth* 2001; 87 : 684–90.

11. Pichot C, Ghignone M, Quintin L. Dexmedetomidine to clonidine: from second to first line sedative agents in the critical care setting. *Journal of Intensive Care Medicine,* 2012; 27 : 219–37.

12. Novaes MA, Knobel E, Bork AM *et al.* Stressors in the ICU: perception of the patient, relatives and healthcare team. *Intensive Care Med* 1999; 25 : 1421–6.

13. Turner JS, Briggs SJ, Springhorn HE, Potgieter PD. Patient's recollection of intensive care unit experience. *Crit Care Med* 1990; 18 : 966–8.

14. Osborne RJ, Joel SP, Slevin MI. Morphine intoxication in renal failure: the role of morphine-6-glucuronide. *Br Med J* 1986; 292 : 1548–9.

15. Breen D, Wilmer A, Bodenham A *et al.* Offset of pharmacodynamic effects and safety of remifentanil in intensive care unit patients with various degrees of renal failure. *Crit Care* 2004; 8 : R21–30.

16. Stundner O, Memtsoudis SG. Regional anaesthesia and analgesia in critically ill patients: a systematic review. *Regional Anaesth Pain Med* 2012; 37 : 537–44.

17. Kress JP, Pohlman A, O'Connor MF, Hall JB. Daily interruption of sedative infusions in critically ill patients undergoing mechanical ventilation. *New Engl J Med* 2000; 342 : 1471–7.

18. Shafer A, White P, Schuttler J, Rosenthal MH. Use of fentanyl infusion in the intensive care unit: tolerance to its anesthetic effects? *Anesthesiology* 1983; 59 : 245–8.

19. Busto U, Sellers E. Pharmacologic aspects of benzodiazepine tolerance and dependence. *J Subst Abuse Treat* 1991; 8 : 29–33.

20. Cammarano WB, Pittet JF, Weitz S *et al.* Acute withdrawal syndrome related to the administration of analgesic and sedative medications in adult intensive care unit patients. *Crit Care Med* 1998; 26 : 676–84.

21. Kress JP, Pohlman AS, Hall JB. Sedation and analgesia in the intensive care unit. *Am J Respir Crit Care Med* 2002; 166 : 1024–8.

22. Ramsay MA, Savege TM, Simpson BR *et al.* Controlled sedation with alphaxolone-alphadolone. *Br Med J* 1974; 2 : 656–9

23. De Jonghe B, Cook D, Appere- De- Veecchi C *et al.* Using and understanding sedation scoring systems : a systematic review. *Intensive Care Med* 2000; 26 : 275–85.

24. Hansen-Flaschen J, Cowen J, Polomano RC. Beyond the Ramsay scale: need for a validated measure of sedating drug efficacy in the intensive care unit. *Crit Care Med* 1994; 22 : 732–3.

25. Sessler CN, Gosnell MS, Grap MJ, *et al.* The Richmond Agitation-Sedation Scale. Validity and reliability in adult intensive care unit patients. *Am J Resp Crit Care Med* 2002; 166, 1338–44.

26. Simmons LE, Riker RR, Prato BS, Fraser GL. Assessing sedation during intensive care unit mechanical ventilation with the bispectral index and the sedation–agitation scale. *Crit Care Med* 1999; 27 : 1499–504.

27. Barr G, Anderson RE, Samuelsson S *et al.* Fentanyl and midazolam anaesthesia for

coronary bypass surgery: a clinical study of bispectral electro-encephalogram analysis, drug concentrations and recall. *Br J Anaesth* 2000; 84 : 749–52.

28. Frenzel D, Greim CA, Sommer C *et al.* Is the bispectral index appropriate for monitoring the sedative level of mechanically ventilated surgical ICU patients? *Intens Care Med* 2002; 28 : 178–83.

29. Carrasco G. Instruments for monitoring intensive care unit sedation. *Crit Care* 2000; 4 : 217–25.

30. Bryan A, Pomfrett CJD, Davidson J *et al.* Functional electrical impedance tomography by evoked response: a new device for the study of human brain function during anaesthesia. *Br J Anaesth* 2011;106 : 428–9.

Chapter

18 Continuous renal replacement therapy

A Ebersohn and Rudi Brits

Renal replacement therapy (RRT) to support critically ill patients with acute kidney injury (AKI) has become routine. It forms a very important part of the combined management of multiorgan failure along with mechanical ventilation and cardiovascular support:

- Severe acute renal failure (ARF) is a common complication in patients with multiorgan failure (10–20% of all critically ill patients) and 70% of these patients will require RRT [1, 2].
- In previous studies mortality rates have been reported to be as high as 33–93% [1,2].
- In contrast, single-organ ARF has a much lower mortality rate – less than 10%.
- AKI is one of the most serious complications in critically ill patients. It occurs in more than one of every twenty patients requiring intensive care unit care [3].
- RRT continues to evolve. Indications for therapy have been well established and new developments, including the development of the complete artificial kidney, look promising.

Renal replacement therapy (RRT)

Renal replacement therapy can be classified as continuous or intermittent. Units differ nationally as well as internationally regarding their preference of therapy. In Europe and Australia continuous renal replacement therapy (CRRT) predominates, while in the USA intermittent replacement therapy (IRT) is preferred.

There are several methods of CRRT, as follows.

Hemofiltration (CRRT)

Continuous veno-venous hemofiltration (CVVH) uses a double lumen venous cannula and a peristaltic pump, which allows higher blood flows and increased membrane surface area, thus higher ultrafiltration rates and better uremic control. Continuous veno-venous hemofiltration produces an ultrafiltrate by maintaining a pressure difference over a highly permeable membrane (convection). Water is pushed across the membrane and carries dissolved solutes (known as solvent drag). A physiological substitution fluid is infused into the patient to maintain hydration status and chemical balance.

In the ICU, CVVH is the most commonly used CRRT. Less common or historical methods of CRRT are as follows:

- Continuous arterio-venous hemofiltration (CAVH) uses the arterio-venous pressure difference across a membrane to continuously produce an ultrafiltrate. Disadvantages

Handbook of ICU Therapy, third edition, ed. John Fuller, Jeff Granton and Ian McConachie. Published by Cambridge University Press. © Cambridge University Press 2015.

include cannulation of both artery and vein, which is associated with a much higher morbidity and also limited solute clearance.

- Slow continuous ultrafiltration (SCUF). Fluid removal by ultrafiltration.
- Continuous veno-venous hemodialysis (CVVHD). Fluid and toxins are removed through a process of diffusion with the use of a dialysate.
- Continuous veno-venous hemodiafiltration (CVVHDF). Widely used in Australia, but less so in other countries. Fluid and toxins are removed through a combination of diffusion, convection and ultrafiltration.

Hemodialysis

Hemodialysis is an intermittent renal replacement therapy (IRT).

- Hemodialysis produces dialysate by counter circulation of the patient's blood and dialysis solution while being separated by a semipermeable membrane. Solutes move down a concentration gradient across the membrane – the process is known as diffusion.
- Treatments are intermittent, 3–4 times per week, each treatment lasting approximately 4 h. However, if IRT is to be used in ICU there is evidence that daily dialysis decreases mortality in medical ICU patients [4].
- IRT is mainly used in the management of end-stage renal failure or single-organ ARF. It is still the preferred method of RRT in the USA. However, even in the USA, CRRT is gaining increasing acceptance in many units.

Advantages of CRRT

- CRRT is slow and "gentle" on the cardiovascular system of these unstable patients. However, despite this, large volumes of fluid can still be removed if required. The continuous removal of fluid creates room for the administration of nutrition and other fluids.
- Adequate uremic control is achieved, even in very severely catabolic patients.
- CRRT may have other advantages, like removal of cytokines and proinflammatory materials (the "middle molecules") from the circulation of the critically ill (see below). This is because of the bigger pore size of the filter membrane.
- Techniques of CRRT are easy to learn.
- IRT is associated with hypotension, which is more severe in those patients with cardiovascular instability.
- Advantages and comparisons are further explored below when discussing controversies.

Indications for starting RRT

Most common indications are:

- Anuria or oliguria (urine volumes less than 200 mL/12 h)
- Hyperkalemia (serum potassium persistently more than 6.5 mmol/L)
- Severe acidemia (pH <7.1)
- Azotemia (urea >30 mmol/L or creatinine >300 mmol/L)
- Pulmonary edema.

Other indications may include:

- Diuretic-resistant cardiac failure
- Anasarca

- Uremic complications (encephalopathy, pericarditis, neuropathy or myopathy)
- Dysnatremia (sodium >160 mmol/L or <115 mmol/L)
- Temperature control (hyper or hypothermia)
- Drug overdose (salicylates, methanol, barbiturates, lithium, amino glycosides, cephalosporin)
- Sepsis.

Timing of CRRT

Most clinicians would prefer to prevent complications arising from the development of uremia and institute CRRT early. In addition, recent studies examining the role of early versus late intervention of renal support are of interest. For example:

- Early initiation of CVVH in a small study of patients with septic shock has been shown to improve hemodynamic and metabolic responses and improve survival [5].
- Early hemofiltration is associated with better than predicted survival in ARF after cardiac surgery [6].
- Despite similarities in injury severity and risk of developing renal failure, survival was increased in the early filtration group in a retrospective review of 100 trauma patients [7].
- Initiation of CRRT within a short time of ICU admission is related to early recovery. Where CRRT is delayed it can cause fluid overload and metabolic derangement, which worsens patient conditions and may affect the outcome [8].
- Data from numerous observational studies have suggested that earlier RRT initiation correlated with improved mortality and renal outcome. This was assessed further in 2011 in a review and meta-analysis [9]. The authors concluded that there was no good evidence for a beneficial effect of early CRRT on mortality. However, various studies have suggested that early CRRT reduces dialysis dependency, reduces duration of renal support and shortens ICU length of stay. However, the evidence for these outcomes is not sufficient to allow firm conclusions to be drawn.

It is advised that early support be instituted in the ICU setting to prevent biochemical decompensation.

Efficacy of CRRT

Size of molecules cleared by CRRTs

Type of molecule	Size	Example	Mode of removal
Small	<500 Da	Urea, creatinine, amino acids	Convection, diffusion
Middle	500–5000 Da	Vit B12, inulin, vancomycin	Convection, diffusion
Low-molecular-weight proteins	5000–50 000 Da	B2 microglobulin, cytokines	Convection or absorption
Large proteins	>50 000 Da	Albumin	Only minimal removal by CRRT

With regards to creatinine and urea clearances; high-volume CVVH may approach clearances associated with intermittent hemodialysis (IHD). Creatinine clearances of 30 mL/min are not unrealistic [10]. Clearance increases with increasing ultrafiltrate volumes and decreases with decreased filter life.

Practicalities

Initial settings

- An adequate pump speed is required, for example, approximately 200 mL/h blood flow through the machine.
- A fluid exchange/ultrafiltrate rate of 20 mL/kg/24 h is recommended (see below).
- Fluid deficits can be set as required (automatically on many modern machines).

Filters (membranes)

As blood comes into contact with the filter (membrane) surface, complement and leukocytes can be activated, therefore triggering the inflammatory and coagulation cascade. The degree of activation is variable, depending on the degree of biocompatibility of the membrane. Greater triggering occurs with bioincompatible membranes and it has been suggested that biocompatible membranes are associated with better outcomes.

Membranes used during RRT can typically be divided into two groups: cellulose-based membranes and synthetic membranes.

- Four randomized, controlled trials have been published comparing the use of biocompatible and bioincompatible membranes in the critically ill patient [11–14].
- Two trials found a significant difference in survival and recovery of renal function in favor of biocompatible membranes.
- A third study did not show any difference, but it must be pointed out that the trial was sponsored by a bioincompatible membrane manufacturer and one of the most potent inducers of complement was used as the biocompatible membrane.
- The fourth study did not show any difference either, but compared a semisynthetic membrane with a synthetic membrane.

Replacement fluid

During RRT a sterile replacement fluid is infused to replace the ultrafiltrate removed by hemofiltration or hemodiafiltration. There are two ways of infusing the replacement fluid:

Pre-dilution:

- Fluid is infused before the filter. It lowers the hematocrit of blood passing through the filter and, therefore, reduces anticoagulant requirements.
- There is 10% less solute clearance compared to the post-dilution method.

Post-dilution:

- Fluid is infused into blood leaving the filter. The concentration of sodium, potassium and glucose can be varied according to the patient's requirements, but the fluid does not contain phosphate, and this may need to be supplemented.

Buffers

The main buffers in replacement fluid are lactate or bicarbonate. A study by Barenbrock *et al.* [15] found bicarbonate buffer solutions to be superior in normalizing acidosis and reduced the incidence of cardiovascular instability in patients with renal failure.

Acetate-buffered solutions are also available, but studies have shown both lactate and bicarbonate buffer solutions to be superior.

Note: lactate-free hemofiltration replacement fluid contains no buffer, so bicarbonate must be infused separately at an appropriate rate to supply this.

Vascular access

Extracorporeal treatments require vascular access and there are two main approaches:

Veno-venous mode

- Most commonly used method in critically ill patients
- Requires cannulation of a large central vein with a double lumen catheter
- A peristaltic pump is used to pump blood through the filter, drawing blood through an "arterial" or outflow limb and returning via a "venous" or inflow limb
- Blood flow is usually between 150 and 200 mL/min.

Arterio-venous mode

- Rarely used
- Requires cannulation of artery and vein, hence higher complication rates
- The arterio-venous pressure gradient drives blood through the circuit
- Blood flow is usually 50–150 mL/min.

Anticoagulation

All forms of RRT expose blood to contact with a nonbiologic surface and therefore, activation of the clotting cascade. Despite coagulation abnormalities often seen in critical care patients, they still require anticoagulation to prevent filter and circuit clot formation during CRRT. No correlation has been found between routine coagulation variables and duration of filter survival. Anticoagulation during hemadialysis can be monitored by the determination of activated clotting times (ACTs). Anticoagulation options include:

- Anticoagulant free
- Continuous pre-filter unfractionated heparin infusion
- Low-molecular-weight heparin
- Sodium citrate
- Regional heparinization
- Prostacyclin and recombinant hirudin.

Anticoagulant free

- Critically ill patients often have deranged clotting, thrombocytopenia or a combination of both. Anticoagulant-free CRRT is made easier with good venous access, good blood flow rates and pre-dilution.

- Tan *et al.* have reported the safe use of CRRT with pre-dilution and no pharmacological anticoagulation in patients with coagulation abnormalities [16].

Continuous pre-filter unfractionated heparin infusion

- Infusion of doses (5–10 IU/kg/h) that does not alter activated partial thromboplastin time
- It may have some unpredictable and undesirable effects on systemic clotting mechanisms
- Infusion doses are adjusted, aiming for an activated clotting time (ACT) of 180–200 s.

Low-molecular-weight heparin

- Reeves *et al.* showed identical filter life, comparable safety, but increased cost when they compared fixed-dose low-molecular-weight heparin (dalteparin) with unfractionated heparin [17].

Regional anticoagulation

- Heparin or sodium citrate. Heparin is infused pre-filter, while protamine is infused post-filter as the neutralizer.
- Sodium citrate may be used as an alternative to heparin in order to avoid heparin-induced thrombocytopenia.
- A technique that involves the prefilter infusion of sodium citrate and post-filter infusion of calcium as a neutralizer.
- Although earlier techniques were associated with metabolic complications, two recent studies with simplified protocols have shown the safe use of citrate anticoagulation [17,18].

Citrate

- Citrate was first reported as an effective anticoagulant in the 1960s by Morita *et al.* [19].
- Citrate is used based on the principle that it avoids systemic anticoagulation. In a North American survey, citrate anticoagulation was used as a method of choice in 13% of patients who received CRRT for AKI in the adult ICU [20].
- The use of citrate anticoagulation will grow in popularity in the near future. The inherent complexities of the method are now reduced since a RRT-dedicated monitor may indeed provide a safe and an easy-to-handle citrate anticoagulation protocol besides standard heparin anticoagulation [21].
- Efficacy and safety of citrate is an important aspect. Most of studies reported longer circuit survival with citrate, but only few studies comparing citrate to heparin were randomized. Circuit life was significantly longer with citrate [22].
- Bleeding complications are a large motivation for the use of citrate as it leads to a regional anticoagulation. It is restricted to extracorporeal circuit and minimizes patient risk of bleeding. The five available randomized studies comparing heparin- to citrate-enrolled patients, excluded those at high bleeding risk [22]. However, bleeding episodes were similar with citrate and heparin in two reports and reduced with citrate in another two.

- Citrate appeared particularly beneficial in the subgroups of patients after surgery, with sepsis or with severe multiorgan failure [23].

Prostacyclin

- Prostacyclin inhibits the interaction between platelets and artificial membranes. It prevents extracorporeal thrombus formation. Heparin is relatively ineffective towards platelets.
- It inhibits fibrin, leukocyte and platelet base microaggregates which might prevent renal, pulmonary and neurological dysfunction.
- A study by Kozek-Langenecker et al. showed that prostacyclins were most effective in prolonging filter life, when coadministered with heparin. Bleeding complications were also less in the group receiving both prostacyclin and heparin than in the group receiving heparin alone [24].

Drug removal

Many of the drugs we administer to patients may be removed during CRRT, including drugs which normally accumulate in renal failure. Some drugs may suffer increased removal. Thus, dosages may have to be increased or decreased, or dosage intervals changed to achieve an adequate therapeutic effect.

A detailed description of the proportional removal of different drugs is beyond the scope of this text. Readers are advised to check the large reference texts available, consult the drug data sheets or take advice from their hospital pharmacy.

Intensity of CRRT in the ICU

The optimal intensity of continuous renal replacement therapy remains unclear. The VA/NIH Acute Renal Failure Trial Network and The RENAL Replacement Therapy Study Investigators showed that mortality at 90 days was not reduced in critically ill patients with acute kidney injury if they received treatment with a higher-intensity continuous renal replacement therapy [25].

The maintenance of a static protocol in a patient with a dynamic condition could result in "dialytrauma." With a dynamic approach, we would match the therapy to the actual necessities for each phase of the illness, limiting losses of valuable substances and improving cost-effectiveness. The study by Ronco et al. clarifies that an adequate dose is important, meaning not too much, but at the same time not too little [26].

The controversy: CRRT or IRT?

No conclusive evidence exists to determine the best form of RRT for critically ill patients. There is, therefore, controversy over which type of RRT should be used in ICU, with practitioners in Europe and Australia increasingly adopting CRRT, while the American nephrologists choose to remain with IRT:

- After adjusting for poor quality and severity of illness, a meta-analysis of 13 studies by Kellum et al. showed that mortality was lower in patients treated with CRRT [27]. The fact that trials have excluded patients with cardiovascular instability from intermittent renal replacement therapy (IRRT) probably supports the use of CRRT in critically ill patients [28].

- A more recent meta-analysis [29], however, was unable to make firm recommendations regarding the superiority of either IRT or CRRT with regard to mortality or recovery of intrinsic renal function, citing methodological concerns with many of the studies.
- The most recent meta-analysis specifically assessed whether IRT or CRRT was associated with likelihood of recovery of intrinsic renal function. They concluded [30] that there was some evidence of less dependence on dialysis after recovery from critical illness in those managed with CRRT. However, this was not based on randomized, controlled trials.
- The French hemodiafe study [31] suggests mortality of approximately 70% in patients in ICU given either CVVHDF or IHD. It is of interest that the IHD groups showed improved survival through the length of the study, that is intermittent dialysis got "better" in critically ill patients with more training, longer duration of treatment and increase in the dialysis "dose." Definitive studies comparing CVVH and IHD remain to be performed.

In addition, there may be other benefits associated with the use of CRRT compared to IRT:

- The rapid fluid shifts and hemodynamic upset associated with dialysis are associated with further ischemic insults to the kidney in animals.
- Creatinine clearance falls after dialysis, but does not after CVVH – presumably because of these shifts [32].
- Computed tomographic (CT) studies of the brain demonstrate changes after dialysis consistent with increased brain water that are not present after CVVH [33].

High-volume hemofiltration?

- The volume of ultrafiltrate may be important. Large volumes of ultrafiltrate (high volume or "aggressive" CVVH) increase creatinine clearance and may remove greater quantities of inflammatory mediators.
- An early large RCT of over 400 patients demonstrated improved survival with high volumes of ultrafiltrate compared to lower volumes [34].
- In a study of over 300 patients from Holland, those managed with high volume CVVH had a mortality of 33% compared with a predicted mortality of 67% given by the Madrid ARF score [35]. A subsequent smaller, randomized study from the same group has, however, failed to confirm these findings.
- The RENAL study compared hemofiltration volumes of 40 mL/kg/h with 25 mL/kg/h. As previously mentioned, there were no improvements in 90-day mortality with high-volume hemofiltration. [25]
- A large randomized trial involving 1124 [36] patients showed no significant difference in two groups, where one group received intensive RRT and the other not such intensive RRT. There was no difference in the duration of treatment or the kidney function improvements.
- A meta-analysis published in 2011 was unable to find any evidence for beneficial effect of high-volume CRRT on mortality [37].
- Overall, renal replacement therapy at 20 mL/kg/h is now recommended [36].

Fluid and electrolyte control

Another controversial area where CRRT may prove to be beneficial is the control of fluid and electrolyte balance:

- Patients with acute respiratory distress syndrome (ARDS) have increased extravascular lung water and in an attempt to improve oxygenation, a negative fluid balance can be introduced. Loop diuretics usually result in the loss of water, but not in a salt diuresis, therefore hypernatremia develops and extravascular lung water remains high. In such circumstances CRRT will normalize sodium levels and remove extravascular water. This often leads to a substantial improvement in gas exchange and lung compliance.

- Some patients in cardiogenic shock post-cardiac surgery might require extracorporeal membrane oxygenation and will usually also require large amounts of clotting factors. In this case CRRT can be used to maintain an even fluid balance by removing fluid while clotting factors are transfused. The development of ARDS and pulmonary edema can be prevented, while factors are infused.

- One study comparing CVVHDF with IRT showed that normalization of sodium, potassium and bicarbonate levels was more frequently achieved with CRRT [38].

- It has been suggested that transfusion requirements may be associated with filter life – frequently clotted filters resulting in greater requirement for blood transfusion.

- A retrospective cohort study was done in Edmonton, Alberta involving 90 children with a median age of 7 months. The study was conducted between 2004 and 2008. Fifty-four of the patients received RRT, where the most common indication was fluid overload. The mortality associated with this treatment was lower than the studies previously and in the adult population [39].

Septic shock, multiorgan failure and RRT

Many patients with ARF have severe sepsis, multiorgan failure and a major systemic inflammatory response. The activation and amplification depends on the release of proinflammatory mediators into the circulation. Targeting the systemic effects of these mediators seems to be a logical goal in the treatment of patients with severe sepsis. Specific single mediators have been targeted, but with disappointing results. Therapies targeting the removal of several circulating inflammatory mediators may prove to be more effective; CRRT is one of these therapies.

- Standard CRRT (exchange rate 1–2 L/h) in early, small studies produced clinical improvement in severe septic shock, independent of fluid balance, but failed to reduce inflammatory mediator plasma concentrations [40].

- Blood purification using high-volume hemofiltration (6 L/min) or coupled plasma filtration with adsorption has been shown to decrease the need for vasopressor therapy in septic shock [41]. The decrease was greater than during standard CVVH. Further, they also showed a significant decrease in plasma levels of C3a, C5a and IL-10. Changes were more striking during the early part of therapy, thus suggesting that the early decline in plasma concentration is due to membrane adsorption as the major removal modality. High-volume hemofiltration (HVHF) increases adsorption because of an increase in transmembrane pressure and larger filtering membrane area. Convective clearance will mainly occur after membrane saturation has taken place through adsorption.

- Other possible explanations for improved hemodynamic parameters are the possibility that other unmeasured vasodilatory solutes are removed during CVVH, causing vasoconstriction and decreased vasopressor requirements. Hypothermia induced by CVVH might also reduce requirements. It is also possible that sedative removal is greater during HVHF, therefore also reducing vasopressor requirements. Cole *et al.* found during their study that more than half of the patients required more sedation [41].
- Protective molecules, such as vitamins and amino acids, might also be removed during HVHF, having a negative effect on an already critically ill patient. No studies have yet been done to look at this effect.
- Overall, a 2011 meta-analysis concluded that neither low-volume nor high-volume CVVH was definitely associated with increased survival in septic shock [42].
- Indeed, CVVH rates as high as 70 mL/kg/h have not been shown to improve outcome in septic shock [43].

Advances in technology

Renal failure continues to be a major source of mortality and morbidity in the critically ill patient. By replacing transport, metabolic and endocrine functions of the kidney one can aim to improve and deliver a more complete form of RRT.

Human renal epithelial cells (RECs) have been isolated and expanded. They have demonstrated differentiated absorptive, metabolic and endocrine functions of the kidney when tested under *in vitro* and preclinical *ex vivo* animal studies. Therapy with RECs may improve morbidity and mortality by altering the proinflammatory state of patients.

Although a very innovative approach for treating renal and inflammatory disease states it may become a ground-breaking, transformative platform to current standard-of-care therapies [44].

References

1. Brivet FG, Kleinecht DJ, Loirat P, Landais PJM. French Study Group on Acute Renal Failure. Acute renal failure in intensive care units – causes, outcome, and prognosis factors of hospital mortality: a prospective, multicentre study. *Crit Care Med* 1996; 24 : 192–8.

2. Guerin C, Girard R, Selli JM *et al.* Initial versus delayed acute renal failure in the intensive care unit: a multicentre prospective epidemiological study. *Am J Resp Crit Care Med* 2000; 161 : 872–9.

3. Uchino S. The epidemiology of acute renal failure in the world. *Curr Opin Crit Care* 2006; 12 : 538–43.

4. Schiffl H, Lang SM, Fisher R. Daily hemodialysis and the outcome of acute renal failure. *New Engl J Med* 2002; 346 : 305–10.

5. Honore PM, Jamez J, Wauthier M *et al.* Prospective evaluation of short-term, high-volume isovolemic hemofiltration on the hemodynamic course and outcome in patients with intractable circulatory failure resulting from septic shock. *Crit Care Med* 2000; 28 : 3581–7.

6. Bent P, Tan HK, Bellomo R *et al.* Early and intensive continuous hemofiltration for severe renal failure after cardiac surgery. *Ann Thorac Surg* 2001; 71 : 832–7.

7. Gettings LG, Reynolds HN, Scalea T. Outcome in post-traumatic acute renal failure when continuous renal replacement therapy is applied early vs. late. *Int Care Med* 1999; 25 : 805–13.

8. Kawarazaki H, Uchino S, Tokuhira N *et al.*; Japanese Society for Physicians Trainees in Intensive Care Clinical Trial Group. Who may not benefit from continuous renal replacement therapy in acute

kidney injury? *Hemodialysis International* 2013; 17 : 624–32.

9. Karvellas CJ, Farhat MR, Sajjad I *et al.* A comparison of early versus late initiation of renal replacement therapy in critically ill patients with acute kidney injury: a systematic review and meta-analysis. *Crit Care* 2011; 15(1) : R72.

10. Brocklehurst IC, Thomas AN, Kishen R, Guy JM. Creatinine and urea clearance during continuous veno-venous haemofiltration in critically ill patients. *Anaesthesia* 1996; 51 : 551–3.

11. Schiffl H, Lang SM, Konig A *et al.* Biocompatible membranes in acute renal failure: prospective case-controlled studies. *Lancet* 1994; 344 : 570–2.

12. Hakim RM, Wingard RL, Parker RA. Effect of dialysis membrane in treatment of patients with acute renal failure. *New Engl J Med* 1994; 331 : 1338–42.

13. Himmelfarb J, Tolkoff, Rubin N, Chandran P *et al.* A multicentre comparison of dialysis membranes in the treatment of acute renal failure requiring dialysis. *J Am Soc Nephrol* 1998; 9 : 257–66.

14. Jorres A, Gahl GM, Dobis C *et al.* Haemodialysis-membrane biocompatibility and mortality of patients with dialysis-dependent acute renal failure: a prospective randomised multicentre trial. *Lancet* 1999; 354 : 1337–41.

15. Barenbrock M, Hausberg M, Matzkies F *et al.* Effects of bicarbonate- and lactate-buffered replacement fluids on cardiovascular outcome in CVVH patients. *Kidney Int* 2000; 58 : 1751–7.

16. Tan HK, Baldwin I, Bellomo R. Continuous veno-venous hemofiltration without anticoagulation in high risk patients. *Int Care Med* 2000; 26 : 1652–7.

17. Reeve JH, Cumming AR, Galagher L *et al.* A controlled trial of low-molecular-weight heparin (dalteparin) versus unfractionated heparin as anticoagulant during continuous venovenous hemodialysis with filtration. *Crit Care Med* 1999; 27: 2224–8.

18. Tolwani AJ, Cambell RC, Schenk MB, Allon M *et al.* Simplified citrate anticoagulation for continuous

renal replacement therapy. *Kidney Int* 2001; 60: 370–4.

19. Morita Y, Johnson RW, Dorn RE, Hall DS. Regional anticoagulation during hemodialysis using citrate. *AM J Med Sci* 1961; 242 : 32–43.

20. Hyman A, Mendelssohn DC. Current Canadian approaches to dialysis for acute renal failure in the ICU. *Am J Nephrol* 2002; 22 : 29–34.

21. Bouman SC. And the winner is: regional citrate anticoagulation. *Crit Care Med* 2009; 37 : 764–5.

22. Monchi M, Berghmans D, Ledoux D *et al.* Citrate vs. heparin for anticoagulation in continuous venovenous hemofiltration: a prospective randomized study. *Intensive Care Med* 2004; 30 : 260–5.

23. Oudemans-van Straaten HM, Bosman RJ, Koopmans M *et al.* Citrate anticoagulation for continuous venovenous hemofiltration. *Crit Care Med* 2009; 37 : 545–52.

24. Kozek-Langenecker SA, Kettner SC, Oismueller C *et al.* Anticoagulation with prostaglandin E1 and unfractionated heparin during continuous venovenous hemofiltration. *Crit Care Med* 1998; 26: 1208–12.

25. RENAL Replacement Therapy Study Investigators. Intensity of continuous renal-replacement therapy in critically ill patients. *N Engl J Med* 2009; 361 : 1627–38.

26. Ronco C, Honore P. Renal support in critically ill patients with acute kidney injury. *N Eng J Med* 2008; 359 : 18.

27. Kellum JA, Angus DC, Johnson JP *et al.* Continuous versus intermittent renal replacement therapy: a meta-analysis. *Int Care Med* 2002; 28 : 29–37.

28. Kenningham J. Controversies in haemofiltration. *CPD Anaesthesia* 2002; 4 : 115–20.

29. Bagshaw SM, Berthiaume LR, Delaney A, Bellomo R. Continuous versus intermittent renal replacement therapy for critically ill patients with acute kidney injury: a meta-analysis. *Crit Care Med* 2008; 36 : 610–7.

30. Schneider AG, Bellomo R, Bagshaw SM *et al.* Choice of renal replacement therapy

modality and dialysis dependence after acute kidney injury: a systematic review and meta-analysis. *Intensive Care Med* 2013; 39 : 987–97.

31. Vinsonneau C, Camus C, Combes A *et al.* Continuous venovenous haemodiafiltration versus intermittent haemodialysis for acute renal failure in patients with multiple-organ dysfunction syndrome: a multicentre randomised trial. *Lancet* 2006; 368 : 379–85.

32. Manns M, Sigler MH, Teehan BP. Intradialytic renal hemodynamics: potential consequences for the management of the patient with acute renal failure. *Nephrol Dial Transp* 1997; 12 : 870–2.

33. Ronco C, Bellomo R, Brendolan A *et al.* Brain density changes during renal replacement in critically ill patients with acute renal failure: continuous hemofiltration versus intermittent hemodialysis. *J Nephrol* 1999; 12: 173–8.

34. Ronco C, Bellomo R, Homel P *et al.* Effects of different doses in continuous veno-venous haemofiltration on outcomes of acute renal failure: a prospective randomised trial. *Lancet* 2000; 356 : 26–30.

35. Oudemans-van Straaten HM, Bosman RJ, van der Spoel JL *et al.* Outcome of critically ill patients treated with intermittent high volume hemofiltration: a prospective cohort analysis. *Int Care Med* 1999; 25 : 814–21.

36. Palevsky P, Hongyuan J, O'Connor TZ *et al.* Intensity of renal support in critically ill patients with acute kidney injury. The VA/NIH Acute Renal Failure Trial Network. *N Engl J Med* 2008; 359 : 7–20.

37. Negash DT, Dhingra VK, Copland M *et al.* Intensity of continuous renal replacement therapy in acute kidney injury in the intensive care unit: a systematic review and meta-analysis. *Vasc Endovascular Surg* 2011; 45 : 504–10.

38. Uchino S, Bellomo R, Ronco C. Intermittent versus continuous renal replacement therapy in ICU: impact on electrolyte and acid–base balance. *Int Care Med* 2001; 27 : 1037–43.

39. Boschee ED, Cave DA, Garros D *et al.* Indications and outcomes in children receiving renal replacement therapy in pediatric intensive care. *J Crit Care* 2014; 29 : 37–42.

40. Van Deuren M, Van der Meer JWM. Hemofiltration in septic patients is not able to alter the plasma concentration of cytokines therapeutically. *Int Care Med* 2000; 26 : 1176–8.

41. Cole L, Bellomo R, Journois D *et al.* High-volume haemofiltration in human septic shock. *Int Care Med* 2001; 27 : 978–86.

42. Latour-Pérez J, Palencia-Herrejón E, Gómez-Tello V *et al.* Intensity of continuous renal replacement therapies in patients with severe sepsis and septic shock: a systematic review and meta-analysis. *Anaesth Intensive Care* 2011; 39 : 373–83.

43. Joannes-Boyau O, Honoré PM, Perez P *et al.* High-volume versus standard-volume haemofiltration for septic shock patients with acute kidney injury (IVOIRE study): a multicentre randomized controlled trial. *Intensive Care Med* 2013; 39 : 1535–46.

44. Buffington DA, Westover AJ, Johnston KA, Humes HD. The bioartificial kidney. *Transl Res* 2014; 163 : 342–51.

Chapter

19
Chronic critical illness

David Leasa

Definition

The hallmark of chronic critical illness (CCI) is respiratory failure requiring prolonged dependence on mechanical ventilation (MV) [1]. A consensus group defined CCI as >21 consecutive days of MV for >6 hours/day [2]. Generally the clinician would recognize a patient with CCI with a constellation of the following characteristics [1,3]:

- Survival of the acute critical illness or injury, but has not yet recovered.
- Continuing need for tracheostomy and feeding tube
- Profoundly weak and deconditioned with myopathy, neuropathy and alterations of body composition, including loss of lean body mass, increased adiposity and anasarca
- Brain dysfunction manifesting as coma or delirium that is protracted or permanent
- Continuing need for vasopressors, inotropes or renal replacement therapy
- Skin breakdown associated with nutritional deficiencies, edema, incontinence and prolonged immobility
- Vulnerability to infection, often with multiresistant microbial organisms, and repeated courses of broad-spectrum antibiotics for ongoing or recurrent infections
- Patient distress from symptoms, including pain, thirst, dyspnea, depression and anxiety, with an inability to communicate effectively.

Outcomes

Patients who have CCI constitute 5–10% of patients with acute respiratory failure, but demand a disproportionate share of intensive care unit (ICU) resources.

- Reports indicate that patients who require MV for ≥21 days account for less than 10% of all mechanically ventilated patients, but occupy 40% of ICU bed days and accrue 50% of ICU cost.

The number of patients receiving prolonged mechanical ventilation (PMV) is growing due to increased patient survival and an aging population, further burdening constrained critical care resources [4].

- The overall 1-year survival for patients with CCI is between 40% and 50% [5].
- Most patients who fail to achieve ventilator independence within 60 days do not do so later.

Handbook of ICU Therapy, third edition, ed. John Fuller, Jeff Granton and Ian McConachie. Published by Cambridge University Press. © Cambridge University Press 2015.

Patients receiving PMV have persistent, profound disability and undergo multiple transitions of care, resulting in substantial healthcare costs [5].

- A prospective cohort study involving five ICUs described trajectories of care and resource utilization for 126 patients receiving PMV. Seventy patients (56%) were alive at 1 year although only 11 (9%) were independently functioning and only 19 (27%) had a good quality of life. Patients with poor outcomes were older, had more comorbid conditions and were more frequently discharged to a post-acute-care facility than patients with either fair or good outcomes.
- While tracheostomy may be the only option available for long-term survival, it can also precipitate physical and psychological discomfort, prolonged immobility and permanent institutionalization. Furthermore, cognitive impairment may prevent them from deciding for themselves and in most cases obligates a surrogate decision-maker.

Both clinicians and surrogates substantially overestimate prospects for recovery and do not anticipate the amount and intensity of caregiving that will be required.

- "ProVent," a mortality prediction model for patients requiring PMV, uses four variables (age, platelet count, and use of vasopressors and hemodialysis), each measured on day 21 of mechanical ventilation, to estimate 1-year survival of patients [6]. This simple model, validated in multiple centers, may help inform discussions of the risk of mortality for the CCI patient.

Reducing the risk of progressing to PMV

Clinicians should be motivated, early in acute critical illness, to prevent or minimize the duration of MV by better maintaining patients' physical and cognitive function [7], hence lessening progression to PMV.

Strategies known to prevent the need for mechanical ventilation include:

- Early goal-directed therapy in the initial treatment of sepsis [8]
- Noninvasive ventilation in selected patients (e.g. COPD, CHF, NMD) [9].

Strategies known to reduce the duration of mechanical ventilation once it has been initiated include:

- Small tidal volumes (6 mL/kg of ideal body weight) in patients with the acute respiratory distress syndrome [10]
- Conservative fluid management in patients with acute lung injury [11]
- Implementing evidence-based, best practice protocols for integrating the management of pain, agitation, and delirium in critically ill patients [12]. This includes: either daily sedation interruption or routine use of a light target level of sedation, an analgesia-first sedation approach and promoting sleep by optimizing patients' environments
- Protocol-driven ventilator weaning using daily spontaneous breathing and awakening trials [13,14]
- Early pulmonary and ambulatory rehabilitation [14,15]
- Protocols to reduce ventilator-associated pneumonia [16].

Care models

Patients with CCI may present a challenge to the "usual" ICU healthcare team. In the fast-paced environment of the ICU, their slow progress can be a source of frustration [17].

- Care programs need to better understand the medical complexities of these patients and adapt the care to meet their specific needs. Many ICUs still rely on input from specialists with limited knowledge and experience in the management of longer-term problems resulting from intensive care [18].
- Management of the CCI population requires a special combination of intensive care and rehabilitative skills, with a context of understanding care for the patient, beyond hospitalization.

Other venues of care have been pursued given the pressure on ICU facilities and the effect on patient flow through blocking of an ICU bed by long-stay patients.

- Venues of care for the CCI patient are varied, depending upon jurisdiction, and include acute care hospitals (both ICU and step-down units), ventilator-dependent rehabilitation units (VDRU), specialized long-term acute care hospitals (LTACH), skilled nursing facilities or even home.
- The CCI patient transition among these venues is frequently punctuated with episodes of acute critical illness and return to ICU [5].
- The nurse–patient and respiratory-therapist–patient ratios are less than continuing care in the ICU, allowing reduced costs.
- Specialist weaning centers, geographically distant from general ICUs, have also been developed to manage patients with PMV. The approach to weaning is usually multiprofessional, involving input from physicians, nurses, respiratory therapists, nutrition specialists, speech therapists, physical therapists, occupational therapists and psychologists.

Quality of life and ventilator independence may be impossible for many patients, particularly those who are older, with multiple comorbidities. However, those with chronic neuromuscular disease/restrictive chest wall disorders [19] can have good long-term survival and quality of life using long-term ventilation (either invasive or noninvasive, continuous or nocturnal). Intensive care units need to develop, or have access to, expertise for managing chronic mechanical ventilation that extends care into community settings [20,21]. They may also need to advocate for, and obtain, the necessary equipment and human resources for safe care outside of the ICU and hospital environments.

Management strategies in CCI
Ventilator support and weaning [22,23]

Patients requiring short-term ventilatory support fall into the easy-to-wean classification [24] and usually do not require a systematic reduction of ventilatory support. Such patients benefit most from early identification of extubation readiness [25]. Patients experiencing PMV present a significantly greater weaning challenge.

A patient's ability to successfully sustain spontaneous ventilation depends upon the balance between the load on the respiratory system (i.e. resistance, compliance and intrinsic PEEP) and how well a patient's respiratory muscles can cope with the imposed load.

Ventilator dependence is usually multifactorial [7]:

- The injured lung (e.g. ARDS, pneumonia) may have abnormal mechanics (e.g. increased airway resistance and decreased compliance), increased dead space and impaired gas exchange.

- The chest wall compliance may be reduced (e.g. obesity, ascites and anasarca).
- There may be limited neuromuscular capabilities that contribute to poor respiratory muscle function (either pre-existing and/or acquired). Immobility/disuse atrophy and critical illness polyneuropathy/myopathy are common.
- Sedating drugs may impair respiratory drive.
- Pre-existing comorbid conditions (e.g. COPD, neuromuscular weakness, heart failure, etc.) may increase load and/or reduce diaphragm capability further.

Weaning protocols reduce the duration of MV and ICU stay in those that wean expeditiously [26]. However, there is no clear consensus on the "best" way to reduce/remove ventilator support in patients that experience PMV. Different weaning methods and models of care may be required. Managing the ventilator is often more "art" than "evidence-based."

- Nocturnal respiratory muscle rest using pressure control ventilation (PCV) has been recommended to promote sleep in ICU patients with acute-on-chronic respiratory failure [27]. Sleep quantity and quality were significantly improved with PCV compared to low-pressure support ventilation (PSV). Frequency/tidal volume ratios were lower during sleep in the PCV group.
- Daily unassisted breathing via tracheostomy mask with full ventilator support at night, compared with systematic reductions in the level of PSV, as tolerated, resulted in shorter median weaning time, although weaning mode had no effect on survival [28]. The superior performance of the tracheostomy mask may have been due to rested respiratory muscles on assist control at night [29] or due to improved clinician ability to judge weaning capability and hence accelerate the weaning process.
- Efforts may be futile until many of the underlying causes of ventilator dependence are reversed, if possible. Some patients may be best managed through earlier planning for long-term mechanical ventilation in the community, either invasively or noninvasively.
- A protocolized weaning approach, specific for the CCI population and facility, should be utilized that incorporates the daily assessment of spontaneous breathing tolerance. This is outlined in Figure 19.1.
- Figure 19.1 shows the stages of the weaning process :

  A = tolerance of spontaneous breathing trials
  B = tolerance of tracheostomy mask trials
  C = tolerance of speaking trials
  D = tolerance of overnight tracheostomy mask trials
  E = transition to decannulation using noninvasive ventilation
  F = tolerance of decannulation.
- The criteria for failure of a spontaneous breathing trial or tracheostomy mask trial are :

  RR >35 breaths/minute for 5 minutes
  SaO_2 ≤90% (unless otherwise indicated)
  HR >140 beats/minute or a sustained change of ±20% from baseline
  Systolic BP <90 or >180 mmHg or a sustained change of ±30% from baseline
  Increased anxiety or diaphoresis
  f/Vt >105 for 5 minutes.

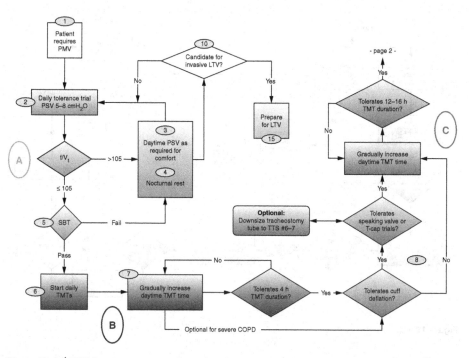

Figure 19.1 *[1] PMV*: Patients requiring prolonged mechanical ventilation ≥21 days with tracheostomy. *[2] Daily tolerance trial of PSV 5–8 cmH₂0*: Screen once or twice daily for the patient's readiness to tolerate T-mask trials. Measure the f/Vt ratio following 2 minutes of PSV 5–8 cmH₂O or at the lowest reachable PSV, if Vt ratio remains >105. *[3] Daytime PSV*: Use a level of PSV during the daytime hours that provides objective respiratory comfort, e.g. target f/Vt ratio ≤90. *[4] Nocturnal rest*: Use a level of PSV or PCV during the night-time hours that provides objective respiratory comfort, e.g. target f/Vt ratio ≤70. *[5] Spontaneous breathing trial (SBT)*: Perform for 30 min using PSV 5–8 cmH₂O/PEEP 5 cmH₂O. See failure criteria of a SBT/TMT. Continue PSV 5–8 cmH₂O for 2–4 hours to accomplish f/Vt ratio <90 before TMT. *[6] Start daily tracheostomy mask trial (TMT)*: First day accept 5–60 (maximum) minutes. See failure criteria of a SBT/TMT. *[7] Gradually increase daytime TMT time*: Aim to increase total duration by 30–60 min daily. Consider multiple TMTs with rest in between. See failure criteria of a SBT/TMT. *[8] Speech language pathologist*: Consider SLP consult to assess swallowing safety. *[9] Overnight TMT*: Use a one-way speaking valve or leave the tracheotomy tube uncapped. Provide oxygen and humidity as required. *[10] Candidate for invasive LTV*: Consider whether patient would best be managed as invasive LTV. *[11] tcpCO₂ and/or AM ABG*: Overnight transcutaneous PCO₂ monitoring and/or early morning ABG. Identify if worsening daytime hypercapnia or nocturnal hypoventilation. *[12] TM × 48 h*: Use tracheostomy mask for 48 hours, if tolerated. Use a one-way speaking valve or leave the tracheotomy tube uncapped. Provide oxygen and humidity as required. *[13] T-Cap × 48 h*: Cap the tracheostomy tube. Further downsize the tracheostomy tube, if necessary. Provide oxygen and humidity as required. Consider repeat blood gases at this time. *[14] Consider trial of full-face mask NIV with T-Cap*: Consider this option if evidence of continued sleep disordered breathing and suspected OSA/OHS ± COPD, diaphragm weakness/paralysis, or neuromuscular weakness. Consider consult to respirology for assistance. Not an option if significant tracheostomy secretions. Process: further downsize the tracheostomy tube, if necessary; cap the tracheostomy tube; provide oxygen and humidity as required. Assess tolerance during the daytime using full-face mask bilevel positive-pressure ventilation starting with: IPAP 10 cmH₂O; EPAP 5 cmH₂O; ST mode; backup 10 breaths/min. *[15] Consider LTV*: Contact the LTV respiratory care facilitator for assistance. *[16] Manageable secretions*: Secretions are considered to be manageable using cough-assist maneuvers once decannulation occurs (e.g. using breathing stacking bag and valve, manually assisted cough, insufflator-exsufflator). *[17] Worsening hypercapnia*: Reassess again. Is there any other modification that can be made to lessen hypercapnia? For example: thoracentesis or pleural drain for pleural effusion; treat respiratory tract infection; modify cardiac medications or bronchodilators, etc.

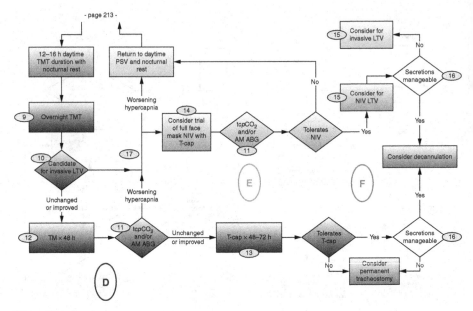

- page 213 -

Figure 19.1 (*cont.*)

Nutritional support [30–32]

Acute critical illness is characterized by catabolism exceeding anabolism.

- Nutrition support attempts to mitigate the breakdown of muscle proteins into amino acids that serve as the substrate for gluconeogenesis.

Recovery from critical illness is characterized by anabolism exceeding catabolism.

- Cumulative energy and protein loss may have become quite severe in the CCI. Loss is secondary to muscle disuse, stress/cortisol-induced catabolism, insulin resistance and other metabolic changes
- Energy expenditure increases significantly
- Nutrition support needs to provide substrate for the anabolic state, during which the body corrects hypoproteinemia, repairs muscle loss and replenishes lost nutritional stores.

Rational goals of nutritional support reflect a balancing of potential benefits of providing sufficient metabolic substrates to minimize further loss of lean body mass against adverse consequences of overfeeding and other risks.

- In the acute phase of critical illness, provide sufficient protein to compensate for hypercatabolism, initially 1.5 g/kg/d and then increased to 2.0 g/kg/d, depending on biochemical tolerance (blood urea nitrogen, ammonia) and clinical requirements (wounds, body composition, organ function). Patients with additional routes of nitrogen loss (renal replacement therapy, decubitus ulcer, high-output ostomy) may require increasing protein to 2.5 g/kg/d.

- In the chronic phase of critical illness, energy expenditure increases significantly and thus increased nonprotein calories (carbohydrates, lipids) should be delivered and sufficient protein should continue to be given. Calorie goals should be set at 25–30 kcal/kg/day.
- Provide intensive insulin therapy to target blood glucose of 7–9 mmol/L. Hyperglycemia (blood sugars >10 mmol/L) should be avoided. Optimal nutrition support is required to avoid the risk of hypoglycemia.
- Supplemental combined vitamins and trace elements, and the use of probiotics should be considered.

Nutrition is provided primarily via the enteral route (EN).

- Small bowel feeding, compared to gastric feeding, with head of the bed elevated to 45° is recommended to reduce the risk of pneumonia.
- A percutaneous endoscopic gastrostomy (PEG) or jejunostomy (PEJ) should be considered if EN is required for a prolonged period of time (>30 d).
- The optimal EN formula should include consideration of fluid and sodium, glycemic and renal status; however, standard EN formulas are sufficient for most patients.
- EN is initially provided continuously, but can alternatively be cycled overnight or provided in boluses to facilitate the timing of physical therapy or other needs.
- Use of immune-enhancing EN formulas in the CCI population requires further study and is not routinely recommended.

Initiation of oral feeding can begin prior to discontinuation of ventilator support if the patient's swallow function is adequate.

- One-way speaking valves have been shown to improve swallow function and reduce the incidence of aspiration while feeding.
- A swallowing evaluation to determine the safety of oral feeding should be done. A dysphagia diet is usually indicated to prevent aspiration, as swallowing dysfunction is common secondary to the effects of intubation and tracheostomy.
- CCI patients who tolerate oral feeding should have a calorie count performed to assess intake, with appropriate reductions in EN subsequently made. Once patients can meet calorie targets solely through the oral route, EN is withdrawn.

Cognitive care [12,33]

Physical and psychological symptom distress is common and severe among patients with CCI.

- Consider the use of both opioid and nonopioid analgesics, as undertreated pain is associated with anxiety, sleep deprivation and delirium.
- Monitor analgesia adequacy with patient self-report, or if not possible, with a validated assessment tool.

Delirium is a disturbance of consciousness characterized by acute onset and fluctuating course of inattention accompanied by either a change in cognition or a perceptual disturbance, so that a patient's ability to receive, process, store and recall information is impaired.

- Monitor all patients for delirium, even those who are calm and not agitated. If you don't look for delirium you won't often find it! Validated tools include: the Intensive

Care Delirium Screening Checklist (ICDSC) and the Confusion Assessment Method-ICU (CAM-ICU).

- Identify and remove, if possible, delirium risk factors (e.g. benzodiazepine use, infection, immobilization).
- Use nonpharmacologic interventions to promote sleep, as sleep deprivation is detrimental and may contribute to the development of delirium (e.g. controlling light and noise, clustering patient care activities, and decreasing stimuli at night to protect patients' sleep cycles).
- The longer patients are delirious, the more cognitive dysfunction during their first year following hospital discharge.

Physiotherapy [34,35]

Early mobilization facilitates mental and physical recovery of critically ill patients receiving MV [36]. Less rigorous evidence is available studying the chronic phase of critical illness, when the patient is already cachectic, profoundly weak and debilitated.

Physiotherapy modalities in the CCI patient aim to: apply therapeutic tools to decrease bed rest complications and ventilator dependency, facilitate functional recovery and improve health status and quality of life. Sedation interruption and sedation protocols that avoid oversedation are crucial to best engage patients in these modalities. Potential modalities aim to:

- Treat muscle weakness
  - Postures (e.g. semirecumbent positioning, regular changes in posture)
  - Passive mobilization (e.g. daily passive movement of all joints)
  - Assisted mobilization (e.g. sitting on the edge of the bed, standing, transferring to a chair and ambulation using a ventilator with/without customized mobility aids)
  - Active limb exercise (e.g. kicking out legs while sitting, bedside cycle ergometers, lifting weights)
  - Neuromuscular electrical stimulation (NMES allows for passive muscle contraction via electrodes placed on the skin over the target muscle groups)
  - Respiratory muscle training (benefits still controversial).
- Manage airway secretions
  - Cough augmentation (e.g. manually assisted cough, manual hyperinflation with breath stacking, mechanical insufflation-exsufflation)
  - Secretion mobilization (e.g. positioning and postural drainage, percussion and vibrations, continuous rotational therapy using specialized beds, chest-wall oscillation therapy).

Patient communication [37,38]

Many CCI patients may be too debilitated or delirious to effectively communicate. However, given its importance as an important source of symptom distress, efforts to facilitate communication should be undertaken. This may enable patients to express their emotions and thoughts to family, and participate in discussions of treatment goals and preferences.

Techniques and tools can assist the CCI patient to communicate.

- Allow speech with the tracheostomy cuff deflated while on MV. To improve voice quality: downsize the tracheostomy tube (using with a low profile, tight-to-the-shaft cuff [39]) to enable expiratory flow to reach the vocal cords; use PSV to prolong inspiratory time as a consequence of the intentional leak; delay ventilator cycling, if possible, and apply PEEP to keep airway pressure positive (can use an in-line one-way valve).
- Place a one-way speaking valve or cap, if the patient can intermittently come off MV with the tracheostomy cuff deflated.
- Use an alphabet board or a communication board, to which either the patient or a caregiver can point (with affirmation from the patient through nodding or other signaling).
- If available, use touch screens and specialized keypads that can translate minimal physical pressure into synthesized speech.

Palliative care

Palliative care (PC) is an essential component of comprehensive care for CCI.

- PC is appropriate throughout all stages of the trajectory of an illness, not just the end, which distinguishes it from hospice care [40].
- PC aims to relieve suffering and can be provided at the same time as curative or life-prolonging treatments. Early implementation can enhance the effectiveness of disease-directed treatment for patients with serious and complex illness, while improving the quality of their lives, supporting their families and promoting efficient use of expensive resources.

Core elements of PC in CCI include [41]:

- The alleviation of symptom distress: many symptoms (e.g. pain, dyspnea, nausea and vomiting, fatigue, delirium and constipation) either related to the disease itself or the associated treatments, often go undertreated and negatively impact overall quality of life. Both pharmacological and nonpharmacological methods can be used.
- The communication about goals of care with the patient and/or their surrogate: this can be coordinated using a series of proactive, sensitive and structured discussions about the nature and prognosis of their illness to obtain consensus on therapeutic options that are consistent with the patient's values and preferences. Surrogates often lack knowledge and providing prognostic information may be challenging. Surrogates may not expect either the eventual profound disability or its associated caregiver burden [42] when the decision to proceed with the provision of PMV (i.e. tracheostomy) is made.
- The continuity of care: fragmentation and discontinuity of care tend to increase as critical illness continues over a prolonged period and different care venues, creating obstacles to coordinated, consistent communication. Key information exchanged during family meetings should be documented in the medical record so that all members of the team understand the status of communication and current goals of care.

End-of-life care

The values, preferences and goals of care of the CCI patient (or their surrogate, when appropriate) must be known to guide ongoing therapy, resuscitation wishes and future services (e.g. return to ICU care).

- Aggressive and further attempts at "curative" care may be incongruent with the patients' goals of care.
- Low-burden treatments, provided outside of an ICU, may become more desirable, reducing disruptive and avoidable transitions of care.
- It may be appropriate to suggest withholding or withdrawing life support when the available medical interventions are either unlikely to achieve the goals of care or become unacceptable to the patient [43].

References

1. Nelson JE, Cox CE, Hope AA, Carson SS. Chronic Critical Illness. *Am J Respir Crit Care Med* 2010; 182 : 446–54.

2. Macintyre NR. Management of patients requiring prolonged mechanical ventilation: report of a NAMDRC Consensus Conference. *Chest* 2005; 128 : 3937–54.

3. Carson SS. Definitions and epidemiology of the chronically critically ill. *Respir Care* 2012; 57 : 848–56.

4. Kahn JM, Benson NM, Appleby D et al. Long-term acute care hospital utilization after critical illness. *JAMA* 2010; 303 : 2253–9.

5. Unroe M, Kahn JM, Carson SS et al. One-year trajectories of care and resource utilization for recipients of prolonged mechanical ventilation: a cohort study. *Ann Intern Med* 2010; 153 : 167–75.

6. Carson SS, Kahn JM, Hough CL et al. A multicenter mortality prediction model for patients receiving prolonged mechanical ventilation. *Crit Care Med* 2012; 40 : 1171–6.

7. McConville JF, Kress JP. Weaning patients from the ventilator. *N Engl J Med* 2012; 367 : 2233.

8. Rivers E, Nguyen B, Havstad S et al. Early goal-directed therapy in the treatment of severe sepsis and septic shock. *N Engl J Med* 2001; 345 : 1368–77.

9. Keenan SP, Sinuff T, Burns KEA et al. Clinical practice guidelines for the use of noninvasive positive-pressure ventilation and noninvasive continuous positive airway pressure in the acute care setting. *CMAJ* 2011; 183 : E195–214.

10. The Acute Respiratory Distress Syndrome Network. Ventilation with lower tidal volumes as compared with traditional tidal volumes for acute lung injury and the acute respiratory distress syndrome. *N Engl J Med* 2000; 342(1) : 301–8.

11. Wiedemann HP, Wheeler AP, Bernard GR et al. Comparison of two fluid-management strategies in acute lung injury. *N Engl J Med* 2006; 354 : 2564–75.

12. Barr J, Fraser GL, Puntillo K et al. Clinical practice guidelines for the management of pain, agitation, and delirium in adult patients in the intensive care Unit. *Crit Care Med* 2013; 41 : 278–80.

13. Girard T. Efficacy and safety of a paired sedation and ventilator weaning protocol for mechanically ventilated patients in intensive care (Awakening and Breathing Controlled trial): a randomised controlled trial. *The Lancet* 2008; 371 : 126–34.

14. Thomsen GE, Snow GL, Rodriguez L, Hopkins RO. Patients with respiratory failure increase ambulation after transfer to an intensive care unit where early activity is a priority. *Crit Care Med* 2008; 36 : 1119–24.

15. Bailey P, Thomsen GE, Spuhler VJ et al. Early activity is feasible and safe in respiratory failure patients. *Crit Care Med* 2007; 35 : 139–45.

16. Rewa OO, Muscedere JJ. Ventilator-associated pneumonia: update on etiology, prevention, and management. *Curr Infect Dis Rep* 2011; 13 : 287–95.

17. Roulin M-J, Spirig R. Developing a care program to better know the chronically critically ill. *Intensive Crit Care Nursing* 2006; 22 : 355–61.

18. Subbe CP, Criner GJ, Baudouin SV. Weaning units: lessons from North America? *Anaesthesia* 2007; 62 : 374–80.

19. Pilcher DV, Bailey MJ, Treacher DF et al. Outcomes, cost and long term survival of

patients referred to a regional weaning centre. *Thorax* 2005; 60 : 187–92.

20. Wise MP, Hart N, Davidson C, Fox R *et al.* Home mechanical ventilation. *BMJ* 2011; 342 : d1687–7.

21. Dybwik K, Tollåli T, Nielsen EW, Brinchmann BS. Why does the provision of home mechanical ventilation vary so widely? *Chronic Respir Dis* 2010; 7 : 67–73.

22. MacIntyre NR. Chronic critical illness: the growing challenge to healthcare. *Respir Care* 2012; 57 : 1021–7.

23. Fan E, Zanni JM, Dennison CR *et al.* Critical illness neuromyopathy and muscle weakness in patients in the intensive care unit. *AACN Adv Crit Care* 2009; 20 : 243–53.

24. Boles J, Bion J, Connors A *et al.* Weaning from mechanical ventilation. *Eur Respir J* 2007; 29 : 1033–56.

25. Thille AW, Richard J-CM, Brochard L. The Decision to Extubate in the Intensive Care Unit. *Am J Respir Crit Care Med* 2013; 187 : 1294–302.

26. Blackwood B, Alderdice F, Burns K. Use of weaning protocols for reducing duration of mechanical ventilation in critically ill adult patients: Cochrane systematic review and meta-analysis. *BMJ* 2011; 342 : c7237.

27. Andréjak CC, Monconduit JJ, Rose DD *et al.* Does using pressure-controlled ventilation to rest respiratory muscles improve sleep in ICU patients? *Respir Med* 2013; 107 : 534–41.

28. Jubran A, Grant BJ, Duffner LA *et al.* Effect of pressure support vs unassisted breathing through a tracheostomy collar on weaning duration in patients requiring prolonged mechanical ventilation. a randomized trial. *JAMA* 2013; 309 : 671–7.

29. Kahn JMJ, Carson SSS. Generating evidence on best practice in long-term acute care hospitals. *JAMA* 2013; 309 : 719–20.

30. Doley J, Mallampalli A, Sandberg M. Nutrition management for the patient requiring prolonged mechanical ventilation. *Nutr Clin Pract* 2011; 26 : 232–41.

31. Schulman RC, Mechanick JI. Metabolic and nutrition support in the chronic critical illness syndrome. *Respir Care* 2012; 57 : 958–77.

32. Heyland D, Dhaliwal R, Drover JW, *et al.* Canadian clinical practice guidelines for nutrition support in mechanically ventilated, critically ill adult patient. *JPEN* 2003; 27 : 355–73.

33. Skrobik Y, Chanques G. The pain, agitation, and delirium practice guidelines for adult critically ill patients: a post-publication perspective. *Ann Intensive Care* 2013; 3 : 9.

34. Ambrosino NN, Venturelli EE, Vagheggini GG, Clini EE. Rehabilitation, weaning and physical therapy strategies in chronic critically ill patients. *Eur Respir J* 2012;39 : 487–92.

35. Needham DM, Truong AD, Fan E. Technology to enhance physical rehabilitation of critically ill patients. *Crit Care Med* 2009; 37 : S436–41.

36. Schweickert WD, Pohlman MC, Pohlman AS *et al.* Early physical and occupational therapy in mechanically ventilated, critically ill patients: a randomised controlled trial. *The Lancet* 2009; 373 : 1874–82.

37. Grossbach II, Stranberg SS, Chlan LL. Promoting effective communication for patients receiving mechanical ventilation. *Crit Care Nurse* 2011; 31 : 46–60.

38. Divo MJ, Gartner E, Scinto S. Communication alternatives. In: Ambrosino N, Goldstein R, editors. *Ventilatory Support for Chronic Respiratory Failure.* New York, London: Informa Healthcare, USA, Inc; 2008 : 323–32.

39. McCracken J, Leasa D. Trach tubes designed to maximize safety may increase risk to ventilated patients. *Crit Care* 2010; 14 : 1008.

40. Litrivis E, Smith CB. Palliative care: a primer. *Mt Sinai J Med* 2011; 78 : 627–31.

41. Nelson JE, Hope AA. Integration of palliative care in chronic critical

illness management. *Respir Care* 2012; 57 : 1004–12.

42. Cox CE, Martinu T, Sathy SJ *et al.* Expectations and outcomes of prolonged mechanical ventilation. *Crit Care Med* 2009; 37 : 2888–94.

43. Truog RD, Campbell ML, Curtis JR *et al.* Recommendations for end-of-life care in the intensive care unit: a consensus statement by the American College of Critical Care Medicine. *Crit Care Med* 2008; 36 : 953–63.

Chapter

20

Recognizing and responding to the deteriorating patient

John Kellett, Christian P Subbe and Rebecca P Winsett

Introduction

When medicine was practiced by solitary, independent practitioners, a patient's outcome depended on their doctor's individual availability and ability. Modern medical care, however, is now a complex chain of events in which multiple players of varying skill and abilities are involved. Although huge advances in medical science have been made, their very complexity often makes their implementation prone to serious systems failures and disastrous outcomes. In order to provide a safety net for patients at risk of catastrophic deterioration outside critical care areas hospitals have started introducing rapid response systems (RRS) [1]. Other terms such as outreach teams, medical emergency teams (MET) and patient at risk teams (PART) are often used interchangeably with RRS in the literature. These systems are designed to ensure that patients are promptly and accurately assessed, and appropriately treated as soon as possible.

A RRS includes two principle components:

- One for event recognition (afferent limb) that when triggered activates
- A response (efferent limb) that promptly provides appropriately equipped expertise.

In addition the RRS should provide post hoc process improvement activities and an administration and educational infrastructure to support the entire system.

Background

The premise of rapid response systems has a number of justifications:

- Critical illness requires increased levels of support and staffing.
  The need is not always obvious on admission to hospital and can
  develop as a complication of the initial pathology. In this case patients
  require timely transfer to ICU.
- Patients who don't quite require full critical care might be able to be stabilized during a transient period of instability faster and more cost-effectively outside of critical care.
- Recognition of critical illness or deterioration and response is often unreliable. Rapid response systems aim to improve reliability of response to critical illness.

The impact of a RRS depends on the reliable functioning of the five Rs of rapid response [2] (Figure 20.1):

- Recording of vital signs
- Recognition of abnormality

Handbook of ICU Therapy, third edition, ed. John Fuller, Jeff Granton and Ian McConachie. Published by Cambridge University Press. © Cambridge University Press 2015.

Table 20.1 Causes of afferent limb failure

Failure to record full sets of observations including respiratory rate

Failure to recognize abnormality

Failure to recognize trends in sets of vital signs

Failure to report abnormalities

Failure to escalate through hierarchies

Figure 20.1 The Chain of Survival for the deteriorating patient on a general ward.

Record - Recognize - Report - Respond - Repeat

- Reporting of deterioration
- Response with appropriate treatment.

A breakdown of this safety chain increases the risk of adverse outcomes.

Making the case for rapid response systems

Most modern hospitals provide numerous specialists: cardiologists, diabetologists, specialist nurses for wound care, case managers for discharge planning. It should, therefore, be a logical step to delegate the care of deteriorating patients to specialists. Moreover, critical-care-based skills should support critically ill patients outside of critical care units in the same way that cardiologists support patients outside of coronary care units.

Rapid response teams have evolved to respond to safety challenges arising from physiological deterioration:

- Cardiac arrests are usually preceded by significant physiological abnormalities that have not been acted on in a timely fashion [3,4]. These abnormalities are present in two-thirds of cases for six hours or more [5].
- Afferent limb failure [6] is a frequent cause for failure to rescue a deteriorating patient (Table 20.1). Unscheduled admissions to intensive care are often the end product of prolonged periods of physiological instability with a failure to escalate care due to a number of reasons, often related to human factors [7], with the most frequent causes of failure to rescue being failure of organization, lack of knowledge, failure to appreciate urgency, lack of experience, failure to seek advice and lack of supervision.

Table 20.2 Examples of rapid response team composition and organization

Team	Composition (example)	Call-out criteria (example)	Comments
Medical emergency team	Intensive care physician, medical resident, critical care nurse	Single parameter trigger or staff "worried"	Initially promoted in Australia. Usually no dedicated staff.
Rapid response system	Critical care physician and nurse	Single parameter trigger or staff "worried"	Initially promoted in the US. Different team make-up for different crisis. Often no dedicated staff.
Critical care outreach	Critical care nurse (with or without a critical care resident)	Composite scores of bedside observations (early warning scores)	Exclusive time commitment to the service; might only operate in office hours or 24/7.

- The majority of adverse events occur in patients with previous chronic illness, frailty or other known risk factors [8].
- RRS were initially developed in Australia, the USA [9] and UK [10], albeit with different configurations.
- In the USA rapid response systems have been endorsed by the National Patient Safety Goals of the Joint Commission in 2008 that required "healthcare staff members to directly request additional assistance from a specially trained individual(s) when the patient's condition appears to be worsening" [11].
- Rapid response teams (RRTs) use critical care nurses and physicians, respiratory physiotherapists and hospitalists to respond to patients at risk of catastrophic deterioration [Table 20.2].
- RRT development is in line with greater specialization in all sectors of healthcare.

Clinical research

Despite the clear rationale for RRS, clinical studies and two randomized controlled trials designed to demonstrate their benefits have yielded mixed results:

- A number of pre and post studies from Australia have shown improvement in a range of clinical outcomes [12,13].
- Priestley [14] randomized paired wards in a single center to RRS intervention in an interrupted time series design. Hospital mortality was nearly halved in patients of comparable severity by the introduction of the system.
- The MERIT study [15], a cluster randomized trial of 23 Australian hospitals was unable to show any differences in primary endpoints between the control and intervention patients. This may have been because activation of the RRS in the intervention group was not consistent. Secondary analysis of the MERIT study showed an inverse linear relationship between the number of cardiopulmonary arrests and the number of RRT call-outs [16]. There is, therefore, a need for a relatively high number of call-outs for a RRS to function optimally [17].

- The most recent systematic review of the literature on the impact of RRS found significant evidence for reduction of cardiac arrests and hospital mortality [18].

The afferent limb

Recognition of critical illness is a complex process. This is due to variability in pathology and physiology of patients and psychology of carers. In most cases catastrophic deterioration is signaled by changes in vital signs:

- Tachypnea is the most sensitive marker of deterioration [19], yet it is one of the most frequently missed vital signs [20]. Although increased breathing rate is a sensitive and early indicator of sepsis and other serious illness, on its own it may occasionally reflect the hyperventilation associated with anxiety, whereas deep and regular rapid breathing indicates metabolic acidosis.
- Tachycardia can be a sign of compensation for decreasing cardiac output and hypovolemia, as well as volume overload. Tachycardia from arrhythmia, the most common being atrial fibrillation, can be a life-threatening complication of numerous cardiac conditions.
- Hypotension can be a sign of decreased cardiac output or hypovolemia. In patients with a healthy cardiovascular reserve, cardiac output and blood pressure are usually maintained by increasing tachycardia. Once the heart rate exceeds 130 beats per minute, however, the filling time of the heart becomes so short that blood pressure can no longer be maintained. In older patients or those with heart disease, hypotension will start to develop at much lower heart rates. The ratio between systolic blood pressure and heart rate is called the shock index – once the heart rate exceeds the systolic blood pressure the patient is usually hypovolemic.
- High and low temperature can signal severe infection. Occasionally medications (including antibiotics) produce low-grade fever that is usually not associated with other symptoms (other than fatigue) or other vital sign changes.
- Hypoxia is now considered a vital sign, since oxygen saturation can be so easily measured at the bedside by oximetery. The normal oxygen saturation is >95% on room air and, since it cannot be lowered by conscious breath-holding, always indicates significant pathology. It may or may not be associated with tachypnea and/or breathlessness. Hypoxia that corrects on 24–28% oxygen is usually the result of small ventilation-perfusion mismatches that are common in patients with chronic obstructive pulmonary disease. However, if more than 28% oxygen is required to correct hypoxia then the patient has a major ventilation-perfusion mismatch (i.e. a shunt), or hypoventilation.

Other physiological signs are rarer markers of catastrophic deterioration:

- Bradycardia occurs in complete heart block, electrolyte disorders and intoxication with medication such as digoxin and β-blockers. It also occurs in association with hypertension in patients with raised intracranial pressure (i.e. the Cushing reflex).
- A reduced breathing rate occurs in neuromuscular disease (e.g. muscular dystrophy, motor neuron disease, Guillain–Barré etc.), opiate and other intoxications and, especially if associated with a bounding pulse and obtundation, may indicate carbon dioxide retention.

Table 20.3 Modified early warning score after Subbe *et al.* QJM [22]

	3	2	1	0	1	2	3
Systolic blood pressure (mmHg)	<70	71–80	81–100	101–199		>=200	
Heart rate (bpm)		<40	41–50	51–100	101–110	111–129	>=130
Respiratory rate (bpm)		<9		9–14	15–20	21–29	>=30
Temperature (°C)		<35		35–38.4		>=38.5	
AVPU score				Alert	Reacting to **V**oice	Reacting to **P**ain	Unres-ponsive

- Hypertension is most commonly associated with pain or fear and more rarely with delirium tremens, or a hypertensive crisis.
- Acute alteration in consciousness, unless associated with intoxication, often indicates serious life-threatening illness. Other aspects of mental status such as thought content and quality, as well as behavior, must also be considered. Fluctuations in mental status are almost pathognomonic of delirium, a serious and often life-threatening complication of critical illness.

In order to improve reliability of detection it is recommended that each set of vital signs is compared with a predefined standard either in the form of single parameter triggers or summary scores.

- With either system, a physiological abnormality should trigger an alert of the efferent arm, and changes in physiology should be used to track the progress of the patient.
- All systems using vital signs to activate the efferent system are therefore summarized as track-and-trigger systems.
- In Australia and the USA these are mostly single parameter triggers [21], whereas hospitals in the UK, Ireland, the Netherlands and Denmark tend to use early warning scores (EWS) [22] (Table 20.3).
- In EWS each parameter is graded according to its degree of abnormality, all abnormalities are summarized in a single score, and the value is then compared to a predefined alert threshold.
- A review of the existing literature in 2007 found little evidence to support any of the published models over its competitors [23].
- Since then Prytherch *et al.* have published an EWS (VitalPAC™ Early Warning Score ViEWS) [24] derived from a large database of vital signs from 35 585 consecutive acute medical admissions. ViEWS is a highly discriminative predictor of early in-hospital mortality with an AUROC for 24 h mortality of 88.8% (95% CI 88.0–89.5%).
- As a result, a modified version of ViEWS has been proposed as a National Early Warning Score by the Royal College of Physicians in the UK [25]. The fact that all hospitals will use the same systems is likely to facilitate training, allow benchmarking and assure familiarity to staff. The use of automated recording might improve the recording of vital signs and alert reliability [26].

- However, it must be emphasized that none of the peer-reviewed EWS has been fully validated in prospective clinical trials and in the health systems in which they are employed.
- Other healthcare systems are developing continuous electronic monitoring systems [27], representing a more proactive approach to identifying patient deterioration, based on the premise that physiologic changes can indicate, and perhaps predict, deterioration episodes. Multiple technologies are becoming available for both the measuring of physiologic data and its analysis.

The efferent limb

There is considerable international variation in the number of ICU beds available and, hence, the time sick patients may have to wait before they are admitted to ICU. The start of intensive care, however, does not have to be delayed until an ICU bed becomes available:

- An essential ingredient of the RRS concept is that intensive therapy can be brought to any bedside by the efferent limb of the system.
- RRS aim to improve the care of patients with deteriorating physiology in areas, such as a general medical ward, where this care cannot usually be delivered within the right time frame or skills set on the general floors.
- The efferent limb includes healthcare professionals with critical care skills.
- Examples of service models include medical emergency teams (METs), rapid response teams (RRTs) and critical care outreach services (CCOS).

In addition to the response to physiological crisis, some models advocate active rounding by advanced nurse practitioners on general floors in order to identify patients at risk at an earlier stage, and also use this contact time with general medical and surgical ward nurses as an educational opportunity [28].

Interventions

Interventions by RRS will depend on the make-up and size of the team. However, they are prioritized along the ABCDE (airway, breathing, circulation, disposition, examination/exposure) algorithm promoted by Advanced Cardiac Life Support and similar training systems. They, therefore, fall into:

- Basic interventions
  - Diagnosis e.g. assessing fluid status (with or without bedside ultrasound), ECG interpretation, rhythm diagnosis, interpretation of laboratory data, arterial blood gases
  - Prescription of fluid boluses
  - Prescription of antibiotics
  - Pain and symptom control
  - Establishing a monitoring plan.
- Advanced interventions
  - Insertion of central venous access

- Administration of assisted ventilation on the general floors until a critical care bed becomes available
- Rhythm control, cardio-version, defibrillation.

End-of-life care

End-of-life care is an important part of care provided by rapid response systems [29], especially if the present deterioration is the first significant episode during the hospital stay of a patient with significant comorbidity or a known malignancy.

- If rescue of a patient with deteriorating physiology seems to be very unlikely or, in the case of a dying patient, inappropriate the RRT is likely to recommend a palliative approach and the limitation of interventions to those appropriate to the patient.
- One of the drivers behind this aspect of RRS might be the lack of experienced senior staff on general floors in some healthcare systems and concerns about prognosticating in an increasingly litigious environment.
- Do-not-attempt-cardiopulmonary-resuscitation (DNACPR) orders are, therefore, one possible outcome of interaction with a RRT [30].
- A DNACPR order does not preclude referral to a RRT. Patients who would not be resuscitated or admitted to intensive care might still benefit from fluid resuscitation, review of antibiotics or noninvasive ventilation with palliative intent.

MET syndromes and standard operating procedures

Whilst some deteriorating patients present with a major abnormality of one vital sign that triggers a single parameter calling criteria, many patients have milder abnormalities of several vital signs, which taken together indicate a severely ill patient.

- The management of these patients with multiple abnormalities often requires considerable expertise.
- In order to achieve reliability of responses and outcomes standardization is likely to be advantageous.
- The bulk of rapid response calls are generated by a very limited number of scenarios.
- For these "medical emergency syndrome" scenarios [31] standard operating procedures or care bundles simplify assessment and treatment and can be audited.
- Treatment is only thought to be satisfactory if all parts of the care bundle have been completed or reasons for deviance from compliance with bundles has been documented.

Sepsis is one the most frequent causes for a RRT call out [32]. More patients die of septic shock than of breast and colon cancer together. Because of the complicated criteria for its formal diagnosis recognition is still often a problem and treatment patchy. A simplified set of criteria of the diagnosis allows greater reliability. The "sepsis six" [33] is a shortened care bundle that is easy to teach and measure, and falls into three pairs of interventions:
Sepsis six – care bundle:

1. Give **oxygen** and check for tissue hypoxia by measuring **lactate** (with a lactate over 4 mmol/dL after fluid resuscitation serving as a trigger for the resuscitation bundle).
2. Give **fluids** and measure tissue perfusion by **monitoring urine output** (aiming for a minimum of 0.5 mL/kg/h, i.e. 40 mL per hour for an 80 kg patient).
3. Give **antibiotics** after **taking** two sets of **blood cultures** and other relevant cultures.

Other common MET syndromes include:

- Bleeding: hypotension due to hypovolemia from causes other than bleeding can be caused by diarrhea, vomiting, diuretics and, last but not least, sepsis.
- Atrial fibrillation of new onset: atrial fibrillation is a frequent complication of acute illness, in particular in patients with sepsis or after major surgery. Underlying conditions should be treated, and management should follow the advanced cardiac life support algorithm [34] (www.heart.org/acls). Patients will often revert into sinus rhythm once the cause of the atrial fibrillation has been addressed.
- Respiratory distress is a common reason for a RRT call out. It is probably the most complex scenario, as the underlying cause is often not immediately obvious, but requires a more detailed work-up following principles of management of critical illness.

Decreased level of consciousness

This warrants discussion in more detail. A decreased level of consciousness should trigger a focused assessment and intervention aided by the use of four mnemonics.

- Possible causes :

  AEIOU: Apoplexy, alcohol, Epilepsy, Intoxication, infarction, Overdose, Uremia
  H*3: Hypoglycemia, Hypercalcemia, Hypoxia
- Immediate management:

  4Cs: level of Consciousness including Glasgow coma score, Collateral history, Concomitant injuries and Control of sphincters
  4 Ps: Pupillary reaction, Plantar reflexes, blood Pressure and Pulse.

In the absence of hypoglycemia, hypoxia or another immediately correctable metabolic cause, imaging of the brain is required. Seizures can impair the level of consciousness and the combination of up-going plantar reflexes and generally increased tone might point towards this diagnosis. Imaging is needed to rule out intracerebral bleeding, especially in patients taking anticoagulants and antiplatelet agents, and patients with proven or suspected intracerebral neoplasms. The latter will require timely treatment with steroids and/or neurosurgical interventions. Patients with a decreased level of consciousness should be monitored for airway problems. This will frequently require positioning the patient in the lateral position. A transfer to an area where one-to-one care can be provided should be considered.

ICU outreach post-discharge from critical care

A significant number of patients who have been discharged from ICU develop secondary complications that require a readmission to the critical care service. Discharge from ICU and step down from coronary care, high dependency care and other critical care areas is a significant event in the journey of the critically ill patient. From being previously continuously monitored and watched closely by nurses and doctors the patient now arrives in an area where there is no direct contact with the caring nursing and medical team for several hours at a time. Readmission to ICU has been reduced by the use of critical care outreach teams [35].

Critical care outreach teams support the recovery of the critically ill patient by:

- Introducing themselves to the patient in ICU prior to discharge
- Seeing the patient directly after ICU discharge
- Supporting an appropriate frequency of bedside observations
- Screening and timely referral of patients with post-traumatic stress disorder: depression and post-traumatic stress disorder might affect more than 20% of ICU survivors [36,37].

Measuring impact of rapid response systems

Rapid response systems aim to improve clinical outcomes of critically ill patients outside ICU. This improvement can be measured in three ways: clinical outcomes, processes of care and ensuring that the RRS does not divert resources away from other areas of care (i.e. balancing measures).

Outcomes measures

Outcomes measures are the:

- Number of cardiopulmonary arrests per 1000 admissions
- Number of patients with delayed admission to intensive care
- Number of patients with episodes of prolonged physiological abnormalities without appropriate escalation.

Process measures

Process measures assure that the RRS has functioning afferent and efferent limb and should include the:

- Quality/completeness of bedside observations: every set of bedside observations should have respiratory rate, oxygen saturations, fraction of inspired oxygen, blood pressure, heart rate, temperature and level of consciousness documented.
- Percentage of trigger events according to local guidelines that have been charted, but not escalated to the RRT.
- Number of calls to the RRT and the time delay between a call and the arrival of the RRT at the bedside. It is generally thought that a mature RRS should generate in excess of 30 calls per 1000 admissions in hospitals that do not exclusively deal with low-risk elective patients. If numbers are well below this, the standard of monitoring and percentage of escalated triggers should be reviewed.
- "Score-to-door" time [38] measures effective escalation to intensive care as the time from the first documented abnormal set of bedside observations to the arrival in intensive care or the start of critical-care-style treatments such as administration of inotropic drugs or invasive ventilation. In a multicenter pilot, a score-to-door time of more than four hours was associated with higher APACHE II scores on admission to ICU. This principle is investigated in significantly more detail in the (spot)light study, a multicenter UK study of the pathway that patients take from contact with the RRT to admission to ICU. The study has completed recruitment of several thousand patients [39].

Table 20.4 Outcomes 24 hours after first contact with the **Rapid Response Team**

Location of patient	Positive outcome	Negative outcome
Patient moved to intensive care	Score-to-door time <4 hours	Score-to-door time >4 hours
Patient died	Patient died with input from palliative care services AND/OR with a do-not-attempt resuscitation order	Patient died after cardio-pulmonary resuscitation
Patient remains on the general floors	Patient physiology improved OR do-not-attempt resuscitation order in place	Patient still unstable and triggering local criteria for RRT call-out
Others	Developed unrelated condition	Lost to follow-up

Balancing measures

Balancing measures assure that the intervention of the RRT does not generate inappropriate workload or divert resources. Suggested measures are the:

- Number of unscheduled admissions to critical care
- Number of calls to patients without changes in escalation status.

Audit

For summary review of rapid response teams we have developed the Multidisciplinary Audit EvaLuating Outcomes of Rapid Response (short MAELOR) audit process [40]. This simplifies measurement of performance of a RRT by classifying clinical outcomes 24 hours after first contact with the RRT into positive and negative outcomes (Table 20.4). A mature RRT should be able to achieve in excess of 90% positive outcomes.

Training requirements

Successful RRS flourish in an organizational culture that encourages training at all levels.

- All members of the wider team need a clear understanding of their responsibilities. Team roles and accountabilities must be well described.
- All members of the team need to show willingness to ask for help and advice, and the organizations need to place value on nurses and doctors who call for assistance.

Training of RRTs and staff from general floors is crucial for the functioning of the RRS. Although medical errors can occur as the result of the negligence or incompetence of a single individual, most are the result of system and communication failures involving a number of team members (Swiss cheese model) [41]. Situational awareness, self-awareness and insight into strengths and weaknesses of team members and the hospital system are crucial to avoid errors. It would therefore be wise to train nursing and medical teams together ("those who work together should train together").

Table 20.5 As the organization develops a rapid response system, the model may evolve over time. The following table represents the three tiers of a rapid response system, the type of personnel and key education and experience

Progression of RRS	Type of personnel used	Education and experience
Tier 1		
Early integration of RRS within an organization	Intensivist ICU nurse Respiratory therapist	Value of prevention of code blues outside the ICU Effective RRS team communication Advanced cardiac life support Effective communication in noncritical assessment and treatment Assessment skills based on role within team Simulation and mock drills are beneficial in coordinating and testing team processes
	Change champion	Integrate value of a RRS at all levels of the organization
Tier 2		
RRS with trigger system	ICU nurse Respiratory therapist Intensivist backup Unit (ward) RN	Continue education of value of RRS, communication, assessment skills Intervention protocols Scoring methods, documentation, expectations of using an early warning score or other type of track-and-trigger assessment.
	Change champion	Organizational value of calling early, calling often
Tier 3		
RRS with track and trigger surveillance in place	Surveillance nurse Information Technology	Assessment skills Effective communication Respected relationships with nursing and medical providers

- Training for the rapid response team should include advanced cardiac life support (ACLS) and clinical assessment skills.
- Professional communication protocols such as SBAR [42] improve communication and might be associated with improved mortality [43].
- Simulation training is advantageous to create positive team communication, given that human factors contribute to the majority of adverse incidents [44].

Considerations for the set-up of a service

The set-up of a new system often occurs gradually (Table 20.5). For efficient rapid response systems, training and education occurs at two levels:

1. Training of individuals:
   - Clinical expertise for RRT members to handle situations when arriving on the general floors without previous clinical involvement in a patient's case.

- Preparation of ward nurses to recognize parameters in which to call for rapid response.
2. Preparing the change within the hospital system:
   - Building a rapid response system within the hospital may have been instigated with the intensive care providers, but to integrate a successful system, other organizational departments and leaders must be included.
   - Along with identifying the factors that create the culture to recognize, prevent and call for backup prior to cardiopulmonary arrest, much work is required at the organization level.
   - Once key stakeholders understand the value of the rapid response system, the appropriate implementation, documentation and auditing processes can be created.
   - Key departments would include:
     - Nursing and medical staff education
     - Quality improvement, medical records
     - Finances/billing
     - Human resources
     - Hospitalists
     - General medicine
     - Information technology.

Controversies

- Concern has been expressed that general ward staff may be less diligent if it is known that a RRS backup is available to compensate for their oversights.
- RRS might promote confusion as to who has primary responsibility for the patient or could potentially divert resources away from more effective interventions.
- Despite the improved discrimination of calling criteria and EWS it is clear that abnormal vital signs do not always result in serious adverse events. It has, therefore, been suggested that changes in vital signs, rather than fixed values, identify deteriorating patients more accurately [45,46].
- Finally some authors have suggested that implementation of a rapid response system is, in essence, creating a system of rescue for patients who have been mis-triaged to lower levels of care. Alternative strategies for managing patient flow and optimizing limited critical care resources may prove more cost effective than an entirely new clinical system [47,48].

References

1. Jones DA, DeVita MA, Bellomo R. Rapid-response teams. *N Engl J Med* 2011; 365 : 139–46.

2. Subbe CP, Welch JR. Failure to rescue: using rapid response systems to improve care of the deteriorating patient in hospital. *Clinical Risk* January 2013; 19 : 6–11.

3. Sax FL, Charlson ME. Medical patients at high risk for catastrophic deterioration. *Crit Care Med* 1987; 15 : 510–15.

4. Schein RMH, Hazday N, Pena M *et al.* Clinical antecedents to in-hospital cardiopulmonary arrest. *Chest* 1990; 98: 1388–92.

5. Franklin C, Mathew J. Developing strategies to prevent inhospital cardiac arrest: analysing responses of physicians and nurses in the hours before the event. *Crit Care Med* 1994; 22 : 244–7.

6. Trinkle RM, Flabouris A. Documenting Rapid Response System afferent limb failure and associated patient outcomes. *Resuscitation* 2011; 82 : 810–4.

7. McQuillan P, Pilkington S, Allan A et al. Confidential inquiry into quality of care before admission to intensive care. *Br Med J* 1998; 316 : 1853–8.

8. Ehsani JP, Jackson T, Duckett SJ. The incidence and cost of adverse events in Victorian hospitals 2003–04. *Med J Aust* 2006; 184 : 551–5.

9. 5 Million Lives Campaign. (2008). *Getting Started Kit: Rapid Response Teams.* Cambridge, MA: Institute for Healthcare Improvement.

10. Comprehensive Critical Care. *A Review of Adult Critical Care Services.* London: Department of Health, 2000.

11. http://psnet.ahrq.gov/primer.aspx? primerID=4 (accessed May 2013).

12. Bellomo R, Goldsmith D, Uchino S et al. Prospective controlled trial of effect of medical emergency team on postoperative morbidity and mortality rates. *Crit Care Med* 2004; 32 : 916–21.

13. Bellomo R, Goldsmith D, Uchino S et al. A prospective before-and-after trial of a medical emergency team. *Med J Aust* 2003; 179 : 283–7.

14. Priestley G, Watson W, Rashidian A et al. Introducing Critical Care Outreach: a ward-randomised trial of phased introduction in a general hospital. *Intensive Care Med* 2004; 30 : 1398–404.

15. Hillman K, Chen J, Cretikos M et al. MERIT study investigators. Introduction of the medical emergency team (MET) system: a cluster-randomised controlled trial. *Lancet* 2005; 365 : 2091–7.

16. Chen J, Bellomo R, Flabouris A et al. MERIT Study Investigators for the Simpson Centre; ANZICS Clinical Trials Group. The relationship between early emergency team calls and serious adverse events. *Crit Care Med* 2009; 37 : 148–53.

17. Jones D, Bellomo R, DeVita MA. Effectiveness of the Medical Emergency Team: the importance of dose. *Crit Care* 2009; 13 : 313.

18. Winters BD, Weaver SJ, Pfoh ER et al. Rapid-response systems as a patient safety strategy: a systematic review. *Ann Intern Med* 2013; 158 : 417–25.

19. Subbe CP, Davies RG, Williams E et al. Effect of introducing the Modified Early Warning score on clinical outcomes, cardio-pulmonary arrests and intensive care utilisation in acute medical admissions. *Anaesthesia* 2003; 58 : 797–802.

20. Hogan J. Why don't nurses monitor the respiratory rates of patients? *Br J Nurs* 2006; 15 : 489–92.

21. Lee A, Bishop G, Hillman KM, Daffurn K. The Medical Emergency Team. *Anaesth Intensive Care* 1995; 23 : 183–6.

22. Subbe CP, Kruger M, Rutherford P, Gemmel L. Validation of a modified Early Warning Score in medical admissions. *QJM* 2001; 94 : 521–6.

23. Gao H, McDonnell A, Harrison DA et al. Systematic review and evaluation of physiological track and trigger warning systems for identifying at-risk patients on the ward. *Intensive Care Med* 2007; 33 : 667–79.

24. Prytherch DR, Smith GB, Schmidt PE, Featherstone PI. ViEWS–Towards a national early warning score for detecting adult inpatient deterioration. *Resuscitation* 2010; 81 : 932–7.

25. Royal College of Physicians. *National Early Warning Score (NEWS): Standardising the Assessment of Acute Illness Severity in the NHS. Report of a Working Party.* London: RCP, 2012.

26. Bellomo R, Ackerman M, Bailey M et al. Vital Signs to Identify, Target, and Assess Level of Care Study (VITAL Care Study) Investigators. A controlled trial of electronic automated advisory vital signs monitoring in general hospital wards. *Crit Care Med* 2012; 40 : 2349–61.

27. Tarassenko L, Hann A, Young D. Integrated monitoring and analysis for early warning of patient deterioration. *Br J Anaesth* 2006; 97 : 64–8.

28. Benson L, Mitchell C, Link M *et al.* Using an advanced practice nursing model for a rapid response team. *Joint Commission J Quality Patient Safety* 2008; 34; 743–7.

29. Jones DA, Bagshaw SM, Barrett J *et al.* The role of the medical emergency team in end-of-life care: a multicenter, prospective, observational study. *Crit Care Med* 2012; 40 : 98–103.

30. Chen J, Flabouris A, Bellomo R *et al.* MERIT Study Investigators for the Simpson Centre and the ANZICS Clinical Trials Group. The Medical Emergency Team System and not-for-resuscitation orders: results from the MERIT study. *Resuscitation* 2008; 79 : 391–7.

31. Jones D, Duke G, Green J *et al.* Medical emergency team syndromes and an approach to their management. *Crit Care* 2006; 10 : R30.

32. Dellinger RP, Levy MM, Rhodes A *et al.* Surviving Sepsis Campaign Guidelines Committee including The Pediatric Subgroup. Surviving Sepsis Campaign: international guidelines for management of severe sepsis and septic shock, 2012. *Intensive Care Med* 2013; 39 : 165–228.

33. Daniels R, Nutbeam T, McNamara G, Galvin C. The sepsis six and the severe sepsis resuscitation bundle: a prospective observational cohort study. *Emerg Med J* 2011; 28 : 507–12.

34. www.heart.org/acls (accessed May 2014).

35. Ball C, Kirkby M, Williams S. Effect of the critical care outreach team on patient survival to discharge from hospital and readmission to critical care: non-randomised population based study. *BMJ* 2003; 327 : 1014

36. Davydow DS, Gifford JM, Desai SV *et al.* Depression in general intensive care unit survivors: a systematic review. *Intensive Care Med* 2009; 35 : 796–809.

37. Davydow DS, Gifford JM, Desai SV *et al.* Posttraumatic stress disorder in general intensive care unit survivors: a systematic review. *Gen Hosp Psychiatry* 2008; 30 : 421–34.

38. Oglesby KJ, Durham L, Welch J, Subbe CP. 'Score to Door Time', a benchmarking tool for rapid response systems: a pilot multi-centre service evaluation. *Crit Care* 2011; 15 : R180.

39. https://www.icnarc.org/CMS/ArticleDisplay.aspx?ID=e40e7adc-ad98-df11-8ff6-002264a1a658&root=RESEARCH&categoryID=70422f67-6983-de11-9a46-002264a1a658 (accessed May 2013).

40. Morris A, Owen HM, Jones K *et al.* Objective patient-related outcomes of rapid-response systems: a pilot study to demonstrate feasibility in two hospitals. *Crit Care Resusc* 2013; 15 : 33–9.

41. Reason J. Human error: models and management. *BMJ* 2000; 320 : 768–70.

42. http://www.ihi.org/knowledge/Pages/Tools/SBARTechniqueforCommunicationASituationalBriefingModel.aspx (accessed May 2013).

43. De Meester K, Verspuy M, Monsieurs KG, Van Bogaert P. SBAR improves nurse-physician communication and reduces unexpected death: a pre and post intervention study. *Resuscitation* 2013; 84 : 1192–6.

44. Huseman, K. F. Improving code blue response through the use of simulation. *Journal for Nurses in Staff Development* 2012; 28; 120–4.

45. Kellett J, Wang F, Woodworth S, Huang W. Changes and their prognostic implications in the abbreviated VitalPAC™ Early Warning Score (ViEWS) after admission to hospital of 18,827 surgical patients. *Resuscitation* 2013; 84 : 471–6.

46. Pimentel MA, Clifton DA, Clifton L *et al.* Modelling physiological deterioration in post-operative patient vital-sign data. *Med Biol Eng Comput* 2013; 51 : 869–77.

47. Litvak E, Pronovost PJ. Rethinking rapid response teams. *JAMA* 2010; 304 : 1375–6.

48. Hickey A, Gleeson M, Kellett J. READS: the rapid electronic assessment documentation system. *Br J Nurs* 2012; 21: 1333–6, 1338–40.

Chapter

21

ICU rehabilitation

Linda Denehy and Sue Berney

Improved survival following critical illness in the last two decades has resulted in more patients suffering severe critical illness living beyond hospital discharge. However, many of these survivors report ongoing muscle weakness and poor physical function, as well as neurocognitive and psychiatric symptoms that impact their health-related quality of life.

- Referred to as post-intensive care syndrome (PICS) [1], this constellation of symptoms can impact family roles and responsibilities, participation in social activities and the capacity for return to work (Figure 21.1).
- It can also cause anxiety and depression in family members and carers of survivors (PICS-family), impacting the health-related quality of life of both the survivor and carer [2].

The patient care model of achieving optimal physiological stability through manipulation of fluid, respiratory and renal function on a backdrop of heavy sedation and prolonged bed rest has been challenged as an understanding of the short- and long-term effects of critical illness have emerged. Muscle weakness is the most common impairment of survivors of critical illness and can result in longer-term loss of function. Early rehabilitation, including mobilization of patients who are intubated and ventilated, has been shown to improve strength and functional status, as well as reduce both ICU and hospital length of stay, and can be achieved within an acceptable patient safety profile.

Iwashyna and Netzer provide a conceptual model to guide choice of assessments and rehabilitation after critical illness, anchored in the International Classification of Functioning, Disease and Health (ICF) [3]. Within the ICF model, an assessment might focus on body function and structure (e.g. muscle atrophy or weakness on strength testing), on activity (e.g. performance on 6-min walk testing), and on participation (e.g. activities of daily living) (Figure 21.2). This model is excellent as it allows clinicians to focus on the limitations or disabilities that most affect individual patients and provides a basis for changing assessments to measure progress along the continuum of ICU recovery. This chapter will further explore the proposed mechanisms and sequelae of PICS, interventions that can be used to prevent or treat concomitant limitations and disability, outcome assessments useful to diagnose and monitor progress of rehabilitation (embedded into the ICF model, see Figure 21.2) and the safety guidelines currently proposed for early ICU rehabilitation.

Handbook of ICU Therapy, third edition, ed. John Fuller, Jeff Granton and Ian McConachie. Published by Cambridge University Press. © Cambridge University Press 2015.

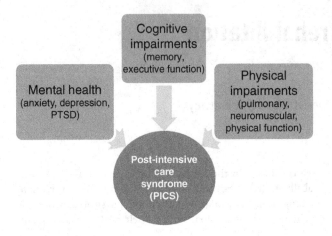

Figure 21.1 Impairments that make up post-intensive care syndrome (PICS). ASD, acute stress disorder; PTSD, post-traumatic stress disorder. (Adapted from [1]).

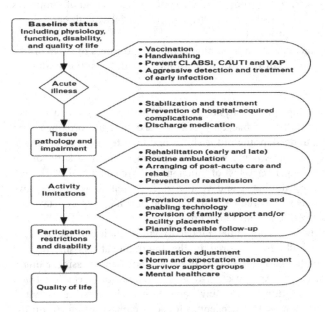

Figure 21.2 Conceptual model of the ICF as it relates specifically to ICU (Reproduced with permission from [3]).

Intensive-care-acquired weakness

Skeletal muscle wasting and weakness are common features in survivors of critical illness [4,5]. Commonly called intensive-care-acquired weakness (ICU-AW), this is a well-recognized clinical problem in patients who are critically ill [1]. Long-term follow-up studies have demonstrated that survivors of critical illness have ongoing severe disability as a result of the muscle wasting and weakness [6] and functional limitations. The majority (up to 25% of muscle mass) of muscle wasting occurs within the first week of admission [7]; therefore, ability to diagnose and target rehabilitation resources early is critical [1,6,8].

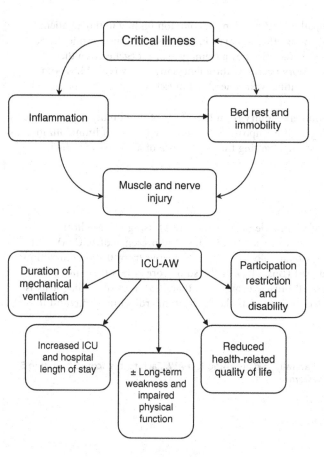

Figure 21.3 Possible mechanisms and sequelae for ICU-AW (Adapted from [8]).

Muscle weakness in the ICU is associated with prolonged mechanical ventilation, delayed rehabilitation and an increased length of stay [4,9]. Intensive care survivors report that loss of function is the most concerning disability up to 12 months after ICU discharge [10].

Definition and mechanisms of ICU-AW

- ICU-AW is defined as weakness secondary to critical illness in the absence of any neurological or metabolic etiology [11].
- Mechanisms that lead to ICU-AW are not well understood, although systemic inflammatory conditions such as sepsis are associated and appear to act synergistically with immobilization to produce more profound weakness than could be expected by bed rest alone (Figure 21.3) [8].
- ICU-AW may be described as either a neuropathy or myopathy or a combination of both, as there is significant overlap observed in critically ill patients with neuropathy and myopathy that may potentially be a continuum of the same disease process [7].

- Critical illness polyneuropathy (CIP) is the most common finding in those patients diagnosed with ICU-AW and is often observed in patients with sepsis, septic shock or multiorgan failure. It is characterized by a primary axonal degeneration that affects motor more than sensory nerves. Critical illness myopathy (CIM) has been described, with patients presenting with generalized muscle weakness, but preserved sensory function.
- Distinguishing muscle and nerve injury from the effects of immobility in the diagnosis of ICU-AW is challenging, as it is impossible to know the impact of immobilization as distinct from critical illness, highlighting the importance of activities to reduce immobility.

Diagnosis of ICU-AW

- Manual muscle testing of 12 muscle groups (Box 12.1) using the Medical Research Council (MRC) scale is used to diagnose the presence of ICU-AW [4]. Each of six muscle groups bilaterally is tested and scored from 0 (no contraction) through 5 (normal strength) (Box 21.2). If the sum score is less than 48/60 (meaning strength across all muscle groups less than 4/5), a positive diagnosis is made. This is currently still accepted as the "gold standard" clinical method to diagnose ICU-AW.

Box 21.1 Muscles tested bilaterally in diagnosing ICU-AW. Each test is scored from 0 to 5 using the Oxford grading system

Arm abduction

Elbow flexion

Wrist extension

Hip flexion

Knee extension

Ankle dorsiflexion

Box 21.2 Oxford grading system for muscle strength

Oxford grading scale

0	No visible contraction
1	Flicker of contraction (no movement of limb)
2	Active movement with gravity eliminated
3	Active movement against gravity
4	Active movement against gravity and resistance
5	Normal strength

- Manual muscle testing requires active participation by the patient, limiting the utility of the test in the critical care setting, as many patients cannot be measured or have a delayed diagnosis that can often not be made until after ICU discharge [12]. As a result detection of weakness using this method is delayed, which may impact rehabilitation planning.
- To improve between-tester reliability, training in the use of the Oxford grading scale is recommended [13].
- The reliability of manual muscle testing has been questioned with poor inter-rater reliability being reported in the ICU [14] and measurement in patients with higher cognitive function improving inter-rater agreement [15].
- Prior to testing, wakefulness and cooperation are assessed, commonly using the five commands developed by De Jonghe [4]. The wakefulness criteria are outlined in Box 21.3.

Box 21.3 Assessment of cooperation as per De Jonghe [4]

Ask the patient in a loud clear voice to do the following activities:
Open/close your eyes
Look at me
Poke out your tongue
Nod your head
Raise your eyebrows

Each one that is performed correctly = 1 point. The criterion is out of five. A minimum of 3 out of 5 is deemed awake

---

The cooperation criteria are most commonly assessed using a sedation scale, for example the Richmond Agitation–Sedation scale or the Riker sedation assessment scale. Different scales may be used in different units.

Assessment of strength and function

Assessment of strength and function in the ICU is essential to document the effectiveness of treatment. Choosing appropriate specific tests in ICU is difficult because of patient (sedation, drips and drains) and environmental (space on floor, equipment) factors.

- While many studies use performance-based tests such as the 6-minute walk test, it is often impossible to perform this type of test in ICU.
- Similarly, tests that require patients to answer questions may also be difficult.
- Since the level of ability of patients is variable, no one method has enough range from easy to difficult tasks to be applicable to all patients, meaning that they often have floor or ceiling effects when applied in ICU [16].
- Few measures of function have been specifically designed for the ICU population, however, with most being drawn from geriatric, neurological and pulmonary rehabilitation cohorts.

- In most cases, therefore, clinically worthwhile changes for measurement tools specific to ICU populations have not been evaluated.
- Often several different tests are used and are changed as the patient improves.

There is a large body of information that describes these tests and their clinimetric properties, although few specifically relate to ICU populations [16]. Table 21.1 explains commonly used tests in the ICU. A brief description follows.

Strength tests (other than MRC)

- **Hand-held dynamometry** may be used to diagnose muscle weakness in the ICU setting in place of MRC. It involves use of a small hand-held manometer to measure muscle strength in kg, used by the clinician to resist the force of contraction. The technique requires patients to actively participate.
- **Grip strength** is measured using a hand-held dynamometer. Recently hand-grip dynamometry has been recommended as a simple and easy surrogate measure for diagnosing ICU-AW. Antigravity muscle strength is required. Ali and colleagues reported that poorer outcomes were related to mortality [17].

Nonvolitional tests of muscle impairment have been advocated to address the implicit problems associated with the diagnosis of ICU-AW. These include muscle biopsies and ultrasound imaging.

- **Muscle biopsies** give insight into mechanisms associated with muscle atrophy and changes in muscle morphology and membrane excitability. A recent paper in *JAMA* [18] examined serial ultrasound and muscle biopsies in patients in the ICU during their first 10 days. The authors found that significant muscle loss occurred within the first 10 days (–17.7 (–25.9–8.1)%) (mean (95% confidence interval)), which was due predominately to proteolysis resulting from changes in muscle RING finger protein 1. The loss of muscle mass correlated with length of ICU stay, extent of organ failure and presence of inflammation, but not with age or nutrition [7,18]. These factors support the notion that ICU-AW results from factors other than just inactivity.
- **Ultrasonography** (US) is a valuable clinical tool for use in both clinical and research settings. It provides information about the muscle architecture and echo-texture that allow early diagnosis of muscle dysfunction. Ultrasonography has a number of beneficial properties: widely accessible in ICUs, performed at the bedside, noninvasive, painless, effort-independent. The nonvolitional nature of this assessment allows early, serial assessment of muscle changes and therefore early recognition of body structure and function changes in the ICU. Early detection may help to identify patients who will most benefit from rehabilitation. Staff can be trained to perform US and it has been demonstrated to be reliable and valid compared with MRI.

Functional tests

Assessment of specific functional activities and attainment of milestones have also been used to assess functional status in the ICU.

- Several tests for use in the ICU are now reported and are described in Table 21.1.

Table 21.1 Commonly used strength and function measures in the ICU

Type of physical function outcome	Description	Psychometrics
Physical Function in the ICU Test (PFIT)		
Denehy et al. [19]	Physical function battery test, scored out of 10 (10 represents best possible function). Four domains: sit to stand assistance level, shoulder flexion strength, knee extensor strength, marching in place cadence.	Correlates moderately with 6-MWT, TUG and MRC-SS. Excellent inter-rater reliability. Responsive to change. Higher PFIT score at ICU admission is predictive of MRC-SS $\geq$ 48, increased likelihood of discharge home, reduced likelihood of discharge to rehabilitation and reduced hospital LOS. Can be used to prescribe exercise intensity.
ICU mobility scale (IMS)		
Hodgson et al. [20]	Consists of 11 levels ranging from 0 (lying in bed) to 10 (walking independently without a gait aid).	Excellent inter-rater agreement (junior/senior physiotherapists and nurses).
Surgical ICU optimal mobility score (SOMS)		
Kasotakis et al. [21]	Scoring system used to determine optimal mobility level in the surgical population. Five levels included: 0 – no activity, 1 – PROM, upright in bed, 2 – sitting up, 3 – standing and 4 – ambulating.	Excellent inter-rater reliability. Scores correlate with hospital mortality and predictive of ICU and acute hospital LOS.
Functional status score for the ICU (FSS-ICU)		
Zanni et al. [22] Thrush et al. [23]	Assessment of physical function based on five tasks: rolling, supine to sit transfer, unsupported sitting, sit to stand and ambulation. Each task scored on a seven-point Likert scale. Score range 0–35 (35 equals complete independence).	Discriminative of discharge destination. Small effect size in small group of chronically critically ill patients [23].
Chelsea critical care physical assessment tool (CPAx)		
Corner et al. [24]	Includes assessment of: respiratory function, cough, bed mobility, supine to SOEOB, dynamic sitting, standing balance, sit to stand, transfer bed to chair, stepping and grip strength.	Moderate to excellent validity. Excellent inter-rater reliability.

Footnotes: LOS = length of stay; MOTS = marching on the spot; MRC-SS = Medical Research Council sum-score; PROM = passive range of motion; 6-MWT = 6-minute walk test; SOEOB = sit on edge of bed; STS = sit to stand; TUG = timed up and go test.

- In addition to these tests, other outcomes such as mortality, length of time on mechanical ventilation, ventilator-free days, ICU length of stay, acute hospital length of stay, and ICU and hospital readmissions are also used as endpoints to measure outcomes.

At ICU discharge or once the patient is discharged to the ward or from the hospital, different tests are common that reflect a higher level of functioning.

- The performance-based tests commonly used to measure higher levels of function are: the 6-minute walk test (6-MWT), timed up and go test (TUG), five times sit to stand test, short physical performance battery (SPPB) and Berg balance scale.
- Patient-reported tests include the instrumental activities of daily living (IADL), functional independence measure (FIM) and the Barthel index.
- Additionally, health-related quality of life measures such as the short form 36 are used as patient-reported outcomes for physical and mental function, as well as overall HRQoL.
- Community-based participation can be measured using (for example) physical activity levels using steps achieved per day measured with an accelerometer [25] and return to work and driving.

This list is not exhaustive and often depends on the country reporting the outcome.

Rehabilitation in the ICU

The aim of the management of patients who are critically ill in ICU should be to minimize exposure to the severity and intensity of critical illness and to promote early rehabilitation [26].

- The definition of what constitutes rehabilitation as opposed to (for example) physical therapy, early ambulation or early mobilization is unclear, with different definitions used by clinicians and researchers or indeed often no definition is provided [27].
- Exercises along a continuum from passive movements to active movements, changes in position such as exercising over the edge of the bed or moving from sitting to standing are considered rehabilitation by some authors [28].
- Others concentrate on early mobilization (walking or marching) as a definition of rehabilitation.

Members of the rehabilitation team in the ICU (physicians, physiotherapists, occupational and respiratory therapist and nurses) need to understand the types of rehabilitation modalities and the safety parameters and monitoring around these in order to provide the best interdisciplinary care [27]. Successful implementation of early rehabilitation programs requires teamwork, culture change and appropriate resource allocation. Physical therapists are key to the success of the implementation of a rehabilitation strategy, as when they are a member of the multidisciplinary team, they provide over 80% of all mobilization activities [29], achieving higher levels of mobilization for patients [30].

- Trials to date report acceptable safety profiles with few adverse events. For example Schweickert [31], Burtin [32] and Denehy [6] in their RCTs of a total of over 350 patients receiving exercise in the ICU reported no serious adverse events during or after exercise intervention. Certainly it is possible that early trials in this area have utilized conservative safety precautions. The limits for safety parameters such as cardiovascular, respiratory and neurological stability are often dependent upon agreed criteria within unit teams. The safety for commencing and for ceasing exercise interventions, as well as the usual precautions, should be established in all units and for all research trials. To date there are no specific published safety guidelines, although some papers have published these within their protocol [33].

- Sedation and cooperation levels of patients are tightly wound up in the rehabilitation process. High levels of sedation prevent early activity in ICU and sedation reduction needs to be targeted for all patients. The changing culture of ICU, highlighted by minimization of sedation, has led to patients, even when requiring mechanical ventilation, being mobilized [34].

- Accurate assessment of level of cooperation, cardiorespiratory reserve and rigorous screening for other factors that could preclude early mobilization is important [35].

- Early ICU rehabilitation is now an evidence-based treatment that should be considered in every critically ill patient from the very beginning of admission to the ICU [27]. There are now many reports that support rehabilitation as a safe and feasible intervention [31,36].

- There are several systematic reviews now available that summarize the efficacy of all or parts of rehabilitation interventions in ICU. As a whole these reviews support the effectiveness of exercise interventions concluding:

  - "Early exercise/PT seems to be the only treatment yet shown to improve long-term PF of ICU survivors" (Calvo-Ayala from 14 studies) [37].
  - "Physical therapy in the ICU appears to confer significant benefit in improving quality of life, physical function, peripheral and respiratory muscle strength, increasing ventilator-free days, and decreasing hospital and ICU stay" (Kayambu from 10 studies) [38].
  - "Physiotherapy intervention that comprises early progressive mobilization is beneficial for adult ICU patients in terms of its positive effect on functional ability, and its potential to reduce ICU and hospital length of stay" (Stiller from 55 studies) [39].
  - "Electrical muscle stimulation is a promising intervention however, there is conflicting evidence for its effectiveness when administered acutely" (Parry from 6 studies) [40].

- A thorough assessment of premorbid health state is essential in determining the likely trajectory of recovery for survivors of a critical illness. The Charlson comorbidity index and the Functional comorbidity index (FCI) can be used to objectively document the extent of premorbid comorbidities. Functional impairment may exist prior to critical illness, and whilst limitations can be worsened as a result of an ICU admission, the patient outcomes cannot necessarily be attributed to the critical illness alone [41]. Figure 21.4 highlights this very well.

- The randomized trials examining in-ICU rehabilitation are shown in Table 21.2. There are also several trials examining rehabilitation after the ICU, demonstrating the importance of the continuum of care of ICU survivors. A description of these is not within the remit of this chapter.

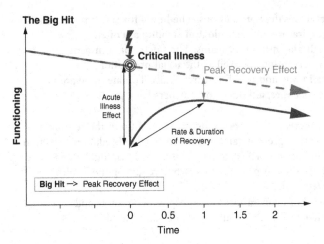

Figure 21.4 The "theoretical trajectory of recovery of an ICU patient after an ICU insult." From [41] with permission. (Reprinted with permission of the American Thoracic Society. Copyright © 2013 American Thoracic Society.)

Rehabilitation interventions

There are many interventions that are prescribed/performed by patients in the ICU. To date there is no evidence that any one or any combination is more effective than another. Studies that report positive effects use different exercise and/or cognitive interventions. More research is required to elucidate the optimal type, intensity and dose of exercise, as well as the timing and frequency. A brief description of the common types of in-ICU exercises is given below.

In-bed exercises

- Electrical stimulation of either single or several muscles (neuromucular electrical stimulation) or associated with a function activity such as cycle ergometry (functional electrical stimulation) are emerging areas of interest. These modes of rehabilitation are attractive as they do not require active patient participation, as other traditional methods of providing rehabilitation. Studies examining the efficacy of electrical stimulation have hypothesized that artificial stimulation of a muscle will protect the muscle from myopathic changes and improve functional outcome [53,54].
- Passive range of motion exercises (PROMS), as well as active exercises, functional activities such as rolling and bridging. There is limited evidence for effectiveness of PROMS.
- Supine cycling using one of the new cycles available. This can be done either passively or with applied resistance through the machine [32].
- Nintendo Wii fit exercises such as tennis assist upper limb movements and indeed can be performed in bed or standing, depending on the patient's ability. These exercises also stimulate cognitive function [55].

Table 21.2 Summary of trials of rehabilitation for patients whilst in the ICU

Study	Intervention	Duration/ frequency/intensity	Key findings
Strengthening			
Zanotti et al. [42]	EMS: 5 mins 8 Hz and 25 mins 35 Hz.	4 weeks, 5 days/ week, up to 30 mins/ session	Intervention group – significant improvements in muscle strength (2.2 versus 1.3, p = 0.02) and reduced number of days to transfer bed to chair (10.8 versus 14.3).
Burtin et al. [32]	Bedside cycle ergometer exercise training commenced day 5 of ICU admission.	20 minutes per day, 5 sessions per week. Passive cycling (20 cycles/minute) if sedated, progressed to active cycling as able (2×10 min bouts, intensity level individualized)	6-MWT distance 196 m (intervention) versus 143 m (controls), p <0.05. No significant difference between groups for quadriceps force. Significant improvement in SF-36 in intervention group.
Gerovasili et al. [43]	Lower limb EMS	55 mins, days 2–9 post-admission, 45Hz	Cross-sectional diameter of the right rectus femoris and vastus intermedius decreased significantly less in intervention subjects compared to control subjects.
Routsi et al. [44]	Lower limb EMS from day 2	55 mins, 7 days/ week, 45 Hz	Significant improvements in intervention group compared with controls for: MRC-SS (58:52), weaning time (1:3 days) and ventilator-free days (4:6 days).
Gruther et al. [45]	NMES	30 mins/day week 1, 60 mins/day from week 2, 5 days/week for 4 weeks, 50 Hz	Improvement in ultrasound measured muscle mass (intervention +4.9% versus control –3.2%, p = 0.013).
Rodriguez et al. [46]	NMES (unilateral brachial biceps and vastus medialis)	30 mins × 2 daily, 100 Hz from enrollment to extubation	Biceps (p = 0.005) and quadriceps (p = 0.034) strength significantly higher on stimulation side at treatment completion.
Ambulation			
Delaney et al. [47]	SOOB, ambulation, incentive spirometry from day 1 post-op.	Subjects advised to ambulate 60–300 m, SOOB and perform regular incentive spirometry	Intervention group – reduced hospital LOS (5.4 versus 7.1 days, p = 0.02).

Table 21.2 (cont.)

Study	Intervention	Duration/ frequency/intensity	Key findings
Muehling et al. [48,49]	Early mobilization	Commenced from surgery evening	Intervention group – significantly reduced post-operative ventilation, complication and hospital (2009) and ICU (2008) LOS.
Strengthening, ambulation			
Nava et al. [50]	P/AROM lower limb, respiratory muscle training, treadmill walking, ambulation, leg ergometer, stairs	× 2 daily, 30–45 mins each. Leg exercises × 2 daily × 30mins, 3 ×/ week. Respiratory: 10mins × 2/day Treadmill: 30mins × 2/day for 3 weeks (70% of incremental enrollment test) Leg ergometer: 20 mins, Borg <6, 15 watts Stairs: 25 ≥ 5 times	Significant improvements in intervention group 6-MWT distance and maximal inspiratory pressure.
Functional mobility, ambulation			
Porta et al. [51]	P/AROM, chest physiotherapy, mobilization, ambulation, arm ergometer.	15 mins chest, 30 mins ROM, 15 mins mobilization, 15 mins ambulation, arm ergometers 20 mins/day, 15 sessions (commenced at 0 W, increased by 2.5 W/ session according to Borg scale.	Intervention group – significant improvements in exercise capacity and endurance testing (ET) and reduced ET dyspnea and muscle fatigue.
Schweickert et al. [31]	PT and OT from recruitment to hospital discharge. Subjects had been on MV for <72 hours. Daily sedation interruption. Unresponsive – PROM exercises for all limbs. Responsive – AA and AROM in supine, bed	Daily. PROM – 10 reps all cardinal directions. Activity progression dependent on patient tolerance and stability.	Independent function at hospital discharge was (C:I) 35%: 59%; intervention group had shorter duration of delirium – 4:2 days, and more ventilator-free days – 21.1:23.5 days.

Table 21.2 (cont.)

Study	Intervention	Duration/frequency/intensity	Key findings
	mobility, transferring to sitting, sitting balance, ADLs, sit to stand transfers, pregait exercises and walking.		
Strengthening, functional mobility, ambulation			
Chiang et al. [52]	Upper (AROM supine and sitting progressed to include weights) and lower limb strength (AROM supine), bed mobility, transfers, standing, ambulation, diaphragmatic exercises.	5 × per week for 6 weeks. Borg scale used to judge intensity and progression (10–11 week 1, 12–13 weeks 2–6) 2 × 10 ROM exercises.	Significant improvements in intervention group in Barthel index and FIM scores, and respiratory and limb muscle strength.
Denehy et al. [6]	Physio: ICU = marching in place, sit to stand, arm/leg active and active resisted movements. Ward/outpatients = cardiovascular, progressive strength and functional.	ICU – MV 1 × 15 mins/day, Weaned 2 × 15mins/day. Intensity ICU – Borg 3–5. Ward – 2 × 30 mins/day progressed to 1 × 60 mins/day. Outpatients – 2 × 60 mins per week for 8 weeks. Intensity ward/outpatients = Borg 4–6, 70% peak walking speed.	No significant differences for 6-MWT or any other outcomes at 12 months after ICU discharge. Rate of change over time in 6-MWT from first assessment were greater in the intervention group.

Footnotes: AA = active-assisted; ADLs = activities of daily living; CSD = cross-sectional diameter; EMS = electrical muscle stimulation; FIM = functional independence measure; LOS = length of stay; MRC-SS = Medical Research Council sum-score; MV = mechanical ventilation; NMES = neuromuscular electrical muscle stimulation; OT = occupational therapy; P/AROM = passive/active range of motion; PT = physical therapy; SOOB = sit out of bed, SF-36 = short form-36; 6-MWT = 6-minute walk test.

Out-of-bed exercises

- These tend to be more functional, such as sitting over the edge of the bed and performing active exercises in this position, transferring to a chair, sitting in the chair, cycling using an arm or leg ergometer in sitting, standing; marching in place or walking away from the bed.

Neurocognitive interventions

Long-term cognitive dysfunction is common after critical illness and may last up to 12 months [56].

- In a land mark study of 821 patients admitted to ICU, the incidence of delirium was 74%, occurred mainly in the first 10 days after admission and was associated with worse global cognition and executive function at 3 and 12 months [56]. These findings were not related to age, sedatives or analgesics. It is not clear if specific interventions provide protection against later neurocognitive dysfunction; however, given the association between delirium and cognitive dysfunction, any treatment that may reduce the incidence of delirium may reduce brain injury.
- Early physical rehabilitation commenced in ICU was shown to reduce the incidence of delirium by 50% [31] and may be a promising intervention, but more research is needed to further test this hypothesis.

Resources

There are several online resources available now to assist ICU health teams to access the latest information about rehabilitation. The most recent and comprehensive of these is called the ICU Recovery Network (IRN). It is a virtual community of clinicians and researchers interested in improving the recovery of critically ill patients, with a particular focus on early rehabilitation and related interventions. The provider of this network (MedConcert or CE City) is providing this service free-of-charge. If you have an iPhone, you can download the "MedConcert" app to view and access the network on your phone. The address is medconcert.com (accessed June 2014).

The future

Improved education of intensivists, rehabilitation specialists, allied health practitioners and nurses regarding the increasing importance of management of sedation and early intervention with rehabilitation is needed. More research is also required that measures results of physical and nonphysical rehabilitation in (and after) ICU; specifically, amount, type and timing of intervention, types of outcome measures, effects on delirium incidence and identification of those who may respond best. As well, international consensus regarding safety parameters and measures of recovery would improve reporting and inform clinical practice guidelines. Randomized trials in this population are difficult to perform, so collaborations between centers would lead to improved research feasibility and subsequently inform the best evidence-based treatments and recovery measures to use at the right stage of the patient's journey.

References

1. Needham DM, Davidson J, Cohen H, *et al.* Improving long-term outcomes after discharge from intensive care unit: report from a stakeholders' conference. *Crit Care Med* 2012; 40 : 502–9.

2. Davidson J, Jones C, Bienvenu O. Family response to critical illness: postintensive care syndrome-family. *Crit Care Med* 2011; 40 : 618–24.

3. Iwashyna TJ, Netzer G. The burdens of survivorship: an approach to thinking about long-term outcomes after critical illness. *Semin Respir Crit Care Med* 2012; 33 : 327–38.

4. De Jonghe B, Sharshar T, Lefaucheur J *et al.* Paresis acquired in the intensive care unit:

a prospective multicenter study. *J Am Med Assoc* 2002; 288 : 2859–67.

5. Schweickert W, Hall J. ICU-Acquired Weakness. *Chest* 2007; 131 : 1541–49.

6. Denehy LSE, Edbrooke L, Haines K *et al.* Exercise rehabilitation for patients with critical illness: a randomized controlled trial with 12 months follow up. *Crit Care* 2013; 17 : R156.

7. Batt J, Dos Santos CC, Herridge MS. Muscle injury during critical illness. *J Am Med Assoc* 2013; 310 : 1569–70.

8. Truong AD, Fan E, Brower RG, Needham DM. Bench-to-bedside review: mobilizing patients in the intensive care unit – from pathophysiology to clinical trials. *Crit Care* 2009; 13 : 216.

9. Stevens R, Dowdy D, Michaels R *et al.* Neuromuscular dysfunction acquired in critical illness: a systematic review. *Intensive Care Med* 2007; 33 : 1876–91.

10. Agard AS, Egerod I, Tonnesen E, Lomborg K. Struggling for independence: a grounded theory study on convalescence of ICU survivors 12 months post ICU discharge. *Intensive Crit Care Nurs* 2012; 28 : 105–13.

11. Griffiths RD, Hall JB. Intensive care unit-acquired weakness. *Crit Care Med* 2010; 38 : 779–87.

12. Connolly BA, Jones GA, Curtis AA *et al.* Clinical predictive value of manual strength testing during critical illness: an observational study. *Crit Care* 2013; 17 : R229.

13. Ciesla N, Dinglas VD, Fan E *et al.* Manual muscle testing: a method of measuring extremity muscle strength applied to critically ill patients. *J Vis Exp* 2011; 50 : 2632.

14. Hough CL, Lieu BK, Caldwell ES. Manual muscle strength testing of critically ill patients: feasibility and interobserver agreement. *Crit Care* 2011; 15(1):R43.

15. Hermans G, Clerckx B, Vanhullebusch T *et al.* Interobserver agreement of Medical Research Council sum-score and handgrip strength in the intensive care unit. *Muscle Nerve* 2012; 45 : 18–25.

16. Elliott D, Denehy L, Berney S, Alison J. Assessing physical function and activity for survivors of a critical illness: a review of instruments. *Aust Crit Care* 2011; 24 : 155–66.

17. Ali NA, O'Brien JM, Jr., Hoffmann S, *et al.* Acquired weakness, handgrip strength, and mortality in critically ill patients. *Am J Respir Crit Care Med* 2008; 178 : 261–8.

18. Puthucheary ZA, Rawal J, McPhail M *et al.* Acute skeletal muscle wasting in critical illness. *J Am Med Assoc* 2013; 310 : 1591–70.

19. Denehy L, de Morton NA, Skinner EH *et al.* A physical function test for use in the intensive care unit: validity, responsiveness, and predictive utility of the physical function ICU test (scored). *Phys Ther* 2013; 93 : 1636–45.

20. Hodgson CL, Berney S, Haines K *et al.* Development of a mobility scale for use in a multicentre Australia and New Zealand: trial of early activity and mobilisation in ICU. *Am J Respir Crit Care Med* 2013; 187 : A1323.

21. Kasotakis G, Schmidt U, Perry D *et al.* The surgical intensive care unit optimal mobility score predicts mortality and length of stay. *Crit Care Med* 2012; 40 : 1122–8.

22. Zanni JM, Korupolu R, Fan E *et al.* Rehabilitation therapy and outcomes in acute respiratory failure: an observational pilot project. *J Crit Care* 2010; 25 : 254–62.

23. Thrush A, Rozek M, Dekerlegand JL. The clinical utility of the functional status score for the intensive care unit (FSS-ICU) at a long-term acute care hospital: a prospective cohort study. *Phys Ther* 2012; 92 : 1536–45.

24. Corner EJ, Wood H, Englebretsen C *et al.* The Chelsea critical care physical assessment tool (CPAx): validation of an innovative new tool to measure physical morbidity in the general adult critical care population; an observational proof-of-concept pilot study. *Physiotherapy* 2013; 99 : 33–41.

25. Denehy L, Berney S, Whitburn L, Edbrooke L. Quantifying physical activity levels of survivors of intensive care: a

prospective observational study. *Phys Ther* 2012; 92 : 1507–17.

26. Hough CL. Improving function during and after critical care. *Curr Opin Crit Care* 2013; 19 : 488–95.

27. Gosselink R, Needham D, Hermans G. ICU-based rehabilitation and its appropriate metrics. *Curr Opin Crit Care* 2012; 18 : 533–9.

28. Morris PE, Goad A, Thompson C *et al.* Early intensive care unit mobility therapy in the treatment of acute respiratory failure. *Crit Care Med* 2008; 36 : 2238–43.

29. Berney S, Haines K, Denehy L. Physiotherapy in critical care in Australia. *Cardiopulm Phys Ther J* 2012; 23 : 19–25.

30. Garzon-Serrano J, Ryan C, Waak K, *et al.* Early mobilization in critically ill patients: patients' mobilization level depends on healthcare provider's profession. *PM R* 2011; 3 : 307–13.

31. Schweickert WD, Pohlman MC, Pohlman AS *et al.* Early physical and occupational therapy in mechanically ventilated, critically ill patients: a randomised controlled trial. *The Lancet* 2009; 373 : 1874–82.

32. Burtin C, Clerckx B, Robbeets C *et al.* Early exercise in critically ill patients enhances short-term functional recovery. *Crit Care Med* 2009; 37 : 2499–505.

33. Denehy L, Berney S, Skinner E *et al.* Evaluation of exercise rehabilitation for survivors of intensive care: protocol for a single blind randomised controlled trial. *T Open Crit Care Med J* 2008; 1 : 39–47.

34. Schweickert WD, Kress JP. Implementing early mobilization interventions in mechanically ventilated patients in the ICU. *Chest* 2011; 140 : 1612–7.

35. Stiller K, Phillips A. Safety aspects of mobilising acutely ill inpatients. *Physiother Theory Pract* 2003; 19 : 239–57.

36. Berney S, Haines K, Skinner EL, Denehy L. Safety and feasibility of an exercise prescription approach to rehabilitation across the continuum of care for survivors of critical illness. *Phys Ther J* 2012; 92 : 1524–35.

37. Calvo-Ayala E, Khan BA, Farber MO *et al.* Interventions to improve the physical function of ICU survivors. *Chest* 2013; 144 : 1469–80.

38. Kayambu G, Boots R, Paratz J. Physical therapy for the critically ill in the icu: a systematic review and meta-analysis. *Crit Care Med* 2013; 41 : 1543–54.

39. Stiller K. Physiotherapy in intensive care: an updated systematic review. *Chest* 2013; 144 : 825–47.

40. Parry SM, Berney S, Granger CL *et al.* Electrical muscle stimulation in the intensive care setting: a systematic review. *Crit Care Med* 2013; 41 : 2406–18.

41. Iwashyna TJ. Trajectories of recovery and dysfunction after acute illness, with implications for clinical trial design. *Am J Respir Crit Care Med* 2012; 186 : 302–4.

42. Zanotti E, Felicetti G, Maini M, Fracchia C. Peripheral muscle strength training in bed-bound patients with COPD receiving mechanical ventilation: effect of electrical stimulation. *Chest* 2003; 124 : 292–6.

43. Gerovasili V. Electrical muscle stimulation preserves the muscle mass of critically ill patients: a randomized study. *Crit Care* 2009; 13 : R161.

44. Routsi C, Gerovasili V, Vasileiadis I *et al.* Electrical muscle stimulation prevents critical illness polyneuromyopathy: a randomized parallel intervention trial. *Crit Care* 2010 : 14 : R74.

45. Gruther W, Kainberger F, Fialka-Moser V *et al.* Effects of neuromuscular electrical stimulation on muscle layer thickness of knee extensor muscles in intensive care unit patients: a pilot study. *J Rehabil Med* 2010; 42 : 593–7.

46. Rodriguez PO, Setten M, Maskin LP *et al.* Muscle weakness in septic patients requiring mechanical ventilation: protective effect of transcutaneous neuromuscular electrical stimulation. *J Crit Care* 2012; 27:319 e1–8.

47. Delaney CP, Zutshi M, Senagore AJ *et al.* Prospective, randomized, controlled trial between a pathway of controlled rehabilitation with early ambulation and diet and traditional postoperative care after

laparotomy and intestinal resection. *Diseases of the colon and rectum* 2003; 46 : 851–9.

48. Muehling BM, Halter G, Lang G *et al.* Prospective randomized controlled trial to evaluate "fast-track" elective open infrarenal aneurysm repair. *L Langenbecks Arch Surg* 2008; 393 : 281–7.

49. Muehling B, Schelzig H, Steffen P *et al.* A prospective randomized trial comparing traditional and fast-track patient care in elective open infrarenal aneurysm repair. *World J Surg* 2009; 33 : 577–85.

50. Nava S. Rehabilitation of patients admitted to a respiratory intensive care unit. *Arch Phys Med Rehabil* 1998; 79 : 849–54.

51. Porta R, Vitacca M, Gile LS *et al.* Supported arm training in patients recently weaned from mechanical ventilation. *Chest* 2005; 128 : 2511–20.

52. Chiang LL, Wang LY, Wu CP *et al.* Effects of physical training on functional status in patients with prolonged mechanical ventilation. *Phys Ther* 2006; 86 : 1271–81.

53. Kho ME, Truong AD, Brower RG *et al.* Neuromuscular electrical stimulation for intensive care unit-acquired weakness: protocol and methodological implications for a randomized, sham-controlled, phase II trial. *Phys Ther* 2012; 92 : 1564–79.

54. Parry SM, Berney S, Koopman R *et al.* Early rehabilitation in critical care (eRiCC): functional electrical stimulation with cycling protocol for a randomised controlled trial. *BMJ* 2012; 2 : e001891.

55. Kho ME, Damluji A, Zanni JM, Needham DM. Feasibility and observed safety of interactive video games for physical rehabilitation in the intensive care unit: a case series. *J Critical Care* 2012; 27(219): e1–6.

56. Pandharipande PP, Girard TD, Jackson JC *et al.* Long-term cognitive impairment after critical illness. *N Engl J Med* 2013; 369 : 1306–16.

22
Palliative care, withholding and withdrawal of life support in the intensive care unit

Lois Champion and Valerie Schulz

Introduction

- Many patients die in the intensive care unit (ICU) either as a result of illness that fails to respond to therapy, or increasingly during withheld or withdrawn therapy [1].
- In the United States more than 25% of healthcare costs are spent in the last year of life and approximately 20% of deaths occur in or after a stay in the intensive care unit [2].
- Canadian hospitals are the location for end-of-life care for 70% of patients and 10–15% have an ICU admission during their final hospital admission [3]. In Ontario in Canada, intensive care units account for ~16% of inpatient expenses, but only ~8% of inpatient days [4].
- Many patients leave the intensive care unit with cognitive and functional morbidity and therefore intensive care has financial, social and personal costs [5,6].
- Quality end-of-life care is recognized as a priority for improving care in the healthcare system. Studies have shown that many patients die in pain or distress, that patients' wishes are not always incorporated into care plans and that communication is vitally important, but not always done well [7–9].

Palliative care

Palliative care referrals take place in communities, hospices and hospitals. Approximately 63% of Canadians die in hospital and, of those, 59% received palliative care [3]. The most common causes of death in Canada are cancer and circulatory disease [3]. Patients approach the end of their lives along trajectories of illness including: organ failure (most common cause of death), terminal illness (including cancer), frailty and sudden death [3], and some die along more than one trajectory simultaneously, for example a patient with metastatic lung cancer who experiences acute exacerbations of severe chronic obstructive lung disease.

Palliative philosophies of care specifically address: pain and symptom management, and consistent communication, including decision-making support for patients and families.

Thus it is increasingly important to address:

- End-of-life (EOL) care in the ICU
- Withholding and withdrawing of therapy
- Optimal care of the dying patient [7,9].

Handbook of ICU Therapy, third edition, ed. John Fuller, Jeff Granton and Ian McConachie. Published by Cambridge University Press. © Cambridge University Press 2015.

Definitions

- **End-of-life care**: the care provided to a person during the final stages of life. There is no exact definition of life's final stages, nor can a person's time of death be predicted with accuracy [10].
- **Life support**: (life-sustaining treatment) is any medical intervention administered to a patient with the goal of prolonging life and delaying death [11].
- **Palliative care**: focuses on pain and symptom relief, caring for the patient as a whole person who is a part of a social network during their experience of illness, while receiving medical treatment and end-of-life care. It includes, but is not limited to hospice care and comfort care near death [11]. Palliative care is an approach to care that improves the quality of life of patients and their families facing the problems associated with life-threatening illness, through the prevention and relief of suffering by means of early identification and impeccable assessment and treatment of pain and other problems, physical, psychosocial and spiritual [12].
- **Withholding of life-sustaining treatment**: to refrain from starting a treatment that has the potential to prolong the life of a person [11].
- **Withdrawal of life-sustaining treatment**: stopping a treatment that has the ability to prolong life after it has been started [11].
- **Physician-assisted suicide**: a practice that permits terminally ill patients to obtain from a physician a prescription for a lethal dose of medication for voluntary self-administration. Physician-assisted suicide is sometime referred to as "assisted suicide," "physician aid-in-dying" or "physician-assisted death" [11].
- **Euthanasia**: The Hastings Center defines euthanasia as "the intentional killing of a patient by a physician, as through the physician's administration of a lethal dose of medication." Euthanasia is permitted in some countries, but is illegal in the USA and Canada [11].

Models for integrating palliative care into ICU care provision

Palliative care can be integrated with critical care in a variety of ways. The models range from the "integrative model" to the "consultative model" of palliative care [13].

- The "integrative model" embeds palliative principles and skills into routine ICU care by training primary ICU staff in palliative care; the advantage is that all patients benefit from basic skills such as communication and symptom management; the disadvantage is training and updating is required for multiple staff members.
- The "consultative model" invites trained palliative providers into the intensive care unit; the advantage is a trained skill-set and role modeling is brought into the ICU, similar to other consultant specialties; the disadvantage is the palliative care teams require adequate staff, ICU-specific skills and knowledge, and acceptance from the ICU team.
- A blend of these models may be the most effective practice, for example the palliative care team can train and support the ICU team, while providing palliative care consultations, assisting with individual patient needs [13].
- As well, the palliative approach to care can be conducted by a team of participants who collectively are skilled in palliative concepts.

Table 22.1 Components of high-quality palliative care in the ICU (adapted from [16–20])

Domains	Characteristics
Communication [16]	• Timely, clear, and compassionate discussion • Involvement of palliative care even with prognostic uncertainty [17] • Identification of standards of care, treatment options and prognosis [18]
Decision-making from patient or SDM and team perspectives	• Identifying the patients' preferences, wishes, goals and values [18] • Participation in goals of care and plan of care discussions [18] • Conducting a family meeting; consider a systematic approach to the family meeting: before the meeting, during the meeting and after the meeting [19] • Resuscitation status/DNR decisions
Care for the patient	• Pain and symptom management [16] • Psychological care [20] • Addressing spiritual, emotional, social, cultural, existential and ethical concerns • Comfort, dignity, personhood and privacy [18]
Caring for the family [18]	• Interprofessional support • Encouraging access to the patient • Grief and bereavement support that can start prior to death • Enable the family to attend to end-of-life legal affairs, funeral arrangements • Transfer patient to local communities/hospice/palliative care where possible and appropriate
Structure and process [20]	• Collaborative development of a palliative support service that compliments and appreciates the uniqueness of each ICU and locally expanding the role of palliative care • Local palliative care champions can assist with this process

Key components of palliative care in ICU [14]

Important components of the palliative approach to care in ICU include:

1. Patient- and family-centered decision-making
2. Communication within the team and with patients and families
3. Continuity of care
4. Emotional and practical support for families
5. Symptom management and comfort care
6. Spiritual support of patients and families
7. Emotional and organizational support for ICU clinicians [15].

Some aspects of palliative care in the ICU are highlighted in Table 22.1 (adapted from references [16–20]).

Framework for ethical decision-making

Benefits for addressing ethical issues routinely may include; patient satisfaction by improving patient-centered care, reducing harm and assisting in conflict resolution [21].

As well, addressing ethical issues improves employee morale, productivity and institutional resource conservation. Law-abiding processes reduce the risk of law suits [21]. A 6-step framework to apply clinical ethical principles includes four integral ethical considerations:

- Patient preferences (from patient, most recent expressed wishes, beliefs and values, or best interests considerations)
- Clinical factors (create a team-based treatment plan)
- Cultural humility (respect individuals and cultures, understand diversity)
- Creating a moral community (follow commitments to healthcare) [21].

Consider involving an ethicist versed in these principles when introducing palliative care and ethically sound programs into the ICU.

Conducting a goal-setting meeting

There are a few fundamental principles to follow when the teams and patients meet to establish a common understanding of current events and a way forward. It is important to recognize these meetings are fundamental in building relationships and trust.

Goals of care and care plans, decision-making process

It is important to focus and clarify goals of care to improve care at the end of life [22]. Decision-making conversations can be considered in three stages; prior, during and after the meeting [23].

Prior to the meeting

Prior to the meeting it is necessary to:

- Decide who should be present, e.g. patient's substitute decision-maker (SDM) [24–26]
- Understand the patient's medical issues and investigations or treatments they may benefit from [27]
- Determine a collaborative opinion of the potential healthcare options to offer
- Review the patient's social situation and advance care planning documents
- Decide the goals of the meeting and the most suitable location for it to occur

During the meeting

During the meeting, after introductions, determine the patient's or SDM's understanding and expectations [24–28], review the medical summary that was prepared prior to the meeting, support the participants if they have an emotional response and provide helpful information [24,29] in terms of prognosis and healthcare options; then, in light of the news, review the patient's or SDM's expressed wishes [21,24] and goals of care.

The next step is to translate the goals into a care plan [23].

- This is a very significant time in the meeting and worth stating openly.
- This marks the point when the decisions are made through a blended lens of reverence toward the individual person being cared for, their health state and the care options.

- Often a consensus on a care plan can be reached in the meeting. Sometimes more information or time to comprehend the situation is required to determine the best care plan [30].
- Periodically, there are fixed discrepancies in opinions on the next steps in the care plan and conflict-resolution strategies are necessary [21,23].
- Ensure there is a follow-up plan, and reassure that the care will continue regardless of the conflict, and involve the palliative care team when appropriate.

After the meeting
After the meeting, document it and follow through on the actions stated during the meeting.
- Components of a family meeting can be found in the tools section of the IPAL-ICU website, "A Guide for Conducting an ICU family Conference" [31].
- It is essential to follow the impact of court cases on how the process of end-of-life decision-making changes
- There is improved family satisfaction with shared decision-making [32].
- Family information leaflets improve family comprehension of diagnosis and treatment, but not patient prognosis [27].

Family meetings to discuss goals of care and care plans can occur anytime after arrival in the ICU and assist in establishing day-to-day care plans. Since the majority of surgical ICU patients survive, withdrawal of life support is not always discussed. However, when decision-making addresses withdrawal of life support, it should be a treatment discussion rather than a breaking bad news discussion [33].

A practical approach to initiating the palliative approach in ICU
Cultural change in ICU practice
Interdisciplinary team participation to establish and sustain new quality initiatives is necessary for cultural change to occur in the ICU setting. This has been demonstrated to decrease the incidence of catheter-related bloodstream infections, and similarly it is expected that interdisciplinary teams will be required to improve the quality of palliative care provided in the ICU. Each team member has an important role in communicating with patients or SDMs, establishing patient prognosis and preferences, and aligning these with care plans. Nurses have strong skills in communicating with patients and families, learning their preferences and following protocols. As well, they may take leadership roles in coordinating family meetings [34].

A practical method to integrate a palliative approach in the ICU calls for time-based strategies:
- Day 0 – admission day
- Day 1 – identify the medical decision-maker, provide the family with information explaining their role, determine the patient's advance directive and resuscitation status, provide pain assessment and optimal management
- Day 3 – offer social-work assistance for practical and emotional support, and spiritual support
- Day 5 – interdisciplinary family meeting [35].

Withholding and withdrawal of life support [29]

Communication

The ICU consultant or delegate and the nurse and/or social worker should meet with the patient and family to discuss goals of care. Communication with the patient and family is a process that begins with patient admission to the ICU and is ongoing throughout the patient's stay in the ICU.

Documentation

Meetings with the patient and/or family to discuss the plan of care must be documented. These notes should include:

- Date and time of the meeting
- Persons present
- A summary of the discussion
- The plan of care decided upon.

Withdrawal of life support protocol

Nursing or social-work role:

- Obtain a quiet and private waiting room for the family if possible
- Offer spiritual support or pastoral care if available.

Nursing role:

- Ensure orders are written by the ICU physician
- Document sedation and analgesia scores if these are used in the ICU
- Ensure that the patient area is as quiet as possible – posting a "Quiet Please" sign at the bedside may be helpful
- Discontinue monitoring (for example, temperature probes, saturation monitors, etc.). If some monitoring is continued (for example ECG monitor) consider monitoring from a central station rather than the bedside. Silence alarms on the bedside monitor that may be distracting and disruptive to the patient and family
- Provide eye, oral and skin care; for example, artificial tears or oral moisture may be helpful for some patients
- Remove unnecessary equipment from the bedside
- Set up the room for easy access for the family if they will be at the bedside; for example:
  - Provide chairs at the bedside
  - Close curtains or doors for privacy
  - Drop bedrails.

Physician role and orders:

- Ensure that appropriate orders are written – for example these may include:
  - Discontinue lab work, radiographs and blood products
  - Discontinue all medications except for medications for sedation and analgesia

- Discontinue enteral feeds or total parenteral nutrition
- Consider removing feeding tubes, C-spine collars etc. – anything that will not contribute to the goal of comfort care.

Sedation and analgesia orders:

- Increasing pre-existing doses of medications may be necessary to ensure comfort (for example, increasing the rate of an opioid infusion)
- Ensure adequate medication is available for sedation and analgesia; for example, orders for narcotics and benzodiazepines as required
- Document reasons for administering medication (for example, signs of agitation, distress, grimacing, gasping respiration, tachypnea (respiratory rate over 20 breaths per minute).

Ventilation orders:

- If the patient is on supplemental oxygen wean or discontinue oxygen
- If the patient is ventilated, consider decreasing the inspired oxygen to 0.21 with PEEP of 0, and changing from an assist-control to a spontaneous mode
- Decide if patient comfort is better supported by removing the endotracheal tube or tracheostomy tube or leaving it in place.

Communication:

- Keep in contact with the patient, family and bedside nurse throughout the process to address any concerns, answer any questions and ensure that the patient is comfortable
- It is important to remember that the dying process may be rapid or take a prolonged period of time. Communicate this to the family and the providing team
- Consult palliative care services to consider a transfer to the palliative care unit after the withdrawal of life support, particularly if the patient survives longer than 24 hours after withdrawal.

Documentation:

- All decision-making discussions should be documented, including date, time, people present and a summary of the discussion.

References

1. Curtis JR, Engelberg RA, Bensink ME, Ramsey S. End-of-life care in the intensive care unit: can we simultaneously increase quality and reduce costs? *Am J Respir Crit Care Med* 2012; 186 : 587–92.

2. Mosenthal AC, Weissman DE, Curtis JR *et al.* Intergrating palliative care in the surgical and trauma intensive care unit: a report from the Improving palliative care in the intensive care unit (IPAL-ICU) project advisory board and the center to advance palliative care. *Crit Care Med* 2012; 40 : 1199–206.

3. Fowler R, Hammer M. End-of-life care in Canada. *Clin Invest Med* 2013; 36 : E127–32.

4. Leeb K, Jokovic A, Sandhu M, Zinck G. CIHI Survey: Intensive care in Canada. *Healthcare Quarterly* 2006; 9(1) : 32–3.

5. Griffiths J, Hatch RA, Bishop J *et al.* An exploration of social and economic outcome and associated health-related quality of life after critical illness in general intensive care unit survivors: a 12-month follow-up study. *Critical Care* 2013; 17 : R100.

6. Nelson JE, Cox CE, Hope AA, Carson SS. Chronic critical illness. *Am J Respir Crit Care Med* 2010; 182 : 446–54.

7. Braun UK, Beyth RJ, Ford ME, McCullough LB. Defining limits in care of terminally ill patients. *BMJ* 2007; 334 : 239–41.

8. Lilly CM, Daly BJ. The healing power of listening in the ICU. *N Engl J Med* 2007; 356 : 513–15.

9. Luce JM. End-of-life decision making in the intensive care unit. *Am J Resp Crit Care Med* 2010; 182 : 6–11.

10. National Institutes of health state-of-the science conference statement on improving end-of-life care. 2004. http://consensus.nih. gov/2004/2004EndofLifeCareSOS024html. htm (accessed August 2013).

11. Berlinger N, Jennings B, Wolf SM. *The Hastings Center Guidelines for Decisions on Life-sustaining Treatment and Care Near the End of Life*, 2nd edn. Oxford: Oxford University Press, 2013.

12. World Health Organization. WHO definition of palliative care. http://www. who.int/cancer/palliative/definition/en/ (accessed August 2013).

13. Nelson JE, Bassett R, Boss RD, et al. Models for structuring a clinical initiative to enhance palliative care in the intensive care unit: a report from the IPAL-ICU Project (Improving Palliative Care in the ICU). *Crit Care Med* 2010; 38 : 1765–72.

14. http://www.capc.org/ipal-icu/ (accessed June 2014).

15. Ho L, Engelberg RA, Curtis JR et al. Comparing clinician ratings of palliative care in the intensive care unit. *Crit Care Med* 2011; 39 : 975–83.

16. Mosenthal AC. Palliative care in the surgical ICU. *Surg Clin North Am* 2005; 85 : 303–13.

17. Mosenthal AC, Murphy PA. Interdisciplinary model for palliative care in the trauma and surgical intensive care unit: Robert Wood Johnson Foundation Demonstration Project for Improving Palliative Care in the Intensive Care Unit. *Crit Care Med* 2006; 34 : S399–403.

18. Nelson JE, Puntillo KA, Pronovost PJ et al. In their own words: patients and families define high-quality palliative care in the intensive care unit. *Crit Care Med* 2010; 38 : 808–18.

19. Novick R, Schulz V. The distinct role of palliative care in the surgical intensive care unit. *Semin Cardiothorac Vasc Anesth* 2013; 17 : 240–8.

20. Adolph MD. Inpatient palliative care consultation: enhancing quality of care for surgical patients by collaboration. *Surg Clin North Am* 2011; 91 : 317–24.

21. Sibbald RW, Chidwick P. Ethical principles and frameworks. In: Hawryluck L, Hodder R, eds. *End-of-Life Communication in the ICU*. Ottawa: CRI Critical Care Education Network, 2008.

22. Kumar G, Markert RJ, Patel R. Assessment of hospice patients' goals of care at the end of life. *Am J Hosp Palliat Care* 2011; 28 : 31–4.

23. Mount Sinai Medical Centre. The Family Goal-Setting Conference. Center to Advance Palliative Care. *The IPAL Project.* 2013. Available at http://ipal-live.capc. stackop.com/downloads/goal-setting-conference-pocket-card-mssm.pdf (accessed January 2013).

24. William Osler Health System. Checklist to meet ethical and legal obligations for patients in intensive care. *William Osler Health System.* Available at http://www. williamoslerhc.on.ca/body.cfm?id=716 (accessed January 2013.

25. Truog RD, Campbell ML, Curtis JR et al. Recommendations for end-of-life care in the intensive care unit: a consensus statement by the American College [corrected] of Critical Care Medicine. *Crit Care Med* 2008; 36 : 953–63.

26. Heyland DK, Cook DJ, Rocker GM et al. Decision-making in the ICU: perspectives of the substitute decision-maker. *Intensive Care Med* 2003; 29 : 75–82.

27. Azoulay E, Pochard F, Chevret S et al. Impact of a family information leaflet on effectiveness of information provided to family members of intensive care unit patients: a multicenter, prospective,

randomized, controlled trial. *Am J Respir Crit Care Med* 2002; 165 : 438–42.

28. Nelson J. Identifying and overcoming the barriers to high-quality palliative care in the intensive care unit. *Crit Care Med* 2006; 34 : S324–31.

29. Center to Advance Palliative Care. Improvement Tools. *The IPAL Project.* 2013. Available at http://www.capc.org/ipal/ipal-icu/improvement-and-clinical-tools (accessed January 2013).

30. Curtis JR, White DB. Practical guidance for evidence-based ICU family conferences. *Chest* 2008; 134 : 835–43.

31. Arnold R, Nelson J. A guide for conducting an ICU family meeting when the patient is unable to participate. *The IPAL Project.* 2010. Available at http://www.capc.org/ipal/ipal-icu/improvement-and-clinical-tools (accessed January 2013).

32. White DB, Braddock CH 3rd, Bereknyei S et al. Toward shared decision making at the end of life in intensive care units: opportunities for improvement. *Arch Intern Med* 2007; 167 : 461–7.

33. Barton E, Aldridge M, Trimble T et al. Structure and variation in end-of-life discussions in the Surgical Intensive Care Unit. *Commun Med* 2005; 2 : 3–20.

34. Nelson JE, Cortez TB, Curtis JR et al. Integrating palliative care in the ICU: the nurse in a leading role. *J Hosp Palliat Nurs* 2011; 13 : 89–94.

35. J E Nelson, C M Mulkerin, L L Adams, P J Pronovost. Improving comfort and communication in the ICU: a practical new tool for palliative care performance measurement and feedback. *Qual Saf Healthcare* 2006; 15 : 264–71.

Chapter

The injured patient in the ICU

23

Neil Parry and W Robert Leeper

- This chapter will focus on the acutely injured and/or post-operative trauma patient.
- There are many similarities in terms of proinflammatory and neuro-hormonal stress state created by both injury and surgery.
- The chapter will be structured into three main segments:
  1. Assessment and initial trauma management. Essentially an ATLS based review of ABCs, e-FAST (extended Focused Assessment of Sonography in Trauma – see below) and select evidence on blood product ratios, tranexamic acid and other important resuscitative pearls.
  2. Intraoperative management. A limited but important section focused on damage-control surgery and the transition back to ICU for ongoing resuscitation.
  3. Post-operative care and ongoing resuscitation. Miscellaneous topics relevant to both trauma and post-operative patients.

Epidemiology

Trauma remains one of the leading causes of death and disability worldwide and is the leading cause of death in children and adults up to age 44. Not surprisingly, care of the traumatically injured patient consumes a great deal of resources.

- The economic burden of unintentional and intentional injuries combined is estimated to be greater than $19.8 billion per year in Canada [1].
- This includes the direct costs to the healthcare system, as well as the indirect costs of reduced productivity due to injury or death.
- Alcohol and other intoxications are common.

Care of the multiply injured trauma patient is likely more closely linked to critical care medicine than any other surgical speciality. Trauma death still follows the classic "trimodal distribution" initially described by Trunkey [2].

- Most deaths (approximately 50%) occur at the scene from major anatomic injury, which results in exsanguination, neurologic and/or respiratory catastrophe.
- An additional 30% die within hours to days from injury from complications of severe hemorrhage or major neurologic dysfunction.

Handbook of ICU Therapy, third edition, ed. John Fuller, Jeff Granton and Ian McConachie. Published by Cambridge University Press. © Cambridge University Press 2015.

- The remainder generally die of multiple organ failure several days to weeks after the initial trauma.

Critical care management can clearly influence the outcome in the later two stages.

Assessment and initial trauma management

The initial assessment of injured patients should follow a uniform algorithm such as the American College of Surgeons Advanced Trauma Life Support (ATLS) course. The sequence and content of the primary survey is abbreviated ABCDE for airway, breathing, circulation, disability and exposure.

Airway

The binary decision of whether or not to take definitive control of a patient's airway is made within moments of the patient's arrival in the trauma bay. This decision can and should be revisited often throughout the course of resuscitation as variables can shift rapidly.

Indications for airway control are straightforward and include:

- Airway obstruction
- Inadequate airway protection associated with facial fractures
- Severe traumatic brain injury evidenced by Glasgow Coma Scale (GCS) <8
- Pending airway compromise as seen with facial burns or cervical hematoma
- Any need for mechanical ventilation to address oxygenation or ventilation failure.

Rapid sequence induction (RSI) and orotracheal intubation is the preferred approach for airway control and reference can be made to Chapter 8 for specifics and details.

- Special considerations include the need for in-line cervical spine (C-spine) stabilization provided by an assistant, for patients with uncleared C-spines.
- One must always assume the patient has a C-spine injury until proven otherwise.
- Airway adjuncts such as the gum-elastic bougie and video laryngoscope must be available as rescue techniques.
- Surgical cricothyrotomy is the final common pathway for failed or unobtainable orotracheal intubation.

C-spine injury

Cervical spine injury may be detected in as many as 10% of all significant blunt trauma patients [3].

- Cervical spines can be cleared in the awake patient on clinical grounds using the Canadian C-spine Rules and when contraindications to clinical clearance exists, radiography is required [4].
- Computed tomography (CT) of the cervical spine is the best imaging modality in the multiply injured patient.
- Controversy still exists regarding the need for further imaging to clear C-spines in obtunded patients with normal CT scans.
- While major North American centers often rely on normal CT imaging, others still perform MRI and/or flexion extension views to rule out ligamentous injury [5–7].

Breathing

Assessing the adequacy of oxygenation and ventilation follows airway in the ATLS primary survey. Clinical assessment with manual palpation for crepitus and auscultation for breath sounds is augmented by pulse oximetry, chest radiography and pleural ultrasound as part of the e-FAST exam.

Supplemental oxygen should be supplied to all victims of major trauma, and mechanical ventilation should be considered when signs of oxygenation or ventilation are impaired.

- A combination of direct trauma and indirect insult from the systemic inflammatory response to trauma may predispose patients to develop acute respiratory distress syndrome (ARDS).
- Therefore, it is reasonable to utilize a lung-protective ventilation strategy in the initial management of trauma patients with severe lung injury; this includes use of low tidal volumes (4–8 mL/kg), plateau pressures less than 30 cm H_2O, and PEEP:FiO_2 matching using a higher PEEP table [8]).

Please refer to the chapter on Acute lung injury and ARDS for advanced ventilation information.

Immediate life-threatening injuries to be identified and managed during the breathing assessment include:

- Open and tension pneumothorax
- Massive hemothorax
- Flail chest + pulmonary contusion.

Management of both hemo- and pneumothoraces is predicated on prompt chest drainage via tube thoracostomy.

- In the setting of tension pneumothorax, pre-thoracostomy decompression using a long (7–10 cm), large bore (14 gauge) needle in the second intercostal space in the mid-clavicular line can be considered as a temporizing maneuver.
- Failure rates of needle decompression have been reported to be as high as 65% [9]. For this reason skilled providers are encouraged to consider rapid tube thoracostomy as a primary option over needle decompression.

Massive hemothorax is typically defined as 1500 mL of blood on initial drainage or >200 mL per hour for the subsequent 2 to 4 hours. Management of massive hemothorax, including consideration of autotransfusion, damage-control resuscitation and selective operative approaches are better considered in the section on Circulation assessment below.

Flail chest is most often defined as greater than three contiguous ribs fractured in two or more places.

- This injury creates a free-floating segment of rib cage which moves paradoxically in opposition to the remainder of the chest wall during respiration.
- The underlying pulmonary contusion associated with flail chest is the major source of hypoxia and morbidity.
- Careful monitoring, multimodal pain control and selective use of ventilation (noninvasive and invasive) are important strategies for managing a patient with flail chest.
- Ultimately many such patients require mechanical ventilation.
- Several trials have been conducted to help identify the patients who will benefit from surgical fixation of flail chest, but the exact criteria remain elusive and further trials are ongoing [10–12].

Circulation

Circulatory assessment and management is perhaps the most important element of trauma resuscitation and the domain in which the majority of lives can be saved. Rapid detection of source of hemorrhage can be difficult, but is essential.

- Assessment begins clinically with assessment of heart rate and blood pressure as well as other signs of perfusion, including pallor, diaphoresis and capillary refill.
- Examination is next performed to identify sources of bleeding such as unilateral decreased breath sounds, an expanding abdomen, an unstable pelvis, an angulated femur or external hemorrhage.
- Treatment is initiated with large-bore peripheral IV access and warmed fluid therapy is begun. Lactated Ringer's is the preferred initial resuscitative fluid, however hypotensive bleeding patients require early transfusion with blood products.

Hypovolemic/hypotensive resuscitation

Landmark work by Bickell and colleagues at Ben Taub Hospital, Houston first demonstrated the potential benefits of a fluid-conservative resuscitation [13].

- Patients suffering penetrating torso trauma (neck/chest/abdomen) who had the availability of a rapid operative intervention achieved a survival advantage when pre-operative fluid therapy was limited and permissive hypovolemia/hypotension was maintained until surgical exposure and hemostasis could be obtained.
- This was predicated on the simple premise of trying not to "pop the clot."

While this study is important, it is critical to consider external validity and applicability to medium- and small-volume centers.

- Not all trauma centers are capable of providing the rapid response times and short injury to intervention times seen at Ben Taub.
- Further, the benefit of the intervention was most pronounced among patients with penetrating cardiac wounds and largely disappeared when these patients were removed from the study.
- Patients with closed head injuries potentially suffer significant secondary neurological injury if hypotension is not promptly treated.
- While the principles of hypovolemic resuscitation are salient, one needs to exercise caution when applying this study to a given local trauma center.

More recently, the term damage-control resuscitation has been used when there is a known surgical source of bleeding. The aim is to use very little, if any, crystalloid and instead use blood products in a 1:1:1 ratio to keep systolic blood pressure <90 mmHg until definitive surgical control of the bleeding can be achieved [14,15].

Blood product ratios and massive transfusion

- Recent military experience would suggest that transfusion in a 1:1:1 (packed red blood cell (PRBC): fresh frozen plasma (FFP): platelets) fashion improves survival in trauma patients suffering from massive hemorrhage [16].

- The military has also promoted the so-called "walking blood banks" and the transfusion of fresh whole blood to improve outcomes over traditional resuscitation composed mainly of packed red blood cells [17].
- While this may not be practical in a civilian setting, the benefits can be approximated utilizing appropriate ratios of PRBC to FFP and platelets.
- Although controversial, the current trend for massive transfusions is to use a ratio of 1:1 or 1:2 for PRBC:FFP, with an adult pack of platelets transfused for every five units of PRBC [18,19]. This essentially results in a 1:1:1 PRBC:FFP:platelets transfusion ratio.

The coagulopathy of trauma is multifactorial, elusive to detect and occurs early after injury.

- The ideal method to quantify coagulopathy has not yet been identified, although many have argued for expanded use of thromboelastography (TEG) in trauma.
- Ultimately we cannot rely on traditional markers of coagulation (INR/PTT) and instead must adhere to predetermined ratios of red cells to plasma and platelets to avoid under- or overtreating during trauma resuscitation.
- An institution-specific massive transfusion protocol (MTP) that reflects this data is a critical component of a safe and successful trauma system [20].

Tranexamic acid

Hemostatic adjuncts have been studied extensively in trauma.

- Systemic treatment with recombinant factor VIIa had shown promise, but has not been shown to improve outcome [21,22].
- Survival advantage was seen in the CRASH II trial of tranexamic acid (TA) when given early (within 3 hours of injury) for patients suffering from or at risk of hemorrhage from trauma.
- Despite the positive findings, caution should be exercised in light of the fact that late administration of TA actually increased mortality [23].

Hemorrhagic sources of shock

Hemorrhage is one of the early principle mechanisms of death and all cases of post-traumatic shock should be considered hemorrhagic until proven otherwise. Death from hemorrhage in adult trauma occurs from bleeding in one or more of five key anatomic locations:

- Chest – massive hemothorax
- Abdomen – intraperitoneal hemorrhage
- Pelvis/retroperitoneum – retroperitoneal hematoma
- Femur – extremity hematoma related to long-bone fractures
- Floor – external hemorrhage.

A combination of clinical exam, e-FAST examination and radiologic imaging should rapidly lead to the diagnosis and initiation of treatment for these conditions. When none of the above sources of hemorrhagic shock are discovered it is likely that an alternate/nonhemorrhagic source is responsible.

Nonhemorrhagic sources of shock
Cardiac
1. Tamponade (obstructive)
   - Clinical diagnosis suspected by injury mechanism and clinical signs of hypotension with *distended* rather than flat neck veins. This must be definitively ruled either in or out with all penetrating injuries to cardiac box (bound laterally by mid-clavicular line, superiorly by clavicles and inferiorly by costal margin).
   - Diagnosis is confirmed with FAST demonstrating pericardial fluid.
   - Positive pericardial FAST mandates operative exploration [24].
   - Emergency department thoracotomy is performed in unstable patients or those who suffer cardiac arrest with <15 min of down time.
2. Blunt cardiac injury
   - Most commonly presents as new-onset arrhythmia
   - Enough force to anterior chest may cause significant right ventricle dysfunction that could lead to cardiogenic shock (acute right heart failure). This is more common in the elderly trauma patient.

Neurogenic shock (distributive)
- Hypotension *and* bradycardia associated with high cervical spine injuries occurs as a result of disruption of sympathetic innervation to the heart and peripheral vasculature
- Treated initially with large volume Ringer's lactate therapy
- Vasopressor and chronotropic agent(s) is appropriate once patient is volume replete. Dopamine with or without norepinephrine is the agent of choice
- Coexisting occult hemorrhage must *always* be ruled out. Patients with acute quadriplegia have notoriously misleading abdominal examinations.

Tension pneumothorax (obstructive)
This remains a clinical diagnosis with absent breath sounds and hyper-resonance on the injured side with tracheal deviation away from the injured side (see above for treatment).

Emergency department (resuscitative) thoracotomy
Performance of an emergency department (reuscitative) thoracotomy (EDT) represents a heroic and maximally invasive effort to salvage a severely injured patient.
- The procedure is performed via a left antero-lateral thoracotomy.
- Principles and objectives of the procedure include pericardotomy to release tamponade, open cardiac massage and finger occlusion of cardiac injuries, cross clamp descending thoracic aorta and control of massive pulmonary hemorrhage with hilar clamping.

Indications for EDT have been recently revised, based on a large multicenter study from the Western Trauma Association (WTA) [25,26]. Indications based on this study are to consider EDT in all cases of post-traumatic cardiac arrest with the following limitations:

- 15 min of CPR time for *penetrating* injuries
- 10 min of CPR time for *blunt* injuries
- Asystole as the presenting rhythm and *no signs* of tamponade.

In patients with asystole as the presenting rhythm who do not have signs of tamponade, or in any patient with CPR times beyond the cutoffs, resuscitation can be terminated.

Disability

Rapid determination of Glasgow Coma Scale (GCS) and pupillary response allows for early assessment of the severity of neurologic injury.

- Noncontrast CT head should be considered in all but the least severe cases of closed head injury [27].
- Signs of intracranial hypertension should be managed aggressively. Simple maneuvers include reverse Trendelenberg positioning and deep chemical sedation, with or without muscle relaxation.
- Mild, temporary hyperventilation (1 hour) down to CO_2 near 30 mmHg is appropriate only as a temporizing maneuver prior to definitive medical and/or surgical therapy. Osmolar therapy with either mannitol or hypertonic saline (HTS) should be instituted early.
- Invasive intracranial pressure (ICP) monitoring should be instituted in all cases of coma with GCS of 8 or less [28].

Brain-directed resuscitation is critical in the hours and days following neurologic injury [28]. Avoidance of hypotension, hypoxia, hyperglycemia, appropriate seizure monitoring and treatment, tailoring care to physiologic measures such as brain oximetry rather than simply cerebral perfusion pressure (CPP) and the emerging role of hypothermia all deserve careful consideration. Early consultation with neurosurgery and/or neuro-ICU specialists is critical. For more details on neurotrauma and ICU management please see the chapter on Neurotrauma.

Exposure

The final aspect of the ATLS primary survey involves exposing the patient for examination by removal of clothing and prompt consideration of environmental/exposure issues, particularly hypothermia. Immediate treatment with warmed blankets, forced air heating systems and warmed IV fluids, as well as maintenance of a high ambient temperature in the trauma bay are recommended.

Advanced assessment

Following the ATLS primary survey a number of adjuncts are completed (chest and pelvic X-ray, FAST, gastric and urinary catheters, ECG, laboratory investigations) and a complete head to toe physical exam is performed (secondary survey).

FAST exam is an adjunct to the primary survey and is well validated [29,30]. Point-of-care ultrasound in the form of the e-FAST (extended-FAST) and the role of CT imaging are advanced assessment techniques in trauma care that merit special attention.

Point-of-care ultrasonography (e-FAST)

- While details of e-FAST are beyond the scope of this chapter, the exam allows providers to rapidly assess for pneumothorax, hemothorax, hemopericardium and hemoperitoneum in a reliable, repeatable and rapid fashion, without leaving the trauma bay or relying on other providers for performance or interpretation.
- Additional qualification to perform bedside echocardiographic assessment for volume status and gross cardiac function is desirable, but not yet standard of care among trauma providers.

Computed tomography (CT)

- A CT scan provides the greatest information about injury pattern and degree of injury for most blunt and selected penetrating trauma patients.
- Whole body CT (WBCT), the so-called trauma "pan scan," refers to CT scanning of the brain, cervical spine, thorax, abdomen and pelvis for blunt multisystem trauma.
- WBCT was studied prospectively by Salim and colleagues (31) and their findings support liberal use of this technique. Despite the absence of overt injury, 18.9% of patients had management change as a result of occult injuries discovered on WBCT. One must weigh the benefit of WBCT against radiation exposure that may infer an increased lifetime risk of blood-borne cancer.

Additional CT images that may be considered in specific clinical scenarios include:

- CT face – in the presence of suspected facial fractures.
- CT head/neck angio – blunt carotid and vertebral injuries are some of the more common and serious missed injuries in trauma. A CT angiogram is the preferred screening modality and guidelines exist for specific injury or patient factors (cervical seatbelt sign, fracture involving transverse foramen, coma without intracranial abnormality) that should prompt investigation [32,34].
- CT cystogram – any significant pelvic fracture, especially in the presence of hematuria, should prompt CT cystogram to rule out bladder injury.

Intraoperative management

Following initial assessment many severely injured patients will require intervention – either surgical, endovascular or both – prior to arriving in the intensive care unit. Although the specific operative and endovascular strategies employed for each injury type are beyond the scope of this chapter, a general review of management principles is pertinent as it informs ongoing resuscitative care in ICU.

Damage-control surgery

- Damage-control surgery (DCS) represents a paradigm shift in operative management.
- The concept of a single operation that accomplished definitive solutions to all injuries is replaced by multiple, abbreviated operations staged in a fashion that prioritizes restoration of metabolic derangements over the performance of complex reconstructive surgery [35,36].

The principle tenets of DCS are:

- Rapid hemorrhage control, e.g. temporary vascular shunts, ligation rather than repair of noncritical vessels, topical hemostatic adjuncts, temporary abdominal packing with adjunctive angioembolization.
- Control contamination, e.g. stapled closure of enteric wounds, GI tract left intentionally in discontinuity, drain or exteriorize urinary, pancreatic and biliary wounds.
- Avoid further injury, e.g. debride dead and devitalized tissue, leave body cavity/ operative sites open to prevent compartment syndrome, terminate surgery early and transition back to ICU to prevent coagulopathy and metabolic failure.

External fixation and angiography

- The role of external fixation and angioembolization as adjunct to surgical hemorrhage control cannot be overstated.
- External fixation is a rapid means of achieving boney alignment and closing down potential spaces in both long-bone and complex pelvic fractures.
- This technique is both rapid and effective and is a natural extension of DCS.
- Angiography with embolization and/or endovascular stenting has become an invaluable management tool for solid organ hemorrhage, hemodynamically unstable pelvic fracture, extremity hemorrhage and traumatic aortic injury.
- Angioembolization can be used as primary therapy for less-injured patients, but also can be used directly following intra-abdominal packing.
- The utility of angiography has become so universal that many trauma operating theatres are now transitioning to a hybrid surgical/endovascular environment [37].

Timing of long-bone fracture fixation

Studies in the 1990s of patients with long-bone fractures showed reduced ARDS and fat embolism with early fracture fixation.

- However, concerns have been raised regarding the associated prolonged surgery in patients with abdominal and head injuries.
- The principle of damage-control orthopedics [38] suggests early temporary fracture stabilization be employed with fracture reduction and stabilization using an external skeletal fixator and later definitive care of all fractures.
- Recent studies, however, suggest that early definitive fracture management may be safe and associated with fewer complications than delayed management after adjusting for patient age and ISS [39].

Post-operative care and ongoing resuscitation
Damage-control resuscitation

- The practical implications of damage-control surgery (DCS) from the point of view of the intensivist are that patients should be expected to return to ICU early, without definitive control of all injuries, and in significant need of prompt and ongoing resuscitation.
- Given the abbreviated nature of the planned ICU resuscitation – often being cut short for return to operating theatre in 12 to 24 hours – this can be thought of quite naturally as damage-control resuscitation (DCR) [40].

- Considerations for DCR in the ICU are similar in many ways to the strategies employed for initial trauma resuscitation, as presented above.

Specifically these include :

Physiologic endpoints of resuscitation

- Physiologic parameters rather than numerically driven endpoints should be the goal.
- Examples include – lactate clearance, normalization of base deficit, $ScvO_2$, and serial echocardiographic assessments *rather* than rigidly targeting a given MAP or CVP.
- Permissive hypotension is therefore a natural extension of this approach, provided perfusion markers are adequate.

Balanced blood product resuscitation (1:1:1)

- Careful monitoring of outputs and balanced replacement of blood loss with appropriate ratios of PRBC:FFP:platelets is favored over high-volume isotonic crystalloid administration.
- All products and fluids should be given via a warming device.

Active rewarming

- Continuous body temperature monitoring via oropharyngeal or rectal probe should be initiated
- Maximize ambient temperature setting in closed ICU bay
- Forced air rewarming devices
- Body surface area exposed for minimum allowable duration for examinations and procedures
- All products and fluids are given via a warming device.

Guided vasopressor and inotrope therapy

- The use of vasopressors and inotropes in the setting of hemorrhagic shock is most often viewed somewhat dubiously by trauma providers.
- However, documentation of post-injury vasoplegia and cardiac dysfunction in the polytrauma patient is both real [41] and likely well suited to appropriate vasopressor and inotrope therapy.
- This can *only* be considered once surgical hemorrhage has been controlled.
- Ideally, this therapy should be guided by traditional markers of cardiac output and tissue perfusion as well as by serial bedside echocardiography to determine fluid responsiveness and guide titration of vasoactive drugs.

Abdominal compartment syndrome

- Abdominal compartment syndrome (ACS) is a common and lethal occurrence following major injury [42,43].
- Open abdominal negative pressure wound therapy (vacuum-assisted closure systems – commercial or homemade) do *not* eliminate the risk of ACS.
- Serial bladder pressure measurements are a requisite for all major trauma and post-operative patients.

- Prompt medical and surgical therapy should be instituted in response to elevated bladder pressures with evidence of end-organ dysfunction.
- For a complete description of assessment and management of ACS please refer to the chapter on ICU patients with GI issues.

Sedation and analgesia

- Traditional pharmacologic agents (narcotics, benzodiazepines, propofol etc.) as per institutional protocol are appropriate for both injured and post-operative patients. Propofol is favored for patients with traumatic brain injury due to its short half-life, which can allow for serial neurologic exminations.
- Minimization of sedation and consideration of sedation interruptions should begin as soon as possible following surgery or trauma [44].
- Use of patient-controlled analgesia (PCA) should be provided whenever feasible for awake and cooperative patients.

Two special forms of analgesia merit particular consideration:

- Epidural analgesia – although controversy exists in both patient groups, epidural analgesia remains an excellent tool for pain control following blunt thoracic trauma [45] and may have benefit for reducing pulmonary morbidity following high- risk elective surgery [46].
- Lidocaine infusion – a growing body of evidence supports its use for both post-operative and post-trauma patients [47]. Careful monitoring for neurologic and cardiac side effects is critical. It may reduce the need for narcotic and sedation substantially and help allay the associated morbidity and mortality of deep sedation [48].

Antibiotic therapy

- Pre-operative and peri-injury antibiotic prophylaxis with appropriate agents (first-generation cephalosporins, vancomycin for MRSA or penicillin allergy, ± anaerobic coverage) have been shown to decrease surgical site infections at mid-line wounds [49].
- Continuation of ABX beyond 24 hours is not indicated and is potentially harmful.
- ABX should only be continued beyond 24 hours under separate, specific indications (e.g. treatment of intra-abdominal sepsis, open fracture, a coexisting pneumonia, etc).

Early enteral nutrition

- Beneficial effects of early enteral nutrition have been seen in many ICU patient populations, but are rarely more pronounced than in trauma and post-surgical patients [50,51].
- Use of early TPN when the GI tract is unavailable is controversial, given evidence of increased mortality when compared to a strategy of gradually increasing enteral feeding as tolerated [52].
- TPN should likely be avoided in all but the most severe cases of GI tract trauma/surgery.
- Aggressive institutional protocols for enteral feeding of post-trauma/surgery ICU patients are appropriate.

- Measurement of "gastric residuals" has been shown to be inappropriate and ineffectual, as it impairs patients from reaching caloric goals without having any impact on rates of VAP or correlation with aspiration risk [53]. Gastric residuals should not be recorded or reported in ICU patients.
- No clear answer regarding pre- versus post-pyloric feeds. If logistically feasible consider post-pyloric feed, but early gastric feeding is likely equally acceptable [54].

Early mobilization

- ICU-acquired weakness (ICU-AW) is a common complication of critical care that increases both length of stay and morbidity for trauma and post-operative patients.
- Early mobilization has become an important strategy to reduce the occurrence and severity of ICU-AW [55].

Trials of early mobilization specific to the polytrauma patient are lacking. However, given the improvement seen in studies focusing on specific injury patterns, as well as benefits in nontrauma ICU patients, it is recommended that [56]:

- Mobilization should begin as soon as definitive repair of orthopedic and/or internal injuries has been obtained.
- Mobilization and early rehabilitation plans should be approached using multidisciplinary, team-based strategies to ensure that allied health, nursing and consulting surgical services buy in to the potential benefits of these initiatives [57].

Thromboembolic prophylaxis

- Prophylactic heparin or low-molecular-weight heparin should be prescribed for *all* major trauma and post-operative patients in ICU, provided that no major contraindication exists. This can begin on day 1 following injury or operation [58].
- Evidence supports the use of low-molecular-weight heparin for trauma patients [59].
- Post-operative patients should receive either low-molecular-weight heparin or low-dose unfractionated heparin, as these two agents appear to be equivalent in terms of DVT rate or incidence of HIT for the general medical/surgical ICU population [60].
- When specific contraindications to anticoagulation exist (e.g. intracranial hemorrhage, solid-organ injury), sequential compression devices and compression stockings should be employed. Compression devices can be added to LMWH for trauma patients at high risk of DVT. Timing of chemical DVT prophylaxis post-solid-organ injury or traumatic brain injury is controversial. However, if there has been no evidence of bleeding or expansion of the hematoma/lesion, chemical DVT prophylaxis can generally be started after 72 hours from admission.
- Use of prophylactic IVC filters for trauma patients is *not* recommended outside of rare circumstances with very high risk of DVT and contraindication to anticoagulation [61]. Most should be reserved for patients with established diagnosis of DVT/PE for whom anticoagulation is contraindicated [62].

Outcome

- Trauma patients in ICU following multiple injuries often have prolonged length of stay and duration of ventilator support.
- Length of stay and mortality are increased in the elderly trauma patient, with less chance of regaining functional independence.
- Young trauma patients have a better overall outcome and a good prospect of rehabilitation.

References

1. SMARTRISK. 2009. *The Economic Burden of Injury in Canada.* SMARTRISK: Toronto, ON.

2. Trunkey DD. Trauma. *Sci Am* 1983; 249 : 28–35.

3. Ross SE, O'Malley KF, DeLong WG *et al.* Clinical predictors of unstable cervical spinal injury in multiply injured patients. *Injury* 1992; 23 : 317–9.

4. Stiell IG, Clement CM, McKnight RD *et al.* The Canadian C-spine rule versus the NEXUS low-risk criteria in patients with trauma. *N Engl J Med* 2003; 349 : 2510–8.

5. Como JJ, Diaz JJ, Dunham CM *et al.* Practice management guidelines for identification of cervical spine injuries following trauma: update from the eastern association for the surgery of trauma practice management guidelines committee. *J Trauma* 2009; 67 : 651–9.

6. Widder S, Doig C, Burrowes P *et al.* Prospective evaluation of computed tomographic scanning for the spinal clearance of obtunded trauma patients: preliminary results. *J Trauma* 2004; 56 : 1179–84.

7. Hennessy D, Widder S, Zygun D *et al.* Cervical spine clearance in obtunded blunt trauma patients: a prospective study. *J Trauma* 2010; 68 : 576–82.

8. The Acute Respiratory Distress Syndrome Network. Ventilation with lower tidal volumes as compared with traditional tidal volumes for acute lung injury and the acute respiratory distress syndrome. *N Engl J Med.* 2000; 342 : 1301–8.

9. Ball CG, Wyrzykowski AD, Kirkpatrick AW *et al.* Thoracic needle decompression for tension pneumothorax: clinical correlation with catheter length. *Can J Surg* 2010; 53 : 184–8.

10. Slobogean GP, MacPherson CA, Sun T *et al.* Surgical fixation vs nonoperative management of flail chest: a meta-analysis. *J Am Coll Surg* 2013; 216 : 302–11.

11. Doben AR, Eriksson EA, Denlinger CE *et al.* Surgical rib fixation for flail chest deformity improves liberation from mechanical ventilation. *J Crit Care* 2014; 29 : 139–43.

12. Marasco SF, Davies AR, Cooper J *et al.* Prospective randomized controlled trial of operative rib fixation in traumatic flail chest. *J Am Coll Surg* 2013; 216 : 924–32.

13. Bickell WH, Wall MJ Jr, Pepe PE *et al.* Immediate versus delayed fluid resuscitation for hypotensive patients with penetrating torso injuries. *N Engl J Med* 1994; 331 : 1105–9.

14. Duchesne JC, Barbeau JM, Islam TM *et al.* Damage control resuscitation: from emergency department to the operating room. *Am Surg* 2011; 77 : 201–6.

15. Cotton BA, Reddy N, Quinton M *et al.* Damage control resuscitation is associated with a reduction in resuscitation volumes and improvement in survival in 390 damage control laparotomy patients. *Annals of Surgery* 2011; 254 : 598–605.

16. Borgman MA, Spinella PC, Perkins JG *et al.* The ratio of blood products transfused affects mortality in patients receiving massive transfusions at a combat support hospital. *J Trauma* 2007; 63 : 805–13.

17. Spinella PC. Warm fresh whole blood transfusion for severe hemorrhage: U.S.

military and potential civilian applications. *Crit Care Med* 2008; 36 : S340–5.

18. Davenport R, Curry N, Manson J *et al.* Hemostatic effects of fresh frozen plasma may be maximal at red cell ratios of 1:2. *J Trauma* 2011; 70 : 90–5.

19. Dente CJ, Shaz BH, Nicholas JM *et al.* Improvements in early mortality and coagulopathy are sustained better in patients with blunt trauma after institution of a massive transfusion protocol in a civilian level I trauma center. *J Trauma* 2009; 66 : 1616–24.

20. Vogt KN, Van Koughnett JA, Dubois L *et al.* The use of trauma transfusion pathways for blood component transfusion in the civilian population: a systematic review and meta-analysis. *Transfus Med* 2012; 22 : 156–66.

21. Hauser CJ, Boffard K, Dutton R *et al.* Results of the CONTROL trial: efficacy and safety of recombinant activated Factor VII in the management of refractory traumatic hemorrhage. *J Trauma* 2010; 69 : 489–500.

22. Boffard KD, Riou B, Warren B *et al.* Recombinant factor VIIa as adjunctive therapy for bleeding control in severely injured trauma patients: two parallel randomized, placebo-controlled, double-blind clinical trials. *J Trauma* 2005; 59 : 8–15.

23. Williams-Johnson JA, McDonald AH, Strachan GG, Williams EW. Effects of tranexamic acid on death, vascular occlusive events, and blood transfusion in trauma patients with significant haemorrhage (CRASH-2): a randomised, placebo-controlled trial. *West Indian Med J* 2010; 59 : 612–24.

24. Rozycki GS, Ballard RB, Feliciano DV *et al.* Surgeon-performed ultrasound for the assessment of truncal injuries – lessons learned from 1540 patients. *Ann Surg* 1998; 228 : 557–67.

25. Burlew CC, Moore EE, Moore FA *et al.* Western Trauma Association critical decisions in trauma: resuscitative thoracotomy. *J Trauma Acute Care Surg* 2012; 73 : 1359–63.

26. Moore EE, Knudson MM, Burlew CC *et al.* Defining the limits of resuscitative emergency department thoracotomy: a contemporary Western Trauma Association perspective. *J Trauma* 2011; 70 : 334–9.

27. Stiell IG, Wells GA, Vandemheen K *et al.* The Canadian CT Head Rule for patients with minor head injury. *Lancet* 2001; 357 : 1391–6.

28. Guidelines for the management of severe traumatic bran injury. The Brain Trauma Foundation. *J. Neurotrauma* 2007; 24 : S1–106.

29. Rozycki GS, Ochsner MG, Jaffin JH, *et al.* Prospective evaluation of surgeons' use of ultrasound in the evaluation of trauma patients. *J Trauma* 1993; 34 : 516–27.

30. Rozycki GS, Ochsner MG, Schmidt JA *et al.* A prospective study of surgeon-performed ultrasound as the primary adjuvant modality for injured patient assessment. *J Trauma* 1995; 39 : 492–500.

31. Salim A, Sangthong B, Martin M *et al.* Whole body imaging in blunt multisystem trauma patients without obvious signs of injury: results of a prospective study. *Arch Surg* 2006; 141 : 468–73.

32. Bromberg WJ, Collier BC, Diebel LN *et al.* Blunt cerebrovascular injury practice management guidelines: the Eastern Association for the Surgery of Trauma. *J Trauma* 2010; 68 : 471–7.

33. Biffl WL, Moore EE, Elliott JP *et al.* The devastating potential of blunt vertebral arterial injuries. *Ann Surg* 2000; 231 : 672–81.

34. Miller PR, Fabian TC, Croce MA *et al.* Prospective screening for blunt cerebrovascular injuries: analysis of diagnostic modalities and outcomes. *Ann Surg* 2002; 236 : 386–93.

35. Moore EE, Burch JM, Franciose RJ *et al.* Staged physiologic restoration and damage control surgery. *World J Surg* 1998; 22 : 1184–90.

36. Rotondo MF, Schwab CW, McGonigal MD *et al.* "Damage control": an approach for improved survival in exsanguinating

penetrating abdominal injury. *J Trauma* 1993; 35 : 375–82.

37. Ball CG, Kirkpatrick AW, D'Amours SK. The RAPTOR: Resuscitation with angiography, percutaneous techniques and operative repair. Transforming the discipline of trauma surgery. *Can J Surg* 2011; 54 : E3–4.

38. Nahm NJ, Como JJ, Wilber JH, Vallier HA. Early appropriate care: definitive stabilization of femoral fractures within 24 hours of injury is safe in most patients with multiple injuries. *J Trauma* 2011; 71 : 175–85.

39. O'Brien PJ. Fracture fixation in patients having multiple injuries. *Can J Surg* 2003; 46 : 124–8.

40. Duchesne JC, McSwain NE Jr, Cotton BA et al. Damage control resuscitation: the new face of damage control. *J Trauma* 2010; 69 : 976–90.

41. Ferrada P, Murthi S, Anand RJ et al. Transthoracic focused rapid echocardiographic examination: real-time evaluation of fluid status in critically ill trauma patients. *J Trauma* 2011; 70 : 56–62.

42. Holodinsky JK, Roberts DJ, Ball CG et al. Risk factors for intra-abdominal hypertension and abdominal compartment syndrome among adult intensive care unit patients: a systematic review and meta-analysis. *Crit Care* 2013; 17(5) : R249.

43. Kirkpatrick AW, Roberts DJ, De Waele J et al. Intra-abdominal hypertension and the abdominal compartment syndrome: updated consensus definitions and clinical practice guidelines from the World Society of the Abdominal Compartment Syndrome. *Intensive Care Med* 2013; 39 : 1190–206

44. Girard TD, Kress JP, Fuchs BD et al. Efficacy and safety of a paired sedation and ventilator weaning protocol for mechanically ventilated patients in intensive care (Awakening and Breathing Controlled trial): a randomised controlled trial. *Lancet* 2008; 371 : 126–34.

45. Simon BJ, Cushman J, Barraco R et al. EAST Practice Management Guidelines Work Group. Pain management guidelines for blunt thoracic trauma. *J Trauma*. 2005; 59 : 1256–67.

46. Liu SS, Wu CL. Effect of postoperative analgesia on major postoperative complications: a systematic update of the evidence. *Anesth Analg* 2007; 104 : 689–702.

47. Vigneault L, Turgeon AF, Côté D et al. Perioperative intravenous lidocaine infusion for postoperative pain control: a meta-analysis of randomized controlled trials. *Can J Anaesth* 2011; 58 : 22–37.

48. Shehabi Y, Bellomo R, Reade MC et al. Early intensive care sedation predicts long-term mortality in ventilated critically ill patients. *Am J Respir Crit Care Med* 2012; 186 : 724–31.

49. Bratzler DW, Dellinger EP, Olsen KM et al. Clinical practice guidelines for antimicrobial prophylaxis in surgery. *Surg Infect (Larchmt)* 2013; 14 : 73–156.

50. Wang X, Dong Y, Han X et al. Nutritional support for patients sustaining traumatic brain injury: a systematic review and meta-analysis of prospective studies. *PLoS One* 2013; 8 : e58838.

51. Doig GS, Heighes PT, Simpson F, Sweetman EA. Early enteral nutrition reduces mortality in trauma patients requiring intensive care: a meta-analysis of randomised controlled trials. *Injury* 2011; 42 : 50–6.

52. Casaer MP, Mesotten D, Hermans G et al. Early versus late parenteral nutrition in critically ill adults. *N Engl J Med* 2011; 365 : 506–17.

53. Reignier J, Mercier E, Le Gouge A et al. Effect of not monitoring residual gastric volume on risk of ventilator-associated pneumonia in adults receiving mechanical ventilation and early enteral feeding: a randomized controlled trial. *J Am Med Assoc* 2013; 309 : 249–56.

54. Davies AR, Morrison SS, Bailey MJ et al. A multicenter, randomized controlled trial comparing early nasojejunal with nasogastric nutrition in critical illness. *Crit Care Med* 2012; 40 : 2342–8.

55. Fan E. Critical illness neuromyopathy and the role of physical therapy and

rehabilitation in critically ill patients. *Respir Care* 2012; 57 : 933–44.

56. Engels PT, Beckett AN, Rubenfeld GD *et al.* Physical rehabilitation of the critically ill trauma patient in the ICU. *Crit Care Med* 2013; 41 : 1790–801.

57. Fan E. A "moving proposition" for the silver day and bronze week in trauma patients. *Crit Care Med* 2013; 4 : 1826–7.

58. Falck-Ytter Y, Francis CW, Johanson NA *et al.* Prevention of VTE in orthopedic surgery patients: Antithrombotic Therapy and Prevention of Thrombosis, 9th ed: American College of Chest Physicians Evidence-Based Clinical Practice Guidelines. *Chest* 2012; 141 : e278S–325S.

59. Cothren CC, Smith WR, Moore EE, Morgan SJ. Utility of once-daily dose of low-molecular-weight heparin to prevent venous thromboembolism in multisystem trauma patients. *World J Surg* 2007; 31 : 98–104.

60. Cook D, Meade M, Guyatt G *et al.* Dalteparin versus unfractionated heparin in critically ill patients. *N Engl J Med* 2011; 364 : 1305–14.

61. Guyatt GH, Akl EA, Crowther M, Gutterman DD, Schuünemann HJ; American College of Chest Physicians Antithrombotic Therapy and Prevention of Thrombosis Panel. Executive Summary: Antithrombotic Therapy and Prevention of Thrombosis, 9th edn: American College of Chest Physicians Evidence-Based Clinical Practice Guidelines. *Chest* 2012; 141 : 7S–47S.

62. Kidane B, Madani AM, Vogt K *et al.* The use of prophylactic inferior vena cava filters in trauma patients: a systematic review. *Injury* 2012; 43 : 542–7.

Neurotrauma

24

Ari Ercole, Jessie R Welbourne and Arun K Gupta

Introduction

As a whole, major trauma is estimated to cost the UK over £3 billion annually in lost economic activity, with a further direct cost to the UK health service of more than £0.3 billion. Of these trauma patients, a substantial number will sustain some degree of central nervous system injury such as traumatic brain injury (TBI) or traumatic spinal-cord injury (SCI). Whilst the improvements in road safety and an aging population are shifting the demographic of trauma patients, these remain diseases of young adulthood with obvious implications for the ongoing long-term care of patients left with serious disabilities. Furthermore, it is increasingly recognized that even relatively minor TBI can lead to neurocognitive deficits with potentially serious personal, social and financial implications.

Traumatic brain injury
General considerations

A number of structural and metabolic features of CNS tissue make it uniquely vulnerable to traumatic insult.

- High cerebral metabolic rate ($CMRO_2$)
- Stringent metabolic substrate requirements with limited local energy reserves
- Cerebral blood flow (CBF) and $CMRO_2$ are normally closely matched and maintained over a wide range of cerebral perfusion pressure (CPP), but this autoregulatory capacity may become precarious after injury
- Maximal displacement of CSF or CSF outflow obstruction (hydrocephalus) will cause a rapid rise in intracranial pressure (Monroe–Kellie doctrine). The compliance of the posterior fossa may be even more limited
- Brain tissue undergoes viscoelastic deformation under acceleration/deceleration with subsequent damage to neuronal and vascular components due to shearing forces
- Finally, CNS tissue has extremely limited capacity for repair: long-term recovery after TBI relies largely on plasticity and functional recruitment of uninjured parts of the brain.

The CPP is a key concept in the critical care of TBI patients and may be calculated as:

$$CPP = MAP - ICP - CVP$$

Handbook of ICU Therapy, third edition, ed. John Fuller, Jeff Granton and Ian McConachie. Published by Cambridge University Press. © Cambridge University Press 2015.

although CVP is often neglected in practice. Similar considerations hold for spinal-cord perfusion pressure. In health, CBF is constant in the face of changes in CPP within the autoregulatory range of approximately $50 < CPP < 150$ mmHg (although this curve relationship may be right-shifted in patients with pre-existing hypertension).

CBF follows a characteristic pattern after injury.

- Initially, global CBF falls and autoregulation is impaired at lower values of CPP due to microvascular dysfunction. Ischemia may occur. Maintaining a normal/adequate CPP is crucial in the early phases after injury, even if ICP is initially relatively normal.
- Ischemia results in energetic ion pump failure and consequent cellular water accumulation. This cytotoxic edema is the dominant mechanism in raising intracranial pressure in the early phase after TBI, excepting where intracranial hematomas are present.
- Between 12 and 24 hours, CBF increases, leading to a state of relative hyperperfusion. ICP is now driven by vascular engorgement due to these increases in CBF and cerebral blood volume (CBV).
- After 48h or so, there is a reduction in integrity of the blood–brain barrier with osmotic and hydrostatic gradients leading to vasogenic edema as a new driver for intracranial hypertension.

Pathology will evolve differently between patients, and multiple processes may coincide at any time point. However, an appreciation of the processes from this stereotypical pattern that are likely to be dominant is helpful in optimizing management and predicting the responses to therapy and the likely course of future events.

Initial assessment and resuscitation

From the above considerations, it is essential to avoid drops in CPP at any point after TBI, even if ICP is not yet raised (or is not yet measured).

- Hypoxia and hypotension (systolic blood pressure <90 mmHg) have been robustly demonstrated as independent predictors of poor outcome after TBI and must therefore be avoided.

The initial assessment and resuscitation of TBI patients may take place in hospital, but is increasingly being undertaken by specialist helicopter or road-deployed prehospital paramedic/doctor critical care. Information from the scene regarding the mechanism of injury is often very helpful in understanding the likely injury pattern and extent of neurological injury that can be expected.

Initial assessment and management of the TBI patient follows an orderly ABCDE trauma approach with catastrophic hemorrhage addressed first.

- It is essential that other injuries are not missed, not least because hypotension from an overlooked hemorrhage source or hypoxia from a poorly managed thoracic injury will have serious implications on TBI outcome.
- Hypotensive resuscitation is contraindicated after TBI.

Traumatic brain injury is classified according to initial Glasgow coma score (GCS);

- Mild: GCS 13–15
- Moderate: GCS 9–12
- Severe: GCS 8 or less.

The GCS may also be affected by alcohol or hypoxia, hypotension, hypoglycemia etc. Intubation often occurs as part of resuscitation; a true "best resuscitated GCS" validated for prognostication is often not available.

Careful note of focal neurological deficits from the scene are important. Pupillary abnormalities are of particular importance. Furthermore, a scene assessment of whether the patient was noticed to move all or some limbs is very helpful if a bony spinal injury is subsequently found on imaging.

Airway compromise is common after TBI, either because of obstruction or failure of airway protection in neurologically obtunded patients.

- Because of the impact of hypoxia, it is important that the airway be secured by endotracheal intubation if it is at risk.
- Anesthesia, intubation and mechanical ventilation also allow physiological control of $CMRO_2$ and $PaCO_2$.

Intubation should take place as part of a rapid sequence intubation routine by an experienced operator.

- TBI patients should be assumed to have a cervical spinal injury until proven otherwise and manual in-line stabilization should be used.
- A difficult intubation should be anticipated.
- Capnography, suction and failed intubation equipment should be immediately to hand.

The choice of induction agent is relatively unimportant, provided that it is used in a manner so as to avoid hypotension. A balanced technique with an opioid to blunt the ICP response to laryngoscopy, in combination with a hypnotic is favored.

- Fentanyl (3 μg/kg) and ketamine (2 mg/kg) are commonly employed in prehospital care, although doses may need to be reduced if the patient is hemodynamically unstable.
- Propofol, etomidate or thiopentone are also recognized agents for induction.
- Ketamine has a favorable hemodynamic profile, may be neuroprotective and its detrimental effect on CBV is irrelevant in mechanically ventilated patients.
- A muscle relaxant should be used and suxamethonium (1–1.5 mg/kg) or rocuronium (1 mg/kg) are common choices, depending on the situation.

Clinical examination may be unreliable or impossible in obtunded patients and urgent whole-body CT imaging should be considered in all patients who have sustained significant trauma. This will generally obviate the need for plain films.

Patients who have sustained significant trauma should be assumed to have also sustained a spinal injury until proven otherwise.

- Therefore all such patients should be immobilized initially. The widespread use of whole-body CT scanning in major trauma has obviated the need for plain films of the cervical, thoracic and lumbar spine, but these will be necessary otherwise.
- CT is highly sensitive for bony injury but ligamentous injury or SCI may occasionally present with little or no radiological abnormality.
- It is dangerous to maintain full spinal immobilization (hard collar, log roll and supine position) for long periods of time in ICU.

- Instead, the spine may be provisionally "cleared" on the basis of CT imaging and three-dimensional reconstructions. Clinical assessment is then deferred until the patient has recovered sufficiently.
- However, where there is doubt, immobilization should be continued and an MRI obtained.

Intensive care management

Guidelines for the management of patients with severe traumatic brain injury have been published [1]. The key aims of therapy are to prevent secondary injury by optimizing oxygen delivery by maintaining CPP, limiting ICP and reducing oxygen consumption by reducing $CMRO_2$.

Reasonable initial physiological targets are:

- ICP <20 mmHg
- CPP 60–70 mmHg
- Best-guess MAP 80 mmHg if ICP/CPP not yet measured
- $SpO_2 \geq 97\%$, $PaO_2 \geq 11$ kPa
- $PaCO_2$ 4.5–5.0 kPa
- T ≤ 37.0 °C
- Blood glucose 6–10 mmol/L.

There is reasonable observational evidence to suggest that outcomes from severe TBI are improved when these patients are managed at specialist neuroscience intensive care centers. This is likely to reflect benefits not only from clinical familiarity from high case load, but also colocation with neurosurgical provision, as well as other specialist services such as advanced neuroradiology, specialist physiotherapy, rehabilitation and so on.

Overview of neuromonitoring

The usual level 3 intensive care monitoring, including invasive arterial blood pressure and central venous catheterization (usually subclavian due to C-spine precautions), is mandatory for severe TBI patients. Additionally, specialist neuroscience intensive care units will employ specific methods for assessing ICP, CPP and the adequacy of cerebral oxygen delivery.

Invasive monitoring carries risks of bleeding or infection and is therefore reserved for patients in whom raised ICP is likely, such as:

- Any TBI patient with GCS <9 and an abnormal CT scan
- TBI patients with GCS <9 and normal CT scans with at least two of:
  - . Age >40 years
  - . Unilateral or bilateral motor posturing
  - . Systolic blood pressure <90 mmHg.

Two methods are most commonly used for ICP measurement:

1. An external ventricular drain (EVD) is a catheter, surgically introduced via a burr hole through the brain parenchyma into the lateral ventricle. The drain is connected to a pressure transducer and manometer device and they have a number of advantages for ICP measurement;

they are reliable and also permit CSF drainage for ICP control. However, the ventricles may be difficult to access when compressed and EVDs are associated with a relatively high rate of ventriculitis.

2. Intraparenchymal microsensors consist of a miniature strain-gauge device introduced either via a bolt or tunneled under a bone flap. They do not permit CSF drainage, but have a low complication rate and may be introduced with other probes through the same bolt.

Invasive probes are typically placed in the right frontal territory since this is noneloquent and generally nondominant cortex.

Intracranial pressure measurements do not guarantee adequate cerebral oxygenation. Measurement of the saturation of venous effluent blood in the jugular bulb by retrograde cannulation of the internal jugular vein allows hemispheric oxygen extraction to be estimated. Jugular saturation below 50% correlates with poor outcome, indicating increased oxygen extraction/inadequate oxygen delivery. The hemispheric nature of this technique and contamination with extracranial blood limits sensitivity and specificity, and it is less commonly used now.

Implantable miniature oxygen sensors are available and may be introduced into the brain tissue through the same bolt as the ICP microsensor. These sensors respond to brain-tissue oxygen tension (P_bO_2) reflecting a balance between cerebral oxygen delivery, $CMRO_2$ and oxygen diffusivity. Values of P_bO_2 below 10 mmHg are suggestive of cerebral ischemia. Sensor positioning is important. If positioned in pericontusional tissue, the recorded P_bO_2 represents a measure of "at risk" brain although such accurate positioning is often difficult to achieve, and the sensor is usually placed in uninjured brain in practice. Readings from a sensor placed within a contusion are clearly not helpful.

Cerebral microdialysis involves placing a fine concentric double lumen tube with a semipermeable membrane into the brain parenchyma. The catheter may be introduced through the same bolt as the ICP and brain-tissue oxygen probes. Perfusate is passed through the catheter, typically at 0.3 µL/min, and the effluent, which has equilibrated with brain chemistry, is sampled hourly. Standard catheters permit the measurement of various biochemical markers – most usefully lactate, pyruvate and glucose. Ratios of lactate to pyruvate >25 suggest impending ischemia. Glucose levels represent a balance between supply and demand – cerebral hypoglycemia below 0.5 mmol/L may lead to waves of cortical depolarization and consequent increases in $CMRO_2$.

Near infrared spectroscopy (NIRS) offers a potentially noninvasive method of assessing cerebral oxygenation. Briefly, the brain is transilluminated by infrared light of different wavelengths using probes placed on the forehead. Differential spectral absorption by oxygenated and deoxygenated hemoglobin allows the inference of cerebral oxygenation. However, the technique is subject to contamination by extracerebral blood (e.g. from scalp vessels), which causes errors.

Management of ICP/CPP

Sustained rises in ICP above 20 mmHg may be harmful and should generally be treated. The management of ICP proceeds in a stepwise progression for which guidelines have been published [1]. This can be protocolized and an example of such a protocol is shown in Figure 24.1.

All patients with or at risk of intracranial hypertension: invasive arterial monitoring, CVP line, ICP monitor +/– brain oxygenation & chemistry monitoring.
• Interventions in stage III to be individualized to clinical picture and multimodality monitoring.
• CPP 70 mmHg set as in initial target, but CPP>> 60 mmHg is acceptable in most patients.
• If monitored; PbO_2 >15 kPa and L/P ratio <25 are 2° targets
Evacuate significant space-occupying lesions (SOL) and drain CSF before escalating medical Rx.
Rx In italics and stages IV and V only with consultant approval.

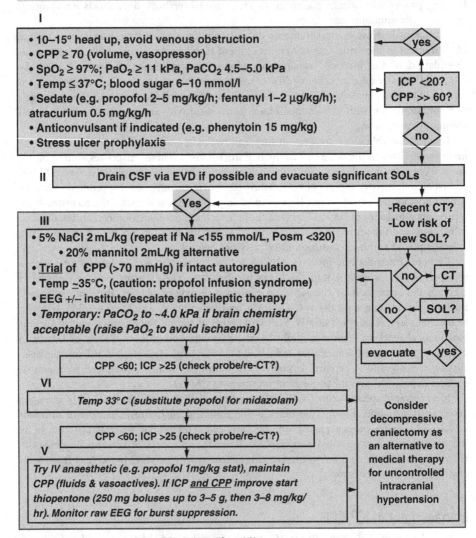

I
• 10–15° head up, avoid venous obstruction
• CPP ≥ 70 (volume, vasopressor)
• SpO_2 ≥ 97%; PaO_2 ≥ 11 kPa, $PaCO_2$ 4.5–5.0 kPa
• Temp ≤ 37°C; blood sugar 6–10 mmol/l
• Sedate (e.g. propofol 2–5 mg/kg/h; fentanyl 1–2 µg/kg/h); atracurium 0.5 mg/kg/h
• Anticonvulsant if indicated (e.g. phenytoin 15 mg/kg)
• Stress ulcer prophylaxis

yes
ICP <20?
CPP >> 60?
no

II Drain CSF via EVD if possible and evacuate significant SOLs

-Recent CT?
-Low risk of new SOL?

Yes

III
• 5% NaCl 2 mL/kg (repeat if Na <155 mmol/L, Posm <320)
 • 20% mannitol 2mL/kg alternative
• Trial of CPP (>70 mmHg) if intact autoregulation
• Temp ~35°C, (caution: propofol infusion syndrome)
• EEG +/– institute/escalate antiepileptic therapy
• Temporary: $PaCO_2$ to ~4.0 kPa if brain chemistry acceptable (raise PaO_2 to avoid ischaemia)

no — CT
no — SOL?
evacuate — yes

CPP <60; ICP >25 (check probe/re-CT?)

VI
Temp 33°C (substitute propofol for midazolam)

CPP <60; ICP >25 (check probe/re-CT?)

V
Try IV anaesthetic (e.g. propofol 1mg/kg stat), maintain CPP (fluids & vasoactives). If ICP and CPP improve start thiopentone (250 mg boluses up to 3–5 g, then 3–8 mg/kg/hr). Monitor raw EEG for burst suppression.

Consider decompressive craniectomy as an alternative to medical therapy for uncontrolled intracranial hypertension

Figure 24.1 Managament of raised ICP. (Adapted from [1].)

Good basic general intensive care measures underpin specific interventions to control raised ICP.

- For all TBI patients, blood pressure should be supported with fluid resuscitation and, where necessary, vasoconstrictors to maintain an adequate CPP between 60–70 mmHg.
- Cerebral venous drainage should be encouraged by nursing in a head up position (unless contraindicated by spinal injury), avoiding jugular venous obstruction from tight endotracheal tube ties or tight-fitting cervical collars and high levels of PEEP (although it is crucial to maintain oxygenation).

Patients should be sedated (e.g. propofol and fentanyl infusions in adults) not only for endotracheal tube tolerance, but also to reduce $CMRO_2$. It may be necessary to use neuromuscular blockade since coughing and gagging cause ICP to increase.

$PaCO_2$ is a key determinant of cerebral vasodilatation and therefore hypercapnia has a significant deleterious influence on ICP.

- However, hyperventilation should also be avoided – it is (transiently) effective in reducing ICP, but the resulting hypocapnia is hazardous since the resultant vasoconstriction may cause cerebral ischemia, and one should aim for a $PaCO_2$ above 4.5 kPa.
- Care should be taken to minimize tidal volumes and airway pressures as far as this is possible to avoid unnecessary lung injury.

Sustained rises in ICP should be acted on promptly. It is important that the basic measures above are in place before escalating therapy. Unexpected changes in ICP may be due to structural problems such as bleeding, exhaustion of CSF reserve or hydrocephalus and will generally prompt a repeat CT head. Seizures, which may not be clinically apparent, should also be considered, particularly if there are spikes in ICP, and an anticonvulsant considered.

A number of neurosurgical interventions may be helpful in controlling raised ICP. Consideration should be given to CSF drainage via an EVD if simple measures are not controlling ICP. In any case, significant discrete space-occupying hematomas causing mass effect should generally be surgically evacuated. Hemorrhagic contusions are more difficult, since although they may appear well circumscribed on CT, they are generally rather ill defined at operation; whether to evacuate them depends on their size and location.

Steroids are associated with increased mortality and should not be routinely used for TBI [2].

Hyperosmolar therapy

Rising ICP may be controlled, at least temporarily, by hyperosmolar therapy aiming to reduce cerebral volume by drawing fluid osmotically from cells.

- Mannitol (e.g. 20%; 0.25–1 g/kg) has traditionally been used.
- However, whilst this agent improves microvascular flow by osmotically reducing erythrocyte and endothelial cell size, the effect that can be exerted on cerebral edema is limited since the osmotic effect can only be exerted via the (intact) blood–brain barrier.
- Furthermore, mannitol exhibits a marked osmotic diuretic effect that is highly undesirable, as it may lead to hypovolemia if volume correction is not instigated.
- Hypertonic saline (e.g. 2 mL/kg of 5% saline, repeated as needed) is superior in both these respects. Serum sodium should not be allowed to increase above 155 mmol/L and osmolarity should be kept below about 320 mOsm/L.

Fluid therapy, feeding and glycemic control

It is important that due care is given to the volume status of TBI patients and this may be unstable in the presence of bleeding from other injuries.

- Hypotonic or glucose-containing solutions must be avoided, however, as they may worsen cerebral edema.
- Isotonic saline or gelatine colloid are used.
- The use of albumin in TBI patients is associated with adverse outcome.
- Clearly hypovolemia secondary to hemorrhage is best treated with blood products (and hemostasis!).

Disordered sodium homeostasis is common after TBI.

- A mild hypernatremia is common (and possibly even desirable).
- However, pituitary dysfunction may lead to diabetes insipidus with consequent dangerous rise in serum sodium, as well as hypovolemia.
- Prompt treatment (e.g. with fluids and desmopressin) is important, but great care should be taken not to correct hypernatremia quickly, as cerebral edema will result.

Hyponatremia is also common and potentially dangerous in terms of worsening cerebral edema. The most commonly cited causes are syndrome of inappropriate ADH secretion (SIADH; typically euvolemic/hypervolemic) and cerebral salt wasting syndrome (CSWS; typically volume depleted).

- Both present with inappropriately high urine osmolarity and distinguishing between the two can be difficult in practice.
- Irrespective of the diagnosis, severe or symptomatic hyponatremia should be corrected with fluid restriction in the first instance.
- Careful use of hypertonic saline is indicated if carefully monitored ensuring the serum sodium concentration is not raised by more than 0.5 mmol/L/h (risk of osmotic demyelination syndrome).
- The ADH antagonist demeclocycline is a second-line therapy.
- CSWS, on the other hand, responds to fludrocortisone: fluid restriction is likely to result in potentially hazardous hypovolemia in this case.

Both hypoglycemia and hyperglycemia are known to be harmful to injured brain. Therefore, blood glucose levels should be tightly controlled at 6–10 mmol/L with a variable-rate intravenous insulin infusion. Targeting the higher end of this range may be appropriate if microdialysis glucose concentrations are worryingly low.

TBI (and trauma patients in general) have high nutritional requirements. Enteral nutrition is usually possible, preferable and should be instituted as early as possible. Impaired gastric emptying is common after head injury, however, and prokinetics may be required.

Temperature control

Mild to moderate therapeutic hypothermia (down to 33 °C) is generally reserved as a rescue therapy for intractable ICP.

- A survival benefit is hard to demonstrate in humans and it is associated with increased risk of infection and harmful hemodynamic and metabolic disturbances.
- Below 35 °C, propofol metabolism may be greatly reduced, causing accumulation and the risk of propofol infusion syndrome – it is best substituted for a benzodiazepine such as midazolam, although sedation may be inferior.
- Rapid rewarming is also known to be harmful and must be avoided.
- Neuromuscular blockade is required to prevent shivering.

Conversely, hyperthermia has an adverse effect on ICP and outcome. Treatment strategies include antipyretics and active cooling.

Other rescue strategies

If ICP remains intractable then EEG burst suppression with thiopentone loading/infusion may be effective by reducing $CMRO_2$ to basal levels. However, this agent accumulates and significant hemodynamic instability may occur, which is highly undesirable. Alternatively, decompressive craniectomy is an effective surgical method of ICP control.

Spinal-cord injury

Although traumatic SCI is rare, its consequences can clearly be devastating and severe injuries will lead to permanent disability. Furthermore, SCI may be initially missed in sedated or obtunded patients and a high index of suspicion must be maintained [3]. As with TBI, high quality acute care aims to maintain perfusion, reduce secondary injury and provide the best substrate for specialist spinal rehabilitation. Even high spinal-cord injuries with severe disability are compatible with excellent patient-assessed quality of life in the longer term.

Neurological injury

Spinal injuries may be described in terms of the stability of any fracture and the degree of cord injury.

- Thoracolumbar stability depends on involvement of anterior, middle and posterior spinal columns [4].
- Fracture/dislocation tends to be most unstable, followed by burst fractures, with wedge fractures being the least unstable.
- Stable injuries include isolated fractures to the transverse processes or spinous processes.

Insult to the spinal cord resulting in a change in the normal motor, sensory or autonomic function may be temporary or permanent. It is described in terms of:

- Neurological level (i.e. the lowest level with normal neurological function)
- Complete injury: absence of both voluntary muscle function and sensation in the lowest S4–S5 segments. This implies there are no significant nerve impulses across the injury site (does not necessarily imply the cord transection).
- Incomplete injury: partial/variable preservation of sacral sensation or motor function. There may be significant function below the level of injury.

The precise distribution of sensory and motor deficits seen after incomplete SCI can be very complex. Clinical assessment is standardized using the ASIA classification [5].

There are two classical phases after SCI:

- Spinal shock phase: flaccid paresis, typically 48 hours, but may last weeks
- Reflex phase: return of sympathetic function and some motor and reflex function, resulting in local spasticity and clonus.

Very little meaningful recovery is to be expected after complete SCI. In contrast, a substantial proportion of patients with incomplete SCI have some meaningful improvement in function by 1 year.

Spinal decompression surgery for unstable fractures will depend greatly on individual risk factors.

- Spinal decompression for cervical SCI before 24 hours as compared to after 24 hours is associated with improved outcome at 6 months [6].
- There is insufficient evidence to draw conclusions about spinal fixation surgery, and prospective, controlled studies are awaited [7].

Unlike TBI, there is some evidence for improved neurological outcome with high-dose steroids [8]. However, there is also significant associated mortality from sepsis (particularly pulmonary) and after TBI [2] and therefore the use of steroids is not common practice in the UK.

Respiratory effects

High spinal-cord injuries may be associated with a variable degree of respiratory compromise, depending on the level and extent of the SCI and on other injuries sustained. It is essential to prevent hypoxia if secondary neurological injury to the spinal cord is to be avoided.

The muscles of respiration are innervated at various levels from the spinal cord. Respiratory function will depend on the level and severity of the SCI.

- Lesions at C1 or 2 result in respiratory paralysis and require the patient to be immediately intubated and ventilated, with long-term ventilation being essential for survival.
- Injuries between C3–5 (phrenic nerve roots) may also necessitate lifelong ventilation, although there is some variation.
- Injuries below C8 will variably spare intercostal function. Adaption to increased use of accessory muscles is a common compensatory mechanism.
- Thoracic and lumbar injuries may still lead to loss of abdominal-wall muscle function with impaired ability for active expiration and cough.

Neurological compromise may increase gradually after the injury with hematoma formation or as cord edema develops and therefore careful, repeated assessment and timely intervention are crucial. Pulmonary injuries or infection may also progress in the period after injury and cause respiratory decompensation. It is better to intervene early in a controlled manner rather than as an uncontrolled emergency. Indications for anesthesia, endotracheal intubation and mechanical ventilation include:

- Hypoxia
- Hypercapnia with associated acidosis or increasing $PaCO_2$ with associated acidosis

- Failure to maintain/protect airway due to depressed consciousness (e.g. due to TBI)
- Low (<20–30% predicted) or falling vital capacity.

All patients with any suspicion of spinal trauma should have a hard cervical collar fitted and be log rolled until the spine may be adequately radiologically and clinically reviewed. An unstable spinal injury requires rapid assessment by a senior spinal surgeon, followed by appropriate surgical or traction fixation.

If emergency intubation is required, this should be performed by an experienced operator with in-line immobilization and full-stomach precautions. Temporarily releasing the cervical collar improves the grade of laryngoscopy. It is essential that hypoxia and hypotension are avoided. Depolarizing neuromuscular blockade is safe in the first 2 or 3 days after SCI but should then be avoided for at least 9 months after the injury, as it may precipitate dangerous hyperkalemia. Awake fiberoptic intubation under topical anesthesia/mild sedation may be an attractive and safer alternative in less-urgent cases if the operator is experienced in the technique.

Spinal injuries that necessitate nursing the patient lying flat markedly increase the risk of pulmonary atelectasis and retention of secretions.

- Morbidity associated with a reduced ability to clear secretions can be significant and the patient should be assessed and treated holistically, taking into account the likely effect of any pre-existing lung disease.
- Surgical fixation of unstable fractures allows upright posture and should be undertaken early.
- Physiotherapy and early tracheostomy allow mobilization of respiratory secretions.
- Care bundles to reduce the risk of developing ventilator-associated pneumonia should be used.

Cardiovascular effects

The initial spinal-cord injury with direct compression of descending sympathetic nerves may cause a large autonomic discharge, producing hypertension and arrhythmias. The resulting increase in afterload may cause left ventricular failure or subendocardial infarction and pulmonary vascular effects.

After this initial phase, lasting minutes, there follows a sudden loss of sympathetic discharge and neurogenic shock – loss of vascular sympathetic tone with reduced systemic vascular resistance and splanchnic pooling of venous blood, with consequent reduction in venous return. Cardioaccelerator impulses arise at T1–T4 so lesions above this level may also cause bradycardia from unopposed parasympathetic tone.

As well as the effects on other organs, the resulting hypotension may reduce spinal-cord perfusion pressure and must be treated aggressively.

- Fluid resuscitation is generally the first-line intervention, but many such patients require infusion of a vasopressor such as noradrenaline once central venous access has been established.
- There are advocates for maintaining a mean arterial pressure of 85 mmHg for the first few days after SCI [9], but this should be individually tailored.
- The presence of other injuries should be ruled out before hypotension is attributed to neurogenic shock.

Appropriate imaging should be performed as symptoms such as pain may not be apparent in insensate patients and tachycardia may be partially masked.

Autonomic dysreflexia may develop particularly in the first 2–4 months post-injury in patients with lesions above T6. Altered neuronal connectivity leads to development of inappropriate sympathetic reflexes in response to noxious stimuli such as pain, constipation or bladder distension.

Features include:

- Hypertension, which may require intervention if severe
- Baroreflex-mediated bradycardia
- Headache, agitation, sweating above the level of the injury, facial flushing and nausea.

Spinal-cord injury above T10 leads to vasodilatation in exercising muscles, with poor compensatory vasoconstriction in areas below the injury. This produces a fall in blood pressure and hypoperfusion with early exhaustion.

Other intensive care considerations

Genito-urinary effects

- Spinal shock phase: loss of bladder sphincter tone and urinary retention
- Reflex phase: desynchronized bladder sphincter contraction; incomplete voiding and vesicoureteric reflux
- Renal calculi, infections and reflux all increase the risk of renal failure. Bladder management with suitable catheter systems and avoidance of distention and dysreflexia is crucial.

Gastrointestinal system

- High incidence of gastroparesis and ileus initially after SCI (especially high cord injury).
- Neurogenic bowel dysfunction. A high fiber diet and osmotic laxatives are required to prevent constipation. Stimulant laxatives and regular digital rectal stimulation may be required to initiate large bowel reflex emptying.

Hematological system

- Anemia (especially normochromic normocytic anemia associated with ulcers and infection).
- Venous thromboembolism risk. Anticoagulation (e.g. warfarinization to an INR of 2–2.5) may be needed and is suggested for 3 months post-injury.

Other effects

- Chronic pain
- Painful reflex spasms. Tizanidine or oral or intrathecal baclofen are commonly used as treatments
- Risk of decubitus ulcers from immobility, lack of sensation and altered skin blood flow. Pressure sores may cause infection, osteomyelitis or precipitate autonomic dysreflexia
- Bone resorption occurs below the lesion. Abnormal joint ossification in 20%
- Thermoregulation affected by loss of shivering and abnormal vasodilation.

Rehabilitation

Participation in therapeutic recreation interventions during inpatient rehabilitation for patients with spinal-cord injury is a positive predictor for functional independence and a return to a productive life after SCI. Early planning for long-term rehabilitation, including a multidisciplinary assessment of the individual patient's needs, should be actively initiated. Initial planning while the patient is still in intensive care is encouraged [10].

References

1. Brain Trauma Foundation Guidelines for the management of severe traumatic brain injury (3rd edn). *J Neurotrauma* 2007; 24 (Supplement 1) : 5–106.

2. Roberts I, Yates D, Sandercock P *et al.* EPC trial collaborators. Effect of intravenous corticosteroids on death within 14 days in 10008 adults with clinically significant head injury (MRC CRASH trial): randomised placebo-controlled trial. *Lancet* 2004; 364 : 1321–8.

3. Hasler R, Exadaktylos A, Bouamra O *et al.* Epidemiology and predictors of spinal injury in adult major trauma patients: European cohort study. *Eur Spine J* 2011; 20 : 2174–80.

4. Denis F. The three column spine and its significance in the classification of acute thoracolumbar spinal injuries. *Spine* 1983; 8 : 817–31.

5. Waring WP, Biering-Sorensen F, Burns S *et al.* 2009 review and revisions of the international standards for the neurological classification of spinal cord injury. *J Spinal Cord Med* 2010; 33 : 346–52.

6. Fehlings M, Vaccaro A. Early versus delayed decompression for traumatic cervical spinal cord injury: results of the Surgical Timing in Acute Spinal Cord Injury Study (STASCIS). *PLoS One* 2012; 7 : e32037.

7. Jones L, Bagnall A. Spinal injuries centres (SICs) for acute traumatic spinal cord injury. *Cochrane Database Syst Rev* 2004; 18 : CD004442.

8. Bracken M. Steroids for acute spinal cord injury. *Cochrane Database Syst Rev* 2002; 3 : CD001046.

9. Vale FL, Burns J, Jackson a B, Hadley MN. Combined medical and surgical treatment after acute spinal cord injury: results of a prospective pilot study to assess the merits of aggressive medical resuscitation and blood pressure management. *J Neurosurg* 1997; 87 : 239–46.

10. Cahow C, Gassaway J, Rider C *et al.* Relationship of therapeutic recreation inpatient rehabilitation interventions and patient characteristics to outcomes following spinal cord injury: the SCIRehab project. *J Spinal Cord Med* 2012; 35 : 547–64.

Chapter	
25	# Acute coronary syndromes

Kala Kathirgamanathan and Jaffer Syed

Epidemiology

Myocardial infarction is a major cause of morbidity and mortality worldwide. With the advent of coronary care units, the mortality has declined. However, coronary artery disease (CAD) continues to remain accountable for one-third of all deaths in those over age 35 [1,2].

The 2010 Heart Disease and Stroke Statistics update for the American Heart Association reported that 17.6 million people in the USA have CAD.

The spectrum of ACS

Acute coronary syndromes (ACS) exist in a spectrum; a continuum that ranges from unstable angina, to NSTEMI (non-ST-elevation myocardial infarction) to STEMI (ST-elevation myocardial infarction) [3,4].

- Myocardial infarction (MI) is defined as a clinical (or pathologic) event caused by myocardial ischemia in which there is evidence of myocardial injury or necrosis. It is accepted that the term MI reflects a loss of cardiac myocytes (necrosis) caused by prolonged ischemia [3].
- The classification as to whether a myocardial infarction is an NSTEMI or a STEMI is entirely based on the electrocardiographic findings. These electrocardiographic changes are also important on a pathologic level, indicating the absence or presence of an occlusive thrombus. The electrocardiogram is a key determinant in diagnosis and the diagnosis of STEMI mandates emergent reperfusion therapy.
- Unstable angina is the presence of unstable ischemic pain, without a rise in biomarkers of necrosis, typically defined by a troponin rise.

Clinical presentation

Chest pain is the most common presenting complaint in patients suffering from myocardial infarction [5]. The description of the pain is important, as typical ischemic pain tends to be aggravated with activity and relieved with rest. The quality of the chest pain is characteristically described using adjectives such as squeezing, crushing and pressure [5]. Associated features may include diaphoresis, nausea, vomiting, symptoms of heart failure or syncope. It is important to remember that not all patients will present with typical chest pain, and

Handbook of ICU Therapy, third edition, ed. John Fuller, Jeff Granton and Ian McConachie. Published by Cambridge University Press. © Cambridge University Press 2015.

diagnosis should be a comprehensive approach, taking into account not only history, but also past history, ECG and biomarker changes.

According to the Rational Clinical Examination series published in *The Journal of the American Medical Association (JAMA)*, the presence of any of the following clinical findings increases the likelihood of MI:

- Patients presenting with chest pain radiating to the left arm, radiating to the right shoulder or radiating to both left and right arms
- Patients presenting with chest pain, diaphoresis, a third heart sound or with hypotension [5].

The presence of any of the following clinical findings decreases the likelihood of MI:

- Patients presenting with chest pain that is described as pleuritic, sharp or stabbing, positional or reproduced by palpation [5].

Diagnosis of ACS

An expert consensus document published in the *European Heart Journal* in 2007 defined acute MI as a rise and/or fall of cardiac biomarkers with at least one value above the 99th percentile of the upper reference limit (URL), together with evidence of myocardial ischemia. Ischemia was defined as:

- Any symptoms of ischemia
- Electrocardiographic changes suggestive of new ischemia
- Development of pathologic Q waves on electrocardiogram
- Imaging evidence of infarction [4].

Imaging evidence would be constituted by the presence of new regional wall motion abnormality, as assessed by echocardiography or new loss of viable myocardium by radionuclide imaging.

Typical ECG appearances of inferior, anterior and posterior MI are shown in Figures 25.1, 25.2 and 25.3, respectively.

By way of contrast, the ECG appearances of diffuse subendocardial ischemia are shown in Figure 25.4.

This consensus document also defines criteria for prior myocardial infarction as:

- The development of new pathologic Q waves, regardless of the presence or absence of symptoms
- Imaging evidence of a region of loss of viable myocardium that is thinned and fails to contract
- Pathologic findings of a healed or healing myocardial infarction.

Management

Those patients presenting with chest pain suspicious for an ACS should be evaluated promptly with immediate history and electrocardiogram.

- The diagnosis of myocardial infarction can be confirmed electrocardiographically and with elevation of serum cardiac biomarkers.
- The history is pivotal in diagnosing unstable angina, as there will be no elevation of cardiac biomarkers.
- Unstable angina, acute STEMI and NSTEMI must be distinguished. Although they often share the common pathophysiology of an unstable atherosclerotic plaque, the

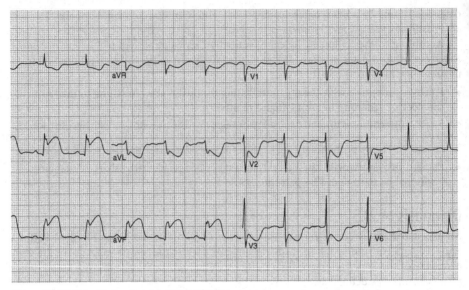

Figure 25.1 Inferior ST elevation myocardial infarction.

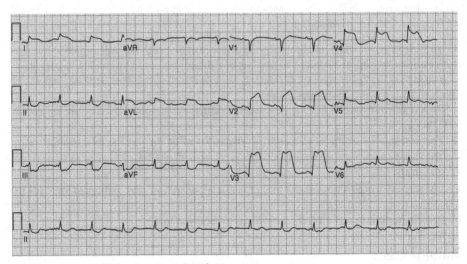

Figure 25.2 Anterior ST elevation myocardial infarction.

management of each entity differs acutely. Regardless of the diagnosis, however, the initial step necessitates expedient recognition, as therapeutic effects are maximized when initiated soon after presentation to hospital.

Once the diagnosis of either UA or acute NSTEMI is made, the acute management of the patient involves the simultaneous achievement of several goals [6].

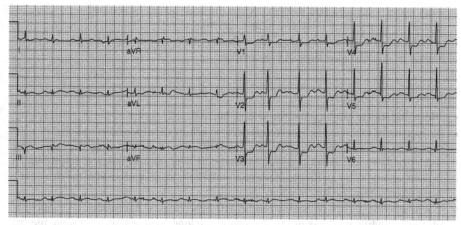

Figure 25.3 Posterior ST elevation myocardial infarction

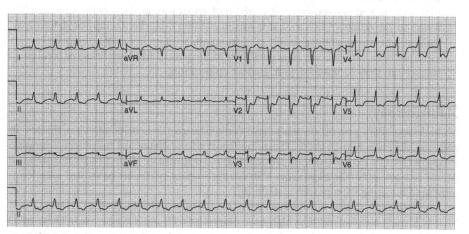

Figure 25.4 Diffuse subendocardial ischemia.

These include:

- Ensuring the patient is in a monitored setting
- Relief of ischemic symptoms
- Monitoring for hemodynamic instability and correction of abnormalities. Patients are often hypertensive and tachycardic, which will both serve to increase oxygen requirements. As such, supplemental oxygen is to be placed on all patients suspected of having an ACS
- Monitoring for dysrhythmia
- Upon initial evaluation, it is important to estimate the patient's risk and decide on whether the patient will necessitate emergent reperfusion, an

early invasive management strategy, versus medical therapy or planned percutaneous coronary intervention at a later time

- Antithrombotic therapies, anticoagulant therapy and other medical therapies should be considered at time of presentation.

Anti-ischemic therapy

- Morphine sulfate can be given for pain or anxiety.
- Nitroglycerin sublingual or intravenous can be administered for relief of ischemic pain. One must be careful to ensure the safe administration of nitrates, as in the case of RV infarction; they may result in severe hypotension. The administration of nitrates in an individual who is on a phosphodiesterase inhibitor is contraindicated if the drug has been taken within the last 24 hours.
- If a patient has previously been on an NSAID other than ASA, consideration should be given to avoiding this class of medications in the long-term setting, as chronic use has been associated with an increased risk of cardiovascular events.
- The 2007 ACC/AHA guidelines recommend that β-blocker therapy should be administered universally to all patients without contraindications. The COMMIT/CCS2 trial is the largest placebo-controlled trial performed with β-blockers in acute MI [7]. Based on the results of this trial, it is reasonable that β-blocker therapy be deferred in patients who are hemodynamically compromised, as mortality may actually be increased with such therapy. Once stability of the patient has been achieved, oral β-blocker can then be initiated with gradual up-titration.

Statin therapy

Multiple secondary prevention trials have demonstrated the benefits of statin therapy in patients who have had an ACS. The third report of the National Cholesterol Education Program (NCEP) Expert Panel on Detection and Treatment of High Blood Cholesterol in Adults recommends that all patients with acute coronary syndrome be treated with long-term lipid-lowering therapy with a statin [8].

Statin therapy should be initiated prior to discharge. The PROVE IT-TIMI 22 and MIRACL trials recommend that high-dose atorvastatin 80 mg daily be used. These trials suggest initiation of initial intensive statin therapy, rather than gradual dose titration upward, provides greater protection against death or major cardiovascular events than does a standard regimen [9,10].

Patients admitted with ACS should have a lipid profile drawn early after admission. Based on changes in the lipid profile, it has been thought to be most accurate in patients with an acute coronary syndrome (ACS) when obtained within hours of hospitalization or in the outpatient setting after at least 1 month has elapsed [11].

Antithrombotic therapy

Antiplatelet therapy is pivotal in the treatment of acute coronary syndromes. This development of atherogenesis is directly related to platelet aggregation. Aspirin therapy is indicated in all patients with ACS, as is a platelet P2Y12 receptor blocker.

Antiplatelet effects have been widely studied.

- In 2002, the Antithrombotic Trialists Collaboration performed a worldwide meta-analysis of randomized trials of antithrombotic therapy. The combined endpoint of nonfatal myocardial infarction, nonfatal stroke or vascular death in patients with unstable angina was significantly reduced by 46% with antiplatelet therapy. There was a 30% reduction in patients with acute myocardial infarction. This analysis also supports the fact that there is no significant difference in efficacy between lower and higher daily doses. However, at initial presentation, patients should be given a 162 mg or 325 mg loading dose of aspirin, prior to continuing with 81 mg daily. The addition of an additional antiplatelet agent was also found to be important, as it resulted in a significantly lowered combined endpoint [12].

- The choice of the second antiplatelet agent is made on an individualized basis and generally left to clinical judgment. However, the second agent should be a P2Y12 receptor blocker. These include agents such as clopidogrel, ticlopidine, prasugrel, ticagrelor and cangrelor.

- The CURE trial [13] compared dual antiplatelet therapy with aspirin and clopidogrel to aspirin alone, in patients with acute coronary syndrome. Based upon this evidence, there is strong recommendation for at least 1 year of dual antiplatelet therapy with both a P2Y12 receptor blocker and aspirin.

- Ticagrelor and prasugrel are both newer agents and evidence to support the use of these drugs comes from comparison studies with clopidogrel. These antiplatelet agents are more potent and have been found to be more efficacious than clopidogrel, but are also associated with a higher bleeding risk. The impetus supporting the development of these agents was the limitations of clopidogrel, which include irreversibility of platelet inhibition, longer time to onset of action and variability of response. Due to the risk of thrombocytopenia, ticlopidine is rarely chosen.

- At the time of presentation, a loading dose of aspirin 162 mg or 325 mg should be administered immediately. This higher dose results in expedient antithrombotic effect due to immediate and almost complete inhibition of thromboxane A2 production. The initial dose should be chewed or crushed to ensure a high blood level, quickly. Subsequent to the initial loading dose, the lower dose of 81 mg must be continued indefinitely for secondary prevention. There has been no evidence to support the notion that higher doses are more efficacious [6].

- The 2013 ACCF/AHA guidelines state that a loading dose of a P2Y12 receptor inhibitor be given as early as possible or at time of primary percutaneous coronary intervention (PCI) to patients with STEMI. They make no recommendations as to favoring one antiplatelet over another and choice of the agent should be individualized, taking into consideration bleeding risk and choosing the agent that best suits each patient's individual risk profile [14].

- For patients who are not at high risk of bleeding, with no planned noncardiac surgery, it is generally recommended that dual antiplatelet therapy be continued for a duration of 1 year, regardless of the type of stent(s) deployed.

- The use of glycoprotein IIb/IIIa inhibitors in patients with STEMI is supported by evidence established prior to the use of dual antiplatelet therapy [14]. In the setting of STEMI, these agents have been used as adjunctive therapy in patients undergoing percutaneous coronary intervention.

Those patients with STEMI who are not in the vicinity of a cardiac catheterization lab, should be administered a thrombolytic agent, provided after clinical review of the risks versus benefits of such therapy, taking into account the relative risks and contraindications for each patient. Thereafter, as with NSTEMI, dual antiplatelet agents must be administered and patients should be considered for invasive risk stratification with coronary angiography.

In the event that there is failure of the thrombolytic agent, arrangements must be made for emergent percutaneous coronary intervention, termed rescue PCI.

Anticoagulation

Anticoagulation must be administered expediently to all patients with acute coronary syndrome.

Anticoagulation used in acute coronary syndromes encompasses several classes of medications. Included are the unfractionated heparins (UFH), low-molecular-weight heparins (LMWH) and the indirect thrombin inhibitors (hirudin, bivalirudin, lepirudin) and fondaparunix, a factor Xa inhibitor.

As with antiplatelet agents, the decision concerning which anticoagulant to use must be individualized to the patient and the anticipated management strategy.

- For example, the risk of heparin-induced thrombocytopenia is greater with administration of UFH, but its relatively short half-life and the reversal of its effect with protamine may be advantageous for patients undergoing invasive angiography and percutaneous coronary intervention.
- LMWH tends to have a more predictable anticoagulant effect and the likelihood of immune-mediated thrombocytopenia is less, while half-life is longer and the effect not reversible [15].
- The decision to use fondaparinux should rely on whether or not the patient has been selected to undergo coronary angiography and PCI. The drug has shown to be of benefit in all groups except those undergoing primary PCI.
- In the OASIS-6 trial [16], Yusuf et al. demonstrated a trend toward worse outcomes with fondaparinux compared to heparin, in patients treated with primary PCI. There was also a higher rate of catheter thrombus, no reflow, dissection or perforation with fondaparinux. However, the addition of UFH with fondaparinux during PCI largely avoided these complications. There was a trend toward fewer severe bleeds with fondaparinux. It is recommended that fondaparinux not be chosen for STEMI patients who will be treated with primary PCI.
- However, in those patients who were not revascularized, fondaparinux significantly lowered the rate of the primary efficacy outcome of death and or reinfarction at 30 days, compared to UFH/placebo. Significant reductions of this endpoint were also seen at the secondary assessment at 9 days and at the 3- or 6-month follow-up. Mortality was also significantly reduced.

Early risk stratification

It is important to evaluate each patient on an individual basis and risk stratify each patient accordingly. Those at the highest risk for further cardiac events or decompensation may benefit from an earlier, more aggressive therapeutic approach [17,18]. The ACC/AHA identifies a number of high-risk features. These include:

- Hemodynamic instability (hypotension, bradycardia, tachycardia)
- Dynamic electrocardiographic changes
- Persistent or accelerating ischemic pain
- Prolonged (more than 20 minutes) and ongoing rest pain
- Sustained ventricular tachycardia
- Pulmonary edema, most likely related to ischemia
- New/worsened murmur of mitral regurgitation
- S3 or worsening rales
- Age greater than 75
- New or presumed new bundle branch block
- Markedly elevated biomarkers (e.g. TnI >0.1 ng/mL)

For those patients with NSTEMI without high-risk features, the optimal timing is uncertain, but the majority will tend to undergo coronary intervention early, within 24 hours.

A number of scores have been developed to help determine risk. These include the TIMI risk score, the GRACE score and the PURSUIT score. The most widely applied score for prognostication is the TIMI risk score [19].

The TIMI risk score is based on seven variables, assessed on presentation:

- Age $\geq$ 65 years
- Presence of at least three risk factors for CHD (hypertension, diabetes, dyslipidemia, smoking or positive family history of early MI)
- Prior coronary stenosis of $\geq$ 50%
- Presence of ST segment deviation on admission ECG
- At least two angina episodes in prior 24 hours
- Elevated serum cardiac biomarkers
- Use of aspirin in the prior seven days (which is probably a marker for more severe coronary disease).

Patients are considered to be at low risk with a score of 1 to 2; intermediate risk with a score of 3 to 4; and high risk with a score of 5 to 7. The TACTICS-TIMI 18 Trial [20] showed that those with a high-risk TIMI score of 5 to 7, as well as those with intermediate scores of 3 to 4, benefited from early invasive approach.

Reperfusion therapy

- Fibrinolytic therapy is not beneficial in patients with non-ST elevation ACS. The ACC/AHA recommend against the routine use of fibrinolytic agents in patients with a non-ST elevation ACS.
- Those presenting with STEMI outside the vicinity of a cardiac catheterization lab should be treated with fibrinolytic therapy, provided there are no contraindications.
- Those who fail thrombolysis must be taken emergently to a cardiac catheterization lab. Failure of thrombolysis is defined as the persistence of unrelenting ischemic chest pain, the absence of resolution of the ST segment elevation,

hemodynamic and/or electrical instability. In these cases of failed reperfusion, rescue percutaneous coronary intervention is likely necessary [21].

Complications of MI

Mechanical complications of myocardial infarction include:
- Cardiac tamponade secondary to left ventricular free wall rupture
- Pseudoaneurysm formation
- Rupture of the interventricular septum
- Acute mitral regurgitation due to partial or full rupture of a papillary muscle.

All mechanical complications constitute emergencies.

The 2004 American College of Cardiology/American Heart Association (ACC/AHA) guidelines on STEMI and CABG recommend emergent surgery, with coronary artery bypass grafting if indicated, for these mechanical complications of an acute MI.
- Early surgical closure is the treatment of choice, even if the patient's condition is stable. Although initial reports suggested that delaying surgery to allow healing of friable tissue improved surgical mortality, it was likely that lower mortality was as a result of selection bias [22].
- The mortality rate for patients with VSD treated medically is 24% at 72 hours and 75% at 3 weeks [23].

As such it is recommended that such patients be considered for urgent surgical repair.
- An intra-aortic balloon pump (IABP) should be inserted as early as possible as a bridge to a surgical procedure, unless there is marked aortic regurgitation. IABP counterpulsation decreases systemic vascular resistance (SVR), decreases shunt fraction, increases coronary perfusion and maintains blood pressure.
- Vasodilators can decrease left-to-right shunt and increase systemic flow by means of reducing SVR; however, caution should be taken, as greater decrease in pulmonary vascular resistance may actually increase shunting. The vasodilator of choice is intravenous nitroprusside, which can be carefully titrated to a mean arterial pressure of 70–80 mmHg.

Other complications include:
- Right ventricular failure, most commonly seen in cases of RV infarction in the setting of inferior myocardial infarction
- LV pump failure, ventricular aneurysms and cardiogenic shock
- Arrhythmic complications are also common in the setting of ischemia.

Pericardial complications

There are several pericardial complications associated with MI. These include:
- Peri-infarct pericarditis
- Pericardial effusion, pericardial effusion with tamponade
- Dressler's syndrome, which is the onset of immune-mediated pericarditis several weeks following myocardial infarction.

Arrhythmic complications

Conduction disturbance is a well-known complication following acute myocardial infarction.

Heart block is a common complication of inferior MI, due to the blood supply to the AV node. During inferior infarction, compromise of blood flow to the AV node may result in heart block. Generally, reperfusion of the culprit vessel should result in resolution of the heart block.

The 2004 ACC/AHA provides recommendations on the indications for temporary pacing in the setting of acute MI.

These indications include:

- Asystole
- Complete heart block
- Alternating right and left BBB or RBBB alternating with LAFB or LPFB
- Mobitz type II second-degree AV block
- Symptomatic bradycardia of any etiology.

Perioperative management of ACS

Diagnosis of perioperative myocardial infarction can be especially challenging, as many such events may be silent. Patients may be asymptomatic in the surgical setting due to sedation or pain medication. If the physician were to rely solely on clinical signs or symptoms, up to 50% of perioperative MIs may be unrecognized [24].

Devereaux *et al.* proposed diagnostic criteria for perioperative myocardial infarction, in those patients undergoing noncardiac surgery. This criterion requires the typical troponin rise and fall and the more rapid rise and fall of CK-MB. Caution must be entertained to ensure that troponin rise is not due to another reason, such as pulmonary embolism. Biomarker rise must be present in association with clinical ischemic signs or symptoms, ECG changes suggestive of injury or infarction, new wall motion abnormality on echocardiography or new fixed defect on radionuclide imaging.

Elective noncardiac surgery after percutaneous coronary intervention

- Between 5 and 10% of patients with coronary stents undergo noncardiac surgery within 1 year of stent implantation [25,26].
- This is an issue of importance because the risks of premature cessation of antiplatelet therapy in a patient with recent stent implantation requiring noncardiac surgery must be carefully weighed against the bleeding risks associated with continuation of these agents.
- For those patients needing to undergo nonelective noncardiac surgery following percutaneous coronary intervention, the cardiac complications are often related to cessation of dual antiplatelet therapy. Complications may include stent thrombosis, acute coronary syndrome and arrhythmia.
- Additionally, surgery places the patient in a prothrombotic state. Surgery causes prothrombotic and proinflammatory effects, which may predispose the coronary circulation to thrombosis at the site of prior stent placement or at other sites of atherosclerotic lesions [27,28].

- There have been observational studies done that suggest that patients undergoing surgery within 6 weeks of stent implantation are at increased risk of myocardial infarction or death [29,30].
- Stent thrombosis carries high rates of morbidity and mortality, leading to high rates of myocardial infarction (50 to 70%) and death (10–40%) [31].
- In effort to minimize adverse cardiovascular events, it would be prudent to delay elective noncardiac surgery until after the minimal recommended duration of dual antiplatelet therapy is completed following coronary stent implantation. For those patients necessitating emergent or life-saving noncardiac surgery, the risks of and benefits must be individualized.

Management of perioperative myocardial infarction

The treatment of a patient who has suffered a perioperative myocardial infarction is similar to that of the general population. The only difference in management relates to the risks of bleeding, given the recent surgical intervention. Risks of bleeding must be weighed carefully when considering therapeutic anticoagulation and antiplatelet therapy. This is an important decision that must be individualized to the patient under consideration.

References

1. Rosamond W, Flegal K, Furie K *et al.* Heart disease and stroke statistics–2008 update: a report from the american heart association statistics committee and stroke statistics subcommittee. *Circulation* 2008;117 : e25–146.

2. Lloyd-Jones D, Adams RJ, Brown TM *et al.* Executive summary: Heart disease and stroke statistics–2010 update: a report from the american heart association. *Circulation* 2010; 121 : 948–54.

3. Alpert JS, Thygesen K, Antman E, Bassand JP. Myocardial infarction redefined–a consensus document of the joint european society of cardiology/american college of cardiology committee for the redefinition of myocardial infarction. *J Am Coll Cardiol* 2000 36 : 959–69.

4. Thygesen K, Alpert JS, White HD, Joint ESC/ACCF/AHA/WHF Task Force for the Redefinition of Myocardial Infarction. Universal definition of myocardial infarction. *J Am Coll Cardiol* 2007; 50 : 2173–95.

5. Panju AA, Hemmelgarn BR, Guyatt GH, Simel DL. The rational clinical examination. Is this patient having a myocardial infarction? *JAMA* 1998; 280 : 1256–63.

6. Wright RS, Anderson JL, Adams CD *et al.* 2011 ACCF/AHA focused update incorporated into the ACC/AHA 2007 guidelines for the management of patients with unstable angina/non-st-elevation myocardial infarction: a report of the American College of Cardiology Foundation/American Heart Association Task Force on Practice Guidelines developed in collaboration with the American Academy of Family Physicians, Society for Cardiovascular Angiography and Interventions, and the Society of Thoracic Surgeons. *J Am Coll Cardiol* 2011; 57 : e215–367.

7. Chen ZM, Pan HC, Chen YP *et al.* Early intravenous then oral metoprolol in 45,852 patients with acute myocardial infarction: randomised placebo-controlled trial. *Lancet* 2005; 366 : 1622–32.

8. National Cholesterol Education Program (NCEP) Expert Panel on Detection, Evaluation, and Treatment of High Blood Cholesterol in Adults (Adult Treatment Panel III). Third report of the national cholesterol education program (NCEP) expert panel on detection, evaluation, and treatment of high blood cholesterol in adults (adult treatment panel III) final report. *Circulation* 2002; 106 : 3143–421.

9. Schwartz GG, Olsson AG, Ezekowitz MD et al. Effects of atorvastatin on early recurrent ischemic events in acute coronary syndromes. The MIRACL study: a randomized controlled trial. JAMA 2001; 285 : 1711–8.

10. Cannon CP, Braunwald E, McCabe CH et al. Intensive versus moderate lipid lowering with statins after acute coronary syndromes. N Engl J Med 2004; 350 : 1495–504.

11. Miller M. Lipid levels in the post-acute coronary syndrome setting: destabilizing another myth? J Am Coll Cardiol 2008; 51 : 1446–7.

12. Antithrombotic Trialists' Collaboration. Collaborative meta-analysis of randomised trials of antiplatelet therapy for prevention of death, myocardial infarction, and stroke in high risk patients. BMJ 2002; 324 : 71–86.

13. Yusuf S, Zhao F, Mehta S et al. Clopidogrel in unstable angina to prevent recurrent events trial investigators: effects of clopidogrel in addition to aspirin in patients with acute coronary syndromes without st-segment elevation. N Engl J Med 2001; 345 : 494–502.

14. O'Gara PT, Kushner FG, Ascheim DD et al. 2013 ACCF/AHA guideline for the management of ST-elevation myocardial infarction: a report of the American College of Cardiology Foundation/ American Heart Association Task Force on Practice Guidelines. J Am Coll Cardiol 2013; 61 : e78–140.

15. Lefkovits J, Topol EJ. Direct thrombin inhibitors in cardiovascular medicine. Circulation 1994; 90 : 1522–36.

16. Yusuf S, Mehta SR, Chrolavicius S et al. Effects of fondaparinux on mortality and reinfarction in patients with acute st-segment elevation myocardial infarction: the OASIS-6 randomized trial. JAMA 2006; 295 : 1519–30.

17. Bertrand ME, Simoons ML, Fox KA et al. Management of acute coronary syndromes: acute coronary syndromes without persistent ST segment elevation; recommendations of the task force of the european society of cardiology. Eur Heart J 2000; 21 : 1406–32.

18. Mehta SR, Cannon CP, Fox KA et al. Routine vs selective invasive strategies in patients with acute coronary syndromes: a collaborative meta-analysis of randomized trials. JAMA 2005; 293 : 2908–17.

19. Antman EM, Cohen M, Bernink PJ et al. The TIMI risk score for unstable angina/ non-st elevation MI: a method for prognostication and therapeutic decision making. JAMA 2000; 284 : 835–42.

20. Cannon CP, Weintraub WS, Demopoulos LA et al. Comparison of early invasive and conservative strategies in patients with unstable coronary syndromes treated with the glycoprotein iib/iiia inhibitor tirofiban. N Engl J Med 2001; 344 : 1879–87.

21. Antman EM, Anbe DT, Armstrong PW et al. ACC/AHA guidelines for the management of patients with ST-elevation myocardial infarction–executive summary: a report of the American College of Cardiology/American Heart Association Task Force on Practice Guidelines (committee to revise the 1999 guidelines for the management of patients with acute myocardial infarction). Circulation 2004; 110 : 588–636.

22. Giuliani ER, Danielson GK, Pluth JR et al. Postinfarction ventricular septal rupture: surgical considerations and results. Circulation 1974; 49 : 455–9.

23. Fox AF, Gkassman EG, Isom OI. Surgically remediable complications of myocardial infarction. Prog Cardiovasc Dis 1979; 107 : 852–5.

24. Devereaux PD, Goldman LG, Yusuf SY et al. Surveillance and prevention of major perioperative ischemic cardiac events in patients undergoing noncardiac surgery: a review. CMAJ 2005; 173 : 779–88.

25. Hawn MT, Graham LA, Richman JR et al. The incidence and timing of noncardiac surgery after cardiac stent implantation. J Am Coll Surg 2012; 214 : 658–66.

26. Berger PB, Kleiman NS, Pencina MJ et al. Frequency of major noncardiac surgery and subsequent adverse events in the year

after drug-eluting stent placement results from the EVENT (Evaluation of Drug-Eluting Stents and Ischemic Events) Registry. *JACC Cardiovasc Interv* 2010, Sep; 3(9) : 920–7.

27. Diamantis T, Tsiminikakis N, Skordylaki A *et al.* Alterations of hemostasis after laparoscopic and open surgery. *Hematology* 2007; 12 : 561–70.

28. Rajagopalan S, Ford I, Bachoo P *et al.* Platelet activation, myocardial ischemic events and postoperative non-response to aspirin in patients undergoing major vascular surgery. *J Thromb Haemost* 2007; 5 : 2028–35.

29. Reddy PR, Vaitkus PT. Risks of noncardiac surgery after coronary stenting. *Am J Cardiol* 2005; 95 : 755–7.

30. Wilson SH, Fasseas P, Orford JL *et al.* Clinical outcome of patients undergoing non-cardiac surgery in the two months following coronary stenting. *J Am Coll Cardiol* 2003; 42 : 234–40.

31. Holmes DR, Kereiakes DJ, Garg S *et al.* Stent thrombosis. *J Am Coll Cardiol* 2010; 56 : 1357–65.

Heart failure

26

Christopher W White, Darren H Freed, Shelley R Zieroth
and Rohit K Singal

Heart failure is a clinical syndrome resulting from inadequate cardiac output and therefore insufficient delivery of oxygen to meet the metabolic demands of the body.

- The prevalence of heart failure in the developed world is approximately 1–2%; however, it increases progressively with age and approaches 10% in those older than 75 years [1,2].
- Acute heart failure (AHF) may occur in a patient without previously diagnosed cardiac dysfunction (*de novo* AHF) or as an acute decompensation of chronic heart failure (ADCHF) [3].
- AHF is the most common cause of hospital admission in patients older than 65 years of age [4], and is associated with a 31% risk of rehospitalization and an 18% risk of mortality within 1 year [5].

Classification of AHF

The European Society of Cardiology guidelines on the diagnosis and treatment of AHF classify it into six categories according to clinical presentation [3,6]:

1. Hypertensive AHF: chest radiograph demonstrates pulmonary edema, preserved left ventricular ejection fraction and high blood pressure.
2. Pulmonary edema: chest radiograph demonstrates pulmonary edema, severe dyspnea accompanied by orthopnea and pulmonary crackles and oxygen saturation <90% on room air prior to treatment.
3. Cardiogenic shock: systemic hypoperfusion as a result of heart failure despite adequate preload and characterized by hypotension (systolic blood pressure <90 mmHg or a drop in mean arterial pressure >30 mmHg), low urine output (<0.5 mL/kg/hour) and a pulse rate >60 beats per minute.
4. Acute decompensated heart failure: history of chronic heart failure, signs and symptoms of heart failure that are mild and do not fulfill the criteria for hypertensive AHF, pulmonary edema or cardiogenic shock.
5. Isolated right heart failure: systemic hypoperfusion, absence of pulmonary congestion with low left ventricular filling pressures, increased jugular venous pressure and hepatomegaly.
6. High-output failure: high cardiac output, usually with a high heart rate, warm periphery and pulmonary congestion, caused by arrhythmias, thyrotoxicosis, anemia, Paget's disease, septic shock or other mechanisms.

Handbook of ICU Therapy, third edition, ed. John Fuller, Jeff Granton and Ian McConachie. Published by Cambridge University Press. © Cambridge University Press 2015.

Characteristics of patients admitted with AHF

Several registries have described the characteristics and clinical outcomes of patients admitted to hospital with AHF [7–11]. The EuroHeart Failure Survey II included 3580 patients (mean age 70 years, 61% male) admitted with AHF [8]. The majority (63%) of patients were admitted with ADCHF and 70% had been hospitalized for AHF within the last 12 months, while 37% were admitted with *de novo* AHF. Acute coronary syndromes, arrhythmias or valvular heart disease precipitated AHF in 89% of patients. Overall hospital mortality was 6.7%; however, among the 4% of patients admitted with cardiogenic shock hospital mortality was 39.6% [8]. One-year mortality for patients who survived to hospital discharge was 21.9% and patients admitted with *de novo* AHF exhibited better 1-year survival compared to those with ADCHF (16.4 versus 23.2%) [12].

Etiology of AHF

Cardiac causes

1. Acute coronary syndromes (1/3 STEMI, 1/3 non-STEMI, 1/3 unstable angina) resulting in:
   - Loss of functional myocytes (impaired cardiac contractility)
   - Papillary muscle rupture and acute mitral regurgitation
   - Ventricular septal defect
   - Free wall rupture.
2. Arrhythmias
   - Supraventricular or ventricular
   - Bradycardic or tachycardic.
3. Valvular heart disease
   - Progression of chronic valvular heart disease (i.e. aortic stenosis)
   - Acute valvular heart disease (i.e. endocarditis, aortic dissection, trauma).
4. Cardiomyopathy (i.e. myocarditis)
5. Cardiac tamponade.

Noncardiac causes

1. Hypertensive crisis
2. Pulmonary embolism
3. Noncompliance with medical therapy
4. Medical causes (alcohol/drugs, renal failure, thyroid disease, anemia, sepsis).

Diagnosis of AHF

Identification of the signs and symptoms of heart failure is important in establishing the diagnosis of AHF.

- Dyspnea, reduced exercise tolerance, orthopnea and paroxysmal nocturnal dyspnea are typical. Exertional dyspnea is the most sensitive (negative likelihood ratio 0.45, 95% CI 0.35–0.67) and paroxysmal nocturnal dyspnea is the most specific symptom (positive likelihood ratio 2.6, 95% CI 1.5– 4.5) [13].

- Pulmonary crackles, an elevated jugular venous pressure and peripheral edema may be evident on physical examination. An elevated jugular venous pressure is the best clinical exam indicator for AHF (positive likelihood ratio 5.1, 95% CI 3.2–7.9) [13].
- Fewer than half of AHF patients present with classic signs and symptoms, which may be difficult to identify and interpret in the obese, the elderly and patients with chronic lung disease [14].
- Therefore, objective testing is an important adjunct to the clinical assessment.

Laboratory testing

- Laboratory testing may help identify precipitants of AHF including anemia, infection, renal failure, electrolyte abnormalities or thyroid disorders.
- Arterial blood gas analysis facilitates assessment of oxygenation, adequacy of ventilation and acid–base balance, and may help identify those patients with respiratory failure or cardiogenic shock requiring urgent intervention.
- Additionally, measurement of mixed venous oxygen saturation aids in determining adequacy of systemic oxygen delivery [3].

Natriuretic peptides

The measurement of biomarkers provides useful diagnostic and prognostic information for patients presenting with signs and symptoms of AHF. B-type natriuretic peptide (BNP) and N-terminal proB-type natriuretic peptide (NT-proBNP) are quantitative markers of cardiac wall stress, which can be used to improve diagnostic accuracy in patients with suspected AHF [15–17]. The levels of natriuretic peptides may also be used to predict in-hospital and 1-year mortality [18,19]:

BNP levels to rule out AHF:

- BNP <100 pg/mL
- NT-proBNP <300 pg/mL

BNP levels to rule in AHF:

- BNP >500 pg/mL
- NT-proBNP >450 pg/mL if age <50 years
- NT-proBNP >900 pg/mL if age 50–75 years
- NT-proBNP >1800 pg/mL if age >75 years.

Troponin

The measurement of troponin is well established for the diagnosis of acute coronary syndromes, and may be used to guide therapy in patients presenting with AHF. Additionally, high-sensitivity assays for troponin T provide prognostic information for patients without acute coronary syndromes admitted with AHF [20].

Electrocardiography

An electrocardiogram should be obtained in all patients with AHF in order to rapidly identify clinical scenarios requiring urgent intervention, such as acute coronary syndromes or arrhythmias requiring pacing, cardioversion or defibrillation. Information regarding the presence of structural heart disease may also be obtained (left ventricular hypertrophy, prior myocardial infarction).

Chest radiography

A chest radiograph should be obtained to identify alternative diagnoses, pulmonary congestion or cardiomegaly.

Echocardiography

- An echocardiogram should be obtained within 72 hours of presentation and aids in establishing the etiologic origin of AHF through assessment of systolic and diastolic function, valvular abnormalities and pulmonary pressures [21].
- Patients presenting with cardiogenic shock require urgent echocardiography to identify acute mechanical abnormalities (ischemic ventricular septal defect, ruptured papillary muscle, free wall rupture, aortic dissection, critical aortic stenosis, cardiac tamponade) requiring immediate intervention.

Coronary angiography

Coronary angiography should be performed immediately in patients with an ST elevation myocardial infarction; however, if coronary angiography is not available then intravenous thrombolytic therapy is recommended [6]. Early coronary angiography should be considered in patients with an acute coronary syndrome and evidence of cardiogenic shock and may be indicated for refractory AHF of uncertain etiology [3,6].

Acute heart failure score

The PRIDE acute heart failure score is a rapid bedside tool that can also aid in the diagnosis of AHF [22]. A total score <6 can be used to rule out AHF (negative predictive value 98%) and a score ≥6 confirms the diagnosis of AHF with 96% sensitivity and 84% specificity [22].

PRIDE acute heart failure score:

- Elevated NT-proBNP (4 points)
- Interstitial edema on chest radiograph (2 points)
- Orthopnea (2 points)
- Absence of fever (2 points)
- Current loop diuretic use (1 point)
- Age >75 years (1 point)
- Pulmonary crackles (1 point)
- Absence of cough (1 point).

Management of AHF

- The initial management of patients with AHF should focus on the identification of reversible causes of heart failure and clinical scenarios requiring immediate intervention (Figure 26.1b).

(a)

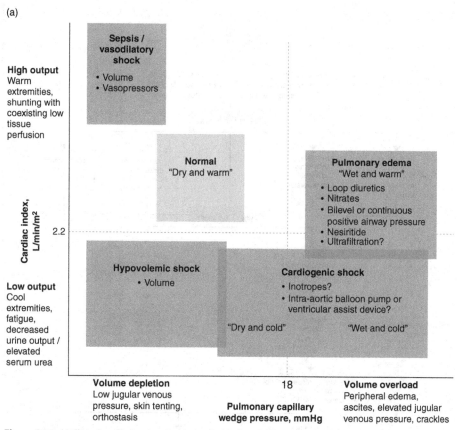

Figure 26.1 (a) Clinical profile (reprinted with permission from [32]) and (b) treatment algorithm (adapted with permission from [6]) for patients with AHF.
[a]noninvasive ventilation (continuous positive airway pressure or noninvasive positive-pressure ventilation), [b]tracheal intubation and positive-pressure ventilation, [c]percutaneous coronary intervention, [d]mechanical complication of an acute coronary syndrome (papillary muscle rupture, ventricular septal defect, free wall rupture), aortic insufficiency resulting from aortic dissection, acute mitral regurgitation, [e]right heart catheterization, [f]mechanical circulatory support.

- Simultaneously, clinical assessment identifying the presence of pulmonary congestion and adequacy of systemic perfusion should be undertaken.
- This information can be used to categorize patients according to clinical profile (Figure 26.1a) and delineate a therapeutic strategy (Figure 26.1b).
- The Forrester diagram was originally developed to group patients presenting with an acute myocardial infarction into clinical profiles according to invasive assessments of systemic perfusion (cardiac index) and pulmonary congestion (pulmonary capillary wedge pressure) [23].
- These clinical profiles have been validated in patients admitted with AHF and can be determined using clinical assessments of systemic perfusion and pulmonary congestion [24].

(b)

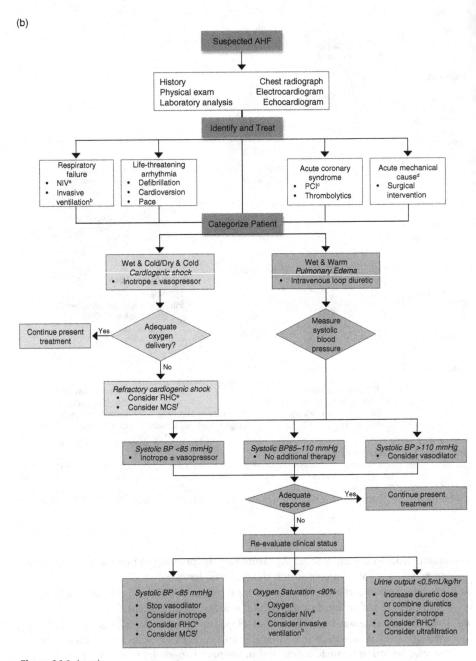

Figure 26.1 (*cont.*)

- The immediate goal in the treatment of AHF is to improve oxygen delivery and minimize oxygen consumption.
- The adequacy of such interventions can be determined by measuring the mixed venous oxygen saturation in a blood sample obtained from a central venous catheter. Therapeutic interventions should be tailored to maintain a mixed venous oxygen saturation >65% [3].
- Measurements of acid–base status and serum lactate also serve as indicators of adequate (or inadequate) oxygen delivery and are useful for trending progress.

Oxygen delivery may be improved through optimization of:
- Heart rate
- Preload
- Afterload
- Cardiac contractility
- Oxygenation
- Hemoglobin concentration.

Oxygen consumption may be minimized by:
- Providing ventilatory support if there is excessive work of breathing
- Minimizing anxiety and pain
- Treating infection and fever.

Diuretics and ultrafiltration

Patients with evidence of pulmonary edema and sufficient systemic perfusion (wet and warm, Figure 26.1A) have an elevated left ventricular end-diastolic pressure, and initial therapy should include an intravenous loop diuretic such as furosemide, bumetanide or torasemide (Figure 26.1B) [21].

- Intravenous loop diuretics promote vasodilation and natriuresis that result in a reduction in right and left ventricular pre-load and alleviation of congestive symptoms [25–27].
- The DOSE trial investigated the impact of continuous versus bolus, and high-dose versus low-dose intravenous furosemide in patients admitted with AHF [28].
- Patients receiving high-dose furosemide experienced greater net fluid loss, relief from dyspnea, and a greater reduction in NT-proBNP at 72 hours; however, more patients experienced an increase in creatinine. There was no significant difference between groups in a composite of death, rehospitalization or emergency department visits.
- This trial suggests that there is no advantage in the routine use of continuous diuretic infusions.
- Diuretic dose should be titrated according to the desired clinical response, and high-dose diuretics can be utilized safely with careful observation of renal function and electrolytes [3].

The addition of a thiazide-type diuretic (metolazone) can be considered for patients with an inadequate response to an intravenous loop diuretic [6]; however, this strategy is associated with a risk of hypokalemia, hyponatremia, hypotension and worsening renal function. There is a need for a large clinical trial examining the safety and efficacy of such an approach [29].

Veno-venous ultrafiltration has also been investigated as an alternative therapy for patients admitted with "warm and wet" AHF.

- The UNLOAD trial randomized 200 patients to ultrafiltration or intravenous diuretics [30]. Ultrafiltration was associated with greater net fluid loss and a reduction in the rate of rehospitalization with AHF.
- However, in the CARRESS-HF trial ultrafiltration did not achieve greater weight loss and was associated with a greater increase in creatinine and adverse events [31].

Given the conflicting results regarding the routine use of ultrafiltration for patients with AHF, it is generally reserved for those patients who are resistant to optimized diuretic therapy [3].

Vasodilators

Patients with "wet and warm" AHF and a systolic blood pressure above 110 mmHg should be considered for treatment with a vasodilator (Figure 26.1B).

- Venodilation causes a reduction in pre-load, pulmonary congestion and myocardial oxygen demand.
- Arterial vasodilation facilitates afterload reduction that further decreases myocardial oxygen demand and increases stroke volume [32].
- Intravenous nitroglycerin, isosorbide dinitrate, nitroprusside and nesiritide can be used effectively as vasodilators [6]. These medications can be titrated to achieve a systolic blood pressure of 100 mmHg for relief of dyspnea in hemodynamically stable patients; however, they should be used with caution in patients with mitral and aortic valve stenosis [6].
- Nesiritide causes venous and arterial vasodilation, enhanced sodium excretion and suppression of the renin-angiotensin-aldosterone and sympathetic nervous systems [33].
- The VMAC trial randomized 489 patients admitted with AHF to nesiritide, nitroglycerin or placebo, and found that nesiritide was associated with a significantly greater reduction in pulmonary capillary wedge pressure and similar dyspnea relief compared to nitroglycerin [34].
- The routine addition of nesiritide to standard therapy in patients admitted with AHF is associated with a modest improvement in dyspnea but increased rates of hypotension [35].
- Nitroglycerin is the preferred vasodilator for patients with an acute coronary syndrome because of its ability to produce a balanced vasodilation of the venous and arterial systems [3].
- Nitroprusside should be reserved for situations where afterload reduction is the primary goal (hypertensive AHF); however, it is limited by the development of cyanide toxicity with prolonged administration [3].

Oxygenation and ventilatory support

- The provision of supplemental oxygen to maintain the arterial oxygen saturation within the normal range (95–98%) is necessary to optimize oxygen delivery and prevent end-organ dysfunction [3].
- Patients with "wet and warm" AHF that remain hypoxemic despite initial oxygen therapy, and those with signs of respiratory failure (accessory muscle use, tachypnea, hypercarbia) require ventilatory support.

Initial ventilatory support for patients in this clinical profile should include a trial of noninvasive ventilation. The two most commonly used methods of noninvasive ventilation are continuous positive airway pressure (CPAP) and noninvasive positive-pressure ventilation (NIPPV) [3].

- CPAP maintains the same positive airway pressure support throughout the respiratory cycle, facilitating pulmonary recruitment and increasing functional residual capacity that leads to decreased work of breathing and an overall reduction in metabolic demand [3].
- NIPPV increases the positive airway pressure to a greater degree during inspiration than during expiration.
- The physiological benefits of NIPPV are similar to that of CPAP; however, the additional positive airway pressure during inspiration results in an incremental reduction in the work of breathing and overall metabolic demand [3].
- A recent meta-analysis of over 3000 patients from 34 randomized controlled trials revealed that the use of noninvasive ventilation reduced the need for endotracheal intubation and in-hospital mortality compared to standard treatment [36].
- Patients who exhibit worsening respiratory failure despite optimized noninvasive ventilation should undergo tracheal intubation and mechanical ventilation (invasive ventilation) [21].
- Additionally, patients with evidence of cardiogenic shock (dry and cold/wet and cold) should be supported with invasive ventilation [21].

Contraindications to the use of noninvasive ventilation include [21,37]:

- Decreased level of consciousness, agitation or high aspiration risk
- Excessive secretions
- Upper airway obstruction and facial injuries or abnormalities.

Inotropes

Inotropic agents increase cardiac contractility and cardiac output at the expense of increased myocardial oxygen demand and risk of arrhythmias.

- The OPTIME-CHF trial randomized 951 patients with AHF and no evidence of cardiogenic shock to a milrinone infusion or placebo in addition to standard therapies [38].
- New-onset atrial arrhythmias, worsening heart failure and symptomatic hypotension requiring intervention occurred more frequently in the milrinone group. There was also a trend towards higher in-hospital mortality in the milrinone group.

- Therefore, routine use of inotropic agents as an adjunct to standard therapy in "warm" patients with AHF is not recommended [21].
- However, "cold" patients with cardiogenic shock and "wet and warm" patients with pulmonary edema refractory to optimal doses of diuretics and vasodilators may require inotropic therapy to prevent end-organ ischemia (Figure 26.1B).

Inotropic support should attempt to minimize the myocardial oxygen demand required to achieve adequate cardiac output and systemic perfusion. Agents that augment cardiac contractility, decrease ventricular filling pressures and afterload, and minimize tachycardia are preferred.

- Dobutamine stimulates β-1 and β-2 receptors and produces a positive inotropic and chronotropic response; however, the chronotropic response is stimulated to a lesser extent than with other catecholamines [3].
- Milrinone and enoximone are phosphodiesterase inhibitors that reduce the degradation of cyclic AMP, causing positive inotropic and lusitropic effects, and a reduction in systemic and pulmonary vascular resistance [39].
- Levosimendan sensitizes myofilaments to calcium and has K-ATP channel-opening effects, resulting in a positive inotropic response and a reduction in systemic and pulmonary vascular resistance [3].
- Agents that cause significant tachycardia and increased afterload are associated with a disproportionate increase in myocardial oxygen consumption and should be avoided if possible (dopamine, norepinephrine, epinephrine); however, when significant hypotension is present these agents may be required to maintain an adequate perfusion pressure [3].

Mechanical circulatory support (MCS)

Patients with cardiogenic shock refractory to maximal medical therapy (Figure 26.1B) should be considered for MCS (Figure 26.2). There is a window of opportunity for rescue therapy with MCS beyond which end-organ injury is irreversible and death is inevitable. Therefore, patient selection and early intervention are important determinants of successful MCS utilization. Mechanical circulatory support is a resource-intensive and complicated therapeutic option that should be provided by a multidisciplinary team comprising heart failure cardiologists, interventional cardiologists, cardiac surgeons, critical care specialists and clinical perfusionists. The overall goal of MCS is to:

- Augment native cardiac output to ensure adequate oxygen delivery and provide an opportunity for end-organ functional recovery
- Decrease ventricular wall stress to minimize myocardial oxygen consumption and provide an opportunity for myocardial recovery.

Intra-aortic balloon counterpulsation is recommended for patients with cardiogenic shock refractory to optimized medical therapy [3].

- While intra-aortic balloon counterpulsation has been shown to prevent reocclusion of infarct-related arteries in patients undergoing cardiac catheterization for acute coronary syndromes [40], the IABP-SHOCK II trial demonstrated that it is not associated with a mortality benefit compared to best medical therapy in patients with acute coronary

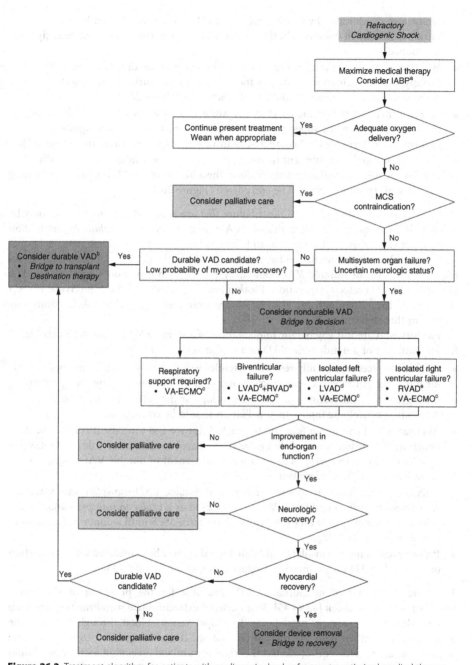

Figure 26.2 Treatment algorithm for patients with cardiogenic shock refractory to optimized medical therapy (adapted with permission from [43]).
[a]intra-aortic balloon pump (counterpulsation), [b]ventricular assist device, [c]veno-arterial extracorporeal membrane oxygenation, [d]left ventricular assist device, [e]right ventricular assist device.

syndromes complicated by cardiogenic shock [41]. Therefore, the routine use of intra-aortic balloon counterpulsation in this patient population has been recently questioned.

- However, for patients with rapidly declining hemodynamics despite maximal medical therapy, prompt initiation of MCS is the only option for survival. Intra-aortic balloon counterpulsation is utilized initially in this scenario (Figure 26.2).
- A recent meta-analysis demonstrated that while percutaneous left ventricular assist devices (VADs) provide superior hemodynamic support, they do not significantly improve short-term survival compared to intra-aortic balloon counterpulsation [42].
- However, if rapid improvement in systemic oxygen delivery does not occur with intra-aortic balloon counterpulsation alone, the addition of a VAD capable of providing full circulatory support should be considered (Figure 26.2).

Patients with established advanced heart failure that are admitted with an ADCHF may be considered for implantation of a durable VAD as a *bridge to transplant* or *destination therapy*, provided that multisystem organ failure is not present, neurologic status is known (i.e. cardiopulmonary resuscitation has not occurred) and the patient's clinical status allows for determination of durable VAD candidacy prior to implantation (Figure 26.2). The HeartMate II (Thoratec Corporation, Pleasanton, CA, USA) and the HeartWare HVAD (HeartWare Inc., Framingham, MA, USA) are examples of durable VADs commonly utilized in this scenario.

Patients who are not eligible for implantation of a durable VAD should be considered for implantation of a nondurable VAD as a *bridge to decision* (Figure 26.2).

- MCS in this scenario rapidly restores systemic perfusion and provides an opportunity for improvement in end-organ function and clinical assessment of neurologic status.
- If progressive multisystem organ failure develops or the patient has suffered a devastating neurologic injury, then palliation should be considered.
- Alternatively, if end-organ function begins to improve and the patient is neurologically intact, native cardiac function should be re-evaluated to determine if device removal is feasible (*bridge to recovery*). A simultaneous assessment of durable VAD/transplant candidacy should be undertaken.
- If native cardiac function does not recover and durable VAD/transplant candidacy is confirmed, then the nondurable VAD can be used as a *bridge to transplantation* or a bridge to a durable VAD that will provide long-term MCS until a donor heart becomes available (*bridge to bridge*).
- If the patient is not a transplant candidate then they may be considered for implantation of a durable VAD for permanent support (*destination therapy*) [43].

There are a number of nondurable VADs available for the provision of short-term MCS as a *bridge to decision* [43,44,45]. Veno-arterial extracorporeal membrane oxygenation (VA-ECMO) utilizes a centrifugal pump to propel venous blood through a membrane oxygenator and return it to the arterial circulation. It can be initiated using peripheral (i.e. femoral artery and vein) or central (i.e. right atrium and ascending aorta) cannulation and provides biventricular and respiratory support.

- The Cardiohelp (Maquet Cardiopulmonary AG, Hirrlingen, Germany) is a miniaturized VA-ECMO circuit optimized for rapid MCS response teams and transport applications.

- The TandemHeart (CardiacAssist, Inc., Pittsburgh, PA) and Impella 2.5, CP and 5.0 (AbioMed Inc, Danvers, MA) devices can be used for percutaneous support of the left ventricle. The TandemHeart can also be modified to provide percutaneous right ventricular support, and other companies are currently developing devices designed specifically for this indication.
- Additionally, a number of different centrifugal pumps can be employed to provide isolated right or left ventricular support via central cannulation. Centrifigal pumps commonly utilized in this senario include the Bio-Pump (Medtronic Inc., Brooklyn Park, MN), CentriMag (Thoratec Corporation, Pleasanton, CA), and the Rotaflow (Maquet Cardiopulmonary AG, Hirrlingen, Germany).

Nondurable VAD selection is based on the degree and duration of hemodynamic support required, the need for biventricular or respiratory support, the clinical senario (i.e. ongoing cardiopulmonary resuscitation, post-cardiotomy), individual patient factors (i.e. size of peripheral vasculature, feasibility of central cannulation) and the availability of interventionalists and cardiac surgeons [43].

The clinical outcomes of patients with refractory cardiogenic shock receiving MCS as a *bridge to decision* has been described by Takayama *et al.* [46].

- Myocardial recovery sufficient to faciliate device removal occurred in 18%, nondurable VADs were used as a *bridge to transplant* in 10% and 26% were transitioned to a durable VAD as a *bridge to transplant* or *destination therapy*.
- Overall hospital survival was 49% and 1-year survival was 46%. Ongoing CPR at the time of MCS initiation was an independent predictor of in-hospital mortality (OR = 5.79, 95% CI 1.3–26.1).
- Multisystem organ failure and neurologic injury accounted for 86% of the in-hospital deaths.

Transition to chronic care

Transition to oral diuretic therapy and afterload reduction should be undertaken as clinical status improves.

- In patients with a reduced ejection fraction not already receiving a β-blocker, ACE inhibitor or mineralocorticoid receptor antagonist (spironolactone, eplerenone), these treatments should be started as soon as possible following resolution of AHF [6].
- Follow-up with cardiology or heart failure specialists should be arranged to tailor outpatient therapy and reduce the need for rehospitalization.

References

1. Mosterd A, Hoes AW. Clinical epidemiology of heart failure. *Heart* 2007; 93 : 1137–46.

2. Redfield MM, Jacobsen SJ, Burnett JC Jr, et al. Burden of systolic and diastolic ventricular dysfunction in the community: appreciating the scope of the heart failure epidemic. *JAMA* 2003; 289 : 194–202.

3. Nieminen MS, Bohm M, Cowie MR et al. Executive summary of the guidelines on the diagnosis and treatment of acute heart failure: the Task Force on Acute Heart Failure of the European Society of Cardiology. *Eur Heart J* 2005; 26 : 384–416.

4. Metra M, Felker GM, Zaca V et al. Acute heart failure: multiple clinical profiles and mechanisms require tailored therapy. *Int J Cardiol* 2010; 144 : 175–9.

5. Tavazzi L, Senni M, Metra M *et al.* Multicenter prospective observational study on acute and chronic heart failure: the one-year follow-up results of IN-HF outcome registry. *Circ Heart Fail* 2013; 6 : 473–81.

6. McMurray JJ, Adamopoulos S, Anker SD *et al.* ESC Guidelines for the diagnosis and treatment of acute and chronic heart failure 2012: The Task Force for the Diagnosis and Treatment of Acute and Chronic Heart Failure 2012 of the European Society of Cardiology. Developed in collaboration with the Heart Failure Association (HFA) of the ESC. *Eur Heart J* 2012; 33 : 1787–847.

7. Abraham WT, Fonarow GC, Albert NM *et al.* Predictors of in-hospital mortality in patients hospitalized for heart failure: insights from the Organized Program to Initiate Lifesaving Treatment in Hospitalized Patients with Heart Failure (OPTIMIZE-HF). *J Am Coll Cardiol* 2008; 52 : 347–56.

8. Nieminen MS, Brutsaert D, Dickstein K *et al.* EuroHeart Failure Survey II (EHFS II): a survey on hospitalized acute heart failure patients: description of population. *Eur Heart J* 2006; 27 : 2725–36.

9. Oliva F, Mortara A, Cacciatore G *et al.* Acute heart failure patient profiles, management and in-hospital outcome: results of the Italian Registry on Heart Failure Outcome. *Eur J Heart Fail* 2012; 14 : 1208–17.

10. Spinar J, Parenica J, Vitovec J *et al.* Baseline characteristics and hospital mortality in the Acute Heart Failure Database (AHEAD) main registry. *Crit Care* 2011; 15 : R291.

11. Yancy CW, Fonarow GC. Quality of care and outcomes in acute decompensated heart failure: The ADHERE Registry. *Curr Heart Fail Rep* 2004; 1 : 121–8.

12. Harjola VP, Follath F, Nieminen MS *et al.* Characteristics, outcomes, and predictors of mortality at 3 months and 1 year in patients hospitalized for acute heart failure. *Eur J Heart Fail* 2010; 12 : 239–48.

13. Wang CS, FitzGerald JM, Schulzer M *et al.* Does this dyspneic patient in the emergency department have congestive heart failure? *JAMA* 2005; 294 : 1944–56.

14. Chiong JR, Jao GT, Adams Jr KF. Utility of natriuretic peptide testing in the evaluation and management of acute decompensated heart failure. *Heart Fail Rev* 2010; 15 : 275–91.

15. Januzzi Jr JL, Camargo CA, Anwaruddin S *et al.* The N-terminal Pro-BNP investigation of dyspnea in the emergency department (PRIDE) study. *Am J Cardiol* 2005; 95 : 948–54.

16. Januzzi, JL, Van Kimmenade R, Lainchbury J *et al.* NT-proBNP testing for diagnosis and short-term prognosis in acute destabilized heart failure: an international pooled analysis of 1256 patients: the International Collaborative of NT-proBNP Study. *Eur Heart J* 2006; 27 : 330–7.

17. Maisel AS, Krishnaswamy P, Nowak RM *et al.* Rapid measurement of B-type natriuretic peptide in the emergency diagnosis of heart failure. *N Engl J Med* 2002; 347 : 161–7.

18. Fonarow GC, Peacock WF, Phillips CO, *et al.* Admission B-type natriuretic peptide levels and in-hospital mortality in acute decompensated heart failure. *J Am Coll Cardiol* 2007; 49 : 1943–50.

19. Michtalik HJ, Yeh HC, Campbell CY *et al.* Acute changes in N-terminal pro-B-type natriuretic peptide during hospitalization and risk of readmission and mortality in patients with heart failure. *Am J Cardiol* 2011; 107 : 1191–5.

20. DA Pascual-Figal, Casas T, Ordonez-Llanos J *et al.* Highly sensitive troponin T for risk stratification of acutely destabilized heart failure. *Am Heart J* 2012; 163 : 1002–10.

21. McKelvie RS, Moe GW, Ezekowitz JA *et al.* The 2012 Canadian Cardiovascular Society heart failure management guidelines update: focus on acute and chronic heart failure. *Can J Cardiol* 2013; 29 : 168–81.

22. Baggish AL, Siebert U, Lainchbury JG *et al.* A validated clinical and biochemical score for the diagnosis of acute heart failure: the ProBNP Investigation of Dyspnea in the Emergency Department

(PRIDE) Acute Heart Failure Score. *Am Heart J* 2006; 151 : 48–54.

23. Forrester JS, Diamond GA, Swan HJ. Correlative classification of clinical and hemodynamic function after acute myocardial infarction. *Am J Cardiol* 1977; 39 : 137–45.

24. Nohria A, Tsang SW, Fang JC *et al*. Clinical assessment identifies hemodynamic profiles that predict outcomes in patients admitted with heart failure. *J Am Coll Cardiol* 2003; 41 : 1797–804.

25. Brater DC. Diuretic therapy. *N Engl J Med* 1998; 339 : 387–95.

26. Nohria A, Mielniczuk LM, Stevenson LW. Evaluation and monitoring of patients with acute heart failure syndromes. *Am J Cardiol* 2005; 96 : 32G–40G.

27. Wilson JR, Reichek N, Dunkman WB *et al*. Effect of diuresis on the performance of the failing left ventricle in man. *Am J Med* 1981; 70 : 234–9.

28. Felker GM, Lee KL, Bull DA *et al*. Diuretic strategies in patients with acute decompensated heart failure. *N Engl J Med* 2011; 364 : 797–805.

29. Jentzer JC, DeWald TA, Hernandez AF. Combination of loop diuretics with thiazide-type diuretics in heart failure. *J Am Coll Cardiol* 2010; 56 : 1527–34.

30. Costanzo MR, Guglin ME, Saltzberg MT *et al*. Ultrafiltration versus intravenous diuretics for patients hospitalized for acute decompensated heart failure. *J Am Coll Cardiol* 2007; 49 : 675–83.

31. Bart BA, Goldsmith SR, Lee KL *et al*. Ultrafiltration in decompensated heart failure with cardiorenal syndrome. *N Engl J Med* 2012; 367 : 2296–304.

32. Allen LA, O'Connor CM. Management of acute decompensated heart failure. *Canadian Medical Association Journal* 2007; 176 : 797–805.

33. Colucci WS. Nesiritide for the treatment of decompensated heart failure. *J Card Fail* 2001; 7 : 92–100.

34. Publication Committee for the VMAC Investigators. Intravenous nesiritide vs nitroglycerin for treatment of decompensated congestive heart failure: a randomized controlled trial. *JAMA* 2002; 287 : 1531–40.

35. O'Connor CM, Starling RC, Hernandez AF, *et al*. Effect of nesiritide in patients with acute decompensated heart failure. *N Engl J Med* 2011; 365 : 32–43.

36. Mariani J, Macchia A, Belziti C *et al*. Noninvasive ventilation in acute cardiogenic pulmonary edema: a meta-analysis of randomized controlled trials. *J Card Fail* 2011; 17 : 850–9.

37. International Consensus Conferences in Intensive Care Medicine: noninvasive positive pressure ventilation in acute Respiratory failure. *Am J Respir Crit Care Med* 2001; 163 : 283–91.

38. Cuffe MS, Califf RM, Adams Jr KF *et al*. Short-term intravenous milrinone for acute exacerbation of chronic heart failure: a randomized controlled trial. *JAMA* 2002; 287 : 1541–7.

39. Colucci WS, Wright RF, Braunwald E. New positive inotropic agents in the treatment of congestive heart failure: mechanisms of action and recent clinical developments. *N Engl J Med* 1986; 314 : 349–58.

40. Ohman EM, George BS, White CJ *et al*. Use of aortic counterpulsation to improve sustained coronary artery patency during acute myocardial infarction: results of a randomized trial. The Randomized IABP Study Group. *Circulation* 1994; 90 : 792–9.

41. Thiele H, Zeymer U, Neumann FJ *et al*. Intraaortic balloon support for myocardial infarction with cardiogenic shock. *N Engl J Med* 2012; 367 : 1287–96.

42. Cheng JM, den Uil CA, Hoeks SE *et al*. Percutaneous left ventricular assist devices vs. intra-aortic balloon pump counterpulsation for treatment of cardiogenic shock: a meta-analysis of controlled trials. *Eur Heart J* 2009; 30 : 2102–8.

43. Sayer GT, Baker JN, Parks KA. Heart rescue: the role of mechanical circulatory support in the management of severe refractory cardiogenic shock. *Curr Opin Crit Care* 2012; 18 : 409–16.

44. Goldstein D, Neragi-Miandoab S. Mechanical bridge to decision: what are the options for the management of acute refractory cardiogenic shock? *Curr Heart Fail Rep* 2011; 8 : 51–8.

45. Westaby S, Anastasiadis K, Wieselthaler GM. Cardiogenic shock in ACS. Part 2: Role of mechanical circulatory support. *Nat Rev Cardiol* 2012; 9 : 195–208.

46. Takayama H, Truby L, Koekort M *et al.* Clinical outcome of mechanical circulatory support for refractory cardiogenic shock in the current era. *J Heart Lung Transplant* 2013; 32 : 106–11.

Chapter 27

Arrhythmias

Umjeet Singh Jolly and Jaimie Manlucu

Introduction

Arrhythmia management in critically ill intensive care unit patients is a common and potentially life-threatening problem [1]. Critically ill patients who develop a cardiac arrhythmia have been found to have longer ICU stays and a higher mortality than those that do not.

- In a review by Goodman *et al.*, critically ill patients who developed a new-onset cardiac arrhythmia had a 36% increase in 4-year mortality. In addition, the same review showed that the median length of stay in the ICU was 7 days longer in a patient who developed an arrhythmia [2].

Arrhythmias are common in the intensive care setting, affecting approximately 20% of the critically ill population [1,3]. This predisposition can be attributed to a number of clinical factors, including extensive fluid shifts, metabolic derangements, medications and the nature and severity of their underlying illnesses, as well as the high demands placed on the heart during this period.

This chapter will focus on the etiology and mechanism of arrhythmia generation in this patient population, as well as provide practical therapeutic tips for the clinician.

Arrhythmogenesis

In order to understand the various mechanisms and therapies of cardiac arrhythmias, one must first understand the cardiac muscle action potential [4] (Figure 27.1):

- An action potential is triggered when the resting membrane potential is partially depolarized by a stimulus to the threshold potential.
- This activates voltage-dependent sodium channels, which allow a rapid influx of sodium. The resultant rapid depolarization is called Phase 0.
- This is followed by Phase 1, early rapid repolarization resulting from inactivation of voltage-gated sodium channels and efflux of potassium from voltage-gated potassium channels.
- In Phase 2, the action potential plateaus as the potassium efflux is balanced by calcium influx.
- Phase 3 marks the rapid repolarization phase, where calcium influx decays, and delayed rectifier potassium channels are activated,

Handbook of ICU Therapy, third edition, ed. John Fuller, Jeff Granton and Ian McConachie. Published by Cambridge University Press. © Cambridge University Press 2015.

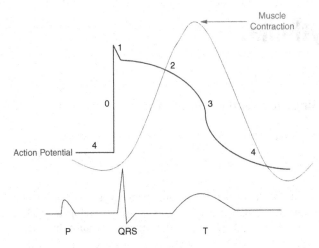

Muscle
Contraction

Action Potential

0 1 2 3 4

P QRS T

Figure 27.1 This is a schematic of the cardiac action potential. Each phase (0–4) is described in detail in the text. The temporal relationship between the action potential and myocardial muscle contraction, as well as between the action potential and the surface electrocardiogram, are illustrated here.

resulting in an efflux of potassium that helps bring the membrane potential back towards baseline.

- Sodium leaves and potassium re-enters the cells during Phase 4 recovery via the Na-K-ATPase pump, until the next stimulus occurs that generates the next action potential.

Antiarrhythmic drugs are classified according to which ion channel they inhibit (Table 27.1). According to the Vaughan Williams classification:

Class I antiarrhythmics block voltage-gated sodium channels. There are three subtypes of Class I antiarrhythmics:

- Class IA (e.g. disopyramide, procainamide, quinidine)
- Class IB (e.g. lidocaine, mexiletine, phenytoin)
- Class IC (e.g. flecainide, propafenone).

All three subtypes are primarily sodium-channel blockers, but have varying degrees of potassium-channel blockade as well.

Class III antiarrhythmics are potassium-channel blockers, which are most commonly used in the setting of structural heart disease. Caution should be taken when using Class III antiarrhythmics in the setting of renal impairment, as all but amiodarone are cleared by the kidneys.

Class II and IV antiarrhythmics encompass all β-blockers and calcium-channel blockers, respectively. These medications are commonly used as rate control agents for atrial arrhythmias and can be used to terminate or prevent AV node-dependent supraventricular tachycardias.

Mechanisms of arrhythmogenesis

There are three main mechanisms underlying cardiac arrhythmogenesis:

- Re-entry
- Abnormal automaticity
- Triggered activity.

Each mechanism can be broadly categorized as abnormalities in impulse formation (abnormal automaticity, triggered activity) or abnormalities in impulse conduction (re-entry). Each mechanism can function on its own or interact with another to initiate and/or perpetuate an arrhythmia.

Table 27.1 Antiarrhythmic medications, side effects and contraindications

Vaughan Williams classification	Mechanism of action and dosing[a]	Indications	Side effects	Contraindications
Class IA • Disopyramide • Procainamide • Quinidine	Na+ channel blockade[b] • Disopyramide (600 mg/day, in 2–4 divided doses)[c] • Procainamide (loading dose 17 mg/kg IV, maintenance 2–6 mg/min IV)[c] • Quinidine (maintenance dose 200–300 mg, 3–4 times a day)	• Procainamide: re-entrant atrial and ventricular arrhythmias • Quinidine: idiopathic VF	• Quinidine: ↑ QTc • Procainamide: ↓ AV conduction, and/or ↑ QTc or QRS, ↓ ionotropy	• Cardiogenic shock • Coronary disease • Heart failure • High-grade AV block • Prolonged QTc
Class IB • Lidocaine • Mexiletine • Phenytoin	Na+ channel blockade[b] • Lidocaine (loading dose 50–100 mg iv over 2–3 min; maintenance dose 1–4 mg/min)[c] • Mexiletine (400–800 mg divided into 2–3 equal daily doses)	• Lidocaine: ischemic VT • Phenytoin in frequently used	• Lidocaine: CNS side effects (e.g. confusion and coma), which must be carefully monitored for	• Cardiogenic shock • High-grade AV block • Liver dysfunction
Class IC • Flecainide • Propafenone	Na+ channel blockade[b] • Flecainide (50–150 mg po BID)[c] • Propafenone (starting dose 150 mg po q8h; maximum 300 mg q8h)	• Atrial arrhythmias	• Should be combined with an AV nodal blocking agent to avoid rapid conduction of slow atrial flutter • Should not be used in patients with significant structural heart disease [13]	• Cardiogenic shock • High-grade AV block • Left ventricular dysfunction • Coronary artery disease [13]

Table 27.1 (cont.)

Vaughan Williams classification	Mechanism of action and dosing[a]	Indications	Side effects	Contraindications
Class II • Atenolol • Bisoprolol • Carvedilol • Metoprolol	β-receptor antagonist • Atenolol (50–100 mg/day) • Bisoprolol (2.5–20 mg/day) • Carvedilol (3.125–25 mg BID) • Metoprolol (50–200 mg BID)	• Effective AV nodal blocking agents • Effective for adrenaline-mediated arrhythmias	• Hypotension, bradycardia	• Cardiogenic shock, High-grade AV block • Severe reactive airway disease
Class III • Amiodarone • Dofetilide • Ibutilide • Sotalol • Dronedarone	K+ channel blockade • Amiodarone (loading dose 150 mg over 10 min; maintenance dose 0.5 mg/min IV) • Dofetilide (250 to 500 mcg po BID)[c] • Ibutilide (1 mg over 10 minutes, or 0.01 mg/kg if less than 60 kg)	• Amiodarone: provides AV nodal blockade acutely when given IV; antiarrhythmic properties take effect after loading dose of 10–14 g over several weeks; good for acute treatment of atrial and ventricular arrhythmias with minimal effects on blood pressure • Sotalol: both β-blockade and Class III properties; useful for atrial and ventricular arrhythmias • Ibutilide: atrial arrhythmias	• Amiodarone: monitor for thyroid, lung, liver, ophthalmic side effects • Sotalol, ibutelide, dofetilide: ↑QTc leading to TdP, especially in renal insufficiency • Dronedarone may increase the risk of death in moderate to severe heart failure [14]	• High-grade AV block, and ↑ QTc • Sotalol and dofetilide: contraindicated in patients with renal impairment • Dronedarone: contraindicated in patients with heart failure • Amiodarone: avoid in patients with liver dysfunction

Class IV	Calcium-channel receptor antagonist	Effective AV nodal blocking agents	Hypotension and bradycardia	High-grade AV block
• Verapamil • Diltiazem	• Verapamil (immediate release 80–160 mg TID) • Diltiazem (immediate release 30–90 mg QID)			• Cardiogenic shock

These agents are also contraindicated in any individual with a known hypersensitivity or allergy to any of these agents.

[a] Dosing information is referenced from the 2013 Compendium of Pharmaceuticals and Specialties (CPS) of the Canadian Pharmacists Association (CPhA) unless specified otherwise.

[b] Class IA, IB, and IC antiarrhythmics also have varying degrees of K+ channel blockade.

[c] Dosing information for these medications is from *Micromedex Healthcare Series* [intranet database], Version 2.0. Greenwood Village, CO: Thomson Healthcare.

Re-entry

Re-entry is a mechanism of arrhythmogenesis in which a depolarizing wavefront propagates continuously in a circuitous path around an anatomic or functional area of conduction block.

- Re-entry is the most common cause of tachyarrhythmias, underlying arrhythmias such as scar-related monomorphic ventricular tachycardia, AV node re-entrant tachycardia, atrioventricular re-entrant tachycardia and atrial flutter.
- Re-entrant arrhythmias are often treated with either Class I or Class III antiarrhythmics.
- Class I antiarrhythmics terminate arrhythmias by inhibiting voltage-gated sodium channels, which depresses Phase 0 depolarization and slows myocardial conduction.
- By inhibiting voltage-gated potassium channels, Class III antiarrhythmics exert their effect by increasing the effective refractory period of the myocardium, which prolongs the repolarization phase and delays the next phase of depolarization.

Abnormal automaticity and triggered activity

Abnormal automaticity and triggered activity are both disorders of impulse formation. Abnormal automaticity refers to accelerated depolarization of atrial and/or ventricular tissue.

- The common reason for this is myocardial ischemia; however, metabolic and electrolyte derangements, as well as digoxin may also be a cause.

Triggered activity refers to abnormal depolarizations either during Phase 2 of the myocardial action potential ("early afterdepolarizations") or during Phase 4 ("delayed afterdepolarizations").

- Early afterdepolarizations (EADs) usually occur in the setting of prolonged repolarization (i.e. long QT), which puts patients at risk for a specific type of polymorphic ventricular tachycardia known as torsades de pointes (TdP).
- Torsades de pointes is a life-threatening tachyarrhythmia, which can be caused by QT-prolonging drugs, hypokalemia, congenital long-QT syndromes and, in some patients, bradycardia.
- Delayed afterdepolarizations (DADs) result from raised intracellular calcium, and can be secondary to digoxin toxicity, ischemia and some inherited arrhythmias [4].

Tachyarrhythmias

Tachyarrhythmias are common in the intensive care unit, and are nine times more common than bradyarrhythmias. Inotropes, the elevated sympathetic tone that often accompanies critical illness, along with a wide range of metabolic disturbances, can create an environment that facilitates the initiation and perpetuation of atrial and ventricular arrhythmias.

Supraventricular arrhythmias

Atrial fibrillation and atrial flutter

- Atrial fibrillation is by far the most common arrhythmia in the intensive care setting, affecting over 10% of critically ill patients.
- It is poorly tolerated in almost 40% of patients who develop it [5].

- Atrial fibrillation is a chaotic arrhythmia whose triggers are thought to come from the pulmonary veins in those with structurally normal hearts.
- The classic ECG appearance usually consists of a disorganized atrial rhythm with no distinct p-waves and an irregularly irregular ventricular response (Figure 27.2a).
- Conversely, atrial flutter is an organized re-entrant arrhythmia that typically circulates along the right atrial cavotricuspid isthmus. Those with prior cardiac surgery or atrial ablation can develop scar-dependent atrial flutter circuits in other areas of the atria, which may have different p-wave morphologies.

The p-waves in typical atrial flutter have a fairly distinct "saw-tooth" appearance. The ventricular response can be either regular (i.e. in a fixed 2:1 or 3:1 pattern) or irregular (Figure 27.2b). When patients are in atrial flutter with rapid ventricular response (i.e. with 1:1 or 2:1 AV conduction), the flutter waves may be difficult to see. In these cases, administration of IV adenosine is very useful, as it will cause transient AV block, which will slow the ventricular rate and unmask the flutter waves (Figure 27.2c). Adenosine is very short-acting, making it a safe and useful diagnostic tool in patients with undifferentiated supraventricular tachycardia.

A thorough search for a correctable precipitating cause should be the initial step in hemodynamically stable patients with atrial fibrillation or flutter, as this can be a physiologic response to an underlying abnormality.

- Any condition that can elevate sympathetic tone, such as pain, trauma, metabolic disturbances, ischemia, heart failure and inotropes can predispose a patient to atrial arrhythmias.
- Identifying and correcting these underlying factors will be much more successful in treating the atrial arrthymia than medical therapy.
- Depending on the cause, ventricular rates may be fairly resistant to rate or rhythm control until the underlying cause is addressed.

If atrial fibrillation or flutter persists after all identifiable precipitants have been corrected, then therapy is indicated to control the arrhythmia and prevent the associated complications. Atrial fibrillation and atrial flutter are usually managed with either a rate- or rhythm-control strategy.

- Unfortunately, the vast majority of critically ill patients are hemodynamically compromised and require vasopressors or ionotropes for blood pressure support.
- The negative inotropic and vasodepressive effects of β-blockers and calcium-channel blockers often preclude the use of a rate-control strategy.
- Digoxin, as a stand-alone agent, has poor efficacy for rate control, especially in a population with elevated sympathetic tone.
- Amiodarone is the most common choice for atrial arrhythmia treatment in the intensive care unit. It is one of the few antiarrhythmics available in intravenous form. During the initial load, amiodarone will mainly have a β-blocking effect with less vasodepressive and negative inotropic effects compared to traditional β-blockers or calcium-channel blockers. Its antiarrhythmic effects are often delayed several days, depending on the method of loading, due to its long half-life.
- The negative inotropic effects of Class IA and IC antiarrhythmics also preclude their use in this setting. They are also contraindicated in patients with coronary artery disease and left ventricular dysfunction.

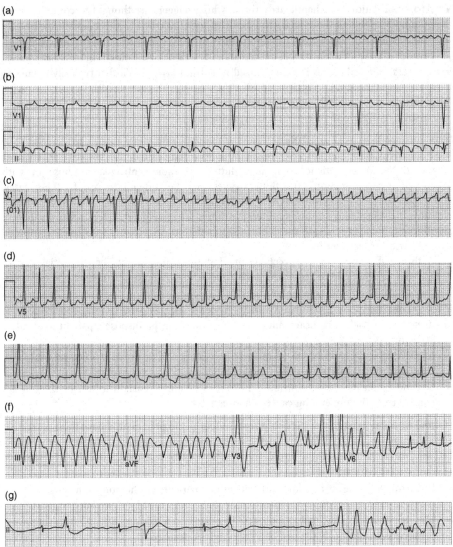

Figure 27.2 Rhythm strips: (a) atrial fibrillation, characterized by the irregularly irregular rhythm, and lack of discernible atrial activity; (b) atrial flutter, with the typical "saw-tooth" flutter waves; (c) the saw-tooth flutter waves in typical atrial flutter are unmasked by the administration of IV adenosine; (d) supraventricular tachycardia (SVT), a regular narrow complex regular rhythm with p-waves seen at the end of each QRS complex; (e) sinus rhythm with intermittent conduction down an accessory pathway (note the short PR interval and the wide, slurred upstroke of the QRS ('delta wave') in the first seven beats compared to the normal PR and narrow QRS in the subsequent nine beats when the accessory pathway stops conducting); (f) atrial fibrillation with pre-excitation. Note the irregularly irregular rhythm and the beat-to-beat variation in QRS width and morphology; (g) a rhythm strip showing the start of TdP. Note the preceding bradycardia and long QT interval prior to the initiation of TdP.

- Lidocaine, a Class IB antiarrhythmic, has minimal hemodynamic side effects, but questionable efficacy in the treatment of atrial fibrillation.
- Class III antiarrhythmics such as ibutilide and sotalol can also be considered, but sotalol is not available in intravenous form, and both drugs are contraindicated in patients with renal impairment due to the risk of torsades de pointes.
- Finally, electrical cardioversion is always a consideration, particularly in the setting of a hemodynamically unstable patient. However, depending on the patient's condition and predisposing factors, the chances of early recurrence is high, regardless of antiarrhythmic therapy.

The other main consideration in the management of atrial fibrillation and atrial flutter is stroke prevention.

- In one study, 2.6% of patients with severe sepsis and new-onset atrial fibrillation suffered an in-hospital stroke [6].
- Depending on the length of time the patient has been in atrial fibrillation, combined with their baseline risk of stroke (as estimated by the $CHADS_2$ or CHADS-Vasc scores) and the presence of structural heart disease, a transesophageal echocardiogram may be required prior to either chemical or electrical cardioversion to rule out left atrial thrombus and reduce the risk of a thromboembolic complication.
- In the weeks following cardioversion, left atrial contractility remains impaired. Therefore, it is recommended that patients be systemically anticoagulated for a period of at least 3 weeks after cardioversion.
- Depending on the patients' comorbidities and bleeding risk, contraindications to anticoagulation often limit the use of a rhythm control strategy in critically ill patients in the ICU [7].

Paroxysmal supraventricular tachycardia

Paroxysmal supraventricular tachycardias (SVT) are a benign group of arrhythmias, which include:

- Atrioventricular re-entrant tachycardias (AVRT)
- AV node re-entrant tachycardias (AVNRT)
- Atrial tachycardias.

They are often regular, narrow complex tachycardias (Figure 27.2d), but the QRS can widen in the presence of aberrancy (i.e. bundle branch block) or antegrade conduction over an accessory pathway.

Both AVNRT and AVRT are AV node-dependent macro re-entrant arrhythmias, which comprise the majority of SVTs.

- AVNRT is due to an extra, slowly conducting pathway that runs through the AV node, alongside the normal "fast pathway" that is present in everyone; the ECG in sinus rhythm is usually normal.
- AVRT is due to a macro re-entrant circuit that involves an "accessory pathway." An accessory pathway is an electrical connection between the atria and the ventricles that is independent of the AV node and native conduction system. In some patients, the presence of an accessory pathway can be seen on an ECG in sinus rhythm. The hallmark findings often consist of a short PR interval (i.e. less than 120 ms) and a wide slurred

upstroke in the QRS (i.e. a delta wave) (Figure 27.2e). AVRT can produce regular narrow complex tachycardias or wide complex tachycardias, depending on whether the circuit is conducting antegrade down the accessory pathway (wide) and retrograde up the AV node, or antegrade down the AV node (narrow) and retrograde up the pathway.

Both types of SVTs are often triggered by conditions of high adrenergic tone, where frequent atrial or ventricular ectopy can initiate tachycardia.

- Termination of these arrhythmias is usually achieved with AV node-blocking agents, such as adenosine, β-blockers or nondihydropyridine calcium-channel blockers.
- In patients who are hemodynamically unstable, adenosine or electrical cardioversion are reasonable first-line therapy.
- Depending on the frequency of recurrence, a routine AV nodal blocking agent or an antiarrhythmic agent may be required.

If a patient with an accessory pathway develops an AV node-independent atrial arrhythmia, such as atrial flutter or atrial fibrillation, AV nodal blockers are contraindicated.

- In the absence of competing conduction down the AV node, the accessory pathway may have the potential to conduct very rapidly to the ventricles.
- Atrial fibrillation in the setting of an accessory pathway ("pre-excited atrial fibrillation") has a distinct electrocardiographic appearance (Figure 27.2f). Competing conduction down both the AV node and accessory pathway results in variable degrees of fusion. This manifests as beat-to-beat changes in QRS morphology.
- First-line therapy is either electrical cardioversion, or an intravenous antiarrhythmic such as procainamide.

Atrial tachycardias are not dependent on the AV node, and are usually automatic, rather than re-entrant in mechanism.

- Therefore, unlike AVRT or AVNRT, they usually do not terminate with AV nodal blockade.
- Depending on the patient's symptoms or hemodynamics, a rate- or rhythm-control strategy can be applied.
- Either β-blockers or nondihydropyridine calcium-channel blockers are appropriate first-line agents to control the ventricular rate, assuming that the patient's blood pressure will tolerate it.
- If not, then electrical cardioversion can be performed.
- Since these tachyarrhythmias often occur in response to the elevated sympathetic tone, the likelihood of recurrence is often high, unless the patient's main issue is addressed and the patient's condition is stabilized.

Ventricular arrhythmias
Ventricular tachycardia
Monomorphic ventricular tachycardia (MMVT) is due to re-entrant activation around an area of myocardial scar. This most often occurs in the context of a previous myocardial infarction.

- β-blockade, while a helpful antiarrhythmic agent in this setting, is often limited because of the commonly tenuous blood pressure.
- In the acute setting, amiodarone and lidocaine can be used.
- Lidocaine is especially helpful for ventricular tachycardia that is thought to be secondary to acute myocardial ischemia; however, one must be mindful of potential central nervous

system (CNS) side effects, particularly if liver function is compromised. The most common CNS side effects include delirium and obtundation; however, coma can also occur. These symptoms are reversible with the discontinuation of lidocaine.

- If the patient is hemodynamically stable, and there is no history of coronary disease or significant left ventricular dysfunction, procainamide can also be considered. Procainamide, a class IA agent, can be given as an intravenous bolus over 5 minutes, or an infusion over 25 to 30 minutes. Careful monitoring for QRS and/or QT prolongation is recommended. Significant prolongation requires discontinuation of the drug to avoid potentially fatal ventricular arrhythmias.

Patients without structural heart disease can develop idiopathic forms of monomorphic ventricular tachycardia. These most often arise from the right or left ventricular outflow tracts or the fascicles (idiopathic LV VT or Belhassen VT). Once cardiac imaging has ruled out any structural abnormalities, the diagnosis usually then rests on QRS morphology.

- For example, right ventricular outflow tract VT usually has a left bundle branch block morphology with a late pre-cordial transition ($\geq$V3) and inferior axis.
- Conversely, idiopathic left ventricular VT has a classic right bundle and left anterior fascicular block morphology.
- Since these ventricular arrhythmias most often occur in young patients with preserved ejection fraction, they are usually well tolerated.
- These arrhythmias usually respond very well to β-blockers and nondihydropyridine calcium-channel blockers.
- Antiarrhythmics are reserved for those with refractory symptoms [8].

Torsades de pointes (TdP)

TdP is a particular type of polymorphic ventricular tachycardia that occurs in the setting of a prolonged QT.

- Since QT prolongation is responsible for the increased risk of TdP, treatment should begin with a search for the underlying cause.
- The differential diagnosis for QT prolongation is vast.
- The causes commonly encountered in the intensive care unit include myocardial ischemia, bradycardia, medications and electrolyte disturbances.

Each of these will be discussed briefly.

1. Myocardial ischemia is a common precipitant for cardiac arrhythmias. This can occur in the setting of an acute plaque rupture (i.e. acute coronary syndrome), or from a supply–demand imbalance in the setting of stable coronary artery disease. Significant ischemia, whether or not it progresses to myocardial infarction, can result in marked QT prolongation, and torsades de pointes. Treatment of TdP is directed at restoration of myocardial perfusion, which usually normalizes the QT interval.
2. In some patients, long QT and torsades can develop as a complication of heart block (Figure 27.2g). Why this occurs remains unclear. However, QT prolongation can be quite dramatic, resulting in recurrent salvos of polymorphic VT and syncope or cardiac arrest. Acute treatment requires an increase in heart rate, either with temporary pacing, or in some cases, an isoproterenol infusion.
3. Medications and electrolyte imbalances are also a frequent cause of prolonged QT in the intensive care setting. Many antipsychotics, antimicrobials, antiemetics, promotility

agents, anesthetic and pain medications are common culprits, particularly in those with an underlying genetic predisposition. A comprehensive list of QT-prolonging drugs can be found at www.torsades.org [9]. Those with (congenital) prolonged QT at baseline are at obvious risk. However, there is also a population of patients with poor repolarization reserve and normal QT intervals at baseline, who are particularly susceptible to QT prolongation and torsades with minor stressors such medication and/or electrolyte imbalances [10].

4. Although profound metabolic imbalances such as hypokalemia, hypocalcemia, hypothermia and hypomagnesemia can cause torsades in isolation, the etiology is most often multifactorial.

Although correction of the underlying cause is the most effective and definitive treatment, there are certain steps that can be taken in the acute phase to stabilize the patient.

- TdP may respond to intravenous magnesium bolus, which can be given acutely.
- In the absence of ischemia or acute infarct, shortening of the QT interval by increasing the heart rate (with either the use of ionotropic agents such as isoproterenol or with temporary pacing), is also an effective way of treating TdP.

Bradyarrhythmias

Bradyarrhythmias in the ICU can be due to:

- Progression of native conduction disease
- Medication toxicity (i.e. overdose of a rate-control agent or antiarrhythmic)
- Metabolic or electrolyte disturbance (e.g. hyperkalemia)
- Excessive vagal tone stimulated by suctioning or adjustment of the endotracheal tube.

The management of hemodynamically significant bradyarrhythmias is to correct any reversible cause. If bradycardia persists, then consideration of temporary pacing should occur.
Bradycardia can be due to sinus node dysfunction and/or heart block.

- Sinus pauses, whether they are spontaneous or due to conversion pauses from atrial fibrillation (i.e. sick sinus syndrome), are usually self-limited and not life-threatening.
- Pacing is usually not urgent, but a more chronic consideration to manage symptoms.
- In the acute setting, the discontinuation of potentially exacerbating medications, such as calcium-channel blockers or β-blockers, can be considered.

The management of bradycardia due to AV block in the acute setting is dependent on the reliability of the escape rhythm.

- In general, a patient with high-grade or complete heart block with a narrow QRS (<120 ms) and a ventricular rate in the 40 to 60 bpm range, is generally safe and does not necessarily require temporary pacing.
- However, a wide QRS with a very slow ventricular rate (<40 bpm) suggests that the escape rhythm is coming from the ventricles or low in the His–Purkinje system, which can be unreliable. In general, a temporary pacing wire is recommended in these patients to protect against asystole, in the event that the escape rhythm fails.
- As discussed previously, there is also a small proportion of patients who develop significant bradycardia-dependent QT prolongation (Figure 27.2g). An urgent

temporary pacing wire is also indicated in these patients to protect against potentially life-threatening torsades de pointes.

- Depending on the clinical scenario, an intravenous isoproterenol infusion can be used to temporize a patient in complete heart block until the placement of a temporary wire can be arranged. Isoproterenol should obviously be avoided in the setting of acute myocardial ischemia or adrenaline-mediated ventricular arrhythmias.

Transvenous pacing can be achieved through a variety of pacing catheters, including a balloon-tipped soft wire or a conventional stiff pacing wire (Figure 27.3). Each of these has particular risks and benefits, which should be considered when selecting a catheter.

- For example, the balloon-tipped soft wire can be inserted without fluoroscopic guidance, in a similar technique to a bedside pulmonary artery (Swan–Ganz) catheter. Capture typically occurs when the wire enters the right ventricle. Proper positioning is confirmed with an ECG (showing an LBBB morphology), as well as a chest X-ray. Rarely, the catheter can end up in the coronary sinus, which is sometimes a less stable position, and may result in atrial pacing or left ventricular pacing (resulting in a right bundle branch block morphology-paced QRS). In general, soft-tipped wires tend to dislodge more easily, particularly in awake or mobile patients.
- On the other hand, although hard wires tend to be much more stable, they require fluoroscopic guidance for placement, and their added stiffness portends a higher perforation risk in the thin-walled right ventricle.

Bradycardia due to simultaneous slowing of the sinus and AV node is usually vagally mediated. This classically manifests as a simultaneous slowing of the sinus rate and prolongation of the PR interval prior to a transient period of heart block or asystole.

- In the intensive care setting, vagal tone is often elevated from direct stimulation of the vagus nerve in the posterior hypopharynx. Common scenarios include bradycardia during deep suctioning, manipulation of an oral airway or endotracheal tube, and severe pain.
- Vagally mediated bradycardia does not require temporary pacing as it is benign and usually self-limited.
- Furthermore, the hypotension seen in vagally mediated bradycardia is often primarily due to a concomitant drop in systemic vascular resistance, which is part of the vagal reflex. As such, artificially increasing the heart rate by temporary pacing does not reliably increase the blood pressure in these situations [11].

Summary

- The development of cardiac arrhythmias is a common complication in the critically ill patient.
- Appropriate management should include an accurate diagnosis of the rhythm disturbance, a thorough search for underlying or contributing factors, correction (when possible) of exacerbating metabolic derangements and administration of the indicated medical therapy or intervention.
- In hemodynamically unstable patients, initiation of advanced cardiac life support (ACLS) protocol as an acute management strategy is an appropriate first step [12].

(a)

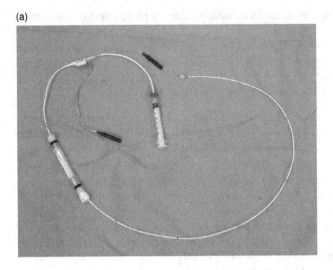

(b)

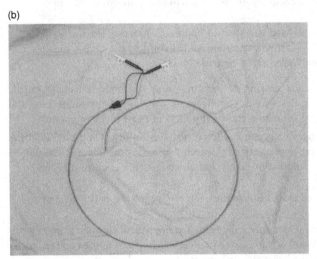

Figure 27.3 Temporary pacing wires: (a) a temporary floating pacing catheter with the balloon inflated with 1.5 mL of air from the syringe. Also note the external sheath that should always be used to maintain sterility of the catheter, particularly if adjustments are made; (b) a stiff temporary pacing catheter, which should be placed under fluoroscopic guidance.

References

1. Knotzer H, Mayr A, Ulmer H, Lederer W et al. Tachyarrhythmias in a surgical intensive care unit: a case-controlled epidemiologic study. *Intensive Care Med* 2000; 26 : 908–14.

2. Goodman S, Weiss Y, Weissman C. Update on cardiac arrhythmias in the ICU. *Curr Opin Crit Care* 2008; 14 : 549–54.

3. Reinelt P, Karth GD, Geppert A, Heinz G. Incidence and type of cardiac arrhythmias in critically ill patients: a single center experience in a medical-cardiological ICU. *Intensive Care Med* 2001; 27 : 1466–73.

4. Libby P. *Braunwald's Heart Disease: A Textbook of Cardiovascular Medicine*, 8th edn. Philadelphia, PA: Saunders Elsevier; 2008.

5. Kanji S, Williamson DR, Yaghchi BM *et al.*
    Canadian Critical Care Trials Group.
    Epidemiology and management of atrial
    fibrillation in medical and noncardiac
    surgical adult intensive care unit patients.
    J Crit Care 2012; 27 : 326.e1–8.

6. Walkey AJ, Wiener RS, Ghobrial JM *et al.*
    Incident stroke and mortality associated
    with new-onset atrial fibrillation in patients
    hospitalized with severe sepsis. *JAMA* 2011;
    306 : 2248–54.

7. Olesen JB, Lip GY, Hansen ML *et al.*
    Validation of risk stratification schemes for
    predicting stroke and thromboembolism in
    patients with atrial fibrillation: nationwide
    cohort study. *BMJ* 2011; 342 : d124.

8. Srivathsan K, Lester SJ, Appleton CP *et al.*
    Ventricular tachycardia in the absence of
    structural heart disease. *Indian Pacing
    Electrophysiol J* 2005; 5 : 106–21.

9. Cahoon WD Jr. Acquired QT
    prolongation. *Prog Cardiovasc Nurs* 2009;
    24 : 30–3.

10. Smithburger PL, Seybert AL, Armahizer
    MJ, Kane-Gill SL. QT prolongation in the
    intensive care unit: commonly used
    medications and the impact of drug-drug
    interactions. *Expert Opin Drug Saf* 2010; 9 :
    699–712.

11. Sud S, Klein GJ, Skanes AC *et al.* Implications
    of mechanism of bradycardia on response to
    pacing in patients with unexplained syncope.
    Europace 2007; 9 : 312–18.

12. Anantharaman V, Gunasegaran K.
    Advanced Cardiac Life Support guidelines
    2011. *Singapore Med J* 2011; 52 : 548–55.

13. The Cardiac Arrhythmia Suppression Trial
    (CAST) Investigators. Preliminary report:
    effect of encainide and flecainide on
    mortality in a randomized trial of
    arrhythmia suppression after myocardial
    infarction. *N Engl J Med* 1989; 321 :
    406–12.

14. Connolly SJ, Camm AJ, Halperin JL *et al.*
    Dronedarone in high-risk permanent atrial
    fibrillation. *N Engl J Med* 2011; 365 : 2268–76.

Chapter

28

The patient with sepsis

Jennifer Vergel Del Dios, Tom Varughese and Ravi Taneja

Sepsis and its sequel, multiple organ dysfunction syndrome (MODS), is the commonest cause of morbidity and mortality in the contemporary ICU. In spite of advances in our understanding of the disease process, the pathophysiology is largely unclear and the mortality remains high, in the range of 30–40%, in critically ill patients. Numerous immunomodulatory agents have been investigated over the last three decades; however, none of these have been successful to date. Perhaps the greatest advance over the last decade has been the development of the Surviving Sepsis Campaign [1] and their recommendations will be the focus of this chapter.

Incidence and causes

An epidemiological study in 2001 suggested that severe sepsis is prevalent in 10% of ICU and 2% of all hospital admissions in the USA [1]. Other developed nations show a similar incidence and it has been suggested that there are over 19 million cases of severe sepsis worldwide annually. The true incidence of sepsis is probably higher due to multiple reasons:

- Most epidemiological studies only count the treated cases of severe sepsis and hence report the treated incidence.
- Data from developing countries may be lacking and scarcity of ICU resources in countries such as the UK and Brazil may also influence the reported incidence of sepsis [2].

Severe sepsis occurs due to both community-acquired and healthcare-associated infections.

- About half the cases are caused by pneumonia.
- Intra-abdominal infections and urinary tract infections are the next most common cause of sepsis. *S. aureus* and *S. pneumoniae* are the commonest isolated Gram-positive pathogens while *E. coli*, *Klebsiella* and *P. aeruginosa* are the commonest Gram-negative pathogens [3].
- A recent study showed that Gram-negative organisms were isolated in 62% of patients, with Gram-positive organisms in 47% and fungi in 19% of patients with severe sepsis [4]. A third of cases have positive blood cultures and a third of patients suspected of having sepsis are culture-negative.

Risk factors for developing sepsis include pre-existing chronic diseases (such as COPD, AIDS and malignancy) and use of immunosuppressive therapy [5].

Development of subsequent organ dysfunction depends on pre-existing organ dysfunction, the genetic makeup of the patient and the timeliness of therapy. The incidence

Handbook of ICU Therapy, third edition, ed. John Fuller, Jeff Granton and Ian McConachie. Published by Cambridge University Press. © Cambridge University Press 2015.

of severe sepsis is higher in infants and the elderly as compared to other age groups, males compared to females and blacks compared to whites.

Terminology, definitions and conceptual challenges

Sepsis terminology has been confusing. For the purposes of this discussion, "infection" is considered a pathological process caused by the invasion of normally sterile tissue, fluid or body cavity by pathogenic or potentially pathogenic mircro-organisms.

The first attempt to homogenize sepsis terminology came about in 1992 following a consensus conference between the American College of Chest Physicians and the Society of Critical Care Medicine [6].

A new concept – "Systemic inflammatory response syndrome (SIRS)" – was proposed. Patients would be considered to have SIRS if they met two or more of the following criteria, in absence of any known causes:

- Temperature – >38 °C or <36 °C
- Heart rate >90 beats/min
- Respiratory rate >20 breaths/min or $PaCO_2$ <32 mmHg
- WBC either >12000 or <4000 or >10% immature band forms.

According to the consensus committee, patients meeting SIRS criteria and having presumed or suspected infection were classed as "sepsis." Patients with sepsis and accompanying organ dysfunction were to be considered as having "severe sepsis." Patients with sepsis and hypotension requiring inotropes and vasopressors were classified as having "septic shock."

The recommendations of SIRS criteria came from expert opinion rather than hard evidence, and in fact all the epidemiological studies on SIRS were published after the term had been coined. The term SIRS has had both supporters and detractors and, for a variety of reasons, has never really been adopted by clinicians at the bedside.

- While the SIRS concept is valid to the extent that a systemic inflammatory response can be triggered by a variety of infectious and noninfectious insults, its main utility has been to allow us to form standard criteria for patient enrollment in research trials, with most enrolling patients with severe sepsis.
- To the clinician at the bedside, a proclamation of SIRS as a diagnosis is not really necessary; but it should lead to an aggressive strategy to rule out ongoing infection, de-escalating antibiotics if no infection is found and appropriate management for any ensuing organ dysfunction.

Despite the definitions outlined above, it was felt that these terms do not allow for accurate characterization and staging of patients with sepsis. This was addressed in the 2001 International Sepsis Definitions Conference [1].

- The definitions laid out earlier were not changed as they were deemed to be helpful.
- However, a staging system, similar to the TNM staging in cancer, was devised and presented as the "PIRO" concept, with the hope that it would serve as a hypothesis-generating model for future research:

P – Predisposition: pre-morbid or genetic factors may influence outcome

I – Infection: site, type and extent of infection

R – Nature and magnitude of the host Response

O – Organ dysfunction.

In our opinion, the PIRO staging serves as a framework for how critical care physicians may manage different facets of this complex disease in the future. Per se, even though it seems preliminary and has limited clinical applications in its current form, it serves to reiterate that clinical outcomes can be affected by patient predisposition, the specific infection and the magnitude of host response that together may affect organ function.

Organ dysfunction

The raison d'être of the ICU is organ dysfunction, the main sequel of sepsis. In fact, most clinical features of sepsis (Table 28.1) can be ascribed to the signs and symptoms of organ dysfunction.

- Earlier it was thought that the main organ systems included the brain, heart, lungs, liver and the kidneys.
- However, in the sepsis field, the endothelium has recently been given credence as a major organ [7].

The two commonly used organ dysfunction scoring systems in adult critically ill patients are the MOD [8] and the SOFA [9] scores. Intuitively, higher scores are associated with increased morbidity and mortality, and resource utilization. However, in practice, they are seldom used to prognosticate patient outcomes at the bedside.

Clinical features and diagnosis

Manifestations of sepsis are varied and depend on many factors, including the initial site of infection, the causative pathogen, pattern of organ dysfunction, health status of the patient and the time taken to initiate treatment. A list of signs and symptoms that could point towards sepsis is appended in Table 28.1.

Organ dysfunction associated with sepsis commonly affects the cardiovascular and respiratory systems.

- Hypotension is the commonest cardiovascular manifestation and is frequently associated with tachycardia and lactic acidosis.
- The classic teaching has been that shock induced by sepsis may present as "warm" shock with warm peripheries and a bounding pulse, as opposed to cardiogenic shock. However, in the authors' opinion, it is rare to see such patients in the contemporary ICU.
- Admissions to the present-day ICU generally tend to occur when patients have more advanced stages of sepsis. Commonly observed signs of shock in the ICU may, therefore, include cool and clammy extremities or delayed capillary refill time with or without peripheral mottling.
- This is commonly associated with a clinical diagnosis of relative hypovolemia based on either low (left- or right-sided) filling pressures or, as per recent trends, a demonstration of IVC collapsibility on bedside ultrasonography.
- Other features may include an elevated mixed venous (SvO_2) or central venous ($ScvO_2$) oxygen saturation accompanied by increased cardiac indices and decreased systemic vascular resistance, as measured by a pulmonary artery catheter.

It should be noted that, in severe cases, it might be difficult to differentiate septic shock from shock due to other causes, as patients at this stage will have cold peripheries, mottling,

Table 28.1 Clinical and laboratory features of sepsis

General

Hyperthermia (core temp >38.3 °C)

Hypothermia (core temp <36 °C)

Decreased capillary refill or mottling

CNS

Altered mental status

CVS

Elevated heart rate (>90 beats/min)

Hypotension (systolic BP <90 mmHg)

Elevated cardiac index

Elevated mixed venous O_2 saturation >70%

Respiratory

Tachypnea, increased work of breathing

Arterial hypoxemia (PaO_2/FiO_2 <300)

Renal

Acute oliguria (<0.5 mL/kg/h)

Splanchnic

Paralytic ileus (absent bowel sounds)

Hyperbilirubinemia

Laboratory

WBC >12 000/mm^3 or <4000/mm^3

or >10% immature forms

Lactic acidosis

Thrombocytopenia

Elevated creatinine

Hyperglycemia

Coagulopathy

Elevated CRP

Elevated plasma procalcitonin

intractable hypotension, marked lactic acidosis and dependence on large doses of vasoactive drugs that may have to be escalated rapidly once they reach a healthcare facility.

- In such cases, it would be common to have mixed or central venous oxygen saturations that are below the normal range and this may reflect poor forward flow or sepsis-associated myocardial depression.

- Perhaps the most critical aspect in the diagnosis of sepsis in the ICU is sepsis-induced tissue hypoperfusion (defined as hypotension persisting after initial fluid challenge or blood lactate concentration ≥ 4 mmol/L).

Respiratory compromise will usually present as acute respiratory distress syndrome (ARDS) and is fully discussed in another chapter.

- Commonly, it presents as hypoxemia, increased work of breathing and V/Q mismatch.
- Chest roentgenography reveals bilateral lung infiltrates which are noncardiac in origin.

The brain and kidneys may be affected and present with altered mental status and oliguria, respectively. Splanchnic hypoperfusion can lead to oliguria, ileus and elevated aminotransferase levels.

Abnormalities in glycemic control, coagulation, adrenal function and thrombocytopenia are all seen in severe sepsis.

Pathophysiology

The pathophysiology of sepsis is complex and remains poorly defined. A complete review is not possible here and the reader is referred to various recent review articles for a detailed explanation [10–15].

Infection triggers a complex and multifaceted host response referred to as inflammation, the primary function of which is to hasten tissue repair and resolution of infection.

The "inflammatory response" in sepsis has been the subject of intense research over the last two decades:

- One of the principal over-riding hypotheses in the pathophysiology of sepsis has been the development of a "dysregulated," "systemic" or "generalized" host response to an infectious insult that may result in bystander host-tissue damage and this in turn leads to organ dysfunction.
- Evidence for this comes mostly from those patients (and animal models) that develop organ dysfunction in conditions that may provoke an inflammatory response in the absence of infection (trauma, pancreatitis, burns, ischemia reperfusion injury).
- While the cardinal clinical manifestations of a local inflammation remain well established – calor (heat), rubor (redness), dolor (pain), tumor (swelling) and function laesa (loss of function), the features of "systemic" or "generalized" inflammation have never been clear.
- Clues to the bedside clinician may generally include high cardiac indices and low systemic vascular resistances associated with evidence of tissue hypoperfusion, especially when there is a strong suspicion of infection.
- The fact that the SvO_2 has classically been elevated in septic shock has led the intensive care community to hypothesize that tissue hypoperfusion is mainly due to failure of oxygen utilization [16].
- It must be emphasized that sepsis, especially in late stages or when associated with cardiac dysfunction, can be associated with decreased $ScvO_2$[17].

The host response in sepsis is characterized by both proinflammatory and anti-inflammatory responses, the duration and magnitude of which vary with time and depend upon many variables, such as the type of the pathogen, its virulence, genetic characteristics of the host and coexisting illnesses.

- In general, proinflammatory responses are necessary for eliminating pathogens and are perceived to cause collateral tissue damage. These include, but are not limited to, leukocyte and complement activation, coagulation and endothelial dysfunction, as well as necrotic cell death.

- Anti-inflammatory responses, on the other hand, play a role in limiting bystander tissue injury and are implicated in increased susceptibility to secondary infections. These may include neuroendocrine regulation and apoptosis of B-cells, CD4+ T-cells and follicular dendritic cells.

- Considerable effort has been spent in quantifying various biomarkers and modulating them in critically ill patients. One of the biggest hindrances to sepsis research has been that most biomarkers show a wide variability in their responses between patients and it is not clear if changes in biomarker levels represent a mere association or a cause and effect phenomenon.

Management

Guidelines proposed by the 2012 Surviving Sepsis Campaign [1] are outlined below. These concepts serve as a core summary of many of the important principles of general management of the critically ill patient in ICU. Many of these outlines are expanded upon in the relevant chapters elsewhere in this text.

Initial resuscitation

Resuscitation should begin as soon as a diagnosis of severe sepsis is made and not be delayed until ICU admission. A protocolized and quantitative resuscitation approach is recommended. Based on a randomized controlled trial into early goal-directed therapy, the following are goals during the first 6 hours of resuscitation [17]:

- Central venous pressure (CVP) 8–12 mmHg
- Mean arterial pressure (MAP) $\geq$ 65 mmHg
- Urine output $\geq$ 0.5 mL/kg/h
- $S_{cv}O_2$ >70% or S_vO_2 >65%.

This strategy, also known as *early goal-directed therapy*, when instituted within the first 6 hours is associated with decreased morbidity and mortality.

- The guidelines also suggest that targeting elevated lactate levels either with or without normalization of $S_{cv}O_2$ levels may help in resuscitation.
- If the goals for $S_{cv}O_2$ or S_vO_2 are not achieved in the first 6 hours, despite adequate intravascular volume resuscitation, then dobutamine can be infused at up to 20 µg/kg/min and transfusion of red blood cells for a hematocrit $\geq$30% may be considered.
- There no longer appears to be benefit in attaining supranormal cardiac indices or oxygen delivery in patients with sepsis.

Caution needs to be exercised when interpreting CVP in critically ill patients:

- Mechanical ventilation, pulmonary hypertension, abdominal distension and tricuspid valve abnormalities may affect the CVP and adequate adjustments may need to be made before a patient is deemed replete with intravascular volume.
- Other indices of intravascular volume status, such as bedside ultrasonography, flow and volumetric indices and microcirculatory changes have been used; however, efficacy of these techniques has not been evaluated systematically yet.

Fluid therapy

Fluids must be given promptly to optimize pre-load as an initial step.

- Crystalloids, and not colloids, are the mainstay of fluid resuscitation.
- This recommendation comes from the results of multiple randomized controlled trials and meta-analyses conducted recently [18,19]. Administration of colloids for resuscitation may be associated with increased requirements for renal replacement therapy.
- Albumin may be used in resuscitation when patients require substantial amounts of crystalloids. The SAFE study showed that albumin administration was safe and as effective as 0.9% saline [20].
- In patients with sepsis-induced hypoperfusion with evidence of hypovolemia, an initial fluid challenge of up to 30 mL/kg of crystalloids or more may be necessary to meet resuscitation targets.
- Efficacy of fluid boluses needs to be assessed on an ongoing basis via their effect on filling pressures, urine outputs and resolution of lactic acidosis.

Vasoactive medications

- Adequate fluid resuscitation is the mainstay of initial sepsis management in the ICU. However, fluids alone will not usually reverse hypotension and tissue hypoperfusion.
- Autoregulation may be lost in various microvascular beds during hypotension, and blood flow may be critically dependent on maintenance of blood pressure. Hence, during the period of fluid resuscitation, critically ill hypotensive patients can and should receive boluses or infusions of vasopressors to sustain cardiovascular stability, especially if the diastolic blood pressure is too low.
- Current guidelines recommend vasopressor therapy initially to achieve a target MAP (mean arterial pressure) of 65 mmHg.
- It should be noted that certain patients, such as those with uncontrolled hypertension, may require higher perfusion pressures to sustain organ perfusion.
- Norepinephrine is the vasopressor of choice for restoration of MAP in the sepsis patient.
- Epinephrine may be added (and potentially substituted for norepinephrine) when an additional agent is required. Epinephrine use may be associated with aerobic lactate production through β_2 receptors and its use may preclude using lactate clearance as a monitoring tool for guiding therapy. However, clinical evidence does not suggest that its use is associated with worse outcomes as compared to norepinephrine [21,22].
- Vasopressin (up to 0.03 U/min) can be added to the above regimen to achieve target MAP. Its use as a sole agent is not recommended.

- Dopamine may be used as an alternative vasopressor, but only in patients with low risk of tachyarrhythmias or bradycardia. Current evidence does not support its routine use [23]. Low-dose dopamine should not be used for renal protection.
- Phenylephrine is not recommended in the management of sepsis, except in extenuating circumstances (norepinephrine-associated dysrhythmias or as salvage therapy). It is, however, used commonly as boluses to sustain life during resuscitation and during procedures such as intubation and mechanical ventilation. A trial of dobutamine is warranted as an adjunct to vasopressor therapy (up to 20 µg/kg/min) in the presence of low cardiac output or with ongoing signs of hypoperfusion, despite adequate intravascular volume and MAP.
- Predetermined supranormal oxygen delivery is not recommended in septic shock. Pulmonary artery or Swan–Ganz catheters have not been shown to improve outcomes and they have not been widely used at our center for many years.

Source control

- Rapid diagnosis is key to source control. Surgical collections and foci of infection (such as intra-abdominal abscesses, cholangitis, pyelonephritis) should be identified and drained as promptly as possible following initial resuscitation. Interventions associated with the least physiological insult should be employed (percutaneous rather than open surgical approaches) for critically ill patients. Intestinal infarction should be diagnosed, excluded and treated as soon as possible. Surgical management of peripancreatic necrosis, however, is best delayed until adequate demarcation of viable tissues has occurred.
- Prompt administration of antibiotic therapy should commence after appropriate cultures have been obtained. In severe sepsis or septic shock, broad-spectrum antibiotic therapy is warranted until the causative organism and its sensitivities have been identified. Antibiotic therapy should be tailored to culture reports as they become available.
- Intravenous catheters suspected of being colonized or infected must be removed as early as possible after establishment of alternate venous access.

Antimicrobial therapy

- The goal is to administer antimicrobials within the first hour of diagnosis. Delay is associated with increased morbidity and mortality. Additional intravenous ports may be required for antibiotics during initial resuscitation of patients.
- Initial empiric therapy should have activity against all pathogens (bacterial, viral or fungal) in doses that will provide adequate concentrations in tissues suspected to be the source of sepsis.
- Choice of antimicrobials depends upon many factors, such as underlying disease, immunosuppression, presence of neutropenia, recent antibiotic use, prevalence of drug-resistant organisms and local susceptibility patterns. Failure to initiate appropriate therapy (for the causative agents subsequently identified) is associated with increased morbidity and mortality. Thus, initiation of broad-spectrum antimicrobials for pathogens most likely responsible is paramount at initial patient contact.

- Combination empiric therapy is recommended for patients with neutropenia and multidrug-resistant pathogens such as *Acinetobacter* and *Pseudomonas* species. A combination of an extended-spectrum β-lactam and an aminoglycoside or fluoroquinolone may be used for pseudomonas bacteremia or severe respiratory failure and shock. β-lactams and macrolides are suggested for streptococcal pneumonia infections.
- Combination therapy when used empirically should not be used for longer than 3–5 days. De-escalation or narrowing the antimicrobial coverage should be considered on a daily basis. It should be remembered that a causative pathogen is not identified in nearly half of patients with severe sepsis. Hence, decisions on continuing antibiotic choices should be made after careful consideration of patients' clinical conditions and response. In general, 7–10 days of antibiotic therapy may be adequate. However, longer courses may be necessary when there is poor patient response, poor source control, immunodeficiency, neutropenia, *S. aureus* bacteremia and some fungal or viral infections. Collaboration with antibiotic stewardship programs is recommended.

Blood products

- The optimum hemoglobin level in the sepsis patient is controversial. The TRICC trial suggested that a restrictive strategy of transfusions (hemoglobin 70–90 g/L) was as effective as a liberal strategy (100–120 g/L) in ICU patients [24]. However, more recently, the Early Goal-Directed Therapy Trial [17] suggested that increased early transfusions along with other management strategies is associated with better outcomes in sepsis patients. It is recommended that a hemoglobin >70 g/L is acceptable once tissue hypoperfusion has resolved and there are no extenuating circumstances (myocardial ischemia, severe hypoxemia, acute hemorrhage). Results from the PROCESS trial may allow for further clarification on this issue. However, it is important to remember that red-cell transfusions may improve oxygen delivery, but without any significant effects on oxygen consumption. Erythropoietin is not recommended for treating anemia in sepsis patients.
- Fresh frozen plasma should not be used to treat coagulopathies in sepsis patients in the absence of bleeding or planned invasive procedures.
- Platelets should be transfused prophylactically for counts <10 000/mm^3 in the absence of active bleeding or when they are <20 000/mm^3 if the patient is at significant risk of bleeding. Platelet counts >50 000/mm^3 are recommended for invasive procedures.

Nutrition

- Evidence is largely inconclusive for the best nutrition strategies. Enteral nutrition, as tolerated, should be started within 48 hours of diagnosis. Low-dose feeding (up to 500 kcal/day) is sufficient for the first week and should be advanced to full caloric requirements in a stepwise fashion.
- Parenteral nutrition, if needed, should be supplemented with intravenous glucose and enteral nutrition, where possible. Current evidence does not support parenteral over enteral nutrition in sepsis patients.
- There is no evidence to support immunonutrition in sepsis.

Glucose control

- A protocolized approach to management of hyperglycemia is recommended.
- Earlier studies showed benefit when insulin infusions were used to control blood glucose between 4.4 and 6.1 mmol/L. However, NICE-SUGAR [25], the largest multicenter randomized trial investigating insulin therapy, compared insulin management of blood glucose levels between 4.5 and 6.0 mmol/L (tight glycemic control) versus conventional control (≤10 mmol/L). The findings demonstrated increased mortality in the tight glycemic control group (27.5% versus 24.9%, P = 0.02) at 90 days.
- Blood glucose should be monitored frequently (1–2 hours) until insulin requirements have stabilized. Results from point-of-care tests (capillary glucose levels) can be inaccurate, especially in the hypoglycemia and hyperglycemia ranges and should be interpreted with caution.
- Hypoglycemia is an independent risk factor for death. Computer-based algorithms may result in tighter glucose control and reduced risk of hypoglycemia. Further research is needed to validate insulin protocols and evaluate the variability of glucose concentrations in sepsis patients.

Renal replacement therapy

- Patients with sepsis who develop acute kidney injury may be treated with either intermittent hemodialysis or continuous renal replacement therapy. There is no convincing evidence to support one method over the other. Traditionally, patients are placed on continuous veno-venous hemofiltration in acute stages of septic shock as renal indices continue to deteriorate in spite of resuscitation.
- Unstable patients may tolerate continuous renal replacement better. There is no evidence to support renal replacement therapy greater than achieving 20–25 mL/kg/h of effluent generation.

Mechanical ventilation of sepsis-induced ARDS patients

General guidelines for managing ARDS need to be followed (see ARDS chapter). Appropriate therapy needs to be instituted early. A conservative fluid strategy is beneficial, but only in the absence of tissue hypoperfusion [26]. Use of pulmonary artery catheters is not associated with improved outcomes [27] and β_2-agonist therapy is not advised in the management of ARDS.

Corticosteroids

Parenteral steroids are not recommended for septic shock if adequate resuscitation can be achieved by fluids and vasopressors [28]. Hydrocortisone may only be used intravenously (200 mg/day) if hemodynamic goals are not achieved. It should be tapered off when vasopressors are no longer required. An ACTH stimulation test is not required to determine the need for corticosteroids.

Screening and infection prevention

Early identification and treatment of sepsis in critically ill patients is associated with improved outcomes.

- Implementation of sepsis screening tools has been associated with performance improvement and decreased mortality [29].
- Obtaining cultures prior to administration of antibiotics is essential to confirm infection and allow de-escalation of therapy as necessary. However, this should not be associated with a delay (>45 min) in starting antimicrobial therapy.
- Two sets of blood cultures (>10 mL in both aerobic and anaerobic bottles) are recommended with at least one drawn percutaneously and the other through each lumen of the vascular access device (unless it is <48 hours old). If the same organism is isolated from both cultures, the likelihood of that organism causing severe sepsis is increased. If the blood culture drawn from the vascular access device is positive more than 2 hours sooner than the peripheral blood culture, it is likely that the vascular device is the source of infection. Quantitative cultures may also help in determining if the vascular catheter is the source of infection.
- Gram stain is useful for respiratory-tract culture specimens; >5 leukocytes/high-powered field and <10 squamous cells/low-powered field are representative of lower respiratory tract samples.
- Biomarkers such as procalcitonin and C-reactive protein may be used to assist clinicians, but, at present, are not recommended for differentiating between states of infection and severe inflammation.
- 1,3 β-D-glucan assay, mannan and antimannan antibody assays are useful when invasive candidiasis are suspected.

Supportive care

- Stress ulcer prophylaxis using proton-pump inhibitors should be given to patients with severe sepsis/septic shock.
- There is no role for selenium, immunoglobulins or any immunomodulatory therapy in sepsis.
- Patients with sepsis are prothrombotic. Prophylaxis for deep-vein thrombosis (DVT) should be provided via subcutaneous low-molecular-weight heparin (LMWH) if there are no contraindications. Patients at a higher risk of bleeding should receive DVT prophylaxis through mechanical devices.
- Sodium bicarbonate should not be used to improve hemodynamics or reduce vasopressor requirements in hypoperfused patients who have lactic acidosis and an accompanying pH ≥7.15.
- Neuromuscular blockers should be avoided, especially in those without ARDS, if possible, although early neuromuscular blockade may have survival advantage without increasing muscle weakness [30].
- It is important to screen all ICU patients for adequate analgesia. The Behavioral Pain Scale (BPS) and Critical Care Pain Observation Tool (CPOT) are recommended as the most valid and reliable methods of screening for pain in patients who cannot verbally communicate, as long as they have intact motor function and no head injuries [31].
- Sedation should be provided to target-specific endpoints, keeping in mind that good analgesia takes priority. It should be monitored through the Richmond Agitation–Sedation Scale (RASS) or Sedation–Agitation Scale (SAS), which are recommended for continuous assessment [31].

Table 28.2 Surviving sepsis campaign bundles

Complete in 3 hours	Complete in 6 hours
• Measure lactate • Blood cultures prior to administration of antibiotics if this does not cause a significant delay (>45 min) in administering antibiotics	• Administer vasopressors for hypotension not responding to initial fluid resuscitation • Target MAP ≥65 mmHg.
• Administer broad-spectrum antibiotics • Administer 30 mL/kg crystalloid for hypotension or lactate ≥4 mmol/L	• For persistent hypotension (despite volume resuscitation) or initial lactate ≥4 mmol/L – measure CVP and $S_{cv}O_2$ • Repeat lactate if initially elevated.

MAP – mean arterial pressure; $S_{cv}O_2$ – central venous oxygen saturation; CVP – central venous pressure

• Goals of care should be discussed with patients and families within 72 hours of ICU admission. End-of-life care plans based on palliative care principles should be initiated where appropriate.

Quality assurance in sepsis management

Development of the Surviving Sepsis Campaign (SSC) has probably been the most crucial step in the evolution of sepsis management. Early diagnosis and therapy are critical for decreasing the morbidity and mortality associated with sepsis [32]. The 2012 SSC guidelines propose 3- and 6-hour targets for meeting clinical endpoints (Table 28.2).

• Management of sepsis requires a multidisciplinary approach. Collaboration with different specialties improves outcome. Intensive care clinicians should pursue local endeavors to develop educational sessions and develop streamlined pathways for expediting management of sepsis patients.
• Continuing medical education sessions and local guidelines can help with continuous quality improvement.
• Data collection and performance review provide valuable feedback and may help modify physician behavior, as well as improve outcomes and cost effectiveness of managing sepsis in the ICU.

Conclusions

Sepsis and multiple organ dysfunction are the commonest cause of morbidity and mortality in intensive care. Prompt resuscitation and supportive care remain the cornerstones of therapy, as all immunotherapies investigated to date have failed to improve outcome. Future advances may come through a better understanding of host–pathogen interactions and how this can be affected by predetermined genetic variability and coexisting disease.

References

1. Dellinger RP, Levy MM, Rhodes A et al. Surviving sepsis campaign: international guidelines for management of severe sepsis and septic shock : 2012. *Crit Care Med* 2013; 41 : 580–637.

2. Adhikari NK, Fowler RA, Bhagwanjee S, Rubenfeld GD. Critical care and the global burden of critical illness in adults. *Lancet* 2010; 376 : 1339–46.

3. Opal SM, Garber GE, LaRosa SP et al. Systemic host responses in severe sepsis

analyzed by causative microorganism and treatment effects of drotrecogin alfa (activated). *Clin Infect Dis* 2003; 37 : 50–8.

4. Vincent JL, Rello J, Marshall J et al. International study of the prevalence and outcomes of infection in intensive care units. *J Am Med Assoc* 2009; 302 : 2323–9.

5. Angus DC, Wax RS. Epidemiology of sepsis: an update. *Crit Care Med* 2001; 29 : S109–16.

6. Bone RC, Balk RA, Cerra FB et al. Definitions for sepsis and organ failure and guidelines for the use of innovative therapies in sepsis. The ACCP/SCCM Consensus Conference Committee. American College of Chest Physicians/ Society of Critical Care Medicine. *Chest* 1992; 101 : 1644–55.

7. Hack CE, Zeerleder S. The endothelium in sepsis: source of and a target for inflammation. *Crit Care Med* 2001; 29 : S21–7.

8. Marshall JC, Cook DJ, Christou NV et al. Multiple organ dysfunction score: a reliable descriptor of a complex clinical outcome. *Crit Care Med* 1995; 23 1638–52.

9. Vincent JL, Moreno R, Takala J. The SOFA score to describe organ failure/dysfunction. *Int Care Med* 1996; 22 : 707–10.

10. Marshall JC. Inflammation, coagulopathy, and the pathogenesis of multiple organ dysfunction syndrome. *Crit Care Med* 2001; 29 : S99–106.

11. Hotchkiss RS, Karl IE. The pathophysiology and treatment of sepsis. *N Engl J Med* 2003; 348 : 138–50.

12. van der Poll T, Opal SM. Host-pathogen interactions in sepsis. *Lancet Infect Dis* 2008; 8 : 32–43.

13. Takeuchi O, Akira S. Pattern recognition receptors and inflammation. *Cell* 2010; 140 : 805–20.

14. Levi M, van der PT. Inflammation and coagulation. *Crit Care Med* 2010; 38 : S26–34.

15. Angus DC, van der Poll T. Severe sepsis and septic shock. *N Engl J Med* 2013; 369 : 840–51.

16. Singer M. The role of mitochondrial dysfunction in sepsis-induced multi-organ failure. *Virulence* 2013; 5 : 66–72.

17. Rivers E, Nguyen B, Havstad S et al. Early goal-directed therapy in the treatment of severe sepsis and septic shock. *N Engl J Med* 2001; 345 : 1368–77.

18. Myburgh JA, Finfer SA, Bellomo R et al. Hydroxyethyl starch or saline for fluid resuscitation in intensive care. *N Eng J Med* 2012; 367 : 20:1901–11.

19. Perel P, Roberts I, Ker K. Colloids versus crystalloids for fluid resuscitation in critically ill patients. *Cochrane Database Syst Rev* 2013; 2 : CD000567.

20. Finfer S, Bellomo R, Boyce N et al. SAFE Study Investigators. A comparison of albumin and saline for fluid resuscitation in the intensive care unit. *N Engl J Med* 2004; 350 : 2247–56.

21. Annane D, Vignon P, Renault A et al. Norepinephrine plus dobutamine versus epinephrine alone for management of septic shock: a randomised trial. *Lancet* 2007; 370 : 676–84.

22. Myburgh JA, Higgins A, Jovanovska A et al. A comparison of epinephrine and norepinephrine in critically ill patients. *Intensive Care Med* 2008; 34 : 2226–34.

23. De Backer D, Aldecoa C, Njimi H, Vincent JL. Dopamine versus norepinephrine in the treatment of septic shock: a meta-analysis. *Crit Care Med* 2012; 40 : 725–30.

24. Hébert PC, Wells G, Blajchman MA et al. A multicenter, randomized, controlled clinical trial of transfusion requirements in critical care. Transfusion Requirements in Critical Care Investigators, Canadian Critical Care Trials Group. *N Engl J Med* 1999; 340 : 409–17.

25. Finfer S, Chittock DR, Su SY et al. Intensive versus conventional glucose control in critically ill patients. *N Engl J Med* 2009; 360 : 1283–97.

26. Wiedemann HP, Wheeler AP, Bernard GR et al. Comparison of two fluid-management strategies in acute lung injury. *N Engl J Med* 2006; 354 : 2564–75.

27. Wheeler AP, Bernard GR, Thompson BT et al. Pulmonary-artery versus central venous catheter to guide treatment of acute lung injury. *N Engl J Med* 2006; 354 : 2213–24.

28. Sprung CL, Annane D, Keh D et al. Hydrocortisone therapy for patients with septic shock. *N Engl J Med* 2008; 358 : 111–24.

29. Levy MM, Dellinger RP, Townsend SR et al. The Surviving Sepsis Campaign: results of an international guideline-based performance improvement program targeting severe sepsis. *Intensive Care Med* 2010; 36 : 222–31.

30. Papazian L, Forel JM, Gacouin A et al. Neuromuscular blockers in early acute respiratory distress syndrome. *N Engl J Med* 2010; 363 : 1107–16.

31. Barr J, Fraser GL, Puntillo K et al. Clinical practice guidelines for the management of pain, agitation, and delirium in adult patients in the intensive care unit. *Crit Care Med* 2013; 41 : 263–306.

32. Jones AE, Shapiro NI, Trzeciak S et al. Lactate clearance vs central venous oxygen saturation as goals of early sepsis therapy: a randomized clinical trial. *J Am Med Assoc* 2010; 303 : 739–46.

Acute kidney injury

RT Noel Gibney

What was known as acute renal failure is now called acute kidney injury (AKI). This change in terminology has been adopted to focus attention on a broader spectrum of injury, ranging from a minor change in serum creatinine or a brief period of oliguria to complete anuria requiring renal replacement therapy (RRT).

Traditionally, acute renal failure was defined as a decline in renal function such that nitrogenous waste accumulates in the circulation and manifests as uremia. In the past, studies on acute renal failure used many different diagnostic criteria and, consequently, it was difficult to compare results across studies, across patient populations and across interventions.

- Because of this, the Acute Dialysis Quality Initiative (ADQI) group developed the RIFLE (Risk, Injury, Failure, Loss, End-stage) criteria in 2004 to classify AKI [1].
- Since then, RIFLE has been validated in a large number of studies encompassing more than 500 000 patients with different underlying disease processes causing AKI.
- In an effort to improve sensitivity and specificity, the AKIN (Acute Kidney Injury Network) criteria and recent KDIGO (Kidney Disease: Improving Global Outcomes) modifications of RIFLE were developed and introduced an absolute increase of 26.5 µmol/L (0.3 mg/dL) to the diagnostic criteria for stage 1 disease, in addition to the 50% increase option published in RIFLE [2]. Staging of AKI is shown in Table 29.1.

Incidence of AKI

Using the KDIGO definitions, AKI occurs in one in five adults and one in three children admitted to hospital worldwide [3]. AKI is more prevalent in (and a significant risk factor for) patients with chronic kidney disease (CKD). Individuals with CKD are especially susceptible to AKI which, subsequently, may promote the progression of the underlying CKD [4].

The incidence of AKI also varies across critically ill populations depending on type of ICU and the populations served.

However, using the RIFLE and AKIN criteria, approximately 60% of critically ill patients admitted to an ICU develop at least RIFLE I class or AKIN Stage 1 AKI and 5–10% of ICU patients require the initiation of renal replacement therapy [5].

Causes of AKI

- Prerenal azotemia is the most common cause of AKI, accounting for over 50% of causes of AKI and is now termed fluid-responsive AKI.

Handbook of ICU Therapy, third edition, ed. John Fuller, Jeff Granton and Ian McConachie. Published by Cambridge University Press. © Cambridge University Press 2015.

Table 29.1 Staging of AKI (KDIGO modification of AKIN)

Stage	Serum creatinine	Urine output
1	1.5–1.9 times baseline increase known or presumed to have occurred within the previous 7 days Or $\geq$0.3 mg/dL ($\geq$26.5 µmol/L) increase within 48 hours	<0.5mL/kg/h for 6–12 hours
2	2.0–2.9 times baseline	<0.5 mL/kg/h for $\geq$12 hours
3	3.0 times baseline Or Increase in serum creatinine to $\geq$4.0 ($\geq$353.6 µmol/L) Or Initiation of renal replacement therapy Or In patients <18 years, decrease in eGFR to <35 mL/min per 1.73m²	<0.3 mL/kg/h $\geq$24 hours Or Anuria for $\geq$12 hours

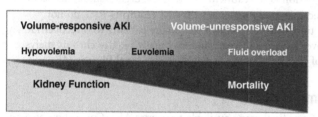

Figure 29.1 Development and clinical course of AKI.

- Severe sepsis and septic shock are the most common causes of RIFLE F or AKIN Stage 3 AKI.
- Other causes of AKI include circulatory shock, major surgery, cardiac dysfunction, trauma, liver failure and nephrotoxic agents, including radiocontrast material [5].
- In addition, patient comorbidities and characteristics influence whether AKI develops following a particular injury.

Pathogenesis of AKI

A conceptual model for the development and clinical course of AKI is shown in Figure 29.1. AKI includes both volume-responsive and volume-unresponsive conditions. These are not mutually exclusive, and a patient may progress from one to the other.

- This figure depicts a closing "therapeutic window" as injury evolves and kidney function worsens.
- Mortality increases as kidney function declines [2].

A number of processes resulting in AKI involve ischemia or sepsis, causing a complex interaction of various cell types within the kidney.

- Epithelial cell injury mediates functional alterations through direct failure of the cells to transport ions and molecules, or indirectly by mediating a decrease in GFR.

- Epithelial cells also influence the function of endothelial cells by releasing chemokines, cytokines and other soluble mediators.
- Interactions between endothelial cells and leukocytes contribute to continued hypoxia, inflammation and further epithelial cell injury and dysfunction [6].

Numerous therapeutic targets have been identified that prevent or limit ongoing injury. Additional approaches to improve repair and minimize fibrosis and vascular dropout will also be critical in limiting the development of CKD and transition from CKD to end-stage renal disease as a consequence of ischemic AKI in patients at high risk [6].

Impact and outcomes of AKI

It is now clear that even minor degrees of AKI, as evidenced by small increases in serum creatinine concentration or transient oliguria, predict immediate and long-term adverse outcomes. Many studies have now shown a significant increase in morbidity and mortality with only Stage 1 AKI and a dramatic step-wise increase in mortality with increasing AKI severity.

- The major clinical value in these new staging and classification systems is the importance of early recognition and treatment before frank organ failure has occurred.
- While it is well recognized that many patients with AKI requiring RRT do not recover their kidney function, it is now evident that many patients who recover kidney function develop CKD over subsequent years and eventually require chronic dialysis, likely as a consequence of residual damage and progressive renal fibrosis [4].

Diagnosis and assessment of AKI

Once established, there is no specific therapy available to reverse AKI. Consequently, early recognition of AKI is vital in order to treat any reversible causes, such as hypovolemia or obstructive uropathy.

- The possibility of AKI should be considered if there is oliguria in a patient at risk of AKI either by virtue of comorbidities or diagnosis.
- The challenge in using creatinine or urea serum levels to diagnose AKI is that they do not become elevated for many hours following kidney injury, which may limit the time available during which injury may be limited or reversed.
- In addition, the concentration of creatinine and other biomarkers in blood may be reduced by hemodilution in patients receiving aggressive fluid resuscitation.
- It has been proposed that the finding of new proteinuria and cellular casts or the presence of novel biomarkers such as NGAL or KIM-1 in the urine may allow the diagnosis of AKI at an earlier phase [7].

An approach to the patient with AKI is outlined in Figure 29.2 [2].

- A clinical history should be obtained from the patient, or if they are confused or comatose, from family or friends.
- This should include the history of the presenting illness, existing conditions and prescribed and over-the-counter medications.
- Vital signs should be obtained.
- Physical examination should determine the level of consciousness and degree of hydration of the patient. Peripheral perfusion should be assessed. Air hunger with rapid

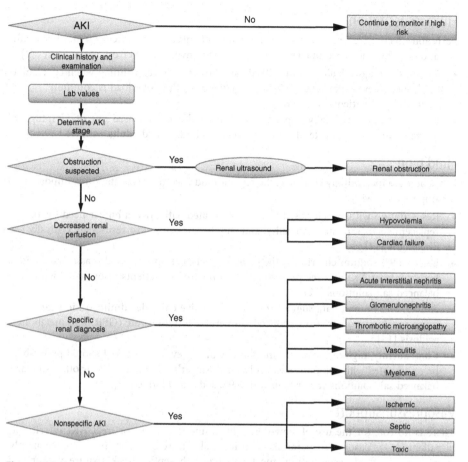

Figure 29.2 Approach to the patient with acute kidney injury (modified from [2])

deep respirations (Kussmaul respirations) should suggest metabolic acidosis while rapid shallow breathing combined with orthopnea should suggest pulmonary edema. Signs of congestive cardiac failure should be sought. The skin should be examined for signs suggestive of vasculitis or endocarditis.

- Laboratory tests should include: urinalysis, including microscopy, hemoglobin, white blood cells, platelets, peripheral blood smear, serum electrolytes, urea and creatinine levels, blood cultures and arterial blood gases.

Prevention and treatment of AKI

It is critical to recognize specific reversible or treatable causes of AKI, such as obstructive nephropathy or specific diseases such as glomerulonephritis, interstitial nephritis, crystal nephropathy, vasculitis or microangiopathies [8]. If any of these are present or suspected, urology, nephrology and/or rheumatology should be consulted. Once AKI is recognized, nephrotoxic drugs should be avoided, or, where possible, guided by drug levels.

Fluid resuscitation

Early and effective fluid resuscitation to achieve euvolemia and normotension may reverse the elevation in urea and creatinine levels in patients with hypovolemia from many causes [2].

- One of the major challenges in critical care, however, is determining when euvolemia has been achieved, particularly in septic patients, as fluid overload is common in critically ill patients with AKI.
- Fluid overload in critically ill patients is associated with increased rate of AKI, higher mortality and a lower rate of renal recovery in children and adults with AKI [9,10].

Fluid type

It has become increasingly clear that the type of fluid used for resuscitation is important in treating patients with AKI.

- Resuscitation with starch-based fluids is associated with AKI, a higher need for renal replacement therapy and mortality, and should not be used to resuscitate critically ill patients [11].
- Use of 0.9% sodium chloride as the primary resuscitation fluid is also associated with a higher rate of AKI and the need for RRT, compared to patients resuscitated with balanced salt solutions [12].
- Animal and human data suggest that such excessive chloride administration can cause renal vasoconstriction, reduced glomerular filtration rate (GFR) and metabolic acidosis [13].
- Consequently, high-risk patients and those with any evidence of AKI should preferably be resuscitated with solutions such as lactated Ringer's, Plasma Lyte A or other similar balanced salt solutions rather than with 0.9% sodium chloride [12].

Vasopressor support

There is no role for the use of "low-dose" dopamine to prevent or treat AKI in critically ill patients [14]. Vasomotor paralysis is an integral feature of septic shock. Consequently, in addition to fluid resuscitation, most patients with septic shock require vasopressor support to maintain an adequate systemic vascular resistance for organ perfusion [15].

- It is not known which vasopressor is most effective for prevention or treatment of AKI in patients with septic shock [16].
- However, dopamine may not be effective in patients with severe or prolonged septic shock and may result in arrhythmias [16].
- Some studies have suggested a higher rate of AKI in septic shock patients treated with phenylephrine [17].
- Most patients are treated with norepinephrine or epinephrine. Vasopressin is frequently used to reduce the dose of norepinephrine.
- However, there is not enough evidence currently to recommend one vasopressor agent over another.
- Whichever agent is used should be titrated to achieve a minimum mean arterial blood pressure of 65 mmHg [15].
- If following adequate fluid resuscitation and vasopressor therapy, a patient's urinary output has not increased, consideration should be given to increasing the target blood pressure, particularly if the patient was hypertensive previously [2].

Inotropic support

- Kidney function requires both adequate renal blood flow and perfusion pressure. Critically ill patients with primary cardiac disease and myocardial dysfunction caused by other causes, primarily sepsis often have severe cardiac dysfunction and require treatment with positive inotropic agents such as dobutamine [18].
- Milrinone, a pulmonary arterial vasodilator and inotrope, should be considered if there is primarily right ventricular failure associated with pulmonary hypertension.
- Inotropic therapy may be guided by clinical response or, more accurately, by sequential measurements of central venous oxygen saturation and lactate levels or by pulse wave contour analysis or pulmonary artery catheterization.

Diuretics

Some studies have suggested worse outcomes in patients with AKI treated with diuretics [19]. As a consequence there has been reluctance to use diuretics.

- However, there are no animal or human studies that conclusively show evidence of a decrease in renal blood flow or an elevation in biomarkers of kidney injury following use of diuretics.
- The careful use of titrated diuretics to minimize or reverse fluid overload in patients with ARDS and AKI has been associated with improved survival [20].
- In fluid-overloaded patients with AKI, several studies have demonstrated that more aggressive use of loop diuretics to achieve greater volume removal is associated with improved outcomes [20,21].
- In addition, a recent randomized controlled trial compared titrated diuretic therapy with ultrafiltration for patients with acute decompensated heart failure and AKI (acute type 1 cardiorenal syndrome) and found diuretic therapy superior [22].

Glycemic control with intravenous insulin

A landmark study and a number of subsequent studies found improved survival and lower rates of AKI in critically ill surgical patients in whom glucose control was tightly maintained in the range of 4.0–6.1 mmol/L [23].

- However, more recent studies have found no benefit, particularly in critically ill medical patients, and a high rate of significant hypoglycemia when targets for glucose levels are less than 6 mmol/L [24].
- Consequently, a number of organizations have developed clinical practice guidelines that vary in the recommended levels at which glucose should be maintained. These range from a low limit of 6.1 mmol/L to a high limit of 11.1 mmol/L [25].

Syndromes associated with AKI
Contrast nephropathy

The use of intravenous radiocontrast material for angiography or enhanced CT scans may be associated with the development of AKI, most often in patients with pre-existing chronic kidney disease or diabetes mellitus.

- Contrast nephropathy is the third leading cause of hospital-acquired AKI [26].
- Although it has been defined in many different ways, contrast nephropathy is defined as an increase of 44.2 μmol/L (0.5 mg/dL) in serum creatinine or a 25% increase from baseline up to 5 days post-procedure.
- Although most cases do not cause oliguria and renal function usually returns to normal after 7–10 days, some patients require renal replacement therapy and up to 30% suffer some degree of permanent loss of renal function [27].
- It is proposed that the renal damage is caused by alterations in intrarenal hemodynamics with an initial vasodilatation and subsequent vasoconstriction causing renal medullary ischemia.
- It has also been shown that the risk of contrast nephropathy increases with the volume of contrast used and with the relative osmolarity of the agents used, with less contrast nephropathy seen with lower osmolarity and iso-osmolar agents.
- It has been suggested that when agents with higher osmolarity are used, the higher viscosity may cause a reduced blood flow in the arterioles and capillaries in the renal medulla.
- The risk is much higher in patients with diabetes and vascular disease [27].

Many different strategies for prevention of contrast nephropathy have been studied, including hydration, n-acetylcysteine, sodium bicarbonate, fenoldopam and theophylline but, to date, only hydration has been conclusively shown to be effective [28].

Abdominal compartment syndrome

Abdominal compartment syndrome occurs when abdominal hypertension results in organ dysfunction.

- The normal intra-abdominal pressure is 5 mmHg or less. Intra-abdominal hypertension refers to a sustained intra-abdominal pressure above 12 mmHg. Intra-abdominal perfusion pressure is the mean arterial pressure minus the intra-abdominal pressure and is ideally maintained above 60 mmHg.
- Abdominal compartment syndrome is an IAP sustained above 20 mmHg that is associated with a new organ dysfunction that may include AKI, bowel and hepatic ischemia, pulmonary restriction and hypotension.
- Renal dysfunction is initially manifest by oliguria as the IAP increases and subsequently by a progressive increase in serum creatinine levels that is often initially masked by the large volume of resuscitation fluid [29].

Most cases of ACS occur in patients who have had aggressive fluid resuscitation, particularly patients following major trauma, burns and abdominal surgery. Since most of these patients were already critically ill, ACS is often missed, and consequently it is important to have a high index of suspicion in patients at risk and measure bladder pressure on a regular basis.

Management of ACS includes minimization of fluid infusions, percutaneous drainage of peritoneal and pleural fluid collections, and maintenance of intra-abdominal perfusion pressure above 60 mmHg by vasopressors.

Consideration of surgical decompression must be considered if supportive therapy is not effective. Early initiation of renal replacement therapy should also be considered for aggressive fluid removal [29].

Tumor lysis syndrome

Tumor lysis syndrome is caused when masses of tumor cells suddenly lyse with release of potassium, phosphate and nucleic acids. It may happen spontaneously with certain malignancies, but most often occurs soon after initiation of chemotherapy. The released nucleic acids are metabolized to uric acid, which may precipitate in the renal tubules. In addition, the hyperphosphatemia may also result in the precipitation of calcium phosphate in the renal tubules, both resulting in AKI. Tumor lysis syndrome-related AKI is often accompanied by lactic acidosis and rapidly developing hyperkalemia due to the rapid release of potassium from tumor cells and the acidosis causing extracellular potassium shift.

Tumor lysis syndrome is most likely to occur in certain malignancies, particularly those with a high tumor burden and high chemosensitivity.

- It may be prevented by aggressive hydration to achieve a urine output ≥2 mL/kg/h to minimize tubular deposits of uric acid and calcium phosphate. If there is concern regarding fluid overload, furosemide may be used to maintain the desired urine output [30].
- Allopurinol is a hypoxanthine analog that competitively inhibits xanthine oxidase and blocks the conversion of the metabolism of hypoxanthine and xanthine to uric acid. While this effectively reduces the production of uric acid, it does not reduce the level if it is already elevated. In addition, allopurinol therapy increases levels of xanthine and hypoxanthine and may result in xanthine crystal nephropathy and AKI.
- Pretreatment with recombinant urate oxidase (rasburicase) promotes rapid metabolism of uric acid to allantoin, which is more water soluble. Rasburicase and standard hydration therapy has been shown to be more effective than allopurinol and standard hydration therapy in reducing the incidence of tumor lysis syndrome and associated AKI following chemotherapy in high-risk children and adults [30,31].

Patients with tumor lysis syndrome-associated AKI often require early initiation of RRT because of rapidly progressive hyperkalemia, acidosis and pulmonary edema [31].

Rhabdomyolysis

Rhabdomyolysis occurs following the breakdown of skeletal muscle and release of myocyte contents. These include the heme pigment, myoglobin, enzymes, creatine kinase (CK), lactic dehydrogenase, glutamic oxalacetic transaminase and electrolytes, particularly potassium and phosphorus.

- Rhabdomyolysis has many causes and ranges in severity from mild asymptomatic increases in CK levels to life-threatening with massive elevation in CK levels, myoglobinuria, AKI and, possibly, death.
- The most common causes of rhabdomyolysis in adults are drugs (illicit and prescribed), alcohol abuse, trauma, neuroleptic malignant syndrome (NMS), seizures, immobility with pressure necrosis and metabolic muscle diseases. The many causes of rhabdomyolysis are outlined in Table 29.2.
- The diagnosis of rhabdomyolysis should be sought in patients at risk and considered in patients with dark "tea-colored" urine. It may be confirmed by the finding of CK levels that are elevated ten times above the normal upper level.

Table 29.2 Causes of rhabdomyolysis

Trauma
Excessive muscular activity
Drugs and toxins
Hyperthermia
Muscle ischemia
Electrolyte and endocrine abnormalities
Metabolic muscle diseases
Viral myositis
Connective tissue disorders

Acute kidney injury occurs in patients with rhabdomyolysis and myoglobinuria due to a combination of precipitation of the heme pigment, myoglobin, in the renal tubules, direct tubular toxicity caused by lipid peroxidation and by myoglobin scavenging nitric oxide resulting in renal medullary vasoconstriction.

In most patients with rhabdomyolysis, AKI may be prevented by early and effective hydration with crystalloid solutions.

- Fluids should be infused to achieve a urine output of 2 mL/kg/h.
- Bicarbonate-containing fluids have been recommended with the goal of alkalinizing urine to make myoglobin more soluble. However, it is virtually impossible to alkalinize the urine in patients with severe rhabdomyolysis and available studies show little extra benefit of bicarbonate infusion over adequate resuscitation with isotonic crystalloid.
- While, traditionally, mannitol was advised in the treatment of myoglobinuria, this is no longer advised as there are no studies that suggest benefit, and mannitol may result in further kidney injury.

In patients with massive muscle damage, as may occur following reperfusion of a crushed limb, the degree of rhabdomyolysis may be massive and result in rapid-onset life-threatening hyperkalemia and metabolic acidosis.

- It is therefore critical that potassium-containing fluids not be used to resuscitate these patients.
- If severe AKI has already occurred and there is no output in response to fluid resuscitation, care should be taken to avoid fluid overload and early intermittent hemodialysis initiated.
- Once stabilized, the patient should be assessed clinically and with measurements of compartment pressure for the possibility of a muscle compartment syndrome. If a compartment syndrome is confirmed, orthopedic surgery should be consulted for consideration of a fasciotomy [32–34].

AKI in liver disease

Renal dysfunction occurs in patients with acute liver failure (ALF) and with acute-on-chronic liver failure (ACLF).

Table 29.3 Criteria for HRS

Cirrhosis with ascites
SCr >130 μmol/L
Absence of shock
No improvement in SCr (decrease <130 μmol/L after 2 days following diuretic withdrawal and volume expansion with albumin. The recommended dose of albumin is 1 g/kg/day up to 100 g/day)
Absence of parenchymal kidney disease as indicated by proteinuria <500 mg/day, microhematuria (<50 rbc/hpf) and/or abnormal renal ultrasound
No current or recent treatment with nephrotoxic drugs

In fulminant ALF, such as occurs following acetaminophen overdose, oliguria often occurs early in the course due to a combination of hemodynamic instability and inflammatory mediators, often combined with sepsis.

- While fluid resuscitation is important, it is vital to avoid fluid overload, particularly with crystalloid, as cerebral edema may be fatal in these patients.
- For this reason, it is important to initiate vasopressor therapy early to maintain an adequate renal perfusion pressure and to consider a higher target blood pressure.
- Albumin adsorbs a number of circulating toxins in liver failure and may be a valuable addition to the fluid resuscitation regime [35].

Ammonia levels correlate well with the risk of development of cerebral edema in patients with ALF, particularly when ammonia levels are in excess of 150 μmol/L.

- In this situation, early initiation of continuous renal replacement therapy (CRRT) should be considered with the dose titrated to keep the ammonia level below 100 μmol/L [36].

Hepatorenal syndrome (HRS) is characterized by functional renal failure in patients with advanced cirrhosis and has a poor prognosis, with most patients dying within 28 days of onset unless they receive a liver transplant.

- The criteria for HRS are outlined in Table 29.3, indicating that the diagnosis of HRS is one of exclusion, so investigations should be performed to rule out other common causes of AKI [37].
- The pathogenesis of HRS involves marked intrarenal arteriolar vasoconstriction and peripheral arterial vasodilatation, mainly in the splanchnic vessels.
- In patients with previously stable ACLF, the most common etiology of deterioration in liver function causing HRS is sepsis, usually caused by spontaneous bacterial peritonitis.
- Management includes diagnostic paracentesis sending the ascitic fluid for analysis and culture, followed by initiation of broad-spectrum antibiotics, typically, ceftriaxone.
- Most patients with HRS due to sepsis are intravascularly hypovolemic and require fluid resuscitation, which should include a significant component of albumin of 1 g/kg/day up to a maximum of 100 g/day [33].

- Tense ascites can cause intra-abdominal hypertension and should be drained by large volume paracentesis of 4–6 liters with the ascites replaced with albumin 8 g for every liter of ascites drained [38].
- Use of vasopressors such as norepinephrine, vasopressin and terlipressin to increase MAP, combined with paracentesis and albumin infusion is effective to increase renal perfusion in some patients with HRS [39].
- However, the only definitive treatment for HRS is orthotopic liver transplant.

Conclusions

- AKI is common in hospitalized patients and is associated with high mortality.
- Early recognition is vital in order to identify potentially reversible causes.
- Fluid resuscitation is a vital part of the management of AKI.
- Fluids containing hydroxyethyl starch should be avoided.
- Balanced salt fluids should be used for resuscitation.
- Nephrotoxic agents should be discontinued.
- Patients should be resuscitated to clear hemodynamic endpoints, avoiding fluid overload.
- Vasopressors and inotropes should be used to maintain renal perfusion and blood flow.

References

1. Bellomo R, Ronco C, Kellum JA et al. Acute renal failure – definition, outcome measures, animal models, fluid therapy and information technology needs: the Second International Consensus Conference of the Acute Dialysis Quality Initiative (ADQI) Group. Crit Care 2004; 8 : R204–12.

2. Kellum JA, Lameire N. KDIGO Clinical Practice Guideline for Acute Kidney Injury. Kidney Inter 2012; 2 1–138.

3. Susantitaphong P, Cruz DN, Cerda J et al. World incidence of AKI: a meta-analysis. Clin J Am Soc Nephrol 2013; 8 : 1482–93.

4. Wald R, Quinn RR, Luo J et al. University of Toronto Acute Kidney Injury Research Group. Chronic dialysis and death among survivors of acute kidney injury requiring dialysis. JAMA 2009; 302 : 1179–85.

5. Uchino S, Kellum JA, Bellomo R et al Beginning and Ending Supportive Therapy for the Kidney (BEST Kidney) Investigators. Acute renal failure in critically ill patients: a multinational, multicenter study. JAMA 2005; 294 : 813–8.

6. Himmelfarb J, Joannidis M, Molitoris B et al. Evaluation and initial management of acute kidney injury. Clin J Am Soc Nephrol 2008; 3 : 962–7.

7. Cruz DN, Bagshaw SM, Maisel A et al. Use of biomarkers to assess prognosis and guide management of patients with acute kidney injury. Contrib Nephrol 2013; 182 : 45–64.

8. Joannidis M, Druml W, Forni LG et al. Prevention of acute kidney injury and protection of renal function in the intensive care unit. Intensive Care Med 2010; 36 : 392–411.

9. Bouchard J, Soroko SB, Chertow GM et al. Fluid accumulation, survival and recovery of kidney function in critically ill patients with acute kidney injury. Kidney Inter 2009; 76 : 422–7.

10. Fortenberry JD, Paden ML, Goldstein SL. Acute kidney injury in children: an update on diagnosis and treatment. Pediatr Clin North Am 2013; 60 : 669–88.

11. Zarychanski R, Abou-Setta AM, Turgeon AF et al. Association of hydroxyethyl starch administration with mortality and acute kidney injury in critically ill patients requiring volume resuscitation: a systematic review and meta-analysis. JAMA 2013 20; 309 : 678–88.

12. Yunos NM, Bellomo R, Hegarty C *et al.* Association between a chloride-liberal vs chloride-restrictive intravenous fluid administration strategy and kidney injury in critically ill adults. *JAMA* 2012; 308 : 1566–72.

13. Yunos NM, Kim IB, Bellomo R, *et al.* The biochemical effects of restricting chloride-rich fluids in intensive care. *Crit Care Med* 2011; 39 : 2419–24.

14. Kellum JA, M Decker J. Use of dopamine in acute renal failure: a meta-analysis. *Crit Care Med* 2001; 29 : 1526–31.

15. Dellinger RP, Levy MM, Rhodes A *et al.* Surviving sepsis campaign: international guidelines for management of severe sepsis and septic shock: 2012. *Crit Care Med* 2013; 41 : 580–637.

16. De Backer D, Biston P, Devriendt J *et al.* Comparison of dopamine and norepinephrine in the treatment of shock. *N Engl J Med* 2010; 362 : 779–89.

17. Plataki M, Kashani K, Cabello-Garza J *et al.* R. Predictors of acute kidney injury in septic shock patients: an observational cohort study. *Clin J Am Soc Nephrol* 2011; 6 : 1744–51.

18. Rivers E, Nguyen B, Havstad S *et al.* Early goal-directed therapy in the treatment of severe sepsis and septic shock. *N Engl J Med* 2001; 345 : 1368–77.

19. Grams ME, Estrella MM, Coresh J, *et al.* Fluid balance, diuretic use, and mortality in acute kidney injury. *Clin J Am Soc Nephrol* 2011; 6 : 966–73.

20. Liu KD, Thompson BT, Ancukiewicz M, *et al.* Acute kidney injury in patients with acute lung injury: impact of fluid accumulation on classification of acute kidney injury and associated outcomes. *Crit Care Med* 2011; 39 : 2665–71.

21. Nadeau-Fredette AC, Bouchard J. Fluid management and use of diuretics in acute kidney injury. *Adv Chronic Kidney Dis* 2013; 20 : 45–55.

22. Bart BA, Goldsmith SR, Lee KL *et al.* Ultrafiltration in decompensated heart failure with cardiorenal syndrome. *N Engl J Med* 2012; 367 : 2296–304.

23. van den Berghe G, Wouters P, Weekers F, *et al.* Intensive insulin therapy in the critically ill patients. *N Engl J Med* 2001; 345 : 1359–67.

24. Finfer S, Chittock DR, Su SY, *et al.* Intensive versus conventional glucose control in critically ill patients. *N Engl J Med* 2009; 360 : 1283–97.

25. Qaseem A, Humphrey LL, Chou R, *et al.* Use of intensive insulin therapy for the management of glycemic control in hospitalized patients: a clinical practice guideline from the American College of Physicians. *Ann Intern Med* 2011; 154 : 260–7.

26. Katzberg RW, Haller C. Contrast-induced nephrotoxicity: clinical landscape. *Kidney Int* Suppl 2006 : S3–7.

27. Mehran R, Nikolsky E. Contrast-induced nephropathy: definition, epidemiology, and patients at risk. *Kidney Int Suppl* 2006 : S11–15.

28. Van Praet JT, De Vriese AS. Prevention of contrast-induced nephropathy: a critical review. *Curr Opin Nephrol Hypertens* 2007; 16 : 336–47.

29. Mohmand H, Goldfarb S. Renal dysfunction associated with intra-abdominal hypertension and the abdominal compartment syndrome. *J Am Soc Nephrol* 2011; 22 : 615–21.

30. Coiffier B, Altman A, Pui CH, *et al.* Guidelines for the management of pediatric and adult tumor lysis syndrome: an evidence-based review. *J Clin Oncol* 2008; 26 : 2767–78.

31. Cairo MS, Coiffier B, Reiter A, Younes A. Recommendations for the evaluation of risk and prophylaxis of tumour lysis syndrome (TLS) in adults and children with malignant diseases: an expert TLS panel consensus. *Br J Haematol* 2010; 149 : 578–86.

32. Vanholder R, Sever MS, Erek E, Lameire N. Rhabdomyolysis. *J Am Soc Nephrol* 2000; 11 : 1553–61.

33. Melli G, Chaudhry V, Cornblath DR. Rhabdomyolysis: an evaluation of 475 hospitalized patients. *Medicine (Baltimore)* 2005; 84 : 377–85.

34. Anton KA, Williams CD, Baker SK, Philips PS. Clinical perspectives of statin-induced rhabdomyolysis. *Am J Med* 2006; 119 : 400–9.

35. Bernal W, Auzinger G, Dhawan A, Wendon J. Acute liver failure. *Lancet* 2010; 376 : 190–201

36. Slack AJ, Auzinger G, Willars C *et al.* Ammonia clearance with haemofiltration in adults with liver disease. *Liver Int* 2013; 34 : 42–8.

37. Slack AJ, Wendon J. The liver and kidney in critically ill patients. *Blood Purif* 2009; 28 : 124–34.

38. Moore KP, Aithal GP. Guidelines on the management of ascites in cirrhosis. *Gut* 2006; 55 Suppl 6 : vi1–12.

39. Gluud LL, Christensen K, Christensen E, Krag A. Systematic review of randomized trials on vasoconstrictor drugs for hepatorenal syndrome. *Hepatology* 2010; 51 : 576–84.

30

Acute lung injury and ARDS

Raj Nichani, MJ Naisbitt and Chris Clarke

Definition of acute respiratory distress syndrome

- The syndrome formerly known as adult respiratory distress syndrome (ARDS) was first described in 1967.
- ARDS is a syndrome characterized by the development of noncardiogenic pulmonary edema resulting in acute hypoxia, bilateral chest infiltrates and respiratory distress.
- The consensus diagnostic criteria for ARDS were finally reached in 1994 with the publication of American European Consensus Criteria (AECC) [1]. Controversy, however, persisted around the reliability and validity of this definition, and as a result its use has recently been superseded. The 2012 Berlin definition of ARDS [2] addresses many of the shortcomings of the original AECC definition, yet is itself only marginally better at predicting mortality when compared to the AECC definition.

Diagnosis

The original AECC criteria (Table 30.1) differentiate acute lung injury (ALI) from ARDS simply by the PaO_2/FiO_2 or shunt fraction. Acute lung injury was characterized by less severe degrees of hypoxia and higher PaO_2/FiO_2 ratios. Additional criteria assessed the presence of bilateral infiltrates on CXR and the absence of a cardiac cause, as confirmed by a low pulmonary capillary wedge pressure (PCWP) or absence of left atrial hypertension. The AECC criteria allowed simple application to clinical trials and provided a degree of uniformity. They did not take into account the level of positive end-expiratory pressure (PEEP) applied, which in turn can influence the degree of recruitment and oxygenation. These criteria also fail to define a specific time cutoff for diagnosis of ARDS and do not stratify ARDS study populations with regard to severity of disease.

The 2012 Berlin definition of ARDS (Table 30.2) specifically takes into account time of onset of ARDS and clarifies the origin of edema whilst abandoning the use of PCWP. In addition, there is more clarity on the interpretation of chest imaging, and the oxygenation scores take into account the use of PEEP. The previous definition of ALI has been abandoned in favor of stratifying ARDS into a spectrum of mild, moderate and severe categories.

An alternate diagnostic score is the Murray lung injury score (LIS) [3], which is widely used in the literature There are four components to the LIS, however not all need to be assessed. A score between 1 and 4 is assigned for:

Handbook of ICU Therapy, third edition, ed. John Fuller, Jeff Granton and Ian McConachie. Published by Cambridge University Press. © Cambridge University Press 2015.

Table 30.1 AECC criteria

Criteria	Oxygenation	Chest radiograph	Pulmonary artery wedge pressure
ALI	PaO_2/FiO_2 ≤300 mmHg (regardless of PEEP level)	Bilateral infiltrates	<18 mmHg when measured (or no clinical evidence of left atrial hypertension)
ARDS	PaO_2/FiO_2 ≤200 mmHg (regardless of PEEP level)	Bilateral infiltrates	<18 mmHg when measured (or no clinical evidence of left atrial hypertension)

Table 30.2 Berlin criteria

Timing	Within 1 week of a known clinical insult or new or worsening respiratory symptoms
Chest imaging	Bilateral opacities not fully explained by effusions, collapse or nodules
Origin of edema	Respiratory failure not fully explained by cardiac failure or fluid overload
Oxygenation	Mild PaO_2/FiO_2 >200 mmHg or ≤ 300 mmHg with PEEP or CPAP ≥5 cmH_2O Moderate PaO_2/FiO_2 >100 mmHg or ≤200 mmHg with PEEP ≥5 cmH_2O Severe PaO_2/FiO_2 ≤100 mmHg with PEEP ≥5 cmH_2O

- Degree of hypoxia
- Lung infiltrates
- Level of PEEP
- Pulmonary compliance.

The total score is divided by the number of components assessed to give the LIS. A LIS >2.5 denotes ALI/ARDS, and a score ≥3 indicates severe disease.

Pre-dispositions to ARDS

Simply seen as a diffuse and overwhelming inflammatory reaction of the pulmonary parenchyma, almost any cause of shock or neutrophil activation can trigger the syndrome:

- The initial insult can be directly injurious to the pulmonary epithelium (e.g. aspiration or pneumonia).
- Alternatively the injury can result as part of an extrapulmonary systemic inflammatory process (e.g. sepsis).

Although there is undoubtedly overlap, the distinction is a focus of interest and there may be implications for ventilation strategies. Gattinoni has proposed that ARDS may be divided into pulmonary ($ARDS_p$) and extrapulmonary ($ARDS_{exp}$) lung injury [4].

- Patients with $ARDS_p$, typically complicating pneumonia, have stiff lungs and exhibit minimal recruitment with PEEP.
- $ARDS_{exp}$ patients have much greater chest wall stiffness, which correlates with the increased intra-abdominal pressure. $ARDS_{exp}$ patients exhibit significant recruitment with PEEP.

Table 30.3 Direct and indirect predispositions to ARDS

Direct lung injury	Indirect lung injury
Gastric aspiration	Sepsis
Severe pneumonia/pulmonary infection	Pancreatitis
	Hypovolemic shock
Smoke inhalation	Trauma
Pulmonary contusion	Fat embolism syndrome
Near-drowning	Burns
	Massive transfusion
	Transfusion-related acute lung injury (TRALI)
	Post-cardiopulmonary bypass

Although these concepts are exciting, studies looking at "medical" and "surgical" ARDS do not confirm Gattinoni's findings.

The primer or trigger for ARDS does affect outcome:

- The prognosis of ARDS following aspiration or trauma is better than that of ARDS complicating sepsis.
- Multiple or combined pulmonary and extrapulmonary insults confer drastically increased mortality.

Pre-dispositions to ARDS split into pulmonary and extrapulmonary causes (Table 30.3).

Incidence

The precise incidence of ARDS is not clear, as uniformity on diagnostic criteria has varied.

- One study estimated the crude incidence of ARDS at around 59 cases per 100 000 population per year in the US [5].
- Data from the UK ICNARC database suggests an estimated prevalence of approximately 70 cases per 100 000 [6].
- Certain pre-morbid factors, such as a history of alcohol abuse and increased severity of critical illness confer a significantly higher incidence of ARDS.

Pathophysiology

Acute respiratory distress syndrome has classically been described by three phases after the initial injury [7]:

1. Exudative phase
2. Proliferative phase
3. Fibrotic phase.

These phases are not distinct and the sequence of events is not fully understood.

- The initial injury to the alveolar epithelium can be direct or endothelially mediated.
- Rapid sequestration and activation of neutrophils as part of an inflammatory cascade involving numerous cytokines, chemokines, complement

activation, arachidonic acid metabolites and activation of the coagulation cascade leads to interstitial and alveolar edema.

- There is intra-alveolar release of superoxide radicals, proteases and other oxidants.
- Normal alveolar physiology is disrupted with the inhibition of surfactant production, destruction of type I alveolar cells and proliferation of type II cells. This results in alveolar collapse and derecruitment and increased vascular permeability. These changes are not uniform throughout West's gravitational zones and there may be areas of consolidation and alveolar collapse with near-normal lung adjacent to each other. This has been confirmed on computerized tomographic (CT) scan with the posterior dependent regions more extensively affected [8].
- Functionally, the patient may have a very limited area available for effective gas exchange, an important element of Gattinoni's "baby lung" hypothesis.
- ARDS is characterized by abnormal lung mechanics. Abnormal lung mechanics are classically demonstrated using static pressure–volume (PV) loops. It must be emphasized that obtaining these curves is essentially a research procedure involving the use of the "supersyringe" or multiple inert gas analysis (MIDGET) and these loops are not equivalent to the dynamic PV loops displayed by modern ventilators. Although PV loops have contributed much to our understanding of ARDS, unfortunately the values of the inflection points on the curve may vary depending on the technique used to obtain the curve [9].
- Collapsed, flooded, open-diseased and near-normal alveoli coexist throughout the lung. Each alveolus will have its own recruitment pressure and level of ventilation/perfusion mismatch related to the extent of disruption to its normal physiology and architecture and that of its neighbors (interdependence).
- Later stages of ARDS are characterized by the migration of myofibroblasts to the alveolar side of the basement membrane and disorganized deposition of collagens. There is subsequent organization of the exudates and abnormal lung repair of the pulmonary capillary membrane with fibrosis.
- Resolution of ARDS is slow. The alveolar edema is cleared and pulmonary membranes are remodeled. The regulation of this process is thought to be humoral.

Clinical features

- After an initial latent period of up to 72 hours, ARDS is a progressive disease.
- A predisposing factor followed by severe hypoxia refractory to oxygen therapy, increasing respiratory distress and reducing pulmonary compliance.
- Chest radiographs may show the classical whiteout picture of diffuse alveolar edema. The radiological appearance often lags behind the clinical picture and degree of hypoxia.
- The fibroproliferative stages of ARDS may disrupt the pulmonary capillary bed, increasing vascular resistance, leading to pulmonary hypertension and progressive right ventricular dysfunction.

Management

The management of the syndrome remains supportive and the importance of treating the predisposing condition cannot be overemphasized.

- The mainstay of management is currently centered on ventilation strategies that reduce ventilator-induced lung injury, possibly reducing the severity of ARDS [10] (discussed below). Assisted spontaneous ventilation and noninvasive positive-pressure ventilation are often sufficient to manage mild forms of ALI and resolving ARDS.
- Ventilator-associated pneumonia [11] and fibroproliferation can be difficult to differentiate between. Acute deterioration in a patient with ARDS should prompt thorough investigation. Pneumothoraces may only be detectable on CT scanning.
- Regular microbiological review, bronchoalveolar lavage and CT of the chest [12] play an important role.
- Many novel therapies have been tried, but little evidence supports their routine use.

Ventilation strategies

The two key components of current ventilation strategies are limitation of tidal volume (and airway pressure) and alveolar recruitment. Limitation of tidal volume with "permissive hypercapnia" was a landmark advance in our management of ARDS. During the 1990s the emphasis shifted from a concept of "barotrauma" to one of "volutrauma." Both these terms are now obsolete and have been replaced by a wider concept of ventilator-induced lung injury (VILI).

The open lung concept

- Traditional ventilation strategies employing low levels of PEEP and large tidal volumes (10–12 mL/kg predicted body weight) may be seen to overdistend compliant areas, whilst possibly not fully recruiting collapsed or flooded alveoli. "Shear stress" may exist between alveoli with differing recruitment pressures. Due to alveolar interdependence, shear stress can be dramatically increased where near-normal alveoli abut upon diseased alveoli [13].
- PV loops also demonstrate an upper inflection point (flattening of the PV curve). At this point there is near maximal recruitment and increasing overdistention of alveoli. Maximal inspiratory pressure should therefore be limited to just below this level. The AECC recommended limitation of transalveolar pressure to <35 cmH$_2$O.
- Limiting inspiratory pressure below the upper inflection point (UIP) and setting PEEP above the lower inflection point (LIP) is an attractive theory often referred to as open-lung ventilation.
- The ALVEOLI study undertaken by the ARDSNetwork attempted to delineate the importance of recruitment by PEEP in a low tidal volume strategy, but was terminated early due to lack of efficacy at its first interim analysis [14].
- Meta-analysis demonstrates that high levels of PEEP may be beneficial in severe ARDS and the ARMA ARDS network tidal volume trial utilized a ladder in which increasing needs for FiO$_2$ were matched to escalating levels of PEEP (FiO$_2$ 0.8 equating to 20–24 cmH$_2$O PEEP).

Limiting lung volumes

- Hickling, in retrospective and later prospective papers in the early 1990s demonstrated a significant decrease in mortality when tidal volume (and airway pressure) was limited [15].

The gold standard ventilation strategy was established by the ARDSNetwork study [10]:

- A group of 861 patients with ARDS were randomized to two groups: one receiving traditional tidal volumes of 12 mL/kg; the second low tidal volumes of 6 mL/kg (lowered to 4 mL/kg where necessary to achieve target airway pressure). Mortality in the traditional group was 39.8% at 28 days in comparison to 31% in the low-volume ventilation group.
- However, three other trials showed no improvement in outcome with protective strategies [16–18].
- Amato *et al.* also showed a relative-risk reduction in mortality with low tidal volume ventilation, but the mortality in the traditional group was unexpectedly very high (71%), limiting data interpretation [19].
- Comparison of the five trials shows that the two trials that showed benefit had greater differences in tidal volume and airway pressure between the groups than the three negative trials. The implication from these studies was that in the pursuit of normal blood gases, clinicians in the trials with negative benefits had inadvertently caused more VILI and increased the mortality of ARDS.
- An intriguing research observation is the demonstration that low tidal volume strategies may beneficially alter the pattern of inflammatory mediator release in the lung [20]. We have known for 20 years that the majority of ARDS patients die not of hypoxia, but of multiple organ failure. The concept that a traditional ventilatory strategy causes further release of inflammatory mediators with ongoing inflammation has been termed "biotrauma."

Lung recruitment

- Reversed I:E ratio ventilation can be utilized and frequently results in intrinsic or auto-PEEP, allowing alveolar recruitment. Prolonged inspiration may allow recruitment of alveoli with long time constants.
- Currently there is a resurgence of interest in airway pressure release ventilation (APRV), which has the potential to achieve lung protection goals whilst maximizing recruitment. Evidence of benefit remains elusive.

Despite recent advances in lung-protective ventilation strategies, critical oxygenation is commonplace in severe ARDS:

- Recruitment maneuvers involving the application of high continuous positive airway pressures for 30 s, intermittent sighs or large tidal volumes may improve oxygenation and lung mechanics, and can be useful following ventilator disconnection.
- The use of recruitment maneuvers has, however, not yet been shown to positively influence mortality outcomes in patients with ARDS. However, they have been shown to be beneficial in reducing the incidence of refractory hypoxia and use of rescue therapies if used as part of a combined strategy along with protective lung ventilation and high levels of PEEP [21].
- Recruitment maneuvers are not without risk. Hypotension and a fall in cardiac output resulting from a reduction in venous return can occur as a result of raised intrathoracic pressures. There is also the potential to cause barotrauma.

- Recruitment is an inspiratory maneuver. Positive end-expiratory pressure is applied in expiration. Response to a recruitment maneuver could indicate the need to apply more PEEP.

Hypercapnia

- Ventilation with low tidal volumes presents problems related to an inability to clear carbon dioxide. This is particularly problematic in patients with cranial injury.
- A degree of respiratory acidosis is tolerated, the so-called permissive hypercapnia. Intriguingly acidosis is protective to the lung in animal models. No consensus exists on the level of hypercapnia that is acceptable and it is of note that the protocol of the ARDSNet trial corrected the acidosis by infusing sodium bicarbonate.
- Infusion of bicarbonate has its own problems and should be administered slowly (if at all) to prevent worsening of intracellular acidosis and increased requirement for excretion of carbon dioxide.
- Extracorporeal CO_2 removal devices may have a role in treating hypercapnia associated with protective lung ventilation strategies. The first-generation devices used arterial access with associated risks such as lower-limb ischemia, bleeding, infection and vessel damage [22]. Whilst some of these problems can be minimized by ultrasound-guided assessment of cannula size to vessel diameter and the development of pumped systems, evidence of benefit is lacking. Current UK NICE guidance is that they should only be used in the setting of close governance frameworks and ongoing clinical trials.

In summary, an overall ventilator strategy derived chiefly from the ARDSNetwork group is presented in Table 30.4.

Adjuvant therapy
Fluid restriction

Once any period of shock has subsided, collective experience has shown that a conservative approach to fluid administration should be adopted. Substantial improvements in oxygenation are possible by achieving aggressive fluid deficits using diuretics or renal replacement technologies. Additional improvements may be possible through the coadministration of human salt-poor albumin.

- The FAACT trial [23] demonstrated that patients treated with a conservative fluid strategy had improved oxygenation parameters and a reduction in the duration of mechanical ventilation, as compared to those on the liberal fluid strategy.
- Administration of excessive fluid is likely to be detrimental to lung function. In the UK CESAR trial patients randomized to the treatment center for consideration of ECMO (but in whom ECMO was not instituted) were run "dry" with high hemoglobin levels resulting in improved mortality, despite mean LIS >3.5. The CESAR trial is further discussed below.

Prone positioning

Ventilation in the prone position may improve oxygenation in some patients allowing the reduction of inspired oxygen and PEEP. The exact mechanism is unclear, but:

Table 30.4 ARDSNet ventilatory strategy. Adapted from [13]

Variable	Setting	Comment
Ventilator mode	Volume-assist control	Pressure-controlled modes are in widespread use in many centres
Tidal volume (mL/kg)	6	Reduced if necessary to keep plateau pressure <30 cmH$_2$O
Plateau pressure	<30 cmH$_2$O	
Rate	6–35	High rates may have generated auto-PEEP
I:E ratio	1:1 to 1:3	
Oxygenation target		
PaO$_2$ (kPa)	7.3–10.7	
SpO$_2$ (%)	88–95	
PEEP and FiO$_2$	Set according to a predetermined table	Range 5–24 cmH$_2$O

- The prone position may increase functional residual capacity (FRC)
- It may increase recruitment of previously "protected" lung zones
- There is redistribution of alveolar edema
- There is a decrease in the physiological shunt.

Previous studies reported beneficial effects in oxygenation, but no improvement in outcome [24,25]. However, further systematic review and meta-analysis suggest a survival benefit in those with severe hypoxemia [26]. Moreover, a recently published randomized trial in patients with severe ARDS has shown a significant reduction in 28-day and 90-day mortality in patients randomized to a protocol including early and relatively long periods of proning with no significant adverse effects [27].

- Proning is not without logistical and clinical pitfalls (pressure sores, facial edema, nerve damage, tube and line displacement, and decompensation on return to the supine position).
- Whether proning is to be used not only as a rescue therapy for patients with severe hypoxia, but as an integral part of a protocolized management plan with early severe ARDS will depend to a large extent on the local experience of individual units.

High-frequency oscillatory ventilation

High-frequency oscillatory ventilation (HFOV) may be regarded as an extreme form of lung-protective ventilation.

High-frequency oscillatory ventilation oscillates the lung around a constant mean airway pressure, usually higher than that applied in conventional ventilation. The pressure swings are attenuated before reaching the alveoli and HFOV may prevent VILI, reduce "biotrauma" and may be useful in the presence of air leak. Tidal volume is usually in the range of 1–3 mL/kg [28].

Two recently reported randomized trials have assessed the efficacy of oscillation in ARDS.

- The OSCAR trial [29] compared HFOV against conventional ventilation in patients with moderate to severe ARDS (PaO_2/FiO_2 ratio ~200 mmHg). Although HFOV did improve oxygenation, this did not translate into a survival benefit, with no difference in the primary outcome of 30-day mortality between groups, 41.7% in the HFOV arm versus 41.1% in the conventional arm.
- The OSCILLATE trial also assessed patients with moderate to severe ARDS. This trial showed a statistically significant higher mortality in the HFOV group, 47% versus 35% in the control group. The control group in this trial received higher levels of PEEP and lower tidal volumes, as compared to those in the OSCAR trial and this may have contributed to the lower mortality in the control arm. Patients in the HFOV arm in this study were more likely to receive vasopressors, neuromuscular blockers and require more sedation.

High-frequency oscillatory ventilation is still used as a form of rescue therapy in patients with severe ARDS. Its role in the treatment of ARDS is now under increasing scrutiny, however, with some authors suggesting that it may be harmful in this situation.

Inhaled nitric oxide

Theoretically the administration of inhaled nitric oxide (iNO) to the ARDS patient is an attractive one:

- There is selective vasodilatation in ventilated lung areas redistributing blood to ventilated regions and improving the shunt fraction.
- The subsequent reduction in pulmonary arterial hypertension may allow improvements in right ventricular dysfunction.

Four prospective randomized, controlled studies demonstrated that iNO significantly increased oxygenation for up to 24 h, but no differences in outcome were detectable between the iNO and control groups. One study reported that patients treated with iNO had a greater requirement for renal replacement therapy [31]. A large study of almost 400 patients concluded that iNO was associated with short-term oxygenation improvements, but had no substantial impact on the duration of ventilatory support or mortality [32]. Further systematic reviews have confirmed transient oxygenation benefits, but no overall mortality benefit with its use [33,34].

Extracorporeal membrane oxygenation (ECMO)

The CESAR trial [35] aimed to assess the safety and efficacy of ECMO, as compared to conventional ventilation in the treatment of severe ARDS.

- Inclusion criteria included adult patients with severe but reversible respiratory failure (LIS >3).
- Exclusion criteria include prolonged high-pressure and high-inspired-oxygen ventilation, intracranial hemorrhage or other contraindications to heparinization.

Patients were randomized to receive either consideration of treatment by ECMO and transfer to a specialist ECMO center or to conventional management in local hospitals.

Sixty-three percent (57/90) of patients in the former group survived to 6 months without disability, compared to 47% (41/87) of those conventionally managed.

- Of note only 75% of patients in the consideration of treatment by ECMO group actually received ECMO and patients in this group were more likely to be treated with standard lung-protective strategies, protocolized care and to receive steroids and liver support with molecular albumin recirculating system (MARS).

- The intervention arm patients transferred to the treatment center that were deemed not to need ECMO had an associated survival rate of 80% (14/17), substantially better survival that the ARDSNet trial. Why might this be so? In a personal communication, one of the trial authors reported that, as part of the process of readying a patient for ECMO, they routinely transfused their patients to a higher Hb to improve O_2 carriage, as on ECMO, oxyhemoglobin saturations run at 80–85%. In combination with other confounding therapies (iNO, positional changes and aggressively promoting a negative fluid balance) they often successfully bridged a patient through to improvement and ECMO was then not required to meet treatment goals.

- This trial result suggests that patients with severe ARDS exposed to evidence-based protocolized care, including ECMO, may have improved combined functional and mortality outcomes. It is also hypothesis-generating as to whether regional pulmonary failure treatment centers are effective in the treatment of severe ARDS.

Drug therapies

Neuromuscular blockers

A recent multicentre randomized trial [36] showed that a short course of therapy (48 hours) with cisatracurium in patients with early, severe ARDS improved the adjusted 90-day survival rate and increased the number of ventilator-free days without increasing the subsequent risk of muscle weakness. It is postulated that neuromuscular blockade may help by improving patient–ventilator interactions and reducing lung inflammation. Recent meta-analysis of this and other trials by the same investigatory team appears to confirm their findings.

$β_2$ agonists

- There was a theoretically attractive rationale for the use of β-agonists in ARDS demonstrated in the 2006 BALTI trial [37]. Extravascular lung water was reduced through the administration of IV salbutamol. This is thought to be mediated by promoting fluid clearance across the alveo-capillary membrane through cAMP upregulation, hence improving pulmonary mechanics. $β_2$ agonists are also postulated to have "anti-inflamatory" properties.

- The ARDSNetwork group randomized 282 patients to treatment with nebulized albuterol or placebo [38]. They were unable to demonstrate any increase in ventilator-free days or decrease in mortality and the trial was terminated for futility.

- Subsequently the UK BALTI-2 trial was published [39]. In this multicenter RCT patients were randomized to 7 days treatment with intravenous salbutamol or placebo. The trial was stopped at the second interim analysis when an increase in 28-day mortality with intravenous salbutamol was demonstrated.

Thus, there is no rationale for "routine" inhaled β-agonists in ARDS and intravenous β-agonists are harmful. β-agonists have joined an increasing group of drugs, n-acetylcysteine, ketoconazole and surfactant, that have shown initial promise but failed to subsequently demonstrate clinical benefit.

Steroids in ARDS

Steroids through their anti-inflammatory mechanism of action have been postulated to reduce inflammation and fibroproliferation in ARDS. A small series and a subsequent small RCT showed an outcome advantage not confirmed in larger trials.

In a randomized trial of 180 patients with ARDS, the administration of methyl prednisolone between 7 to 28 days post-onset did not improve 60-day survival [40]. Methyl prednisolone, however, did improve cardiorespiratory physiology, leading to an increase in ventilator-free days and shock-free days. Patients treated with methyl prednisolone were more likely to be able to progress to ventilator independence, but conversely also more likely to need the reinstitution of ventilatory support. While there appears to be no increase in infectious complications associated with steroid use, there does appear to be an increased severity of neuromuscular weakness in patients in the steroid arm. It is important that patients are infection-free prior to consideration of commencement of methyl prednisolone. Patients who were reventilated had a poor outcome, and institution of steroids more than 14 days after the onset of ARDS seemed to worsen outcome.

Outcome

In the NHLI institute trial of 1974–1977, survival was 11%. The mortality of ARDS appears to have progressively declined in subsequent decades. Extracorporeal oxygenation trials demonstrated a survival of 45% by 1991 and 63% of patients in the 2009 CESAR treatment group survived [35]. In the ARDSNet trial mortality was 31% in the low-volume ventilation group. The UK OSCAR [29] trial had a 41% mortality in the conventional arm and the recent PROSEVA prone trial [27] demonstrated a mortality of 32.5% in the control arm. This improved mortality undoubtedly reflects a greater understanding of lung-protective ventilation strategies. There have also been multiple improvements in the global quality of supportive care through innovations such as ventilator care bundles, daily checklists, improved fluid management and increased specialist intensivist input in critical care units. The effect of these positive confounding variables is undoubtedbly significant.

References

1. Bernard GR, Artigas A, Brigham KL et al. The American–European Consensus Conference on ARDS: definitions, mechanisms, relevant outcomes and clinical trial co-ordination. Am J Respir Crit Care Med 1994; 149 : 818–24.

2. The ARDS definition task force. Acute respiratory distress syndrome: the Berlin definition. J Am Med Assoc 2012; 307 : 2526–33

3. Murray JF, Matthay MA, Luce JM et al. An expanded definition of the adult respiratory distress syndrome. Am Rev Respir Dis 1998; 138 : 720–3.

4. Gattinoni L, Pelosi P, Suter PM et al. Acute respiratory distress syndrome caused by pulmonary and extrapulmonary disease. Different syndromes? Am J Respir Crit Care Med 1998; 158 : 3–11.

5. Rubenfeld GD, Caldwell E, Peabody E et al. Incidence and outcomes of acute lung injury. New Eng J Med 2005; 353 : 1685–93.

6. Management of severe refractory hypoxia in critical care in the UK in 2010 – Report from the expert group. http://www.wyccn.

nhs.uk/Emergency%20Planning,%20incl.%
20Flu/Mngmnt%20of%20Severe%
20Refractory%20Hypoxia%20in%20CC%
20in%20UK%202010.pdf (accessed July
2014).

7. Wright JL. The pathology of ARDS.
In: Russell JA, Walley RW, editors.
Acute Respiratory Distress Syndrome.
Cambridge: Cambridge University
Press; 1999.

8. Gattinoni L, Pelosi P. Pathophysiologic
insights into acute respiratory failure. *Curr
Opin Crit Care* 1996; 2 : 8–12.

9. Dreyfuss D, Saumon G. Pressure–volume
curves: searching for the grail or laying
patients with ARDS on proscruste's bed?
Am J Respir Crit Care Med 2001; 163 : 2–3.

10. Brower RG, Matthay MA, Morris A et al.
Ventilation with lower tidal volumes as
compared with traditional tidal volumes
for acute lung injury and the acute
respiratory distress syndrome. *New Eng
J Med* 2000; 342 : 1301–8.

11. Markowicz P, Wolff M, Djedaini et al.
Multicenter prospective study of ventilator
associated pneumonia during acute
respiratory distress syndrome. *Am J Respir
Crit Care Med* 2000; 161 : 1942–8.

12. Presenti A, Tagliabue P, Patroniti N et al.
Computerised tomography scan imaging in
acute respiratory distress syndrome. *Int
Care Med* 2001; 27 : 631–9.

13. Moloney ED, Griffiths MJD. Protective
ventilation of patients with acute
respiratory distress syndrome. *Br J Anaesth*
2004; 92 : 261–70.

14. The ARDS Clinical Trials Network;
National Heart, Lung and Blood Institute;
National Institutes of Health. Effects of
recruitment manoeuvres in patients with
acute lung injury and the acute respiratory
distress syndrome ventilated with high
positive endexpiratory pressure. *Crit Care
Med* 2003; 31 : 2592–7.

15. Hickling KG, Walsh J, Henderson S et al.
Low mortality rate in adult respiratory
distress syndrome using low volume
pressure limited ventilation with
permissive hypercapnia; a prospective
study. *Crit Care Med* 1994; 22 : 1568–78.

16. Stewart TE, Meade MO, Cook DJ et al.
Evaluation of a ventilation strategy to
prevent barotraumas in patients at high
risk for acute respiratory distress
syndrome. *New Eng J Med* 1998; 338 :
355–61.

17. Brower RG, Shanholtz CB, Fessler HE et al.
Prospective, randomized, controlled
clinical trial comparing traditional versus
reduced tidal volume ventilation in acute
respiratory distress syndrome patients. *Crit
Care Med* 1999; 27 : 1492–8.

18. Brochard L, Roudot-Thoraval F, Roupie E
et al. Tidal volume reduction for
prevention of ventilator-induced lung
injury in acute respiratory distress
syndrome. *Am J Respir Crit Care Med* 1998;
158 : 1831–8.

19. Amato M, Barbas C, Medeiros D et al.
Effect of a protective ventilation strategy on
mortality in the acute respiratory distress
syndrome. *New Eng J Med* 1998; 338 :
347–54.

20. Ranieri VM, Suter PM, Tortorella C et al.
Effect of Mechanical ventilation on
inflammatory mediators in patients with
acute respiratory distress syndrome: a
randomised controlled trial. *J Am Med
Assoc* 1999; 282 : 54–61.

21. Meade MO, Cook DJ, Guyatt GH et al.
Ventilation strategy using low tidal
volumes, recruitment maneuvers and high
positive end-expiratory pressure for acute
lung injury and acute respiratory distress
syndrome: a randomised controlled trial.
J Am Med Assoc 2008; 299 : 637–45.

22. NICE interventional procedure guidance
428. Extra corporeal membrane carbon
dioxide removal. guidance.nice.org.uk/
ipg428 (accessed June 2014).

23. The National Heart, Lung and Blood
Institute Acute Respiratory distress
Syndrome (ARDS) Clinical Trials network.
Comparison of two fluid management
strategies in acute lung injury. *New Eng
J Med* 2006; 354 : 2564–75.

24. Gattinoni L, Tognoni G, Presenti A et al.
Effect of prone positioning on the survival
of patients with acute respiratory failure.
New Eng J Med 2001; 345 : 568–73.

25. Taccone P, Pesenti A, Latini R *et al.* Prone positioning in patients with moderate and severe acute respiratory distress syndrome: a randomised controlled trial. *J Am Med Assoc* 2009; 302 : 1977–84.

26. Sud S, Friedrich JO, Taccone P *et al.* Prone ventilation reduces mortality in patients with acute respiratory failure and severe hypoxemia: systematic review and meta-analysis. *Intensive Care Med* 2010; 36 : 585–99.

27. Guérin C, Reignier J, Richard J-C *et al.* Prone positioning in severe acute respiratory distress syndrome. *N Engl J Med* 2013; 368 : 2159–68.

28. Derdak S, Mehta S, Stewart TE *et al.* High frequency oscillatory ventilation for acute respiratory distress syndrome in adults. *Am J Respir Crit Care Med* 2002; 166 : 801–8.

29. Young D, Lamb S, Shah S *et al.* High Frequency Oscillation for Acute Respiratory Distress Syndrome. *New Eng J Med* 2013; 368 : 806–13.

30. Ferguson ND, Cook JC, Guyatt GH *et al.* High-Frequency Oscillation in Early Acute Respiratory Distress Syndrome. *New Eng J Med* 2013; 268 : 795–805.

31. Afshari A, Brok J, Møller AM, Wetterslev J. Inhaled nitric oxide for acute respiratory distress syndrome (ARDS) and acute lung injury in children and adults. *Cochrane Database Syst Rev.* 2010 Jul 7;(7): CD002787.

32. Taylor RW, Zimmerman JL, Dellinger RP *et al.* Low-dose inhaled nitric oxide in patients with acute lung injury: a randomized controlled trial. *J Am Med Assoc* 2004; 291 : 1629–31.

33. Adhikari NKJ, Burns KEA, Friedrich JO *et al.* Effect of nitric oxide on oxygenation and mortality in acute lung injury: systematic review and meta-analysis. *BMJ* 2007; 334 : 779.

34. Ashrafi A, Brok J, Møller AM *et al.* Inhaled nitric oxide for acute respiratory distress syndrome and acute lung injury: a systematic review with meta-analysis and trial sequential analysis. *Anesth Analg* 2011; 112 : 1411–21.

35. Peek GJ, Mugford M, Tiruvoioati R *et al.* Efficacy and economic assessment of conventional ventilatory support versus extracorporeal membrane oxygenation for severe adult respiratory failure (CESAR): a multicentre randomised controlled trial. *Lancet* 2009; 374 : 1351–63.

36. Papazian L, Forel J-M, Gacouin A *et al.* Neuromuscular blockers in early acute respiratory distress syndrome. *New Eng J Med* 2010; 363 : 1107–16.

37. Perkins GD, McAuley DF, Thickett DR, Gao F. The beta-agonist lung injury trial (BALTI): a randomized placebo-controlled clinical trial. *Am J Respir Crit Care Med* 2006; 173 : 281–7.

38. Matthay MA, Brower RG, Carson S *et al.* Randomized, placebo-controlled clinical trial of an aerosolized β-agonist for treatment of acute lung injury. *Am J Respir Crit Care Med* 2011; 184 : 561–8.

39. Gao Smith F, Perkins GD, Gates S *et al.* Effect of intravenous β-2 agonist treatment on clinical outcomes in acute respiratory distress syndrome (BALTI-2): a multicentre, randomised controlled trial. *Lancet* 2012; 379 : 229–35.

40. The National Heart, Lung and Blood Institute Acute Respiratory Distress Syndrome (ARDS) Clinical Trials Network. Efficacy and safety of corticosteroids for persistent acute respiratory distress syndrome. *New Eng J Med* 2006; 354 : 1671–84.

The patient with gastrointestinal problems

Biniam Kidane and Tina Mele

The most common gastrointestinal (GI) disorders encountered in patients admitted to the ICU will be reviewed in this chapter.

Gastrointestinal bleeding

Critically ill patients are at particular risk for developing stress-induced ulcers in the upper GI tract and hypotension-induced ischemia of the colon.

- Gastrointestinal bleeding is classified into upper GI bleeding (blood source proximal to the ligament of Treitz) or lower GI bleeding (blood loss distal to ligament of Treitz).
- This classification is useful, as the two sources usually have different presentations, require different investigations and ultimately, different treatment strategies.

Upper GI bleeds

- The majority of GI bleeds in critically ill patients are due to an upper GI source.
- An upper GI bleed usually presents as hematemesis or coffee-ground emesis. Occasionally, a rapid upper GI bleed can present as bright red blood per rectum.
- Ulcers in the stomach and/or duodenum and gastroesophageal varices are the most common causes of significant upper GI bleeding that require ICU admission.
- Other causes of upper GI bleeding include stress gastritis, esophagitis, Mallory–Weiss tear, angiodysplasia, including gastric antral vascular ectasia (GAVE), Dieulafoy's lesion and mass lesions.
- Urgent esophagogastroduodenoscopy for an acute upper GI bleed is often diagnostic and has potential therapeutic capabilities.

Lower GI bleeds

- A lower GI bleed usually presents as melena or bright red blood per rectum.
- Lower GI bleeds most likely to produce significant bleeding that requires ICU admission are usually due to diverticula or angiodysplasia. Other causes include neoplasia or colitis.
- Colonoscopy for an acute lower GI bleed is often difficult due to active bleeding or an inadequately prepped colon impairing adequate visualization.
- A tagged red blood cell (RBC) scan or angiography are alternative investigations to localize the site of the lower GI bleed. A tagged RBC scan will detect bleeding

Handbook of ICU Therapy, third edition, ed. John Fuller, Jeff Granton and Ian McConachie. Published by Cambridge University Press. © Cambridge University Press 2015.

>0.1 mL/min, but does not offer any therapeutic options. Angiography is more accurate than an RBC scan at localizing the site of bleeding, but will only detect bleeding >0.5 mL/min. Angioembolization is a potential therapeutic option during angiogram, but does carry a risk of colonic ischemia.

Management of gastrointestinal bleeding in the ICU

General principles of management

- First and foremost, ensure the patient has a patent airway which can be a particular concern in patients with massive upper GI bleeding.
- Re-establish intravascular volume via large bore peripheral intravenous access (at least 18 gauge) with crystalloid fluids initially. A patient who is tachycardic has lost at least 20% of total blood volume. Hypotension indicates the patient has lost at least 40% of total blood volume.
- RBC transfusion should be considered for hemoglobin ≤70 mg/dL [1].
- Transfuse platelets when values are below 50 000/mm^3 in an actively bleeding patient.
- Correct or reverse any coagulopathy and discontinue any antiplatelet or anticoagulant medications.
- Arrange for endoscopy to confirm source of bleeding.
- Institute definitive treatment based on etiology.

Stress-induced ulceration

Critically ill patients are at increased risk for developing stress ulcers in the stomach and duodenum.

- Mechanical ventilation >48 hours and coagulopathy are the two major risk factors for developing stress ulcers. Other risk factors include hypotension, sepsis, liver failure, renal failure, severe burns, organ transplantation and trauma [2].
- Prophylaxis therapy includes either histamine-2 receptor antagonists (H2RAs) or proton-pump inhibitors (PPIs). The latter have been shown to be superior to H2RAs in reducing the incidence of upper GI bleeding in critically ill patients [3].

Gastroesophageal varices

- Varices are the source of bleeding in 50 to 90% of cirrhotic patients with upper GI bleeding.
- Treatment options include medications, endoscopy, balloon tamponade, transjugular intrahepatic portosystemic shunting (TIPS) and surgery.

Medications

Vasopressin and terlipressin

- Vasopressin directly constricts mesenteric arterioles and decreases portal venous inflow, which leads to reduced portal pressures. Vasopressin will achieve initial hemostasis in 60 to 80% of patients, but has minimal effects on rebleeding risk and does not improve survival from active variceal hemorrhage [4]. Furthermore, vasopressin has potentially significant risks due to its extrasplanchnic vasoconstrictive effects and resultant myocardial, cerebral, bowel and limb ischemia. Thus, vasopressin has been replaced by somatostatin or its analog, octreotide.

- Terlipressin, a synthetic analog of vasopressin, has a sustained effect on portal pressure and blood flow and thus is preferred in countries where it is available, since it is the only pharmacologic treatment associated with a reduction in mortality compared with placebo [4].

Somatostatin and octreotide

- Somatostatin inhibits the release of vasodilator hormones, indirectly causing splanchnic vasoconstriction and decreased portal inflow. However, it has a short half-life and disappears within minutes of a bolus infusion. Somatostatin has an increased probability of achieving initial control of the bleeding and an absence of side effects compared to vasopressin or balloon tamponade [5].
- Octreotide, a long-acting analog of somatostatin, is given as a 50 µg bolus followed by a continuous infusion of 50 µg/h.

Infection and use of prophylactic antibiotics

- Bacterial infections occur in up to 20% of patients with cirrhosis hospitalized with GI bleeding; up to an additional 50% develop an infection while hospitalized.
- Most common sites include: urinary tract infections (12–29%), spontaneous bacterial peritonitis (7–23%), respiratory infections (6–10%) and primary bacteremia (4–11%).
- Antibiotic prophylaxis is associated with decreased mortality, bacterial infections, rebleeding risk and days of hospitalization. Thus, antibiotic prophylaxis is recommended in any patient with cirrhosis and GI hemorrhage [6]. Common treatment regimens include oral norfloxacin (400 mg twice daily), intravenous ciprofloxacin or intravenous ceftriaxone (1 g/day).

Endoscopic therapy

Endoscopic therapy is the definitive treatment of choice for active variceal hemorrhage. Two modes of endoscopic treatment are commonly used, sclerotherapy and variceal band ligation:

- Sclerotherapy involves injection of a sclerosant solution into the varices through an injection needle placed through an endoscope.
- Variceal band ligation involves placing small elastic bands around varices in the distal esophagus.
- Endoscopic treatment is successful in 80–90% of patients. If unsuccessful, a second attempt at endoscopic control can be considered. If bleeding persists, balloon tamponade or transjugular intrahepatic portosystemic shunt (TIPS) should be considered.

Balloon tamponade

- Achieves short-term hemostasis and temporary stabilization of patients until more definitive treatment can be instituted.

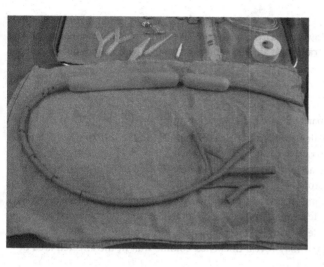

Figure 31.1 Minnesota tube used for balloon tamponade.

- Temporary control of variceal bleeding with balloon tamponade is achieved in 30–90% of patients. Initial control of active bleeding and patient stabilization with balloon tamponade must be followed by a definitive therapy such as endoscopy or TIPS.
- Pressure can be applied to varices by balloon inflation and traction on the tube.

Two commonly used tubes are available:

- Sengstaken–Blakemore tube: an esophageal balloon, a gastric balloon and a gastric aspiration port
- Minnesota four-lumen tube: esophageal and gastric balloons, esophageal and gastric aspiration ports (Figure 31.1)

Transjugular intrahepatic portosystemic shunt (TIPS)

- Decompression of the portal venous system is achieved by passing a needle catheter via the transjugular route into the hepatic vein, advanced through the liver parenchyma to the intrahepatic portion of the portal vein.
- Hemostasis is achieved in the majority of patients with refractory variceal hemorrhage.

Surgery

Rarely, surgery may be considered when variceal bleeding has been refractory to all other measures. There are two basic types of operation: shunt operations and nonshunt operations.

- Nonshunt operations generally include either esophageal transection (the distal esophagus is transected and then stapled back together) or devascularization of the gastroesophageal junction.
- Several shunt operations have been described, all of which aim to decompress the portal venous system.

- Both portal decompressive surgery and esophageal transection are highly effective in achieving hemostasis. However, portal decompressive surgery alters vascular anatomy, complicates future liver transplant surgery, and is associated with a 40 to 50% incidence of encephalopathy.

Ischemic colitis

Critically ill patients are at particular risk due to compromised arterial supply to the colon.

- This usually occurs in patients with atherosclerotic disease in the setting of hypotension in combination with vasoactive drugs.
- Patients develop crampy abdominal pain followed by passage of bright red blood or dark blood mixed with stool.
- If ischemia continues to progress, abdominal distension and peritonitis develop. This is usually accompanied by fever, leukocytosis and elevated serum lactate levels.
- Abdominal X-rays may demonstrate "thumbprinting," indicating submucosal edema.
- A CT scan of the abdomen may reveal thickened colonic wall in the affected area or pneumatosis intestinalis.
- All segments of the colon can be affected, but the majority of cases are in the "watershed" segments, which include the splenic flexure and rectosigmoid junction.
- The majority of patients have mild–moderate ischemia that is reversible with supportive measures.
- Patients with transmural ischemia will require urgent laparotomy for resection.

Clostridium difficile infection

The range of disease associated with *Clostridium difficile* infection (CDI) can range from mild *C. difficile*-associated diarrhea to severe fulminant or toxic colitis.

Although several clinical parameters have been used to classify CDIs, there are currently no widely accepted consensus definitions.

- Clinical parameters used to classify CDIs include evidence of acute kidney injury, fever, severe abdominal pain and hypoalbuminemia [7].
- Some studies have used management in an ICU as a sufficient criterion for severe CDI [8].
- Almost all definitions include the criterion of increased leukocyte count above 15 000 or 20 000 cells/μL [7].
- Although the classic presentation of CDI is diarrhea, patients with moderate-severe CDI can present with lack of diarrhea or even constipation, due to the ileus induced by the CDI [9].
- These issues are important with respect to both diagnosis and management in the ICU setting.

Diagnosis

The major risk factors for CDI include: recent use of antibiotics, older age (≥60) and use of proton-pump inhibitors (PPIs) [10,11].

- CDI can occur up to 3 months following cessation of antibiotic; the highest risk is during the time period of actual antibiotic use and the first month thereafter [8].

- Given that most ICU patients: (1) are currently or have recently been on antibiotics, (2) tend to be older and (3) are receiving PPIs, CDI should be considered as part of the differential diagnosis in an ICU patient with significant leukocytosis with or without evidence of diarrhea.

Medical management

- Oral metronidazole (500 mg three times daily) is the first-line therapy for CDI.
- Due to metronidazole's biliary excretion and to the effect of the entero-hepatic circulation, intravenous metronidazole (500 mg every 8 hours) can be used effectively, especially in a setting where oral metronidazole cannot be given or is not tolerated [12,13].
- Oral vancomycin (125 mg up to 500 mg four times daily) can be used as first-line therapy for ICU patients with CDI, whether or not they meet all criteria for moderate-severe CDI based on several observations:
  - Metronidazole has a much higher failure rate than vancomycin in moderate-severe CDI [7,14].
  - A growing body of literature suggests that earlier surgical intervention is associated with better outcomes [15,16]. Thus, it would be prudent to use the antibiotic with the highest likelihood of successful CDI eradication as a first-line agent rather than delay time to surgery with multiple rounds of antibiotic attempts.
  - Intravenous vancomycin is not effective as it is not excreted by the colon; however, oral/enteral vancomycin is not absorbed systemically and thus produces high levels in the colon. For this reason, intracolonic vancomycin (via enema) has also been shown to be effective [17,18].
- Duration of antibiotic therapy should be at least 10–14 days [7].
- If there is ongoing need for use of other antibiotics, CDI therapy should be continued for at least 1 week after the cessation of the other antibiotics [7].

Surgical management

Indications for surgical intervention include: perforation, toxic megacolon, peritonitis and/ or rapidly progressive CDI that is unresponsive to optimal antibiotic therapy [19].

- Traditionally, the definitive surgical management of severe CDI has been subtotal colectomy with end ileostomy [19,20]. However, patients with severe CDI requiring surgery have an approximately 50% mortality [19,20].
- Recent observational studies have suggested that a better alternative may be creation of loop ileostomy and intraoperative colonic lavage with polyethylene glycol through the ileostomy followed by post-operative vancomycin through the ileostomy [16]. This approach resulted in lower morbidity and mortality, as compared to subtotal colectomy with only minimal risk of a salvage subtotal colectomy [16].
- In any case, there is increasing evidence to suggest that earlier surgical intervention (i.e. within 48 hours of failure of medical management) is associated with lower morbidity and mortality. Thus, early surgical consultation is recommended when CDI is diagnosed in the ICU patient.

Intra-abdominal hypertension (IAH) and abdominal compartment syndrome (ACS)

The normal intra-abdominal pressure (IAP) in the ICU population is 5–7 mmHg; IAP should be measured as follows:

- At end-expiration
- Completely supine
- With absent abdominal muscle contractions
- Via bladder (i.e. foley catheter) with installation of saline (max 25–50 mL)
- Transducer zeroed at level of mid-axillary line.

Intra-abdominal hypertension is defined as sustained IAP >12 mmHg. Abdominal compartment syndrome is defined as sustained IAP >20 mmHg, *and* new organ dysfunction or failure:

- Renal failure: oliguria despite volume repletion
- Respiratory failure: difficulty ventilating, elevated peak airway pressures, hypercarbia, hypoxemia refractory to oxygen and PEEP
- Cardiovascular instability
- Metabolic acidosis despite resuscitation
- Intracranial hypertension.

Primary ACS is due to disease originating in the abdomen and/or pelvis (e.g. hemoperitoneum, pancreatitis) and usually requires early surgical/percutaneous intervention. Secondary ACS is due to increasing IAH due to disease originating outside of the abdomen and pelvis (e.g. sepsis, massive fluid resuscitation).

Risk factors for IAH/ACS:

- Decreased abdominal wall compliance (e.g. major trauma/burns, high intrathoracic pressures)
- Increased intraluminal contents (e.g. ileus)
- Increased abdominal contents (e.g. ascites, hemoperitoneum)
- Capillary leak (e.g. sepsis, pancreatitis, massive transfusion/resuscitation)

If ≥2 risk factors for IAH/ACS, measure IAP
If IAH present, continue serial measurement of IAP.

Medical management of IAH/ACS [21,22]

1. Nasogastric tube ± rectal tube (especially if ileus/Ogilvie's is the etiology of IAH):
   - Consider advanced decompression (via endoscopy)
2. Limit fluid volume:
   - Consider hypertonic saline and colloids
   - Consider diuresis
3. Sedation and analgesia
4. Optimize positioning:
   - Avoid prone position
   - Consider reverse Trendelenburg.
5. Consider using neuromuscular relaxant drugs.

Surgical management of ACS [21,22]

1. Percutaneous drainage of intra-abdominal fluid, blood or abscess
2. Surgical decompression:
   - Opening of abdomen
   - Evacuation of intra-abdominal fluid, blood or abscess
3. Preventative strategy:
   - Patients that are undergoing laparotomy and are at high risk for IAH/ACS should be considered for leaving the abdomen open.

Acute pancreatitis

- Acute inflammation of the pancreas that presents with acute onset of severe epigastric pain and elevated pancreatic enzymes, amylase and/or lipase. The severity of the disease ranges from mild to the severe, necrotizing form that carries a mortality of up to 45%.
- Most attacks are mild in severity and resolve within 5–7 days.

Etiology

The majority of cases (~70%) can be attributed to gallstones or alcohol abuse. Other common causes include:

- Traumatic: post-endoscopic retrograde cholangiopancreatography (post-ERCP), abdominal trauma, surgery
- Metabolic: hypertriglyceridemia, hypercalcemia
- Drug-induced: thiazide diuretics, azathioprine, mercaptopurine
- Infection: mumps, rubella, hepatitis, Epstein–Barr virus, cytomegalovirus
- Ischemic: following hemorrhagic shock, CABG, vascular surgery
- Autoimmune/vasculitis
- Idiopathic accounts for ~10% of cases.

Predicting severity of disease

Several scoring systems exist to predict severity of acute pancreatitis.

- Each system has their limitations, but most have been shown to be better predictors of disease severity than clinical judgment.
- Newer scoring systems incorporating CT findings (e.g. based on degree of necrosis) exist. However, their test characteristics have not been shown to be superior to clinical scoring systems like APACHE II. Furthermore, CT evidence of pancreatic necrosis may be delayed and thus limits the triaging capabilities of CT-based scores.

The most accepted scoring systems are: Ranson's criteria (Table 31.1) and APACHE II score:

- Most widely used and accepted scoring system for pancreatitis in the ICU population
- Very good positive predictive value and moderate negative predictive value
- Can predict the rise and fall of disease

Table 31.1 Ranson's criteria

	Nonbiliary	Biliary
At admission		
Age (yr)	>55	>70
White cell count	>16 000 cells/mm^3	>18 000 cells/mm^3
Blood glucose	>11.1 mmol/L	>12.2 mmol/L
Lactate dehydrogenase (LDH)	>350 U/L	>400 U/L
Aspartate aminotransferase (AST)	>250 U/L	>250 U/L
Within 48 hours		
Calcium	<2 mmol/L	<2 mmol/L
PaO$_2$	<60 mmHg	<60 mmHg
Base deficit	>4 mEq/L	>5 mEq/L
Fluid sequestration	>6 L	>4 L
Decrease in hematocrit	≥10%	≥10%
Increase in blood urea nitrogen	>1.8 mmol/L despite fluid resuscitation	>1.8 mmol/L despite fluid resuscitation

One point is awarded for each factor. A score of <3 is associated with 0–3% mortality while scores between 3 and 6 are associated with 11–15% mortality. Scores ≥6 are associated with 40% mortality.
Adapted from Ranson JHC, Rifkind KM, Roses OF *et al. Surg Gynecol Obstet* 1974; 139 : 69–81.

- Main limitations are the poor predictive ability in the first 24 hours and also that it is somewhat cumbersome to calculate

C-reactive protein (CRP), as a stand-alone test, is among the most useful in tracking the severity of acute pancreatitis. The caveat is that CRP is a nonspecific acute-phase reactant and an increase may reflect other processes (e.g. ventilator-associated pneumonia).

Management
- Fluid resuscitation is perhaps the most critical element due to profound third-space losses associated with pancreatitis. If cardiac function is adequate, IV maintenance rates of 250 mL/h are recommended for the first 48 hours. Although changes in blood urea nitrogen (BUN) over the first 24–48 h of treatment are good predictors of mortality, most advocate continued fluid resuscitation despite improvements in BUN [23]. Fluids should be titrated to maintain urine output greater than 0.5 mL/kg/h
- Adequate analgesia
- ERCP should be performed within 72 hours for patients with a persistent retained stone
- Organ support as required (i.e. renal replacement therapy, mechanical ventilation).

Current controversies in management

Feeding

- Traditionally, parenteral feeding was the preferred method of delivering nutrition in order to "rest the gut." Evidence now shows better outcomes (decreased mortality, organ failure, septicemia and need for surgery) with enteral nutrition compared to parenteral feeding.
- Early enteral feeding is recommended within 24 hours of diagnosis of severe pancreatitis or admission to ICU.
- Post-pyloric or ideally jejunal (i.e. naso-jejunal or gastro-jejunal) feeds are preferable to nasogastric feeds, if feasible. However, nasogastric feeds may be equivalent in patients without gastric outlet obstruction [24].

Antibiotics

- Infection of necrotic pancreas often develops late and is more common with biliary etiology.
- Subsequent sepsis is associated with a high mortality. Bacterial translocation is thought to be important in the pathogenesis as Gram-negative organisms are isolated in 75% of cases.
- Use of prophylactic antibiotics is controversial, with supporting evidence on either side.
- If aspiration of pancreatic fluid collections shows evidence of infection, empiric followed by directed antibiotic use is indicated. Carbapenems are the empiric antibiotics of choice.
- There is no role for antibiotics in sterile pancreatic necrosis.
- In the absence of culture-proven infection, retroperitoneal air or gas in pancreatic bed on CT imaging may justify use of antibiotics.
- If prophylactic antibiotics are used, most sources agree that carbapenems are the first choice and that duration of antibiotics should be limited to <2 weeks.

The role of surgery

- Pancreatic necrosectomy is indicated for: (1) infected necrosis or (2) symptomatic sterile necrosis (intolerance of enteral feeds).
- Necrosectomy is best performed in the late phase of pancreatitis, ideally >3–4 weeks after onset, at which point the inflammatory/vascular intra-abdominal reaction has settled down and necrotic areas of pancreas have demarcated themselves. This allows for more effective surgical debridement. Furthermore, delayed necrosectomy allows for clinical stabilization and treatment of early organ dysfunction/failure.
- Cholecystectomy should be performed in patients with gallstone pancreatitis once the pancreatitis has resolved and ideally, prior to being discharged home.

Acute mesenteric ischemia

In general, acute mesenteric ischemia is associated with mortality rates in excess of 60% [25]. There are four major causes:

1. Superior mesenteric artery (SMA) embolism
   - Mostly caused by embolization from thrombus in left atrium, left ventricle or heart valves.

2. Superior mesenteric artery thrombosis
   - Mostly due to acute-on-chronic thrombosis in an atherosclerotic patient.
3. Mesenteric vein thrombosis
   - Mostly due to hypercoagulable states (i.e. Factor V Leiden, prothrombin mutation, protein C/S deficiency, antiphospholipid antibody, paroxysmal nocturnal hemoglobinuria, myeloproliferative disease), portal hypertension, pancreatitis, major abdominal infections or trauma.
4. Nonocclusive mesenteric ischemia (NOMI)
   - Mostly due to splanchnic hypoperfusion and vasoconstriction, usually in the setting of an atherosclerotic patient [26].

Superior mesenteric artery embolism and NOMI are most common causes and account for approximately 75% of cases [27]. Nonocclusive mesenteric ischemia is a significant concern in the ICU as splanchnic hypoperfusion is a common consequence of the hypotension and peripheral vasoconstriction associated with shock state, as well as the vasoactive medications used to treat the shock state.

Nonocclusive mesenteric ischemia (NOMI)

Occurs as a result of mesenteric vasospam (i.e. peripheral vasoconstriction) in an attempt to redirect blood flow centrally (i.e. to perfuse brain and heart) [27]. It usually requires a chronic predisposition or a "first hit."

- This is usually atherosclerotic disease with some degree of thrombosis in the mesenteric arterial tree.

The "second hit" is acute or subacute and results in a general hypoperfused state, such as:
- MI or arrhythmias, resulting in cardiogenic shock
- Aortic insufficiency
- Following cardiac surgery, especially those using cardiopulmonary bypass with long aortic cross-clamp times [28]
- Use of vasopressors.

Nonocclusive mesenteric ischemia can be associated with up to 70% mortality [29].
- This is likely a reflection of delay in diagnosis and the poor prognosis of patients at risk of NOMI. Thus, early diagnosis is crucial.

Diagnosis

- Classically, abdominal pain out of proportion with clinical findings and concomitant metabolic acidosis should be considered acute mesenteric ischemia, until proven otherwise.
- NOMI may present, however, with minimal or no abdominal pain.
- Presentation may be limited to abdominal distension and ileus.
- The best aid to early diagnosis is having awareness of those at risk of NOMI.
- Laboratory evidence of anion gap metabolic acidosis is important. Bloodwork may also show increased serum lactate and other signs of acute phase reaction (leukocytosis, thrombocytosis).

- A CT scan with IV contrast or CT angiography should be performed if AMI is suspected [30].
- Mesenteric angiography allows for diagnosis and potential treatment of NOMI. However, it does not allow cross-sectional evaluation of the viscera and state/extent of the bowel ischemia (e.g. bowel wall enhancement, intramural pneumatosis, portal venous gas) and thus is often not the best first test.

Treatment

- Resuscitation with IV fluids and broad-spectrum antibiotics
- Limit use of vasoconstrictive agents. It must be balanced against the need to maintain adequate blood pressure and central perfusion.

Angiography:

- Allows for correction of pathology in occlusive embolic disease (i.e. embolectomy)
- In NOMI, use of intra-arterial papaverine (vasodilator) has been reported [29] in the acute setting and for up to 5 days with an in-dwelling angio-catheter.

Surgery:

- Should not be delayed if there is any evidence of infarction (i.e. peritonitis and metabolic acidosis) or perforation.
- Bowel resection with return for second-look laparotomy and delayed anastomosis is associated with better outcomes [31]. A second-look laparotomy and delayed anastomosis allows for ischemic segments of bowel to declare themselves as viable or nonviable (and thus requiring further resection).

Acute colonic pseudo-obstruction (Ogilvie's syndrome)

Acute colonic pseudo-obstruction, also referred to as Ogilvie's syndrome, is a disorder characterized by dilatation of the colon in the absence of an anatomic lesion that obstructs the flow of intestinal contents.

Etiology

Acute colonic pseudo-obstruction is most commonly associated with the following conditions:

- Nonoperative trauma
- Infection (pneumonia, sepsis most common)
- Cardiac conditions: myocardial infarction or heart failure
- Obstetric or gynecologic disease, Cesarean section (even without bowel injury), normal vaginal delivery and spinal anesthesia used during childbirth or surgery
- Abdominal/pelvic surgery
- Neurological conditions such as Parkinson's disease, spinal-cord injury, multiple sclerosis, Alzheimer's disease
- Orthopedic surgery
- Opiate administration
- Electrolyte abnormalities.

An increasingly recognized association of acute colonic pseudo-obstruction is chemotherapy, especially vincristine and other medications (e.g. all-*trans* retinoic acid and methotrexate) used in the treatment of a variety of malignancies, including hematological malignancies such as acute myeloid and lymphoblastic leukemias [32].

Pathogenesis

The precise mechanism by which colonic dilation occurs in these patients is unknown. The clinical association with retroperitoneal pathology or trauma, spinal anesthesia and pharmacological agents suggests an impairment of the autonomic nervous system. Interruption of the parasympathetic fibers from S2 to S4 leaves an atonic distal colon and a functional proximal obstruction [33].

Clinical manifestations

Abdominal distention is the most common presenting complaint. Patients can also develop nausea, vomiting, abdominal pain, constipation and, paradoxically, diarrhea. On physical examination, the abdomen is distended and tympanic.

- Peritoneal signs are absent in the early stages of the disease; if they develop, they suggest impending perforation.

Diagnosis

The diagnosis of acute colonic pseudo-obstruction can be made only after excluding the presence of toxic megacolon or mechanical obstruction.

Laboratory evaluation

There are no pathognomonic laboratory findings in patients with acute pseudo-obstruction. Laboratory evaluation may reveal leukocytosis, which may be due to the patient's underlying illness or represent impending perforation.

- Metabolic abnormalities, such as hypokalemia, hypocalcemia and hypomagnesemia, are present in more than 50% of patients [34].

Imaging

Plain and upright abdominal radiographs show a dilated colon, often from the cecum to the splenic flexure, and occasionally to the rectum.

- A CT scan of the abdomen is required to confirm the diagnosis and exclude mechanical obstruction and toxic megacolon.

Treatment

The objectives of treatment are:
- Relief of discomfort
- Prevention of perforation or ischemia.

General measures

- Supportive care with removal of precipitants is the first step in the management of patients with acute colonic pseudo-obstruction. Conservative therapy can be instituted provided that there is no pain, extreme (>12 cm) colonic distension or evidence of perforation
- Serial physical examinations and plain abdominal radiographs (every 12 to 24 hours) to measure the colonic diameter and determine which patients may need colonoscopic decompression or surgery [35]
- Treat underlying reversible diseases, such as infection or congestive heart failure
- Bowel rest – oral intake should be avoided with intravenous fluids for hydration
- Correct electrolyte imbalances (particularly hypomagnesemia, hypocalcemia and hypokalemia)
- Insert a nasogastric tube and initiate intermittent suction
- Insert a rectal tube and attach to gravity drainage
- Discontinue unnecessary medications, especially opiates, sedatives and those with anticholinergic side effects
- Patients should be positioned and rotated to right or left lateral decubitus positions each hour.

Pharmacologic agents

Several reports have demonstrated that neostigmine, an acetylcholinesterase inhibitor, may be effective in producing rapid colonic decompression [36,37].

- The standard dose in adults is 2.0 mg IV with cardiovascular monitoring [38].
- Decompression in response to neostigmine has been achieved in 80 to 100% of patients.
- Time to clinical response is short. In a controlled trial of 21 patients with acute colonic pseudo-obstruction treated with neostigmine, the median time to response was 4 minutes (range 3 to 30) [37]. Prompt decompression was observed in 11 patients (91%) who received neostigmine compared to none receiving placebo. Post-operative patients tend to have a favorable response to neostigmine, while patients with electrolyte imbalance or those using antimotility agents have been associated with a poor response [39].
- Side effects may vary. Symptomatic bradycardia requiring atropine may occur. The most frequent adverse effect was mild to moderate crampy abdominal pain. Excessive salivation, vomiting, bronchospasm and hypotension have also been reported.
- Neostigmine should therefore be used with caution in patients with known bronchial asthma, underlying bradyarrhythmias, recent myocardial infarction or receiving concurrent therapy with β-blockers. Atropine should be available at the bedside, patients should be kept supine on a bedpan and should receive continuous electrocardiographic monitoring with vital signs for 30 minutes, and continuous clinical assessment for 15 to 30 minutes [38].
- The reported recurrence rate after neostigmine ranges from 5 to 33%. Anecdotal experience suggests that recurrence may also be treated with repeat administration of neostigmine with the usual precautions (especially cardiovascular monitoring) [38].

Decompression

- Decompression in patients with Ogilvie's syndrome may consist of endoscopic decompression with or without placement of a decompression tube, or percutaneous tube cecostomy. The latter procedure is more invasive, involving a combined endoscopic and radiographic approach, and is usually reserved for those who fail initial endoscopic decompression.
- The role of decompression in patient management remains controversial. Success rates for endoscopic decompression in uncontrolled series vary from 69 to 90% [40].
- There is no colonic diameter which mandates decompression; the rate of dilation is probably more important than the absolute diameter of the colon [40]. Nevertheless, an attempt at colonoscopic decompression is indicated when supportive measures have failed and the colonic diameter has progressed to 11 to 13 cm or there is evidence of clinical deterioration.
- Recurrence requiring repeated colonoscopic decompression occurs in approximately 40% of patients after initial successful decompression.
- A variety of approaches have been developed to manage patients who have failed initial endoscopic decompression. A tube cecostomy involves placing a tube using a combined endoscopic and radiologic approach (fluoroscopic guidance). Percutaneous endoscopic cecostomy can be effective for treatment for both acute colonic pseudo-obstruction and neurogenic bowel, when other more conservative measures have failed [41,42].

Surgery

Surgery is rarely required. It is reserved for patients who fail medical and endoscopic management, and for those who develop signs of peritonitis or perforation. The type of operation will depend upon the findings at surgery.

References

1. Villanueva C, Colomo A, Bosch A et al. Transfusion strategies for acute upper gastrointestinal bleeding. New Engl J Med 2013; 368 : 11–21.

2. Cook D, Heyland D, Griffith L et al. Risk factors for clinically important upper gastrointestinal bleeding in patients requiring mechanical ventilation. Canadian Critical Care Trials Group. Crit Care Med 1999; 27 : 2812–7.

3. Alhazzani W, Alenezi F, Jaeschke RZ et al. Proton pump inhibitors versus histamine 2 receptor antagonists for stress ulcer prophylaxis in critically ill patients: a systematic review and meta-analysis. Critical Care Medicine 2013; 41 : 693–705.

4. Ioannou G, Doust J, Rockey DC. Terlipressin for acute esophageal variceal hemorrhage. Cochrane Database Syst Rev 2003(1):CD002147.

5. Imperiale TF, Teran JC, McCullough AJ. A meta-analysis of somatostatin versus vasopressin in the management of acute esophageal variceal hemorrhage. Gastroenterology 1995; 109 : 1289–94.

6. Garcia-Tsao G, Sanyal AJ, Grace ND et al. Prevention and management of gastroesophageal varices and variceal hemorrhage in cirrhosis. Hepatology 2007; 46 : 922–38.

7. Cohen SH, Gerding DN, Johnson S et al. Clinical practice guidelines for Clostridium difficile infection in adults: 2010 update by the society for healthcare epidemiology of America (SHEA) and the infectious diseases society of America (IDSA). Infect Contr Hosp Epidemiol 2010; 31 : 431–55.

8. Kelly CP. Immune response to Clostridium difficile infection. Eur J Gastroenterol Hepatol 1996; 8 : 1048–53.

9. Kelly CP, Pothoulakis C, LaMont JT. Clostridium difficile colitis. *New Engl J Med* 1994; 330 : 257–62.

10. Leffler DA, Lamont JT. Treatment of Clostridium difficile-associated disease. *Gastroenterology* 2009; 136 : 1899–912.

11. Kwok CS, Arthur AK, Anibueze CI et al. Risk of Clostridium difficile infection with acid suppressing drugs and antibiotics: meta-analysis. *Am J Gastroenterol* 2012; 107 : 1011–9.

12. Bolton RP, Culshaw MA. Faecal metronidazole concentrations during oral and intravenous therapy for antibiotic associated colitis due to Clostridium difficile. *Gut* 1986; 27 : 1169–72.

13. Friedenberg F, Fernandez A, Kaul V et al. Intravenous metronidazole for the treatment of Clostridium difficile colitis. *Dis Colon Rectum* 2001; 44 : 1176–80.

14. Bartlett JG. The case for vancomycin as the preferred drug for treatment of Clostridium difficile infection. *Clin Infect Dis* 2008; 46 : 1489–92.

15. Dallal RM, Harbrecht BG, Boujoukas AJ et al. Fulminant Clostridium difficile: an underappreciated and increasing cause of death and complications. *Ann Surg* 2002; 235 : 363–72.

16. Neal MD, Alverdy JC, Hall DE et al. Diverting loop ileostomy and colonic lavage: an alternative to total abdominal colectomy for the treatment of severe, complicated Clostridium difficile associated disease. *Ann Surg* 2011; 254 : 423–7.

17. Apisarnthanarak A, Razavi B, Mundy LM. Adjunctive intracolonic vancomycin for severe Clostridium difficile colitis: case series and review of the literature. *Clin Infect Dis* 2002; 35 : 690–6.

18. Shetler K, Nieuwenhuis R, Wren SM, Triadafilopoulos G. Decompressive colonoscopy with intracolonic vancomycin administration for the treatment of severe pseudomembranous colitis. *Surg Endosc* 2001; 15 : 653–9.

19. Lamontagne F, Labbe AC, Haeck O et al. Impact of emergency colectomy on survival of patients with fulminant Clostridium difficile colitis during an epidemic caused by a hypervirulent strain. *Ann Surg* 2007; 245 : 267–72.

20. Longo WE, Mazuski JE, Virgo KS et al. Outcome after colectomy for Clostridium difficile colitis. *Dis Colon Rectum* 2004; 47 : 1620–6.

21. Malbrain ML, Cheatham ML, Kirkpatrick A et al. Results from the International Conference of Experts on Intra-abdominal Hypertension and Abdominal Compartment Syndrome. I. Definitions. *Intensive Care Med* 2006; 32 : 1722–32.

22. Cheatham ML, Malbrain ML, Kirkpatrick A et al. Results from the International Conference of Experts on Intra-abdominal Hypertension and Abdominal Compartment Syndrome. II. Recommendations. *Intensive Care Med* 2007; 33 : 951–62.

23. Tenner S. Initial management of acute pancreatitis: critical issues during the first 72 hours. *Am J Gastroenterol* 2004; 99 : 2489–94.

24. Al-Omran M, Albalawi ZH, Tashkandi MF, Al-Ansary LA. Enteral versus parenteral nutrition for acute pancreatitis. *Cochrane Database Syst Rev* 2010(1):CD002837.

25. McKinsey JF, Gewertz BL. Acute mesenteric ischemia. *Surg Clin North Am* 1997; 77 : 307–18.

26. Wilcox MG, Howard TJ, Plaskon LA et al. Current theories of pathogenesis and treatment of nonocclusive mesenteric ischemia. *Digest Dis Sci* 1995; 40 : 709–16.

27. American Gastroenterological Association Medical Position Statement: guidelines on intestinal ischemia. *Gastroenterology* 2000; 118 : 951–3.

28. Garofalo M, Borioni R, Nardi P et al. Early diagnosis of acute mesenteric ischemia after cardiopulmonary bypass. *J Cardiovasc Surg* 2002; 43 : 455–9.

29. Bassiouny HS. Nonocclusive mesenteric ischemia. *Surg Clin North Am* 1997; 77 : 319–26.

30. Taourel PG, Deneuville M, Pradel JA et al. Acute mesenteric ischemia: diagnosis with contrast-enhanced CT. *Radiology* 1996; 199 : 632–6.

31. Ward D, Vernava AM, Kaminski DL *et al.* Improved outcome by identification of high-risk nonocclusive mesenteric ischemia, aggressive reexploration, and delayed anastomosis. *Am J Surg* 1995; 170 : 577–80.

32. Xie H, Peereboom DM. Ogilvie's syndrome during chemotherapy with high-dose methotrexate for primary CNS lymphoma. *J Clin Oncol* 2012; 30 : e192–4.

33. Ogilvie WH. William Heneage Ogilvie 1887–1971. Large-intestine colic due to sympathetic deprivation. A new clinical syndrome. *Dis Colon Rectum* 1987; 30 : 984–7.

34. Jetmore AB, Timmcke AE, Gathright JB, Jr *et al.* Ogilvie's syndrome: colonoscopic decompression and analysis of predisposing factors. *Dis Colon Rectum* 1992; 35 : 1135–42.

35. Johnson CD, Rice RP, Kelvin FM *et al.* The radiologic evaluation of gross cecal distension: emphasis on cecal ileus. *Am J Roentgenol* 1985; 145 : 1211–7.

36. Loftus CG, Harewood GC, Baron TH. Assessment of predictors of response to neostigmine for acute colonic pseudo-obstruction. *Am J Gastroenterol* 2002; 97 : 3118–22.

37. Ponec RJ, Saunders MD, Kimmey MB. Neostigmine for the treatment of acute colonic pseudo-obstruction. *New Engl J Med* 1999; 341 : 137–41.

38. Saunders MD, Kimmey MB. Systematic review: acute colonic pseudo-obstruction. *Aliment Pharmacol Ther* 2005; 22 : 917–25.

39. Mehta R, John A, Nair P *et al.* Factors predicting successful outcome following neostigmine therapy in acute colonic pseudo-obstruction: a prospective study. *J Gastroenterol Hepatol* 2006; 21 : 459–61.

40. Sloyer AF, Panella VS, Demas BE *et al.* Ogilvie's syndrome: successful management without colonoscopy. *Digest Dis Sci* 1988; 33 : 1391–6.

41. Saunders MD. Acute colonic pseudo-obstruction. *Best Pract Res Clin Gastroenterol* 2007; 21 : 671–87.

42. Ramage JI, Jr., Baron TH. Percutaneous endoscopic cecostomy: a case series. *Gastrointest Endosc* 2003; 57 : 752–5.

Chapter

32 The comatose patient: neurological aspects

G Bryan Young

To be fully conscious one needs to be both awake and aware.

- Alertness is a function of the ascending reticular activating system (ARAS) in the rostral brainstem tegmentum (from the mid-pons through the mid-brain) and then the thalamus and its projections through the cerebral white matter to the cerebral cortex. This allows for an eyes-open vigilant state, including arousability, and spontaneous wake and sleep cycles.
- Awareness depends on the integrity of integrated cerebral gray matter structures and their interconnecting fibers running through the white matter. Awareness has multiple inter-related functions, including sensation, perception, attention, memory, attention (with selectivity), emotions, judgement, motivation and planned action, with various interconnected anatomical loci.
- To be aware one needs to be awake. One can be awake, but not aware in the vegetative and minimally conscious states; this implies severe dysfunction of the above-mentioned, integrated "higher" functions and structures.

Coma is unarousable unconsciousness and implies dysfunction of the ARAS. There are many causes (alluded to below in broad categories). Within coma there are grades of unconsciousness ranging from brain death to nearly rousable states. These are captured in the Glasgow Coma Scale [1] and FOUR scoring [2] systems shown below (Tables 32.1 and 32.2).

- For the GCS a score of 8 or less is usually taken as coma. Usually eye opening is minimal.
- The FOUR scoring system is applied in a similar manner to the GCS, with the best score taken for each of the categories and the sum of these determined. The system has the advantage or being applicable to intubated patients. A score of 0 is compatible with brain death. Only the eye and motor scores address consciousness: 3 or better for eye and 4 for motor function are compatible with consciousness.

The approach to the acutely unresponsive patient

The approach can be divided into history, examination and tests. As in the clinical approach to all neurologic disorders, the initial step is to localize the problem, then to determine the etiology. Therapy is then targeted for the etiology. The issue of prognostication often follows (see later).

- History: the history can help localize the problem, as well as provide a story of the tempo or course of the illness, thus addressing both the localization *and* the cause.

Table 32.1 Glasgow Coma score

Eyes	Does not open eyes	1
	Opens eyes to painful stimuli	2
	Opens eyes to voice	3
	Opens eyes spontaneously	4
Verbal	No sounds	1
	Incomprehensible sounds	2
	Inappropriate words	3
	Confused, disoriented	4
	Converses normally	5
Motor	No movements	1
	Decerebrate response (extension)	2
	Decorticate response (flexion)	3
	Withdrawal	4
	Localizes	5
	Obeys	6
Total of best score from the three categories		

Table 32.2 The FOUR score system

Eye response	Eyelids closed with painful stimulation	0
	Eyelids open with painful stimulation	1
	Eyelids open with vocal stimulation	2
	Eyelids open but no tracking	3
	Eyelids open and tracking or blinking to command	4
Motor	No response to painful stimulation or generalized myoclonic seizures	0
	Extensor posturing to stimulation	1
	Flexor/decorticate response to stimulation	2
	Localizes to the painful stimulus	3
	Gives "thumbs up" or peace sign to command	4
Brainstem reflexes	Absent pupillary, corneal and cough reflexes	0
	Absent pupillary and corneal reflexes	1
	Pupillary or corneal reflexes present	2
	One pupil wide and fixed	3
	Pupillary and corneal reflexes present	4
Respirations	Breathes at ventilator rate or apnea	0
	Breathes above the ventilator rate	1
	Not intubated and breathes irregularly	2
	Not intubated with Cheyne–Stokes respirations	3
	Not intubated and breathes normally	4

A description of the acute behavioral change is usually available from the ambulance attendants and persons living with the patient. Was the problem a disturbance in alertness or a change in behavior? Was it a sudden collapse or a gradual and progressive or fluctuating change? Were there any preceding incidents or illness, e.g. head injury, drug ingestion, fever or headache? Were there focal features, e.g. a hemiparesis or aphasia, which preceded the loss of consciousness? What chronic conditions were present, e.g. cancer, diabetes, epilepsy, autoimmune diseases, or cardiac, pulmonary, hepatic or renal impairment? What medications was the patient taking? Was there a history of drug or alcohol abuse? What were the details of the collapse – falling limply versus like a tree? Were there convulsive movements? Did anyone feel for a pulse?

- The neurological examination: the degree of obtundation, using the Glasgow Coma score (GCS) or FOUR score if desired, is determined. Observe spontaneous movements and response to stimulation. If the patient remains unresponsive one applies progressively increasing stimuli, starting with calling the patient's name then applying somatic stimulation. Cranial nerve examination can help localize the lesion to specific cranial nerves or the brainstem. Check for gaze preference or palsy (using oculocephalic (doll's eyes) or caloric testing), pupillary reactivity and size. The corneal reflex if unilaterally absent can be localizing, but both corneal reflex being present or absent can reflect the degree of ARAS depression from an overwhelming metabolic disorder or a drug overdose. The combination of intact pupillary and absent oculovestibular reflexes raises the possibility of Wernicke encephalopathy, but the same phenomenon can be seen with a wide variety of sedative and analgesic drugs, as well as antihistamine overdoses [3]. The presence of nystagmus with caloric testing is strongly supportive of psychogenic unresponsiveness. One should always check for vertical eye movements, as lesions of the thalamus or rostral brainstem can abolish vertical, but not horizontal eye movements.
- Motor tone is assessed by passively moving the patient's limbs and noting the resistance to movement. Patients with neuroleptic malignant syndrome, malignant hyperthermia or serotonin syndrome typically have marked, persistent increased resistance to movement. Patients with other causes of encephalopathy, when comatose, may have flaccid tone, but encephalopathic patients with metabolic or septic causes often show a fluctuating, velocity-dependent increase in tone (the resistance increases with the speed of movement) known as *gegenhalten* or paratonic rigidity. In Parkinsonian rigidity (commonly produced by neuroleptic medications or metoclopramide) the resistance is present throughout the range of movement and is not as velocity-dependent as in *gegenhalten*. In spasticity there is a velocity-dependent increase in tone and then a release as the muscle spindles fire, causing flaccidity (clasp-knife effect). It is useful to note the motor responses to stimulation. The lack of movement on one side of the body or hemiplegia indicates a central cause for the paralysis. Purposeful movements in which the arm moves to the stimulus, often pushing it away or crossing the mid-line, indicates a lighter level of consciousness and an intact motor system on the side with movement. Decerebrate (upper and lower limb extension) or decorticate (upper limbs flexed at the elbows) were thought to indicate lesions below or above the red nucleus in the mid-brain, respectively, but in humans both can occur with deep cerebral lesions, and the type of posturing can alternate over time.

- In the less obtunded patient, the presence of postural-action tremor (with the upper limbs held up against gravity and/or moving to a target), asterixis (flapping tremor caused by the loss of postural tone as the patient holds the upper limbs out and extends the wrists) and multifocal myoclonus are strongly suggestive of a toxic or metabolic encephalopathy.
- Routine blood and urine testing: routine testing of serum glucose, electrolytes, magnesium, calcium, phosphate, urea and creatinine, and arterial or capillary blood gases are usually worthwhile. Urine is commonly sent for glucose, protein and cell counts, but bacterial culture and drug screening (usually with specific drugs in mind) are commonly indicated. Serum drug concentrations, checking for alcohol or drug intoxications or for compliance of maintenance drugs, e.g. anticonvulsant levels are often performed. Blood gas determination can help narrow the differential diagnosis (e.g. a metabolic acidosis is commonly due to increased lactate (as in sepsis or hypoperfusion), ketones, uremic toxins or some exogenous agents such as methanol or propylene glycol). Point-of-care testing often obviates the need to administer glucose intravenously; if the latter is done, it is wise to give thiamine simultaneously to prevent Wernicke encephalopathy.
- Lumbar puncture (LP): in the acutely comatose patient LP is used to rule out CNS infection or subarachnoid hemorrhage. Less commonly, meningeal cancer can present with loss of consciousness. A CT head before LP is usually done, as unexpected mass lesions, (e.g. cerebral or cerebellar abscess) can coexist with bacterial meningitis, making the LP dangerous. Subarachnoid hemorrhage can be detected by CT in over 95% of cases [4]. Other contraindications include coagulopathy and infection near or over the proposed puncture site.
- Neuro-imaging in the acute setting: neuro-imaging is necessary in all cases of disorders of consciousness except for cases in which a nonstructural cause of coma is readily identified, e.g. hypoglycemia reversed by an infusion of glucose. Even in metabolic, toxic or infectious cases, neuro-imaging is often advisable to exclude cerebral edema, associated traumatic lesions or a cerebral abscess or empyema. Computed tomographic (CT) scanning is usually available and is generally sufficient to make decisions about the safety of doing a lumbar puncture. One of the most common indications for neuro-imaging in the ER is for stroke. Hemorrhagic stroke is readily detected on CT. However, ischemic stroke may be missed in very acute infarction. Subtle gray-white differentiation can be helpful in showing ischemic damage affecting the cortex, insula and basal ganglia. Recently, the American Academy of Neurology recommended diffusion-weighted MRI over CT for the assessment of acute ischemic stroke [5]. This allows for clearer delineation of the infarcted vascular territory.
- Neurophysiological testing: EEG can be invaluable in confirming seizures as a cause of coma and is worth considering when a patient fails to waken after a convulsive seizure or after a reasonable time following a surgical procedure on the brain, and when the obtundation seems greater than expected after traumatic brain injury. Up to 20% of patients comatose after brain injury are having nonconvulsive seizures [6]. A single 20-minute EEG will capture fewer than 15% of these; continuous recordings of 24–48 hours are required to capture more than 80% [7]. Facial myoclonus or spontaneous nystagmus can be clues that seizures are occurring, but these features are found in a minority of nonconvulisve seizures. When the etiology is not apparent it is wise to have

Table 32.3 Classification of status epilepticus (10)

Generalized status epilepticus
1. Tonic-clonic
2. Tonic (e.g. in Lennox–Gastaut)
3. Clonic (infants and children)
4. Myoclonic status (bilaterally symmetrical jerks, mainly with acute/subacute brain disorders, including post-anoxic/ischemic injury)
5. Absence
6. Nonconvulsive generalized status (NCSE) in ICU

Partial status epilepticus
1. Simple partial (including epilepsia partialis continua)
2. Complex partial status epilepticus
3. NCSE with localization-related seizures, including transitional forms

an EEG performed. Other electrophysiological testing, e.g. somatosensory evoked potentials are used mainly for prognostic purposes.

Therapy

- The patient is supported in airway, breathing and circulation while the testing proceeds.
- If there is a suspicion of hypoglycemia, 50 mL of 50% glucose is administered preceded by thiamine (usually 50 mg IM) to prevent Wernicke encephalopathy.
- It is wise to lower a core temperature of over 40 °C to prevent cerebellar damage: usually cooling with fans and tepid sponging are used.
- Definitive therapy is dictated by the revealed etiology.
- Management of status epilepticus is discussed in greater detail later in this chapter.

Status epilepticus

Status epilepticus (SE) is defined as seizures that continue for more than 30 minutes or occur intermittently over 30 minutes without recovery between seizures. Table 32.3 gives a classification of the varieties of SE.

Virtually any type of seizure disorder can evolve into SE if it continues long enough. There is good evidence that all but absence (petit mal) SE can lead to further brain damage. Such damage begins in about 30 minutes in convulsive and by 60 minutes in nonconvulsive SE – hence the importance of prompt control.

- Pathophysiologically there is an increase in N-methyl-D-aspartate (glutamate) receptors and a downregulation of γ-amino-butyric acid (GABA)-A receptors on the neuronal membrane in SE. This favors further excitatory activity [8].
- Since benzodiazepines facilitate the GABA-A receptor, these agents can quickly lose their effectiveness in stopping SE that has persisted for extended amounts of time [9].

The goals of management in status epilepticus are:
1. Ensuring adequate vital functions (oxygenation and perfusion)
2. Stopping the seizures
3. Preventing recurrent seizures
4. Predicting and preventing systemic complications.

A careful search for the underlying cause should always be pursued if this is not apparent at the outset. Of course, any reversible causes should also be addressed urgently. For practical purposes we shall concentrate on the aspect of stopping the seizures.

- To ensure the seizures, including nonconvulsive seizures (which often evolve from convulsive seizures) are stopped and to assure a desired pharmacological effect it is strongly recommended that continuous EEG monitoring be done, especially when the patient does not awaken after initial SE treatment or in refractory or super-refractory SE (see below). The goals of EEG monitoring are to ensure that seizures are stopped. If seizures are still breaking through, the usual strategy is to induce a burst-suppression pattern, with epochs of generalized flattening (suppression) of cortical activity at least for several seconds on every screen. If this fails to stop the seizures, some neuro-intensivists aim for complete suppression of the EEG for 24 hours or more and then remove the anesthetic drug to see if seizures recur. If they do, then anesthesia is reinstituted [10].
- Initial drug therapy: randomized, controlled studies showed that lorazepam 2 mg intravenously was more effective than diazepam or phenytoin in stopping seizures as first-line treatment [11,12]. A more recent study showed that 10 mg of midazolam (in adults) was at least as effective as lorazepam [13]. This has some practical value when intravenous access is not immediately feasible.
- Since lorazepam and midazolam have fairly short durations of actions, a loading dose with a standard antiepileptic drug is usually administered immediately following the benzodiazepine. Phenytoin at 15–20 mg/kg (or the prodrug fosphenytoin in the same phenytoin equivalents), valproate (30–60 mg/kg) or phenobarbital (15 mg/kg), each given intravenously, are the most commonly administered agents and, if effective, will prevent seizures into the next day, when maintenance doses are started [10].
- Refractory SE is defined as failure of the first two agents to work, i.e. a benzodiazepine and either phenytoin, valproate or phenobarbital. By this stage the patient should be intubated in the ICU and an anesthetic agent is then used. Most commonly intravenous propofol or midazolam are used. The anesthetic agents pentobarbital or thiopental are next in line. Ketamine (commonly 1–1.5 mg/kg loading dose followed by an infusion at 0.5 mg/min) is also a good choice, as it addresses the increase in excitatory transmission in SE, while the other agents prop up the compromised inhibitory system [10].
- Super-refractory SE is defined as SE that fails to be controlled by anesthetic agents after 24 hours. In this situation, usually the anesthetic agents are continued, often with the aim to suppress all cerebral cortical activity for a time (say 24 hours or more). Other therapies that are based on case series rather than controlled trials include: hypothermia (usually 32–34 °C), surgical options (e.g. cortical resection if the seizures are focal or regional in origin) or even electroconvulsive therapy [14].
- Standard antiepileptic drugs: not more than three are commonly used while anesthetic agents are given and are there to help with the acute seizures and to prevent breakthrough seizures when the anesthesia is stopped.

The prognosis of SE is heavily dependent on etiology, but duration and refractoriness are also important. For SE in general the mortality is at least 10%. For refractory and super-refractory seizures, over 40% of patients die in the acute phase [14]. Survivors are often left with severe memory problems mixed with other deficits. It is very difficult to prognosticate accurately while the patient is still in SE. It is strongly recommended that such prognostic determinations wait until the SE has resolved and the patient is off anesthetic drugs [10].

Anoxic-ischemic encephalopathy after cardiac arrest

There is a delay between the time of the cardiac arrest and cell death. The following changes occur:

- Anaerobic glycolysis leads to an accumulation of hydrogen, phosphate and lactate, all of which result in intracellular acidosis [15].

- Intracellular ionized calcium concentration increases from increased calcium, as well as glutamate release and activation of NMDA channels, which also allow sodium and chloride influx, leading to hyperosmolarity, followed by water influx and neuronal death [15]. The calcium activates intracellular proteases causing intracellular damage to various organelles.

- Restoration of circulation leads to the formation of oxygen-derived free radicals, which can cause additional damage [16].

- In addition, apoptosis, due to caspase-3 activation in neurons and oligodendroglia in the cerebral neocortex, hippocampi and striatum, can contribute to cell death, although this has been shown only in perinatal models of anoxia-ischemia [17].

- Different brain regions and specific neuronal populations appear more susceptible to hypoxic-ischemic injury, especially the hippocampus, the Purkinje cells of the cerebellum and the pyramidal cells of the neocortex.

The neurological morbidity and mortality in patients resuscitated from cardiac arrest is improved by the use of hypothermia, cooling the patient to between 32 and 34 °C for 24 hours [18,19]. Prognostic guidelines based on literature that antedated the use of hypothermia were formulated in 2006 [20]. Although these require modification for patients treated with hypothermia, they can still be applied to those who were not hypothermic.

After the patient is sufficiently stabilized and confounders (circulatory shock, sedative drugs and paralyzing agents) are removed or accounted for, prognostic determination is undertaken.

Prognostic determination of cardiac arrest survivors not treated with hypothermia [20]

After 24 hours, if a patient has absence of all brainstem reflexes, motor responses and apnea, ancillary testing can be used to confirm a diagnosis of brain death. In patients who remain comatose, but have a less severe neurological insult, clinical signs and electrophysiological tests can be used to establish a poor prognosis. The clinical signs that predicted poor neurological outcome were myoclonus status epilepticus (bilaterally synchronous muscle twitches that are primarily axial, i.e. face, platysma, trunk, diaphragm and proximal limbs) on day one (false-positive rate, or FPR 0%, CI 0–8.8), absence of the pupillary light reflex or corneal reflex on day three (FPR 0%, CI 0–3), and best motor response of extension or worse on day three (0%, CI 0–3) [20]. Somatosensory evoked potentials (SSEPs) completed on days 1 to 3 that demonstrate bilateral absent N20 responses (negative peak (N) at 20 ms) also predicted poor outcome (FPR of 0.7%, CI 0–3–7). Neuron-specific enolase greater than 33 ug/L on days 1 to 3 was also a negative prognosticator (FPR 0, CI

0–3). The practice parameters allow a physician to identify a patient who will definitely have a poor neurological outcome; however, it is important to note that many patients without any of these criteria will also have a poor outcome [20].

Prognostic determination after hypothermia

- Neurological examination: the pupillary light reflexes, corneal reflexes and motor response have reduced accuracy for predicting poor neurological outcome. Rossetti and colleagues [21] prospectively studied a cohort of post-arrest patients undergoing therapeutic hypothermia (TH) to evaluate the American Academy of Neurology practice parameters. When examined 72 hours after the arrest, they found TH affects the accuracy of several of the variables used in the practice parameter algorithm. They found higher false-positive rates (FPRs) for predicting mortality for absence of pupillary reactivity (FPR 4%), presence of axial myoclonus (FPR 3%) and best motor response of extensor or worse (FPR 24%). Al Thenayan and colleagues [22] found that motor response, specifically extension or worse, was not prognostically reliable at day three following TH. In their respective review 14 patients had delayed return of the motor response, as late as day 6 post-arrest, and two of these patients had favorable outcomes. [22]. We have encountered a patient treated with TH who lacked motor response until day 21 post-arrest (unpublished data).
- Axial myoclonus may be cortical in origin, having an EEG correlation, or reticular, meaning originating from the brainstem, and having a variable EEG correlation. Until recently, the presence of axial myoclonus has been considered uniformly fatal [20]. Recent case reports of good outcome despite axial myoclonus suggest that TH may modify the outcome of a small but significant number of patients who develop status myoclonus after resuscitation from cardiac arrest 23–25]. It is important to note that the presence of axial myoclonus is still suggestive of poor neurological outcome, but should not be used in isolation to prognosticate.
- Characteristics of the cardiac arrest, specifically anoxia time (the time to initiation of CPR) and total arrest duration, are often brought up in discussions of post-arrest prognosis. Goldberger and colleagues [26] respectively reviewed a cohort of 64 339 patients who suffered in-hospital cardiac arrest, and had neurological outcome data available for 8724 patients. They found that the duration of resuscitation did not affect neurological outcome. Favorable outcome occurred in 81% of resuscitation times of less than 15 min, 80% for durations between 15 and 30 minutes and 78% for resuscitation lasting greater than 30 minutes [26]. The Brain Resuscitation Clinical Trial 1 Study Group [27] found that anoxia time greater than 5 minutes and total resuscitation time exceeding 20 minutes independently predicted mortality. However, it is important to note that the presence of prolonged anoxia time or CPR exceeding 20 minutes did not preclude a favorable neurological outcome. Of 245 patients, 41 with anoxia time exceeding 5 minutes had a cerebral performance category of 1 or 2 at outcome assessment. Similarly, 48 of 311 patients with resuscitation times exceeding 20 minutes also had a favorable outcome [27].
- Similarly, age is not a reliable determinant of outcome [28].
- Somatosensory evoked responses: Tiainen and colleagues [29] evaluated SSEPs in post-arrest patients randomized to TH or standard care at the time. Although TH resulted in delayed latencies of the waveforms, 100% of patients with bilaterally absent N20

responses, regardless of whether they underwent TH, had poor neurological outcome [29]. Leithner and colleagues [30] found a slightly lower predictive value in the setting of TH. They had 36 patients with bilaterally absent N20 responses post-arrest; 35 had poor outcome and 1 patient regained consciousness [30]. While median nerve SSEPs can still be used to accurately predict outcome, the false-positive rate is not zero, again emphasizing that in the post-hypothermia era, no test should be used in isolation.

- The EEG may be used to prognosticate in the post-arrest period, but one must be aware of its sensitivity to multiple confounders, including sedation, hypothermia and multiorgan failure. The American Academy of Neurology practice parameters found that generalized suppression to less than 20 μV, burst suppression with epileptiform bursts and periodic complexes on a flat background were all associated with poor outcome, but had insufficient accuracy on their own [20]. Additional EEG patterns that are often considered malignant include status epilepticus, alpha coma, theta coma, spindle coma, triphasic waves and burst suppression with nonepileptifom bursts. Recently, EEG reactivity has received increased attention. This reactivity is defined as a change in frequency or amplitude that occurs in response to verbal or noxious stimuli. Al Thenayan and colleagues [31] retrospectively reviewed the EEG of 29 patients post-arrest and found that 17 out of 18 patients who lacked EEG reactivity did not regain conscious awareness [31]. In a prospective series of 34 patients conducted by Rossetti and colleagues [32], a nonreactive background had a positive predictive value of 100%. In addition, all the survivors had EEG reactivity and 74% of these patients had a favorable neurological outcome. They also found that nonreactivity had an FPR of 7% for predicting mortality following cardiac arrest. Up to 30% of post-arrest patients may develop status epilepticus. While often associated with poor outcomes, this same series found that epileptiform activity on the first EEG recording predicted poor outcome with FPR of 9% [25]. Aggressive antiepileptic treatment should be administered to these patients until other criteria suggest poor outcome. In summary, the EEG can aid in prognostication, both for favorable and unfavorable outcomes, but must be considered in context with other established prognostic indicators as the positive predictive value is insufficient to use in isolation.

- Biomarkers: several biomarkers have shown potential for prognostication post-arrest. The use of biomarkers is appealing as it does not require patient transport to radiology, nor are the levels affected by sedation.

- The American Academy of Neurology practice parameters recommended using a serum neuron-specific enolase (NSE) concentration cutoff of 33 μg/L to accurately predict poor outcome [20]. Results from studies in the post-hypothermia era have challenged the accuracy of this cutoff. Fugate and colleagues [33] found that following TH, using this recommended cutoff had an unacceptably high FPR of 29% for poor outcome. Daubin and colleagues [34] measured serum NSE at 24 and 72 hours post-arrest and found that a serum level of 97 μg/L was needed to achieve a 100% positive predictive value. A meta-analysis, which included studies with and without TH, found that the reported cutoff to achieve reliable prediction varied from as low as 5μg/L to as high as 91 μg/L [35]. At this time further research is needed to determine the post-hypothermia cutoff level for NSE.

- S100B is a calcium-binding protein secreted by glial and Schwann cells. It may also act as a cytokine resulting in neuronal apoptosis. It has a biological half-life of 2 hours.

Results from a meta-analysis suggest the cutoff level for S100B to predict poor neurological outcome also varies, ranging from 0.7–5.2 μg/L [35]. Other biomarkers that require further research before they can be useful clinically for prognostication include creatine kinase BB isoenzyme, glial fibrillary acidic protein and brain-derived neurotrophic factor. The lack of availability of biomarkers at many medical centers and the conflicting evidence over serum cutoff measurements that predict poor outcome with 100% specificity currently limit the use of biomarkers in post-arrest prognostication, at least for now.

Improving prognostic accuracy in the hypothermic era

Identifying those patients who will have poor neurological outcomes has become increasingly difficult.

- Ensuring the presence of at least two negative prognosticators can improve prognostic accuracy [36]. In addition, it allows for the use of some prognostic signs, such as EEG and MRI, which have good, but not perfect, predictive ability.
- Rossetti and colleagues [21] found that the presence of at least two of: absence of at least one set of brainstem reflexes, myoclonus, unreactive EEG and bilaterally absent N20 responses on SSEPs had a positive predictive value of 100% for poor neurological outcome.

It is useful to consider the factors that may indicate a *favorable* outcome, usually defined as the ability to obey commands, indicating the return of awareness. These include localization on motor examination, minimal to no diffusion restriction on MRI and EEG reactivity [21]. Further research is needed to clarify the effect of hypothermia on current prognostic signs and also to help differentiate those patients who will have near complete neurological recovery from those who will have moderate disability.

Some general statements regarding prognostic determination and discussions of level of care

- Prognosis depends on establishing the diagnosis with certainty.
- Potentially reversible brain conditions, e.g. sepsis or hepatic failure, should not be used to determine the overall prognosis based only on the neurological aspects.
- Features of the examination, neuro-imaging (especially MRI) and neurophysiological testing can be used to help determine the severity and permanence of brain damage.
- Prognostication should follow established guidelines whenever possible.
- When the prognosis is uncertain, more time should be allowed and repeated evaluations performed.

Doctors in ICUs tend to overestimate poor outcomes and underestimate good outcomes, especially on the first day in ICU [37]. Furthermore, some families express doubt about the accuracy and sincerity of doctors giving prognostic opinions and management suggestions. Yet, what "experts" say to families and to fellow physicians and other care givers has enormous influence. There is a need for accuracy, honesty, frankness, consideration/acknowledgment and patience in discussions that involve possible end-of-life discussions.

References

1. Teasdale G, Jennett B. Assessment of coma and impaired consciousness: a practical scale. *Lancet* 1974; 7872 : 81–4.

2. Wijdicks EF, Bamlet WR, Maramattom BV et al. Validation of a new coma scale: the FOUR score. *Ann Neurol* 2005; 58 : 585–93.

3. Morrow SA, Young GB. Selective abolition of the vestibular-ocular reflex by sedative drugs. *Neurocrit Care* 2007; 6 : 45–8.

4. Tong DM, Zhou YT. Predictors of the subarachnoid hemorrhage of a negative CT scan. *Stroke* 2010; 41 : e556–7.

5. Schellinger PD, Bryan RN, Caplan LR et al. Evidence-based guideline: the role of diffusion and perfusion MRI for the diagnosis of acute ischemic stroke: report of the Therapeutics and Technology Assessment Subcommittee of the American Academy of Neurology. *Neurology* 2010; 75 : 177–85.

6. Vespa PM, Nuwer MR, Nenov V et al. Increased incidence and impact of nonconvulsive seizures after traumatic brain injury as detected with continuous EEG monitoring. *J Neurosurg* 1999; 91 : 750–60.

7. Claassen J, Mayer SA, Kowalski RG, et al. Detection of electrographic seizures with continuous EEG monitoring in critically ill patients. *Neurology* 2004; 62 : 1743–8.

8. Wasterlain CG, Hiu H, Naylor DE et al. Molecular basis of self-sustaining seizures and pharmacoresistance during status epilepticus: the receptor trafficking hypothesis revisited. *Epilepsia* 2009; 50 (Suppl 12) : 16–18.

9. Kapur J, Macdonald RL. Rapid seizure-induced reduction of benzodiazepine and Zn2+ sensitivity of hippocampal dentate granule cell GABA-A receptors. *J Neurosci* 1997; 17 : 7532–40.

10. Hunter GRW, Young GB. Status epilepticus: a review, with emphasis on refractory cases. *Can J Neurol Sci* 2012; 39 : 157–69.

11. Alldredge BK, Gelb AM, Isaacs SM et al. A comparison of lorazepam, diazepam, and placebo for the treatment of out-of-hospital status epilepticus. *N Engl J Med* 2001; 345 : 631–7.

12. Treiman DM, Meyers PD, Walton NY et al. A comparison of four treatments for generalized convulsive status epilepticus. *N Eng J Med* 1998; 339 : 792–8.

13. Silbergleit R, Durkalski V, Lowenstein D, et al. Intramuscular vs. intravenous therapy in prehospital status epilepticus. *N Eng J Med* 2012; 366 : 591–600.

14. Shorvon S, Ferlisi M. The treatment of super-refractory status epilepticus: a critical review of available therapies and a clinical treatment protocol. *Brain* 2011; 134 : 2802–18.

15. Busl KM, Greer DM. Hypoxic-ischemic brain injury: pathophysiology, neuropathology and mechanisms. *NeuroRehabilitation* 2010; 26 : 5–13.

16. Greer DM. Mechanisms of injury in hypoxic-ischemic injury: implications to therapy. *Semin Neurol* 2006; 26 : 373–9.

17. Hee Han B, D'Costa A, Black SA et al. BDNF blocks caspase-3 activation in neonatal hypoxia-ischemia. *Neurology of Disease* 2000; 7 : 38–53.

18. Barnard SA, Gray TW, Buist MD et al. Treatment of comatose survivors of out of hospital cardiac arrest with induced hypothermia. *N Eng J Med* 2002; 346 : 557–63.

19. Hypothermia after Cardiac Arrest Study Group. Mild hypothermia to improve the neurologic outcome after cardiac arrest. *N Eng J Med*; 346; 557–63.

20. Wijdicks EFM, Hijdra A, Young GB et al. Practice parameter: prediction of outcome in comatose survivors after cardiopulmonary resuscitation (an evidence-based review): report of the Quality Standards Subcommittee of the American Academy of Neurology. *Neurology* 2006; 67 : 203–10.

21. Rossetti AO, Oddo M, Logroscino G et al. Prognostication after cardiac arrest and hypothermia: a prospective study. *Ann Neurol* 2010; 67 : 301–7.

22. Al Thenayan EA, Savard M, Sharpe M, et al. Predictors of poor neurologic

outcome after induced mild hypothermia following cardiac arrest. *Neurology* 2008; 71 : 1535–37.

23. Chen CJ, Coyne PJ, Lyckhom LJ, *et al.* A case of inaccurate prognostication after the ARCTIC protocol. *J Pain Symptom Manage* 2012; 43 : 1120–5.

24. Lucas JM, Cocchi MN, Salciccioli J, *et al.* Neurologic recovery after hypothermia in patients with post-cardiac arrest myoclonus. *Resuscitation* 2012; 83 : 265–9.

25. Rossetti AO, Oddo M, Liaudet L *et al.* Predictors of awakening from postanoxic status epilepticus after therapeutic hypothermia. *Neurology* 2009; 72 : 744–9.

26. Goldberger ZD, Chan PS, Berg RA, *et al.* Duration of resuscitation efforts and survival after in-hospital cardiac arrest: an observational study. *Lancet* 2012; 380 : 1473–81.

27. Brain Resuscitation Clinical Trial 1 Study Group. A randomized clinical study of cardiopulmonary-cerebral resuscitation: design, methods and patient characteristics. *Am J Emerg Med* 1986; 4 : 72–86.

28. Rogove HJ, Safar P, Sutton-Tyrrell K, Abramson NS. Old age does not negate good cerebral outcome after cardiopulmonary resuscitation: analyses from the brain resuscitation clinical trials. The Brain Resuscitation Clinical Trial I and II Study Groups. *Crit Care Med* 1995; 23 : 18–25.

29. Tiainen M, Kovala TT, Takkunen OS, Roine RO. Somatosensory and brainstem auditory evoked potentials in cardiac arrest patients treated with hypothermia. *Crit Care Med* 2005; 33 : 1736–40.

30. Leithner C, loner CJ, Hasper D *et al.* Does hypothermia influence the predictive value of bilateral absent N20 after cardiac arrest. *Neurology* 2010; 74 : 965–9.

31. Al Thenayan EA, Savard M, Sharpe M, *et al.* Electroencephalogram for prognosis after cardiac arrest. *J Crit Care* 2010; 25 : 300–4.

32. Rossetti AO, Urbano LA, Delodder F *et al.* Prognostic value of continuous EEG monitoring during therapeutic hypothermia after cardiac arrest. *Crit Care* 2010; 14(5) : R173.

33. Fugate JE, Wijdicks ER, Mandrekar J *et al.* Predictors of neurologic outcome after cardiac arrest. *Ann Neurol* 2010; 68 : 907–14.

34. Daubin C, Quentin C, Allouch S, *et al.* Serum neuron-specific enolase as predictor of outcome in comatose cardiac-arrest survivors: a prospective cohort study. *BMC Cardiovasc Disord* 2011; 11 : 48–61.

35. Shinokzaki K, Oda S, Sadahiro T *et al.* S-100B and neuron-specific enolase as predictors of neurological outcome in patients after cardiac arrest and return of spontaneous circulation: a systematic review. *Crit Care* 2009; 13(4) : R121.

36. Zingler VC, Krumm B, Bertsch T *et al.* Early prediction of neurological outcome after cardiopulmonary resuscitation: a multi-modal approach combining neurchemical and electrophysiological investigations may provide higher prognostic certainty in patients after cardiac arrest. *Eur Neurol* 2003; 49 : 79–84.

37. Rocker G, Cook D, Sjokvist P, *et al.* Clinical predictions of intensive care unit mortality. *Crit Care Med* 2004; 32 : 1149–54.

Chapter 33

The obstetric patient in the ICU

Carlos Kidel and Alan McGlennan

Introduction

The approach and management of the obstetric patient in intensive care presents particular challenges that often differ from the "general" ICU patient. Whilst admissions are rare, they usually arise from disorders specific and unique to pregnancy. An appreciation of this pathology along with physiological differences in this patient group is important when caring for an obstetric patient on the ICU.

Changes in pregnancy

When treating pregnant patients, it is important to be aware of the physiological changes that take place during pregnancy. These occur under the influence of hormonal and mechanical alterations. The main hormone responsible for this is progesterone, which causes smooth-muscle relaxation, bronchodilation, vasodilatation and reduced transit time in the gastro-intestinal tract. Mechanical change is produced by compression from the enlarging uterus.

Whilst almost all organs undergo some changes, for the purpose of the management in ICU the most significant are those to the cardiovascular, respiratory and renal systems, so these will be highlighted in more detail below.

Respiratory system

- The partial pressure of carbon dioxide in arterial blood is "reset" to 4 kPa during the first trimester. This persists throughout the pregnancy and results in a respiratory alkalosis.
- The alkalosis is driven by an increase in sensitivity of the respiratory center under the influence of progesterone. Minute ventilation is increased by 40–45%.
- Functional residual capacity (FRC) reduces progressively throughout the pregnancy. This is due to an increase in intra-abdominal pressure and pressure from the gravid uterus on the diaphragm. By term, FRC can be reduced by up to 80% and, whilst it does not impinge on closing capacity in the upright position, it can do when supine.
- Oxygen demands increase progressively as a result of metabolic activity. By term they will have increased by 35% above pre-pregnancy levels. The placenta accounts for 40% of total oxygen uptake by the gravid uterus at this stage.
- Chest wall compliance is reduced by 30%, but there is no change in lung compliance. This results in a parallel, but slightly smaller decrease in total compliance.

Handbook of ICU Therapy, third edition, ed. John Fuller, Jeff Granton and Ian McConachie. Published by Cambridge University Press. © Cambridge University Press 2015.

- There is generalized progesterone-driven bronchodilation.
- Increased risk of regurgitation and aspiration.
- Difficulties in bag-mask ventilation and intubation can occur secondary to:
  . Airway and mucosal edema
  . Mucus secretion
  . Nasal congestion
  . Increased BMI
  . Large breasts may obstruct the handle of a laryngoscope when inserting the blade into the mouth.

Reduced oxygen reserves coupled with increased oxygen demand make potential difficult intubation and ventilation all the more important to consider.

Cardiovascular

- Blood volume increases throughout pregnancy by 45–50% by term. Both red cell mass and plasma increase, but the latter to a greater extent, resulting in a physiological anemia.
- Vascular smooth muscle relaxes under the influence of progesterone. This reduces systemic vascular resistance and serves to accommodate the increase in blood volume and results in a fall in systolic and diastolic blood pressure.
- Heart rate, stroke volume and therefore cardiac output all increase. Most of the 40–50% increase is achieved by 20 weeks gestation and is directed to the uterus.
- Mechanical compression from the uterus on the aorta or vena cava causes aortocaval compression when the patient is in the supine position. This can occur from 16 weeks gestation. Venous return can occur via azygous, lumbar and paraspinal veins.
- The uteroplacental circulation lacks autoregulation. Periods of systemic hypotension compensated for by vasoconstriction can result in reduced uteroplacental perfusion and fetal hypoxia.

Renal

- Renal plasma flow and glomerular filtration rate (GFR) increase progressively throughout pregnancy and are 50–60% greater by term compared to pre-term levels. This has an impact on the clearance of certain drugs.
- There is increased clearance of creatinine, urea, urate and excretion of bicarbonate, which results in lower plasma levels than in the non-pregnant population.
- Raised GFR increases the filtered levels of glucose and protein to a point where the reabsorption is overwhelmed, resulting in glycosuria and proteinuria.
- Raised progesterone and the activation of the renin–angiotensin–aldosterone system produces water retention and reduced plasma osmolality. This has an impact on the volume of distribution of certain drugs.

Maternal critical care epidemiology

It is worthwhile examining why maternal critical care has recently become an area of interest. Firstly, data requiring maternal morbidity hasn't really been aggregated until relatively recently. Secondly, media interest in the care of the pregnant woman has risen.

Next, critical care is expanding in its remit exponentially. Lastly, the ability to manage all maternity ill-health by midwives and obstetricians has lessened, especially in the UK.

Critical care can mean many different things to many different people. It is sensible to start here with a few definitions. Although somewhat arbitrary, the standard definitions in the UK have emanated from the Intensive Care Society [1]. These rank the care using a numerical scale, whereby level 0 is normal ward care (and therefore in parallel normal maternity care). Next is level 1, which is reserved for those patients at risk of deterioration. These risks could be solely maternal (such as epilepsy) or obstetric (such as placenta previa). Level 2 is for patients who require invasive monitoring or a single-system support. Patients with arterial lines, for instance, or requiring vasoactive infusions to treat hypertension would fit here. As can be inferred, this can be quite a range of patient interventions and actually take place in a variety of locations – in high dependency units or intensive care units or indeed on the labor ward itself. Lastly, mothers requiring respiratory support or multiple-system intervention are placed in level 3. In the UK this is almost exclusively performed in intensive care areas.

If we take the definition of critical care as a patient requiring either level 2 or level 3 care, then the amounts of patients treated can be unclear. Trying to delineate the pathologies is also difficult. However, an idea can be gleaned from data that looks at women who die, women admitted to ICU facilities and women who develop severe morbidity.

In the UK there are robust data regarding women who die. These are collated in the "triennial" reports that have been administered by various agencies. The last published report looked at the years 2006 to 2008 [2]. Overall there were 261 maternal deaths and 2 291 493 maternities. This gave a maternal mortality rate of 11.4 per 100 000 maternities. The crude incidence doesn't really tell us too much, however looking at the leading causes of death does: indirect (that is, unrelated, but exacerbated by pregnancy) cardiac and indirect neurological pathologies were the commonest causes, followed by maternal sepsis, eclampsia and then thrombus. Obstetric pathology is represented, but at a lower rate than has been described traditionally.

It can be argued that the causes of death and the pathologies that lead to them are not representative of the critical care burden. Data exists from ICNARC (Intensive Care National Audit and Research Centre) that looked into admissions to general adult intensive care facilities in the child-bearing population [3]. Essentially this was looking at level 3 care only and comparing currently or recently pregnant women with women of a similar age. Multiple reports have been made, but using the data from around the time of the previous triennial report (2007) there were 260 ICU admissions per 100 000 maternities; 18.5% were reported as "currently pregnant" and 81.5% were "recently pregnant." Overall, 61% were admitted for obstetric reasons. The top five causes of admission were more predictably obstetric: sepsis, hemorrhage, ARDS, epilepsy and eclampsia. To reiterate, many of the deadly cardiac and neurological pathologies do not form much of the maternal ICU workload.

However, this data looks only at level 3 women. To get an idea of the need for critical care provision we have to also consider pathology that may render a patient in need of level 2 care, but not necessarily ICU admission. Unfortunately this work has not been done. The closest to this is the work of the Scottish Confidential Audit of Severe Maternal Morbidity. As the name suggests this was not UK wide, rather confined to Scotland. This group has reported on multiple years, but looking at data contiguous with the above, there were 580 episodes of severe maternal morbidity per 100 000 maternities [4]. A close look at the pathologies that were used for inclusion illustrates that they deserved their label of "severe": anaphylactic shock, coma, pulmonary edema – but other pathologies that would not necessitate an ICU admission were also included (e.g. the commonest cause – hemorrhage; as well as liver and renal dysfunction and anesthetic problems). As the definition of severe morbidity does not include all those who would require level 2 care, I believe this number under-represents the need for critical care provision.

As can be seen, a pyramid of pathology is being described. Death is a rare event and the pathologies reflect this. Intensive care admission is around 20 times more common and the causes tend towards the more traditional. Severe maternal morbidity illustrates that outside of the ICU there is still a lot of critical care, with hemorrhage representing the majority. To answer the question of how common is the need for critical care in the maternity population, unfortunately some guess-work is required. I believe level 3 and level 2 (either delivered on the labor ward, HDU or ICU) will be required in some degree in 1000 per 100 000 maternities and that hemorrhage will be by far the greatest cause of this, followed by renal and liver dysfunction, sepsis, eclampsia and pulmonary edema.

Obstetric conditions resulting in ICU admission

Pre-eclampsia and eclampsia

The National Institute for Health and Care Excellence (NICE) is a nondepartmental public body of the Department of Health in the UK. It produces evidence-based guidance on several aspects of medical care and practice in the form of guidelines. For the diagnosis and management of pre-eclampsia, the Royal College of Obstetricians and Gynaecologists (RCOG) refers to the NICE publication on pre-eclampsia [5], which forms the basis of the steps outlined below.

Whilst there is more than one definition for hypertension in pregnancy, RCOG and NICE agree on a systolic blood pressure greater than 140 mmHg or diastolic greater than 90 mmHg. Hypertension accompanied with proteinuria after the 20th week of gestation is defined as pre-eclampsia and complicates 5–8% of pregnancies. It is a multisystem disease and is a major cause of maternal death worldwide.

The precise mechanism for pre-eclampsia is poorly understood, but there is impaired trophoblast invasion of the uterine spiral arteries, which prevents the normal increase in blood flow to the placenta. There is local release of endothelial thromboxane, activation of platelets, reduction in nitric oxide and vascular sensitivity to angiotensin. The result is placental hypoperfusion with more generalized systemic vasoconstriction and reduced organ perfusion.

These patients are frequently relatively hypovolemic and vasoconstricted. They have a low colloid osmotic pressure with a raised hydrostatic pressure which predisposes the development of edema.

Untreated pre-eclampsia can develop into seizures (eclampsia) and death.

Features of severe pre-eclampsia

- Severe hypertension and proteinuria or mild to moderate hypertension with proteinuria with one of the following:
  - Severe headache
  - Visual disturbance (blurring or flashing)
  - Epigastric pain or vomiting
  - Papilledema

- Signs of clonus
- Liver tenderness
- HELLP syndrome (see below)
- Platelet count <100 ×10^9/L
- Abnormal liver enzymes (ALT or AST raising to >70 IU/L).

Management of severe pre-eclampsia and eclampsia

- Control hypertension: oral labetalol is first line with a goal of achieving diastolic blood pressure at 80–100 mmHg and systolic <150 mmHg. Other antihypertenisves to consider include hydralazine and nifedipine. A cautious fluid bolus should be considered when using the vasodilating hydralazine in these hypovolemic patients. Angiotensin-converting enzyme inhibitors or antiangiotensin receptor agents should be avoided because of their fetotoxic effects.
- Prevention and control of seizures: intravenous magnesium sulfate 4 g over 5 minutes followed by 1 g/h for 24 h. Further doses of 2–4 g can be given over 5 minutes for recurrent seizures. The use of phenytoin or diazepam is not advised.
- Fluid management in these patients has been controversial. The risk of volume overload in a patient with low oncotic pressure resulting in pulmonary and cerebral edema must be weighed up against hypotension arising from administration of vasodilators without volume replacement.
- Urea and electrolytes, along with liver enzymes should be monitored to assess renal or hepatic involvement.
- Early delivery may be indicated and is determined by the obstetric team responsible for the patient.

HELLP syndrome

Hemolysis, Elevated Liver enzymes and Low Platelets complicates 10 to 20% of cases of severe pre-eclampsia and is believed to be on the spectrum of pre-eclampsia. Patients present with abdominal pain, nausea and malaise.

- Key features are thrombocytopenia (<100 000/mm^3), microangiopathic hemolytic anemia with schistocytes, elevated lactate dehydrogenase (>600 IU/L) and elevated transaminases.
- Complications include renal failure, disseminated intravascular coagulation, pulmonary edema, pleural effusions, ARDS, cerebral edema and placental abruption.
- Treatment is largely supportive with delivery of the placenta being the definitive treatment. Although corticosteroids may be given to aid fetal lung development in pre-eclampsia, dexamethasone or betamethasone are not advised for the treatment of HELLP syndrome.

Venous thromboembolism (VTE)

Deaths arising from thrombosis and thromboembolism have fallen since the mid-1990s to a level of 0.79 per 100 000 maternities [2], the majority of these occurring in the post-partum period, especially after cesarean section. Whilst the incidence should have increased though improved diagnosis, it has in fact declined. This has been attributed to more aggressive thromboprophylaxis.

Pregnancy predisposes to VTE because of increased venous stasis, endothelial injury and an increase in coagulation factors [6]. The venous stasis is a result of progesterone-induced increases in venous capacitance and venacaval obstruction from the gravid uterus. Endothelial injury occurs at the uteroplacental surface at delivery. There is an increase in factors I, II, VII, VIII and X; a decrease in the coagulation inhibitor protein S; an increase in resistance to activated protein C; impaired fibrinolysis attributable to an increase in plasminogen activator inhibitors; and activation of platelets [7].

Risk factors for VTE in pregnancy include:

- Previous VTE
- Recent surgery
- Older age
- Obesity
- Thrombophilia
- Bed rest
- Dehydration
- Pre-eclampsia.

Diagnosis

Diagnosis of VTE in pregnancy can be difficult. However, the latest CMACE report [2] states that the mothers that died of VTE had clinical signs suggestive of VTE. The issue is further complicated by the recent NICE guidance on diagnosis of VTE [8], which advocates the use of D-dimer. This frequently gives a false-positive result in pregnancy and is therefore of limited use. A sensible approach, however, would be to use the principles of this guidance, where clinical suspicion can trigger Doppler ultrasound of the leg. Where this is negative, but the clinical suspicion is high, further imaging can be organized. Chest X-ray serves to exclude alternative diagnoses. Ventilation-perfusion (V/Q) scans have been a traditional test for pulmonary embolism in pregnancy. The gold standard for diagnosis of pulmonary embolism in nonpregnant individuals is computed tomography pulmonary angiograms (CTPA). Spiral chest computed tomography has increased in popularity because of the high diagnostic yield. It is also considered to be the most cost-effective initial diagnostic test in the diagnosis of pulmonary embolism in pregnant women. The data below provides estimates of fetal radiation dose for different radiological investigations. Given the recommended fetal radiation exposure is less than 5 rad, these figures should tip the clinician's mind in favor of investigating suspected VTE using definitive imaging, albeit with a relatively small radiation dose.

Estimates for fetal radiation dose are as follows [6,9]:

- Chest radiograph: <0.001 rad
- V/Q scan   <0.001 rad
- Pulmonary angiogram   <0.05 rad
- Chest CT scan   <0.016 rad.

Treatment

Warfarin is avoided until the post-partum period because it crosses the placenta causing fetal hemorrhage and malformations. In contrast, unfractionated heparin or low-molecular-weight heparins do not do this, so are the treatment of choice. They have the added benefit of being shorter acting and easier to reverse in the event of a catastrophic hemorrhage. Low-molecular-weight heparins are easier to administer, have fixed dosing, do not require monitoring and are associated with a lower incidence of osteoporosis and thrombocytopenia than heparin.

Massive pulmonary embolism can present with symptoms of right ventricular failure secondary to embolic obstruction.

- Initial measures include placing the patient in the left lateral position to alleviate any venacaval obstruction and improve venous return.
- Hemodynamic support should be provided in the form of intravenous fluids and vasopressors, although the latter may cause uterine artery vasoconstriction.
- Delivery of the fetus should always be considered.
- The use of potent fibrinolytic drugs may be employed, but may result in massive hemorrhage.
- Radiological clot dispersion or open embolectomy should be considered as options, if available.

Amniotic fluid embolism (AFE)

Amniotic fluid embolism is a syndrome characterized by abrupt cardiorespiratory collapse and coagulopathy occurring during labor or immediately post-partum. The 2006–2008 CMACE report [2] describes 13 maternal deaths directly attributable to AFE, which gives a mortality rate of 0.57 per 100 000 pregnancies. The UK Obstetric Surveillance System collects data on AFE on a prospective basis and gave an incidence of 2.0 per 100 000 pregnancies for the period 2005–2009; 20% of women with AFE died in this series, which is a dramatic improvement from traditional data. The majority of patients with AFE die within the first hour and 85% of those surviving go on to have permanent neurological impairment [9].

The condition is triggered when amniotic fluid enters the maternal circulation. The exact pathophysiology is unclear, but current opinion appears to favor an immune basis rather than an embolic one. Amniotic fluid containing fetal antigens stimulates a cascade of endogenous immune mediators, producing an anaphylactoid-type reaction in the mother. Two phases are described [10]:

- Phase 1: the amniotic contents trigger the release of vasoactive substances causing pulmonary artery vasospasm and pulmonary hypertension. This results in raised right ventricular pressure and right ventricular failure leading to hypoxemia and hypotension.
- Phase 2: if phase 1 is survived, left ventricular failure and pulmonary edema occur. Further release of biochemical mediators triggers disseminated intravascular coagulation (DIC), leading to massive hemorrhage and uterine atony.

There is no single diagnostic test for AFE. The presence of fetal squames in maternal blood samples is neither sensitive nor specific as a diagnostic tool. Diagnosis continues to be made on clinical grounds and although it can easily be confused with other causes of maternal collapse, the treatment is largely the same.

The cornerstones of management are early recognition, early resuscitation and delivery of the fetus. Senior multidisciplinary support should be sought early. There is no "cure" as such and treatment should be supportive.

Maintaining oxygenation may involve tracheal intubation and ventilation. Rapid intravenous filling along with vasopressors to maintain cardiac output and ensure adequate perfusion may be required. Disseminated intravascular coagulation being a feature of AFE should be expected and restoration of normal coagulation under the guidance of hematologists should be sought. Surgical intervention may be required to control hemorrhage. Delivery of the baby should take place as soon as is safe if AFE occurs pre-partum. If cardiopulmonary resuscitation is in place, delivery should occur within 5 minutes. Most patients require admission to ICU.

Amniotic fluid embolism is no longer regarded as a condition with near universal mortality. Higher-quality supportive multidisciplinary care can result in good outcomes for mother and baby.

Major obstetric hemorrhage

The UK incidence of major obstetric hemorrhage is 4.7 per 1000 births, with uterine atony being the commonest cause [11]. The 2006–2008 CMACE report, however, describes nine maternal deaths from obstetric hemorrhage giving an overall mortality of 0.39 per 100 000 maternities [2]. The reason for such a large discrepancy between incidence and mortality is due, largely, to good multidisciplinary management.

The following is not a full account of how to manage hemorrhage per se, but will serve to highlight some of the unique differences in the obstetric patient compared to in the general population.

In assessing and treating a bleeding obstetric patient, it is worth noting the following.

- The extent of bleeding may be underestimated because it is concealed (in bedclothes, between legs, within the abdomen or in the vagina).
- Bleeding from the uteroplacental bed can be torrential and difficult to control.
- Moderate bleeding can rapidly develop into major hemorrhage.
- They may tolerate significant blood loss, despite significant decrease in circulating volume.
- Hypotension and tachycardia in this setting represents severe hypovolemia.
- Coagulopathy be may the underlying cause or arise from dilution and develop into a secondary contributory factor.

Massive obstetric hemorrhage is defined as blood loss of >1500 mL, a decrease in hemoglobin >4 g d/L or acute transfusion requirement of >4 units [12]. It can be classified as antepartum (APH) which corresponds to bleeding between 24 weeks gestation and birth. Post-partum hemorrhage (PPH) refers to bleeding occurring after birth. It is further subdivided into primary: from birth to 24 h after delivery and secondary: 24 h to 6 weeks. Causes of antepartum hemorrhage include:

- Placenta previa: where the placenta implants on or very near to the cervical os
- Placenta accreta, increta and percreta arise when the placenta abnormally invades varying degrees of the myometrium
- Placental abruption: there is premature separation of the placenta from the endometrium

- Uterine rupture: rare, but can be fatal to mother and baby
- Splenic and renal artery aneurysm rupture: very rare.

Causes of post-partum hemorrhage include:
- Uterine atony is responsible in 80% of cases
- Trauma to the perineum, cervix and vagina
- Retained placenta
- Coagulopathy; may be primary or secondary
- Uterine inversion is rare, but can cause cardiovascular compromise through blood loss and autonomic stimulation. Early reduction of the uterus is required.

Management

The general management of hemorrhage is not covered here. However, specific treatments that apply to these patients will be included. They can be divided into pharmacological, surgical and radiological.

Pharmacological

- Oxytocin: causes smooth (uterine) muscle contraction, so particularly useful in treating atony. Normally given in a slow bolus of 5 units followed by an infusion. It can cause tachycardia and hypotension.
- Ergometrine: causes smooth (uterine) muscle contraction and vascular smooth muscle. It is given via the intravenous or intramuscular route as 250 or 500 µg. It can cause hypertension, so should be avoided in pre-eclampsia. Vomiting is a common side effect.
- Prostaglandin $F_2.\alpha$ (carboprost) is used if oxytocin or ergometrine have been ineffective, and atony is believed to be the cause. A 250 µg intramuscular dose is given. It can cause flushing, hypertension and bronchospasm, so is avoided in asthma.

Surgical

- Manual removal of placenta if this is the cause
- Uterine packing
- Uterine and hypogastric artery ligation
- B-lynch suture to provide uterine compression
- Hysterectomy.
- Balloon tamponade

Radiological

- Depending on facilities and staff available, patients can be transferred to an interventional radiology suite for selective embolization of pelvic vessels.

The principles in managing massive obstetric hemorrhage are generally the same as managing other massive hemorrhages; namely resuscitation with volume, cessation of bleeding and replacement of hemoglobin, clotting factors and platelets. There are, however, some important differences in the assessment of volume loss, the causes of bleeding and the treatment.

Nonobstetric complications

There are numerous nonobstetric conditions that could result in a patient being admitted to ICU. In general, the principles for managing these patients are the same as for the nonpregnant population. There are, however, some considerations which should be taken into account.

Sepsis

The latest CMACE report for 2006–2008 revealed sepsis as the leading direct cause of maternal death in the UK. Deaths arising from Group A Streptococcal (GAS) infections have been increasing over the last ten years. Contamination of the perineum is more likely when a woman or close family contacts have sore throats or upper respiratory tract infections, as the organism may be transmitted from the nose or throat via her hands to the perineum. This latest report describes 13 women dying from these infections and identifies substandard care in many of these cases, particularly a lack of recognition of sepsis [2]. Other causes of sepsis include urinary tract infection, chorioamnionitis and endometritis following cesarean section [7]. The general principles of managing sepsis in this population are the same as with the general population, as highlighted in the sepsis chapter.

Respiratory infections

Causative pathogens of community-acquired pneumonia are, largely, similar to those in nonobstetric patients. Complications of pneumonia include maternal death, premature delivery and low birth weight.

Pregnancy has an impact on cell-mediated immunity. This results in a decrease in T-helper cells, reduced natural killer cell activity and reduced lymphocyte proliferation [7]. These individuals are therefore more likely to contract and suffer from viral infections. This is supported by the finding that influenza causes disproportionately more deaths in the pregnant population during influenza epidemics [13]. This predisposition to develop a viral respiratory infection may be complicated further by a secondary bacterial infection.

Antivirals, even if given early, may reduce the duration of the illness, but have not been shown to affect the course of any respiratory failure.

When treating patients with respiratory failure, there is the theoretical advantage of delivering the baby, because many of the physiological respiratory changes described previously are reversed following delivery. There is little evidence to support this theory, but this lack of evidence may indeed be due to the scarcity of such incidence and the obvious difficulties in performing a true randomized, controlled trial. Each case should be judged individually in conjunction with obstetricians and pediatricians. If delivery is to be performed, it is important to note that neuromuscular blocking agents and sedatives such as opiates may have crossed the placenta.

Trauma

Major trauma involving obstetric patients has marked differences in different countries:
- Gun shot wounds, while once rare outside of the USA are increasing in incidence. The same is true of penetrating trauma.

- Road traffic accidents are the most common cause of trauma deaths in the western world [14].

Various countries have organized their trauma provision differently. Larger trauma units are becoming the norm. However, this occasionally forces the first responder to deal with patients outside of their normal remit.
The following points serve as a reminder in these circumstances:

- Resuscitation of the mother with adequate fluids and oxygenation is of course beneficial to the fetus.
- Aortocaval compression is frequently forgotten in these cases due to worries about spinal injury.
- Suspicion of fetal–placental damage must be high even for trivial sounding trauma. This should be investigated with kick-charts, cardiotocography and ultrasound to rule out abruption.
- Domestic violence as the potential root cause of non-RTA incidents must be addressed immediately following the emergency treatment.
- Anti-D treatment should be considered even in minor trauma.

Cardiopulmonary arrest

The management of a pregnant patient in cardiac arrest has some important differences from nonpregnant individuals. The effect of the gravid uterus, as previously described, can reduce venous return and causes upward displacement of the diaphragm. This can clearly hinder any efforts to resuscitate these patients. Placing the patient in the left lateral position would improve venous return, but providing chest compressions in this position is challenging. Chest compressions are therefore delivered with the patient tilted to the left 30°. Many obstetric units have a "wedge" that can be placed under the patient to achieve this.

The single most important intervention in these situations is to deliver the fetus. The "4-minute rule" has been used to describe the time frame in which perimortem cesarean delivery should have started following arrest, with the aim to achieve delivery within 5 minutes.

Advanced life support treatment and procedures such as drugs and their timing, placement of hands for chest compressions and positioning of defibrillator pads should be followed as per published guidelines for nonpregnant adults.

The care of the parturient in critical care

Slightly under 20% of parturient admissions to critical care are still pregnant. This will make some difference to their treatment. For instance, aortocaval compression must be attended to – usually by tilting the patient in the left lateral position. This can be done by altering the angle of the bed, but just as easily by the use of a "Cardiff wedge." Pregnant women will need particular attention to pharmaceutical dosing – a relative hemodilution and alteration of liver physiology can cause a larger dose requirement (e.g. for suxamethonium (succinylcholine)). However, the contracture of various compartments, like the functional residual capacity and the epidural space (by back pressure in the epidural veins) may require less medicine (e.g. with local anesthetics). Historical use, familiarization, fetal concerns and a lack of rigorous testing has led to a reduced pharmacopeia for pregnant women. Hence, critical care areas may have to avail themselves of medicines not commonly used there – for instance, hydralazine, ergometrine, oxytocin and carboprost. Fluid balance, although clearly important in critical care, can be of the utmost importance, especially when the admission has PET as a primary component. Critically ill pregnant women can carry to term. Spontaneous delivery is, however, frequently premature, especially with ongoing critical illness and, in particular, sepsis. Therefore, it is essential when planning critical care services for these women that the department avails themselves of basic obstetric equipment. It is important to note at this point that current resuscitation guidelines advise that an emergency cesarean section is performed 5 minutes after cardiac arrest in a parturient. It is self-evident that a proper obstetric (with a named clinician) and midwifery plan is enacted for each patient that is admitted to critical care areas. Central to these will be a plan for fetal surveillance, which will include daily heart monitoring and regular growth estimation by ultrasound. Thromboprophylaxis is an important area for all inpatients, but arguably more so for parturients due to their procoagulant status. There is a comprehensive set of NICE guidelines that addresses this and many other issues [15].

In the post-partum period, many of these requirements are lessened; however, it is worth noting a few things:

- The benefits of breast-feeding should be emphasized, while recalling that the transmission of drugs to the newborn must be taken into account.
- Continued obstetric and midwifery care is essential to ensure anti-D assays and administration are carried out, that venous thromboprophylaxis is still addressed and to make a plan for return to the labor ward.

References

1. Levels of critical care for adult patients. *Standards and Guidelines.* ICS, London 2009 http://www.ics.ac.uk/ics-homepage/guidelines-standards/ (accessed July 2014).

2. Special Issue: Saving Mothers' Lives: Reviewing maternal deaths to make motherhood safer: 2006–2008. The Eighth Report of the Confidential Enquiries into Maternal Deaths in the United Kingdom. *BJOG* 2011; 118(Supl S1) : 1–203. http://onlinelibrary.wiley.com/doi/10.1111/bjo.2011.118.issue-s1/issuetoc (accessed June 2014).

3. Female admissions (aged 16–50 years) to adult, general critical care units in England Wales and Northern Ireland, reported as "currently pregnant" or 'recently pregnant'. 1 January 2007 to 31 December 2007. ICNARC, 2009. www.oaa-anaes.ac.uk/assets/_managed/editor/File/Reports/ICNARC_obs_report_Oct2009.pdf (accessed June 2014).

4. *Scottish Audit of Severe Maternal Morbidity: 6th Annual Report. Reproductive Health Programme.* NHS QIS, Scotland 2008. www.nhshealthquality.org/nhsqis/files/SCASMM_REP_APR10.pdf (accessed June 2014).

5. *Hypertension In Pregnancy: The Management of Hypertensive Disorders During Pregnancy.* NICE clinical guideline 107. NICE, London 2011. http://www.nice.org.uk/nicemedia/live/13098/50418/50418.pdf (accessed June 2014).

6. Shapiro JM. Venous thromboembolism in pregnancy. *J Intensive Care Med.* 2001; 16 : 22–8.

7. Shapiro JM. Critical Care of the Obstetric Patient. *J Intensive Care Med* 2006; 21 : 278–86.

8. *Venous Thromboembolic Diseases: The Management of Venous Thromboembolic Diseases and the Role of Thrombophilia Testing.* NICE clinical guideline 144. NICE, London 2012. http://www.nice.org.uk/nicemedia/live/13767/59720/59720.pdf (accessed June 2014).

9. Winer-Muram HT, Boone JM, Brown HL, *et al.* Pulmonary embolism in pregnant

patients: fetal radiation dose with helical CT. *Radiology* 2002; 224 : 487–92.

10. Dedhia JT, Mushambi MC. Amniotic Fluid Embolism. *Contin Educ Anaesth Crit Care Pain* 2007; 7 (5) : 152–6.

11. Brace V. Learning from adverse outcomes—major haemorrhage in Scotland in 2003–05. *BJOG* 2007; 114 : 1388–96.

12. Shevell T, Malone FD. Management of obstetric hemorrhage. *Semin Perinatol* 2003; 27 : 86–104.

13. Bridges CB, Harper SA, Fukuda K, *et al.* Prevention and control of influenza. *MMWR Morbid Mortal Wkly Rep.* 2003; 52 : 1–36.

14. Johanson R, Cox C, Grady K, Howell C. *Managing Obstetric Emergencies and Trauma: The MOET Course Manual.* London: RCOG Press; 2003.

15. *Intrapartum Care: Care of Healthy Women and Their Babies During Childbirth.* NICE, London 2007. www.nice.org.uk/guidance/CG55 (accessed June 2014).

Chapter 34

The critically ill asthmatic

Ian M Ball

Incidence

Asthma is a worldwide problem, affecting approximately 300 million people [1]:

- The prevalence of people afflicted with asthma ranges from 1–18% of the population in various countries [2].
- The World Health Organization estimates that asthma accounts for 15 million disability-adjusted life years lost annually [2].
- This represents 1% of the global disease burden.
- The monetary costs, and days lost from work due to asthma are significant [3,4].

There are 250 000 deaths worldwide from asthma [2]:

- Asthma mortality is 40% higher for females than males, and three times higher in blacks than in whites.
- The death rate due to asthma is increasing [5,6].

Pathophysiology

Asthma is an inflammatory disease of the small airways caused by a spectrum of mediators [5] released in response to: allergen exposure, air pollution, infections and poor compliance with treatment. Many asthma exacerbations have no clearly identifiable cause.

- Autopsies of patients dying of asthma exacerbations demonstrate peripheral airway occlusion by mucous and secretions with inflammatory and epithelial cells, surrounded by hypertrophied smooth muscles, eosinophilic submucosal infiltration and inflamed, edematous bronchial walls [7,8].
- This diffuse airway occlusion causes severe ventilation/perfusion mismatch and hypoxemia [9,10].

Differential diagnosis

The diagnosis may be obvious, but in adults, especially in the absence of a previous history of asthma or failure to respond to appropriate treatment, the following alternatives should be considered:

- Chronic obstructive airways disease
- Left ventricular failure

Handbook of ICU Therapy, third edition, ed. John Fuller, Jeff Granton and Ian McConachie. Published by Cambridge University Press. © Cambridge University Press 2015.

- Upper airways obstruction
- Pulmonary embolus.

Clinical examination

The severity of an exacerbation may be underappreciated by less experienced clinicians. Patients' respiratory status can deteriorate precipitously. As such, frequent serial evaluations by experienced personnel are strongly recommended.

- In general however, patients with severe asthma will have increased work of breathing and appear in distress from the foot of the bed.
- They will sit up, and will answer questions with only a few words at a time. Patients may be agitated or describe a "sense of impending doom."
- Patients with severe asthma exacerbations will be tachypneic and tachycardic.
- Auscultation may reveal expiratory, biphasic wheezes, or a "silent chest," in order of associated increasing disease severity. A silent chest, evidenced by a patient who appears to be working very hard to breathe, but in whom breath sounds are very quiet or absent, portrays pending respiratory arrest. It should be managed aggressively and promptly.
- Pneumothorax should be ruled out with chest radiography.
- Other clinical exam findings suggestive of imminent respiratory arrest include: an alteration in level of consciousness, change from tachycardia to bradycardia and paradoxical thoracoabdominal movement.

Investigations

- Chest radiography should be performed to rule out pneumothoraces, pneumomediastinum, pneumopericardium and subcutaneous emphysema. Atelectasis secondary to excessive secretions and mucous plugging is seen, although this is rare.
- An electrocardiogram is important to detect right axis deviation and other signs of right ventricular strain, as well as to rule out acute myocardial ischemia.
- Serial measurements of peak flow or FEV_1 can help quantify attack severity and monitor response to therapy. Values less than 30% predicted indicate severe attacks.
- Blood gas analysis certainly contributes to the overall diagnostic and management algorithms in severe asthma, but should never be interpreted in isolation. Earlier in an exacerbation, blood gas analysis reveals respiratory alkalosis, which may normalize and convert to a respiratory acidosis in refractory or untreated cases.
- Metabolic acidosis is a very serious finding that suggests impending respiratory arrest. Its etiologies are multifactorial. Severe dynamic hyperinflation increases intrathoracic pressure, thereby decreasing venous return and cardiac output. Right-sided cardiac output may be further reduced by elevated pulmonary artery pressure and increased right ventricular afterload. Large negative intrathoracic pressures during inspiration may cause rapid right ventricular filling, and a leftward shift of the intraventricular septum. This can reduce left ventricular end-diastolic volumes and subsequent left ventricular cardiac output [11,12].
- Other potential mechanisms of metabolic acidosis include: anaerobic metabolism in heavily strained respiratory muscles, profound tissue hypoxemia and decreased hepatic lactate clearance secondary to liver hypoperfusion [13].

Management

Education

Patients with moderate to severe asthma require intensive education regarding prevention, maintenance and exacerbation treatment. Patients need to be followed closely as outpatients, and a plan should be in place for how to recognize disease worsening, how to escalate treatment in the event of exacerbations and when to seek medical attention [14].

Initial treatment

The following measures should be taken immediately:

- Supplemental oxygen titrated to maintain oxygen saturation by pulse oximetry >90%.
- Nebulized β_2-agonists, albuterol 2.5 mg (0.5 mL) in 2.5 mL NS is a standard dosing regimen. Continuous or multiple nebulizations should be administered as the efficacy and duration of β-agonists are inversely related to the degree of severity of the exacerbation [13]. High doses of β-agonists will cause tremors, tachycardia and hypokalemia. These side effects must be weighed against the risk of respiratory failure and potential asthma death prior to de-escalating therapy in the critically ill asthmatic. In particular, the potential risk of tachycardia-induced myocardial ischemia pales in comparison to the immediate life-threatening risk of a severe asthma exacerbation.
- Inhaled β-agonist treatment is at least as good, if not better than, intravenous therapy [13]. While albuterol infusions do not have any proven therapeutic advantage, they clearly cause more systemic absorption and side effects.
- Inhaled β-agonist treatment should be continued until there is clear evidence of improvement, both clinically and on blood gas analysis.

Other aspects of treatment include:

- Systemic corticosteroid therapy, either intravenously or orally (in the critically ill patient, the intravenous route is preferred due to unreliable gut perfusion) [15]. Steroid treatment should be administered promptly, but will take several hours to take effect.
- Ipratropium bromide can be added to albuterol. It is usually administered as 500 μg by nebulizer every 4–6 hours.

Patients with severe asthma should not receive any sedatives that will blunt their respiratory drive or affect their ability to protect their airways.

Response to treatment must be monitored with peak expiratory flow rate (PEFR) and repeat blood gases.

If the patient improves with the above:

- Continue a high-concentration oxygen
- Regular nebulized β_2-agonists (frequency should be titrated to clinical response, but ranges from continuous to every 4 hours)
- Monitor the patient's saturations, blood gases and PEFR closely.

If the patient does not improve in the first 15–30 minutes:

- Continue oxygen
- Give β_2-agonists more frequently (up to 15–30 min or even continuously)
- Continue the ipratropium every 4–6 hours.

Response to treatment must be monitored with PEFR, "clinical" assessment of the patient and blood gas estimations if life-threatening features persist or oxyhemoglobin saturation by oximetry is <92%.

Indications for ICU admission

Intensive care admission is indicated for:

- All patients with moderate to severe asthma exacerbations who are deteriorating despite optimum treatment
- Patients with significant complicating comorbidities that make them intolerant to the physiologic stress of asthma.

Noninvasive ventilation

Reports of noninvasive ventilation (NIV) in acute asthma exacerbations are rare. Due to the low amount of experience and supporting literature, the use of NIV for the critically ill asthmatic is controversial.

There is, however, sound physiologic rationale for a beneficial effect of NIV:

- NIV may offset the increased demand placed on respiratory muscles by asthma-associated positive end-expiratory pressure
- NIV may decrease auto-PEEP [16]
- The PEEP from NIV may improve asthma-induced ventilation-perfusion mismatch [17]
- Bronchodilator delivery to peripheral airways may improved by the coadministration of NIV [18,19]
- NIV may recruit collapsed alveoli [20].

Two observational trials, [21,22] and two small randomized trials [23,24] support the notion that NIV can be used effectively for managing acute, severe asthma exacerbations. NIV use in asthmatic patients, however, should be selective. Soroksky et al. [20] suggest some absolute and relative contraindications.

Absolute contraindications to NIV use:

- Need for immediate endotracheal intubation
- Decreased level of consciousness
- Excess respiratory secretions and risk of aspiration
- Past facial surgery precluding mask fitting.

Relative contraindications to NIV use:

- Hemodynamic instability
- Severe hypoxemia and/or hypercapnia (PaO_2/FiO_2 <200 mmHg, $PaCO_2$ >60 mmHg)
- Poor patient cooperation
- Severe agitation
- Lack of trained or experienced staff.

The downside to application of NIV rather than invasive ventilation in severe asthma exacerbations pertains to delaying the establishment of a definitive airway in a patient with respiratory collapse. Noninvasive ventilation should only be used in critically ill asthmatics in a fully monitored setting by experienced personnel that are able to intubate at a moment's notice.

Indications for intubation

Absolute indications for intubation and mechanical ventilation include:

- Coma
- Respiratory arrest or ineffective respirations
- Exhaustion.

Other considerations for early intubation include:

- Progressive hypoxemia despite increasing inspired oxygen
- Progressive hypercapnia (note that a normal $PaCO_2$ may denote a rising level passing through the normal range as the patient becomes tired)
- Progressive acidosis (respiratory, metabolic or mixed)
- Ineffective cough/inability to clear secretions.

These nonmandatory indications should be used in conjunction with the general state and appearance of the patient.

A physician with extensive experience in airway management should be present for intubation. Ketamine is an excellent choice of induction agent because of its rapid onset and short duration of action, its hemodynamic stability and its bronchodilating properties.

Mechanical ventilation of the asthmatic patient

Similar to most medical conditions, there is a large spectrum of asthma exacerbation severity. In its mildest form, the ventilated asthmatic may be successfully treated with fairly standard ventilator strategies. The focus of this review will be the severe, difficult-to-ventilate asthmatic.

Ventilation strategies in severe asthma [25]

Pressure-limited or volume-limited strategies are both acceptable.

- In pressure-limited modes, the risk of barotrauma and reduced cardiac output from high intrathoracic pressure is reduced, at the potential expense of hypoventilation from low tidal volumes.
- Volume-cycled modes are effective, but airway pressure limits must be set and closely monitored.

Oxygen

The fraction of inspired oxygen should be titrated to correct hypoxemia. Unlike some exacerbations of chronic obstructive pulmonary disease, there is no need to limit oxygen therapy.

Respiratory rate

Setting an appropriately low ventilator rate may be the single most important ventilator strategy, as low rates optimize expiratory time to prevent dynamic hyperinflation.

- In the severe asthmatic, an initial rate of 8–10 breaths per minute is a good starting point
- Like all other parameters, it will likely require titration based on patient response.

Inspiratory to expiratory ratio

The second most important ventilator setting is likely the inspiratory to expiratory (I:E) ratio.

- Standard I:Es in nonasthmatics usually range from 1:2 to 1:2.5.
- In the severe asthmatic, I:Es as high as 1:5 or 1:6 may be required to allow sufficient time for expiration to be completed.
- Similar to the respiratory rate, a starting point of 1:4 that is titrated to patient response is appropriate.
- Low tidal volumes and low respiratory rates have long been known to be associated with improved outcomes, despite moderate hypercarbia and respiratory acidosis [26].

Tidal volumes

Despite the absence of large scale randomized trials comparing tidal volumes in the ventilation of the severe asthmatic, it is very reasonable to use a low tidal volume (6–8 mL/kg) strategy. This will reduce dynamic hyperinflation and barotrauma.

Positive end-expiratory pressure (PEEP)

The optimal PEEP setting in the severe asthmatic is controversial and will likely remain that way, as definitive trials on this topic are methodologically nearly impossible to conduct.

- Theoretically, external PEEP could reduce the work of breathing by reduction of gas trapping through splinted small airways, thereby reducing carbon dioxide production and hence facilitating ventilation.
- The counter argument is that extrinsic PEEP could increase total PEEP and worsen gas trapping, thereby impairing ventilation [27–30].
- Once again, the choice of appropriate PEEP is an example of the need for individualized patient decision-making, frequent patient reassessment and titration of therapy.

Inspiratory flow

Higher inspiratory flow rates (70–100 L/min) will reduce the amount of time spent in the inspiratory phase, allowing a longer expiratory phase, which reduces the risk of dynamic hyperinflation.

- High inspiratory flow times may cause high plateau pressures, so these too require careful monitoring and titration to patient response. Generally a plateau pressure of below 30 cmH_2O should be the target.
- Should clinicians be unable to meet this target, it may be due to severe bronchospasm or dynamic hyperinflation alone, but an evaluation for pneumothorax, mucous plug or endotracheal tube dislodgement should be undertaken.

Permissive hypercapnia

Ventilation with low respiratory rates may lead to overall hypoventilation and hypercarbia. The first step to addressing hypercarbia is ensuring that the patient is adequately sedated, and any fever is treated with antipyretics in an effort to reduce carbon dioxide production.

Respiratory acidosis can be tolerated to a pH of 7.2. Should the pH fall below 7.2, a sodium bicarbonate infusion should be initiated, particularly in the face of any evolving hemodynamic instability [31].

Dynamic hyperinflation

Figure 34.1 illustrates the potential problems of dynamic hyperinflation (progressive air trapping and increases in lung volumes caused by the next breath occurring before the end of expiration) in the asthmatic patient.

- Example A shows a classic example of gas trapping in an asthmatic. The expiratory flow has not returned to baseline prior to initiation of inspiratory flow, with a resultant increase (Example B) in lung volume.
- Example C shows that increasing the I:E ratio allows for completion of expiration prior to initiation of inspiratory flow. The result (Example D) is that lung volume does not increase over time.

Additional medical therapies

Intravenous magnesium sulfate

Magnesium sulfate has bronchodilating properties that make it an appealing treatment in the critically ill asthmatic. It can be administered as boluses or infused. There is some

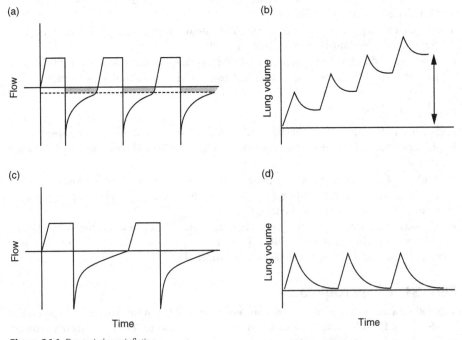

Figure 34.1 Dynamic hyperinflation.

evidence demonstrating a benefit and the risks are small [32,33] (respiratory muscle weakness in an intubated ventilated patient is inconsequential).

Ketamine

In most intubating clinical scenarios there are many appropriate choices of intravenous induction agent. For intubation of the deteriorating asthmatic, ketamine is a clear choice because of its favorable kinetics, hemodynamic stability and, in particular, for its bronchodilatory properties.

There is not a lot of clinical data on the use of ketamine infusions for the management of the mechanically ventilated, refractory asthmatic [34,35].

- It has a fairly benign side-effect profile and there is good rationale for its benefit, in particular when patients are not responding to more traditional treatments.
- A bolus of 0.3–0.5 mg/kg followed by an infusion starting at 0.3–0.5 mg/kg/h, titrated to clinical response may be beneficial.

Heliox

Heliox has a long history of use in asthma, and for patients with airway obstructions such as malignancies.

- It is a blend of oxygen and helium that is usually available in two concentrations: a 20% oxygen/80% helium blend, and a 30% oxygen/70% helium blend.
- Substituting the smaller helium molecule for nitrogen is thought to improve laminar air flow through small airways, thereby reducing turbulence and improving overall ventilation [36,37].
- Although there is no convincing evidence for the benefit of Heliox [38–40], it has little downside, other than the inability to provide higher than 30% oxygen during administration.
- Heliox is likely more beneficial if started early in the course of the management of a severe asthma exacerbation [41].

Volatile anesthetic agents

Inhalational anesthetics are generally reserved for the most extreme cases of severe asthma.

- The most experience with inhalational anesthetics is with isoflurane and sevoflurane.
- These agents are all bronchodilators and have been used successfully for asthma treatment [42–44].
- The downsides to the use of inhalational anesthetics include: lack of intensivist experience (in the nonanesthetist), requirement for a cumbersome anesthetic machine in the space-limited critical care area and the hemodynamic instability that inhalational gases may cause.

Extracorporeal membrane oxygenation (ECMO)

In extreme cases of asthma that are refractory to all of the above therapies, ECMO may be considered. Patients on ECMO require anticoagulation, and bleeding complications are common. Extracorporeal membrane oxygenation is expensive and requires a lot of space and trained personnel. It is only available in specialized centers. The decision to transport a patient with refractory hypoxemia to an ECMO center should not be taken lightly, as any patient sick enough to require ECMO will have a high risk of transport-associated morbidity and even mortality. Extracorporeal membrane oxygenation may save lives in the severe asthmatic refractory to all other therapies [45,46].

References

1. Masoli M, Fabian D, Holt S, Beasley R. The global burden of asthma: executive summary of the GINA Dissemination Committee report. *Allergy* 2004; 59 : 469–78.

2. Beasley R. The Global Burden of Asthma Report, Global Initiative for Asthma (GINA). Available from http://www. ginasthma.org 2004 (accessed June 2014).

3. Papiris S, Kotanidou A, Malagari K, Roussos C. Clinical review: severe asthma. *Critical Care* 2002; 6 : 30–44.

4. Weiss KB, Gergen PJ, Hodgson TA. An economic evaluation of asthma in the United States. *N Engl J Med* 1992; 326 : 862–6.

5. National Heart, Lung and Blood Institute. Guidelines for the Diagnosis and Management of Asthma, Expert Panel Report 2. Bethesda: National Institutes of Health. Publication number 97–4051, 1997.

6. McFadden ER Jr, Warren EL. Observations on asthma mortality. *Ann Intern Med* 1997; 127 : 142–7.

7. Reid LM. The presence or absence of bronchial mucous in fatal asthma. *J Allergy Clin Immunol* 1987; 80 : 415–19.

8. Saetta M, Di Stefano A, Rosina C et al. Quantitative structural analysis of peripheral airways and arteries in sudden fatal asthma. *Am Rev Respir Dis* 1991; 143 : 138–143.

9. Rodriguez-Roisin R, Ballaster E et al. Mechanism of hypoxemia in patients with status asthmaticus requiring mechanical ventilation. *Am Rev Respir Dis* 1989; 139 : 732–9.

10. Roussos CH, Macklem PT. The respiratory muscles. *N Engl J Med* 1982; 307 : 786–97.

11. Manthous CA. Management of severe exacerbations of asthma. *Am J Med* 1995; 99 : 298–308.

12. Levy BD, Kitch B, Fanta CH. Medical and ventilator management of status asthmaticus. *Intensive Care Med* 1998; 24 : 105–17.

13. Corbridge TC, Hall JB. The assessment and management of adults with status asthmaticus. *Am J Resp Crit Care Med* 1995; 151 : 1296–316.

14. Petty TL. Treat status asthmaticus three days before it occurs. *J Intensive Care Med* 1989; 4 : 135–6.

15. Manser R, Reid D, Abramson M. Corticosteroids for acute severe asthma in hospitalized patients. *Cochrane Database Syst Rev* 2001; (1): CD001740.

16. Tokioka H, Saito S, Saeki S et al. The effect of pressure support ventilation on auto-PEEP in a patient with asthma. *Chest* 1992; 101 : 285–6.

17. Broux R, Foidart G, Mendes P et al. Use of PEEP in management of life-threatening status asthmaticus: a method for the recovery of appropriate ventilation-perfusion ratio. *Appl Cardioplum Pathophysiol* 1991; 4 : 79–83.

18. Pollack CV Jr, Fleisch KB, Dowsey K. Treatment of acute bronchospasm with beta-adrenergic agonist aerosols delivered by a nasal BiPap circuit. *Ann Emerg Med* 1995; 26 : 552–7.

19. Brandao DC, Lima VM, Filho VG et al. Reversal of bronchial obstruction with bi-level positive airway pressure and nebulization in patients with acute asthma. *J Asthma* 2009; 46 : 356–61.

20. Soroksky A, Klinowski E, Ilgyev E et al. Noninvasive positive pressure ventilation in acute asthmatic attack. *Eur Respir Rev* 2010; 19 : 115,39–45.

21. Meduri GU, Cook TR, Turner RE, et al. Noninvasive positive pressure ventilation in status asthmaticus. *Chest* 1996; 110 : 767–74.

22. Fernandez MM, Villagra A, Blanch L *et al.* Non-invasive mechanical ventilation in status asthmaticus. *Intensive Care Med* 2001; 27 : 486–92.

23. Soroksky A, Stav D, Shpirer I. A pilot prospective, randomized, placebo-controlled trial of bilevel positive airway pressure in acute asthmatic attack. *Chest* 2003; 123 : 1018–25.

24. Soma T, Hino M, Kida K *et al.* A prospective and randomized study for improvement of acute asthma by non-invasive positive pressure ventilation (NPPV). *Intern Med* 2008; 47 : 493–501.

25. Stather DR, Stewart TE. Clinical Review: mechanical ventilation in severe asthma. *Crit Care* 2005; 9 : 581–7.

26. Darioli R, Perret C. Mechanical controlled hypoventilation in status asthmaticus. *Am Rev Respir Dis* 1984; 129 : 385–7.

27. Kondili E, Alexopoulou C, Prinianakis G *et al.* Pattern of lung emptying and expiratory resistance in mechanically ventilated patients with chronic obstructive pulmonary disease. *Intensive Care Med* 2004; 30 : 1311–18.

28. Tuxen DV. Detrimental effects of positive end-expiratory pressure during controlled mechanical ventilation of patients with severe airflow obstruction. *Am Rev Respir Dis* 1989; 140 : 5–10.

29. Peigang Y, Marini JJ. Ventilation of patients with asthma and chronic obstructive pulmonary disease. *Curr Opin Crit Care* 2002; 8 : 70–6.

30. Rodrigo GJ, Rodrigo C, Hall JB. Acute asthma in adults: a review. *Chest*. 2004; 125 : 1081–102.

31. Menitove SM, Goldring RM. Combined ventilator and bicarbonate strategy in the management of status asthmaticus. *Am J Med* 1983; 74 : 898–901.

32. Rowe BH, Bretzlaff JA, Bourdon C *et al.* Intravenous magnesium sulfate treatment for acute asthma in the emergency department: a systematic review of the literature. *Ann Emerg Med* 2000; 36 : 181–90.

33. Silverman RA, Osborn H, Runge J *et al.* IV magnesium sulfate in the treatment of acute severe asthma: a multicenter randomized controlled trial. *Chest* 2002; 122 : 489–97.

34. Sarma V. Use of Ketamine in acute severe asthma. *Acta Anaesthesiol Scand* 1992; 36 : 106–7.

35. Hemmingsen C, Nielsen PK, Odorico J. Ketamine in the treatment of bronchospasm during mechanical ventilation. *Am J Emerg Med* 1994; 12 : 417–20.

36. Schaeffer EM, Pohlman A, Morgan S, Hall JB. Oxygenation in status asthmaticus improves during ventilation with helium-oxygen. *Crit Care Med* 1999; 27 : 2666–70.

37. Gluck EH, Onorato DJ, Castriotta R. Helium-oxygen mixtures in intubated patients with status asthmaticus and respiratory acidosis. *Chest* 1990; 98 : 693–8.

38. Henderson SO, Acharya P, Kilaghbian T *et al.* Use of heliox-driven nebulizer therapy in the treatment of acute asthma. *Ann Emerg Med* 1999; 33 : 141–6.

39. Tassaux D, Jolliet P, Roeseler J, Chevrolet JC. Effects of helium-oxygen on intrinsic Positive end-expiratory pressure in intubated and mechanically ventilated patients with severe chronic obstructive pulmonary disease. *Crit Care Med* 2000; 28 : 2721–8.

40. Kass JE, Terregino CA. The effect of heliox in acute severe asthma: a randomized controlled trial. *Chest* 1999; 116 : 296–300.

41. Ho AMH, Lee A, Karmakar MK *et al.* Heliox vs air–oxygen mixtures for the treatment of patients with acute asthma: a systematic overview. *Chest* 2003; 123 : 882–90.

42. Otte RW, Fireman P. Isoflurane anesthesia for the treatment of refractory status asthmaticus. *Ann Allergy* 1991; 66 : 305–9.

43. Maltais F, Sovilj M, Gottfried SB. Respiratory mechanics in status asthmaticus: effects of inhalational anesthesia. *Chest* 1994; 116 : 296–300.

44. Rooke GA, Choi JH, Bishop M. The effect of isoflurane, halothane, sevoflurane, and

thiopental/nitrous oxide on respiratory system resistance after tracheal intubation. *Anesthesiology* 1997; 86 : 1294–9.

45. Kukita I, Okamoto K, Sato T *et al.* Emergency extracorporeal life support for patients with near-fatal status asthmaticus. *Am J Emerg Med* 1997; 15 : 566–9.

46. Shapiro MB, Kleaveland AC, Bartlett RH. Extracorporeal life support for status asthmaticus. *Chest* 1993; 103 : 1651–4.

35 Endocrine problems in critical illness

Wael Haddara

This chapter addresses three common problems in critical illness:

1. Hyperglycemic crises: diabetic ketoacidosis (DKA) and hyperosmolar hyperglycemic state (HHS)
2. Glycemic control in critically ill patients
3. Use of corticosteroids in critically ill patients.

Hyperglycemic crises [1]

Diabetic ketoacidosis and hyperosmolar hyperglycemic states occur in patients with insulin deficiency and insulin resistance, respectively. Insulin deficiency is most commonly associated with type 1 diabetes mellitus (DM), but can also occur in patients who have had type 2 DM for many years, as a result of β-cell depletion.

The diagnosis of DKA and HHS is primarily a clinical one based on the history and presentation, and supported by laboratory findings of hyperglycemia, high anion gap acidosis and ketosis (DKA) and hyperglycemia in the absence of acidosis (HHS).

A new diagnosis of DM or insulin omission can be the precipitating cause, but a thorough history and investigation must be undertaken to rule out other precipitants (see Table 35.1).

Indications for admission to ICU

Depending on the hospital's organization of care and availability of laboratory investigations, most patients do not require admission to the ICU for management of DKA or HHS; however, a step down unit or other high intensity unit is recommended. Mortality for patients with HHS is significantly higher than patients with DKA and those patients should be treated with extra care as they tend to be older and have more comorbid conditions [2]. The primary determinant of where the patient is admitted is the availability of rapid turnaround for blood gases and tests, as well as the ability to run insulin by infusion.

Indications for ICU admission include:

- Airway compromise
- Severe acidosis, unless rapidly responsive to fluid therapy
- Hypotension, unless rapidly responsive to fluid therapy
- Hypoxia
- Severe coexisting medical conditions (e.g. heart failure)
- Lower threshold in the elderly patient.

Handbook of ICU Therapy, third edition, ed. John Fuller, Jeff Granton and Ian McConachie. Published by Cambridge University Press. © Cambridge University Press 2015.

Table 35.1 DKA and HHS

	DKA	HHS
Precipitants	New diagnosis of DM Myocardial ischemia/infarction Infection Insulin omission New drugs: atypical antipsychotics, corticosteroids	
Mechanism	Insulin deficiency leading to ketosis; acidosis; glycosuria and poor oral intake leading to volume depletion. Potassium derangements secondary to high urine output and acidosis.	High catecholamine state leading to insulin suppression; insulin resistance leading to severe hyperglycemia; glycosuria and poor oral intake leading to volume depletion; potassium derangements secondary to high urine output.
Patient profile	Type 1 DM or longstanding type 2 DM	Type 2 DM
Clinical presentation	Acidosis; moderate hyperglycemia; decreased level of consciousness; nausea, vomiting and abdominal pain; symptoms of precipitating cause.	No acidosis (unless due to precipitating cause); moderate-severe hyperglycemia; acute kidney injury (AKI) due to volume depletion.
Fluid deficit	~100 mL/kg	~100–200 mL/kg
K deficit	3–5 mEq/kg	4–6 mEq/kg
Na deficit	7–10 mEq/kg	5–13 mEq/kg

Principles of treatment

- ABCs
- Investigate and treat underlying cause(s)
- Treat volume deficit
- Resolve ketoacidosis (DKA) and hyperglycemia (HHS)
- Treat electrolyte deficits.

Patients requiring ICU admission should be approached in the usual manner with emphasis on ABCs and usual ICU care, including strict monitoring of volume in/out, venous thromboembolism prophylaxis and other treatments as necessary for sepsis, myocardial ischemia etc.

Fluid management

In severe DKA/HHS and in patients without comorbidities, a rapid initial rate of fluid replacement is warranted: 1–2 L/h for the first 2 L followed by 500 mL/h for 4 hours and then 250 mL/h for another 4 hours.

- Both 0.9% NS and Ringer's lactate are acceptable choices for resuscitation, with Ringer's theoretically associated with less hypernatremia and less hyperchloremic metabolic acidosis than normal saline.

Insulin

In patients with DKA, start with a bolus of 0.1 U/kg and infusion of 0.1 U/kg/h. Insulin should be continued until the anion gap has normalized. If blood glucose should fall below 14 mmol/L, D5W should be started. The anion gap, not the bicarbonate or the glucose level, is the target for treatment. Intravenous insulin can be discontinued once the anion gap has closed. Patients presenting with DKA must be placed on a regimen that provides them with basal insulin requirements (typically 0.2–0.5 U/kg/day) even if they are not eating. A regimen consisting solely of sliding scale is not acceptable.

Similar insulin regimens can be used in HHS, although the use of insulin is not *strictly* necessary in this population. Fluid replacement alone can reduce glucose levels in HHS.

Potassium

Patients presenting with normal or low potassium should have potassium replaced immediately (20–40 mEq KCl per L of IV fluid). Patients with potassium levels <3.3 mmol/L should receive a bolus and insulin should be withheld until potassium levels are >3.3 mmol/L. Patients who are hyperkalemic should have their potassium replaced once the K levels reach 5.0–5.5 mEq/L.

Other issues

- The use of bicarbonate is not routinely recommended as it may worsen intracellular acidosis.
- There is no evidence supporting the replacement of phosphate.
- However, because of the association with rhabdomyolysis and hypophosphatemia, potassium phosphate may be used when serum phosphate is very low.
- The rates of fluid replacement and drop of glucose may be related to the risk of developing cerebral edema in children, but this is not observed in adults.

Glycemic control in the ICU

Exploration of the optimal glucose levels in critically ill patients date back to the 1990s with a number of studies documenting an association between hyperglycemia and poor outcomes in conditions such as stroke and acute myocardial infarction (AMI).

- DIGAMI [3] was one of the earlier interventional trials and documented a reduction in mortality at 1 year in patients with AMI who were placed on an insulin infusion during their hospitalization to control glucose levels.
- The first major randomized controlled trial (RCT) to document the benefit of intervening in critically ill patients was conducted by Van den Berghe *et al.* in post-cardiac-surgery patients [4]. This trial showed an overall benefit for intensive glycemic control to achieve target glucose levels in the normal range (4–6 mmol/L).

Since that landmark trial, other RCTs have been conducted with varying results.

- A follow-up RCT by the same authors in a medical ICU showed a mortality reduction only in the subpopulation of patients with an ICU stay greater than 3 days [5].

- Other direct RCTs such as VISEP [6] and Glucontrol [7] were stopped early because of an unacceptably high rate of hypoglycemia.
- An RCT conducted at the National Guard Hospital in Riyadh in septic patients only was carried out to completion, but failed to show a reduction in mortality [8].
- Finally, a very large, high-quality multicenter RCT failed to show a mortality benefit to normal glucose targets (4–6 mmol/L) versus a tight target of 6–8 mmol/L. The 90-day mortality was increased in the normal glucose group [9].

Unlike the RCTs, "real-world" implementation and observational studies have demonstrated a net improvement in various outcomes with very tight glucose control. For example, TRIUMPH examined implementation of very tight glycemic control in several ICUs and found a statistically significant reduction in ICU length of stay and a trend towards decreased mortality and costs of care associated with implementation of glucose targets of 4–6 mmol/L [10].

Recent studies have identified hypoglycemia, variability in glycemic control and premorbid diabetic control as likely modulators of the response to tight glycemic control. Hence investigators are focusing on developing insulin algorithms that can help achieve tight glucose targets without hypoglycemia and without large swings in glycemic control. The issue of whether patients with longstanding diabetes or poorly controlled diabetes should be managed with tight levels remains entirely unclear.

In a bid to reconcile the conflicting evidence, current recommendations suggest that *hyperglycemia* in critically ill patients should be avoided, but that normal glucose levels should not be targeted and that *hypoglycemia* can be particularly harmful. Until further evidence is available, most guidelines have adopted the more cautious target levels of 8–10 mmol/L.

In order to achieve these levels, protocolized insulin infusions should be used. Insulin protocols should be tested and routinely assessed for effectiveness and safety, given that hypoglycemia and glycemic variability are associated with major morbidity.

Corticosteroid use in the ICU

Since the late 1980s when high-dose steroid use was conclusively shown not to be of benefit and possibly to be harmful in patients with sepsis and acute lung injury, the use of high-dose steroids in critically ill patients has become limited to specific indications such as interstitial lung disease and inflammatory autoimmune conditions.

However, there has been an ongoing interest in using low-dose (200–300 mg) hydrocortisone per day or equivalent to reverse shock in patients with septic shock.

- In the 1990s, a series of small RCTs examining steroids in septic shock documented shorter duration of shock when steroids were given.
- This was followed by a larger RCT [11] that demonstrated a mortality benefit in patients with refractory septic shock.
- Another large RCT [12] in less severely ill patients failed to document a reduction in mortality.

In reviewing the various studies, there is a significant variation in a number of parameters that make extrapolating a general conclusion difficult. For example, there is a difference in the steroids used (hydrocortisone alone versus hydrocortisone and fludrocortisone), the severity of illness (refractory shock despite adequate fluid resuscitation and pressors versus only requirement for pressors) and the window of time in which the steroids are given (within 1 hour of refractory shock versus 72 hours) [13].

Given the state of the evidence, a number of studies are currently underway to further explore the role of steroids in septic shock:

- Hydrocortisone for Prevention of Septic Shock (HYPRESS – NCT00670254)
- ADjunctive coRticosteroid trEatment iN criticAlly ilL Patients With Septic Shock (ADRENAL) has an estimated enrollment of 3800 patients and an estimated completion date in 2016 (NCT01448109).

Through the last decade there was an interest in defining a population that has relative adrenal insufficiency [14].

- The premise of this pursuit was that patients who are under stress because of critical illness should have very elevated cortisol levels.
- Patients who did not have very elevated levels were postulated to have "relative adrenal insufficiency" and some trials attempted to stratify patients on the basis of a cosyntropin challenge test.

However, defining "relative adrenal insufficiency" was complicated by a number of factors.

- First, there was no particular clinically useful outcome that separated "responders" from "nonresponders" to the cosyntropin challenge test.
- Second, no particular cutoff value could be found for either basal or stimulated cortisol that clearly defined a population at risk.
- Third, it quickly became apparent that the reliability of serum cortisol levels was in question, given the profound metabolic changes that take place during sepsis. The question of whether "total" or "free" serum cortisol should be measured has not been satisfactorily resolved.

For all of those reasons, the quest for defining "relative adrenal insufficiency" as an entity has been essentially abandoned.

Surviving Sepsis Campaign guidelines [15] reconcile these findings by recommending *against* using steroids in septic patients without shock or in patients in whom shock can be reversed using fluids and vasopressors/inotropes. Hence steroids should only be administered in patients with refractory shock, despite adequate fluid resuscitation and use of vasopressors/inotropes.

- When steroids are used a dose of 200 mg hydrocortisone per day in divided doses is sufficient.
- Steroids should be tapered rather than discontinued abruptly once shock is reversed.
- Cosyntropin challenge should not be used.

Measurement of serum cortisol, with or without a cosyntropin challenge test still has a role in patients suspected of having classic adrenal insufficiency. Patients suspected of:

- primary (mostly on the basis of prolonged steroid use or Waterhouse–Friderichsen syndrome)
- or secondary (head trauma, post-pituitary surgery, infiltrative CNS disease etc.) adrenal insufficiency should be treated promptly with stress doses of hydrocortisone, irrespective of the presence of refractory septic shock.

References

1. Goguen J, Gilbert J. Canadian Diabetes Association 2013 Clinical Practice Guidelines for the Prevention and Management of Diabetes in Canada: Hyperglycemic emergencies in adults. *Can J Diabetes* 2013; 37(suppl 1) : S72-6.

2. Huang CC, Kuo SC, Chien TW, *et al.* Predicting the hyperglycemic crisis death (PHD) score: a new decision rule for emergency and critical care. *Am J Emerg Med* 2013; 31 : 830-4.

3. Malmberg K. Prospective randomised study of intensive insulin treatment on long term survival after acute myocardial infarction in patients with diabetes mellitus. DIGAMI (Diabetes Mellitus, Insulin Glucose Infusion in Acute Myocardial Infarction) Study Group. *BMJ* 1997; 314 : 1512-5.

4. Van den Berghe G, Wouters P, Weekers F *et al.* Intensive insulin therapy in critically ill patients. *N Engl J Med* 2001; 345 : 1359-67.

5. Van den Berghe G, Wilmer A, Hermans G *et al.* Intensive insulin therapy in the medical ICU. *N Engl J Med* 2006; 354 : 449-61.

6. Brunkhorst FM, Engel C, Bloos F *et al.* Intensive insulin therapy and pentastarch resuscitation in severe sepsis. *N Engl J Med* 2008; 358 : 125-39.

7. Preiser JC, Devos P, Ruiz-Santana S *et al.* A prospective randomised multi-centre controlled trial on tight glucose control by intensive insulin therapy in adult intensive care units: the Glucontrol study. *Intensive Care Med* 2009; 35 : 1738-48.

8. Arabi YM, Dabbagh OC, Tamim HM *et al.* Intensive versus conventional insulin therapy: a randomized controlled trial in medical and surgical critically ill patients. *Crit Care Med* 2008; 36 : 3190-7.

9. Finfer S, Chittock DR, Su SY *et al.* Intensive versus conventional glucose control in critically ill patients. *N Engl J Med.* 2009 Mar 26; 360(13) : 1283-97.

10. Sadhu AR, Ang AC, Ingram-Drake LA *et al.* Economic benefits of intensive insulin therapy in critically Ill patients: the targeted insulin therapy to improve hospital outcomes (TRIUMPH) project. *Diabetes Care* 2008; 31 : 1556-61.

11. Annane D, Sébille V, Charpentier C *et al.* Effect of treatment with low doses of hydrocortisone and fludrocortisone on mortality in patients with septic shock. *J Am Med Assoc* 2002; 288 : 862-71.

12. Sprung CL, Annane D, Keh D *et al.* Hydrocortisone therapy for patients with septic shock. *N Engl J Med* 2008; 358(2) : 111-24.

13. Moran JL, Graham PL, Rockliff S *et al.* Updating the evidence for the role of corticosteroids in severe sepsis and septic shock: a Bayesian meta-analytic perspective. *Crit Care* 2010; 14 : R134.

14. Cohen J, Venkatesh B. Relative adrenal insufficiency in the intensive care population; background and critical appraisal of the evidence. *Anaesth Intensive Care* 2010; 38 : 425-36.

15. Dellinger RP, Levy MM, Rhodes A *et al.* Surviving sepsis campaign: international guidelines for management of severe sepsis and septic shock: 2012. *Crit Care Med* 2013; 41 : 580-637.

36

The cardiac surgical patient in the ICU

Jeff Granton

Depending on the type of center, the post-operative cardiac surgical patient may be the most frequent critical care admission. They may also be the type of patient with the shortest average length of stay in a critical care unit. In the Canadian province of Ontario there are well over 8000 cardiac surgical procedures (coronary bypass grafting and valve surgery) per year [1]. In addition to this massive volume of cases, the complexity of cases is increasing and novel surgical techniques for cardiac disease are becoming the norm.

It should be noted that the following discussion focuses on the adult cardiac surgical patient. Extrapolation to the pediatric experience may not be appropriate.

Structure of cardiac surgical critical care unit

Given the unique challenges of cardiac surgical patients, these patients are best managed post-operatively in specialized units.

- This allows healthcare providers working with these patients to gain exposure to high volumes of cases and thus acquire and maintain the skills required to provide optimal care.
- It also allows patient safety initiatives, house staff education and research endeavors to be focused on this type of patient.
- There is evidence to suggest that the development of units specializing in the post-operative cardiac surgical patient is an improvement on models of care where these patients are mixed in with a more general critical care unit [2].

The physicians staffing dedicated cardiac surgical units should have advanced critical care training. Beyond this the base specialty of physicians can come from a variety of domains such as cardiac anesthesia, cardiac surgery or internal medicine. It would seem to make the most sense that there is a mix of base specialties to allow the greatest breadth and depth of medical knowledge in the physician group.

The cardiac surgical critical care unit should have full access to all the services of a typical tertiary critical care unit, including invasive and noninvasive ventilation, dialysis, interventional radiology and echocardiography. Physicians staffing the cardiac surgical critical care unit should have advanced perioperative transesophageal echocardiography (TEE) training or have immediate access to personnel that can provide this service 24 hours a day.

Handbook of ICU Therapy, third edition, ed. John Fuller, Jeff Granton and Ian McConachie. Published by Cambridge University Press. © Cambridge University Press 2015.

Pre-operative assessment

Often those staffing the critical care units are not involved in the assessment of cardiac surgical patients pre-operatively. However, certain highly complex cases may require multiple opinions prior to operating, including intensive care physicians.

- Information obtained pre-operatively can certainly help predict the clinical course within the post-operative time period, both acutely and chronically.
- Particular attention should be paid to the pre-operative cardiac investigations, respiratory system, kidney function and age.
- Certainly pre-operative findings, such as poor ventricular function, New York Heart Association class, advanced age, chronic kidney disease and mitral valve disease are predictors of a challenging post-operative course [3].
- Complex surgical procedures and emergency surgery are also associated with greater morbidity and mortality.

There are a variety of risk assessment tools for patients about to undergo cardiac surgery. The EuroSCORE and the Society of Thoracic Surgeons (STS) score are two well-known methods. However, great caution needs to be exercised when using these scoring systems, as they likely apply better to a population of patients versus any individual patient [4].

Transfer of care

One of the most vital moments in any cardiac surgical patient's course is the handover from the operating room team to the critical care unit team.

- Key information about the patient's pre-operative status, issues in the operating room and concerns that surgeons or anesthesiologists may have for the post-operative period all need to be discussed.
- The exchange of this information should be protocolized so details are not missed by those who need to know them.
- A report should come from members of the surgical, anesthesia and operating room nursing teams. It should be delivered to the critical care nurse assigned to the patient and the critical care physician admitting the patient.
- In addition, the contents and the order of information given should be standard. A simple sheet or screen with a list of questions to be answered and checked off when satisfied may assist in accurate information transfer [5].

Fast-track cardiac anesthesia

In the 1980s it was standard to use high doses of narcotics when anesthetizing cardiac surgical patients. However, this often required the patients to be intubated and ventilated for many hours after the cases where completed.

- In an attempt to increase efficiency and reduce costs, while maintaining patient safety, the concept of fast-track cardiac anesthesia (FTCA) was popularized by Cheng *et al.* out of Toronto [6,7].
- In particular, a reduction in the dose of narcotics was undertaken and extubation was earlier than traditional models of care.

Multiple studies have shown FTCA to be safe [8,9].

- Methods of predicting which patients can safely undergo FTCA are available.

- Patients with poor left ventricular function, recent myocardial infarction, previous cardiac surgery, extracardiac vascular disease, emergency operations, kidney dysfunction and complex surgery are not good candidates for fast-track anesthesia [10].

One challenge is defining FTCA.

- It is not clear if the definition is based on time to extubation, e.g. what that time should be to qualify as FTCA.
- Less than 10 hours has been proposed by some [8].
- That being said some patients with straightforward cardiac surgical procedures and a relatively low burden of illness are extubated in the operating room and bypass the critical care unit to the post-anesthetic care unit and then to the cardiac surgery ward. This could be termed ultra-fast cardiac anesthesia.

Post-operative complications

Bleeding

Certainly one of the most common challenges caring for the post-operative cardiac surgical patient is bleeding.

- It is difficult to define an acceptable rate of bleeding as this depends on the patient's hemoglobin, coagulation status, hemodynamic stability and the time frame after surgery is completed.
- However, bleeding from chest or mediastinal tubes that is 200 mL/h or greater may be of concern. Output of 400 mL/h is certainly excessive and may warrant re-exploration of the surgical site.
- Packed red blood cell transfusion is used to keep hemoglobin above 70 g/L; however, in the face of ongoing bleeding targeting this value can be difficult.
- In Canada, just over 40% of cardiac surgical patients are transfused red blood cells [11,12].

Standard principles for treatment of excessive bleeding after cardiac surgery include maintaining normothermia, ensuring proper reversal of intraoperative anticoagulation, frequent laboratory investigations and treating the complications of massive transfusion, such as hypocalcemia and hyperkalemia.

The normalization of a patient's coagulation profile should be a goal (although often difficult to attain) in the bleeding patient. However, it should be noted that normalization need not be values within the standard reference range for coagulation studies.

- Aiming for an INR less than 1.5 and a platelet count of greater than 100 seems appropriate in the face of bleeding.
- Measurement of a fibrinogen level may help guide the use of cryoprecipitate.
- The use of activated factor VIIa has been successful in reducing bleeding; however, given the cost and possible thrombotic complications of the factor VIIa, consultation with a hematologist is likely warranted before its use [13].

The use of blood products in cardiac surgical patients needs to be tempered with the realization that their use is an independent predictor of morbidity and mortality [14,15].

Cardiac tamponade

Tamponade is one of the most common life-threatening circumstances that those caring for cardiac surgical patients face.

- Risks for developing tamponade include coagulopathy, excessive post-operative bleeding and prolonged and/or complex surgical procedures.
- Refractory hypotension, reduced urine output, elevated central venous pressure, low cardiac index (if pulmonary artery catheter in place) and increasing serum lactate may appear together or isolation.
- A high index of suspicion for tamponade is required and early surgical intervention with re-exploration of the surgical site under controlled and sterile conditions is preferred.
- Diagnosis often occurs with the use of TEE. However, failure to indentify tamponade on TEE does not rule out the possibility.

Cardiac arrest

Although rare, cardiac arrest in the post-operative cardiac surgical patient requires a team of healthcare professionals to work efficiently and skillfully. Given the complex nature of treating cardiac arrest in this population, a well-organized plan (including equipment available to reopen the patient's chest) and team training would seem prudent.

- Resternotomy should be performed if clinically appropriate, in particular in clinical circumstances that make hemorrhage or tamponade a possibility [16].
- External chest compressions should begin prior to resternotomy.
- If equipment or personnel are not available to perform a resternotomy, external chest compressions should not be withheld, despite the concern of injury to the recent surgical site [17].
- The pharmacologic management of cardiac arrest should not deviate from standard guidelines unless clinically indicated. However, large doses of drugs such as epinephrine may lead to other complications due to a drastic increase in blood pressure when circulation returns.
- If ventricular fibrillation or ventricular tachycardia is the cause of the cardiac arrest, then chest compressions can be withheld and defibrillation quickly attempted first [16].
- If initial treatments of the arrhythmia have failed, then external compressions and preparation for resternotomy should commence.
- The challenge of "opening the chest" in patients with nonsternotomy cardiac procedures requires a prospective plan of what to do if these patients arrest, including the requirement for sternotomy [16].
- It should be remembered that epicardial pacing wires are often present in cardiac surgical patients and bradycardia or asystole may respond to epicardial pacing. Increasing the pacer output (mA) or converting to an asynchronous mode of pacing may be required.

Arrhythmia

Atrial fibrillation is a common complication after cardiac surgery.

- The rate after coronary artery bypass grafting (CABG) can be over 30% and even higher with valve surgery [18].
- Risks for the development of post-operative atrial fibrillation include advanced age, female, low ejection fraction, left atrial enlargement and surgery other than CABG [19,20].

- Prevention of atrial fibrillation is done routinely by prescription of oral β-blockers [20]. These are typically started on the first post-operative day, if tolerated.
- Short-term use of amiodarone is an alternative medication that can be considered for prophylaxis in prevention of atrial fibrillation. However, this drug is more routinely used to treat atrial fibrillation once it has developed [18,20].
- Sotalol is also a viable option for prophylaxis [18].
- Although the evidence is not completely clear, it seems prudent to supplement magnesium if the measured value is low [18].

Neurological complications

One of the most devastating complications after cardiac surgery is a stroke.

- Thankfully, this is fairly uncommon, with a reported incidence of 1% to 3% [21,22].
- It should be remembered that a significant proportion of ischemic strokes can occur in the post-operative period, in particular in relation to atrial fibrillation [23].
- Patients who emerge from the intraoperative anesthetic and have clinical signs of a lateralizing lesion should undergo a CT of the head, possible MRI and have neurology specialists consulted.
- Interestingly, the actual frequency of cerebral lesions found on screening MRI is far greater than clinically obvious strokes [22].

Seizures are seen at times after cardiac surgery, with a reported incidence of 0.9 to 1.2% [24,25].

- Factors that increase the risk of post-operative seizures include valve surgery, critical state pre-operatively, deep hypothermic arrest and aortic calcification or atheroma [26].
- Treatment of seizures includes the use of benzodiazepines and phenytoin; if hemodynamics are an issue, valproic acid is a reasonable alternative [25].
- Patients with post-operative seizures should have an urgent CT of the head, EEG and neurology consultation.
- In addition, patients with an unexplained loss of consciousness post-operatively should have an EEG performed to rule out nonconvulsive status epilepticus.

Certainly a frustrating issue in the post-operative time frame is delirium.

- It should be remembered that the entity of hypoactive delirium exists and patients need not be agitated and aggressive to be suffering from delirium.
- Risks for the development of delirium include advanced age, stroke, dementia and depression [27].
- Patients with inattention and impaired cognition post-operatively should be screened for delirium and have organic causes ruled out.

Acute kidney injury

The development of acute kidney injury or failure after cardiac surgery is independently associated with an increased incidence of in-hospital mortality and reduced long-term survival [28].

- Typically, the incidence of renal replacement therapy after cardiac surgery is just over 1% [29].
- Patient-related risk factors for the development of kidney injury around the time of cardiac surgery include female gender, diabetes mellitus, peripheral vascular disease, pre-existing kidney disease, poor ejection fraction and congestive heart failure.
- Risks related to the surgery itself include emergency cases, prolonged cardiopulmonary bypass time and "on-pump" surgical cases [29].

Prevention of kidney injury is key. Limiting exposure to contrast for pre-operative angiography and post-operative investigations would be wise. Also simple measures, such as proper treatment of dehydration and cardiogenic shock in the perioperative period will help reduce kidney injury, even well before the operative procedure. Avoiding nephrotoxic medications such as nonsteroidal anti-inflammatory drugs is vital, but often overlooked. Intraoperatively optimizing oxygen delivery, pressure and flow on cardiopulmonary bypass theoretically would be of benefit to post-operative kidney function; however, studies are not clear on this matter [29]. Choosing an off-pump technique for CABG can help reduce kidney dysfunction [29].

If a patient does require renal replacement therapy (RRT) after cardiac surgery this is best done in consultation with a nephrologist.

- The best choice for the method of RRT is not clear.
- The outcome results for continuous RRT versus intermittent hemodialysis are mixed at best.
- However, for unstable patients continuous RRT is certainly better tolerated hemodynamically.

Vasoplegic syndrome

Patients that undergo cardiac surgery often have some form of a systemic inflammatory response. This can manifest itself as profound vasodilation leading to low systemic vascular resistance. These patients can have hypotension that is highly resistant to typical vasoconstrictors, such as norepinephrine and vasopressin. This clinical condition is often referred to as vasoplegia or vasoplegic syndrome. It is important to rule out other causes of hypotension, such as bleeding, hypovolemia, ventricular failure, anaphylaxis and tamponade.

Risk factors for the development of post-operative vasoplegia include:

- Hypotension on cardiopulmonary bypass (CPB)
- Elevated euroSCORE
- Prolonged CPB
- Pre-operative vasopressor requirement and pre-operative use of ACE inhibitors [30].

Treatment includes:

- Fluids and vasoconstrictor medications such as vasopressin, norepinephrine and phenylephrine.
- Refractory cases can be treated with intravenous injection of methylene blue at a dose of 1.5 to 2.0 mg/kg over 20 minutes.
- Repeating the dose or starting an infusion may also be required [31].

Special procedures

Heart transplantation

Over 4000 heart transplants are done worldwide every year, with cardiomyopathy and coronary artery disease being the most common etiologies of heart failure leading to transplant [32].

- These patients can be very challenging to manage in the immediate post-operative period with bleeding and right ventricular dysfunction being particularly problematic.
- Within the first 30 days after transplantation, graft failure, multiorgan failure and noncytomegalovirus infection are the most common causes of mortality [32].
- Right ventricular failure can be treated and possibly prevented by the use of phosphodiesterase inhibitors (such as milrinone), which should improve right ventricular function and lower pulmonary artery pressures.
- The use of inhaled nitric oxide, sildenafil or inhaled prostacyclin may also help reduce pulmonary artery pressures [33,34,35].
- It should also be remembered that these patients will have a denervated heart and that bradycardia will be best treated with pacing or direct-acting β-agonists, while atropine will be ineffective.

Ventricular assist devices

Details regarding the indications and function of ventricular assist devices are described elsewhere in this text. However, when caring for these patients, several issues can arise in the immediate post-operative period.

- Bleeding is of particular concern and can be challenging to manage.
- After bleeding in the post-operative period has subsided, a decision will need to be made in consultation with cardiac surgeons about when and how to begin anticoagulation.
- This decision to anticoagulate postoperatively is often based on specifications of the manufacturer for any given variety of assist device.
- Monitoring of patient blood pressure with nonpulsatile flow devices requires a technique of Doppler measurement and necessitates some training for nursing staff [36].
- The early identification of complications, such as tamponade, requires a high index of suspicion and prompt investigation. Hence, the immediate availability of echocardiography is very helpful.
- Great care needs to be taken with aseptic technique in the post-operative period, as infection is one of the more frequent complications, in particular at the drive line exit [36].
- Cardiac arrest protocols should be laid out in advance with the guidance of cardiac surgeons and the manufacturer.

Emerging surgical techniques

Newer surgical techniques, including transcatheter aortic valve implantation (TAVI), minimally invasive mitral valve surgery and robotically assisted surgery are all gaining popularity.

As with any emerging techniques, education and vigilance of those looking after these patients is key. Plans to deal with issues such as bleeding, re-exploration of surgical site, bradycardia, anticoagulation, duration of mechanical ventilation and cardiac arrest all need to be discussed and understood for each individual procedure.

References

1. Oakes GH, Feindel C, Purdham DM et al. Report on Adult Cardiac Surgery in Ontario. Cardiac Care Network October 2012; 9.

2. Novick RJ, Fox SA, Stitt LW et al. Impact of the opening of a specialized cardiac surgery recovery unit on postoperative outcomes in academic health sciences centre. Can J Anesth 2007; 54 : 737–43.

3. De Cocker J, Messaoudi N, Stockman BA et al. Preoperative prediction of intensive care unit stay following cardiac surgery. Eur J Cardiothor Surg 2011; 39 : 60–7.

4. Granton J, Cheng D. Risk stratification models for cardiac surgery. Semin Cardiothor Vasc Anesth 2008; 12 : 167–74.

5. Zavalkoff SR, Razack SI, Lavoie J, Dancea AB. Handover after pediatric heart surgery: a simple tool improves information exchange. Pediatr Crit Care Med 2011; 12 : 309–13.

6. Cheng DCH. Fast track cardiac surgery pathways: early extubation, process of care, and cost containment. Anesthesiology 1998; 88 : 1429–33.

7. Cheng DC, Karski J, Peniston C, Sandler A et al. Early tracheal extubation after coronary artery bypass graft surgery reduces costs and improves resource use: a prospective, randomized, controlled trial. Anesthesiology 1996; 85 : 1300–10.

8. Myles PS, Daly DJ, Djaiani G et al. A systematic review of the safety and effectiveness of fast-track cardiac anesthesia. Anesthesiology 2003; 99 : 982–87.

9. Silbert BS, Myles PS. Is fast-track cardiac anesthesia now the global standard of care? Anesth Analg 2009; 108 : 689–91.

10. Moll V, Mutlak H, Steudel W. A new scoring system to predict fast-track failure in cardiac surgery. Crit Care Med 2006; 34 : 3034–35.

11. Hutton B, Fergusson D, Tinmouth A et al. Transfusion rates vary significantly amongst Canadian medical centers. Can J Anesth 2005; 52 : 581–90.

12. Bennett-Guerrero E, Zhao Y, O'Brien SM et al. Variation in use of blood transfusion in coronary bypass graft surgery. JAMA 2010; 304 : 1568–75.

13. Warren O, Mandal K, Hadjianastassiou V et al. Recombinant activated factor VII in cardiac surgery: a systematic review. Ann Thorac Surg 2007; 83 : 707–14.

14. Rawn J. The silent risks of blood transfusion. Curr Opin Ansesthesiol 2008; 21 : 664–8.

15. Jakobsen CJ, Ryhammer PK, Tang M et al. Transfusion of blood during cardiac surgery is associated with higher long-term mortality in low-risk patients. Eur J Cardiothor Surg 2013; 42 : 114–20.

16. Soar J, Perkins GD, Abbas G et al. European Resuscitation Council Guidelines for Resuscitation 2010 Section 8. Cardiac arrest in special circumstances: electrolyte abnormalities, poisoning, drowning, accidental hypothermia, hyperthermia, asthma, anaphylaxis, cardiac surgery, trauma, pregnancy, electrocution. Resuscitation 2010; 81 : 1400–33.

17. Vanden Hoek TL, Morrison LJ, Shuster M et al. Cardiac arrest in special circumstances: 2010 American Heart Association guidelines for cardiopulmonary resuscitation and emergency cardiovascular care. Circulation 2010; 122 : S829–61.

18. Koniari I, Apostolakis, Rogkakou C et al. Pharmacologic prophylaxis for atrial fibrillation following cardiac surgery: a systemic review. J Cardiothor Surg 2010; 5 : 121.

19. Helgadottir S, Sigurdsson MI, Ingvarsdottir IL et al. Atrial fibrillation following cardiac surgery: risk analysis and long-term survival. J Cardiothor Surg 2012; 7 : 87.

20. Passannante AN. Prevention of atrial fibrillation after cardiac surgery. *Curr Opin Anesthesiol* 2011; 24 : 58–63.

21. Li Y, Walicki D, Mathiesen C *et al.* Strokes after cardiac surgery and relationship to carotid stenosis. *Arch Neurol* 2009; 66 : 1091–96.

22. Barber PA, Hach S, Tippett LJ *et al.* Cerebral ischemic lesions on diffusion-weighted imaging are associated with neurocognitive decline after cardiac surgery. *Stroke* 2008; 39 : 1427–33.

23. Carrascal Y, A Guerrero. Neurological damage related to cardiac surgery. *The Neurologist* 2010; 16 : 152–64.

24. Koster A, Borgermann J, Zittermann A *et al.* Moderate dosage of tranexamic acid during cardiac surgery with cardiopulmonary bypass and convulsive seizures: incidence and clinical outcome. *Br J Anesth* 2013; 110 : 34–40.

25. Hunter GRW, Young B. Seizures after cardiac surgery. *J Cardiothorac Vasc Anes* 2011; 25 : 299–305.

26. Goldstone AB, Bronster DJ, Anyanwun AC *et al.* Predictors and outcomes after cardiac surgery: a multivariable analysis of 2578 patients. *Ann Thorac Surg* 2011; 91 : 514–18.

27. Rudolph JL, Jones RN, Levkoff SE *et al.* Derivation and validation of a preoperative prediction rule for delirium after cardiac surgery. *Circulation* 2009; 119 : 229–36.

28. Bagshaw SM. The long-term outcome after acute renal failure. *Curr Opin Crit Care* 2006; 12 : 561–66.

29. Gude D, Jha R. Acute kidney injury following cardiac surgery. *Ann Card Anesth* 2012; 15 : 279–86.

30. Levin MA, Lin HM, Castillo JG *et al.* Early on cardiopulmonary bypass and other factors associated with vasoplegic syndrome. *Circulation* 2009; 120 : 1664–71.

31. Shanmugan G. Vasoplegic syndrome: the role of methylene blue. *Eur J Cardiothorac Surg* 2005; 28 : 705–10.

32. Taylor DO, Stehlik J, Edwards LB *et al.* Registry of the International Society for Heart Transplantation: twenty-sixth official adult heart transplant report. *J Heart Lung Transplant* 2009; 28 : 1007–22.

33. DeWet CJ, Affleck DG, Jacobsohn E *et al.* Inhaled prostacyclin is safe, effective, and affordable in patients with pulmonary hypertension, right heart dysfunction, and refractory hypoxemia after cardiothoracic surgery. *J Thorac Cardiovasc Surg* 2004; 127 : 1058–67.

34. Granton J, Moric J. Pulmonary vasodilators: treating the right ventricle. *Anesthesiol Clin* 2008; 26 : 337–53.

35. Stobierska-Dzierzek B, Awad H, Michler RE. The evolving management of acute right-sided heart failure in cardiac transplant recipients. *J Am Coll Cardiol* 2001; 38 : 923–31.

36. O'Shea G. Ventricular assist devices. *AACN Adv Crit Care* 2012; 23 : 69–83.

Care of the organ donor

37

Mowaffaq Almikhlafi and Michael D Sharpe

Introduction

Despite efforts to increase deceased organ donation rates in Canada, recipient waiting lists are increasing and the numbers of patients dying while waiting for an organ continue to increase. It is, therefore, imperative to maximize the number of organs per donor, as well as optimize donated organ function by proper implementation of practice guidelines in donor management to promote better graft outcomes. Overall, this will translate into an increase in the number of organs successfully transplanted [1–3].

This chapter will discuss the physiological changes that occur with neurological determination of death (NDD), originally referred to as "brain death," and will outline general and organ-specific measures for investigating, monitoring and optimizing organ donors.

Physiological changes associated with NDD

Neurological

Neurological determination of death is a result of acute brain injury, either traumatic or nontraumatic, that causes acute intracranial hypertension.

- If not managed early in its course, it may result in cerebral ischemia and subsequent edema that progresses towards herniation of the brain through the foramen magnum.
- The result is progressive ischemia/infarction and worsening cerebral edema to the point that cerebral circulation ceases.

Herniation of the brain usually causes ischemia of different parts of the brainstem, in a rostral-caudal fashion.

- Pontine ischemia results in the classic Cushing response with bradycardia, hypertension and irregular breathing patterns due to mixed sympathetic and vagal stimulation.
- Unopposed sympathetic stimulation is seen, as function of the caudal portion of the medulla is lost.
- Ultimately, all brainstem function ceases and sympathetic denervation ensues with the loss of spinal sympathetic pathways [4].

The following are the effects of NDD on specific organ function [5].

Handbook of ICU Therapy, third edition, ed. John Fuller, Jeff Granton and Ian McConachie. Published by Cambridge University Press. © Cambridge University Press 2015.

Cardiovascular

Serum catecholamine levels increase as a result of the sympathetic surge that accompanies brainstem ischemia, causing profound systemic vasoconstriction.

- This results in an increased mean arterial pressure, which, along with the concomitant tachycardia, increases myocardial oxygen demand, causing myocardial injury in different forms, including subendocardial and scattered transmural ischemic foci.

This autonomic surge is followed by loss of sympathetic tone resulting in significant drop in systemic vascular resistance (SVR).

- Thus, hypotension is commonly a result of this phenomenon rather than from an ischemic myocardium.

Common electrocardiographic changes include changes in ST segments and T-waves, as well as conduction abnormalities and arrhythmias (both atrial and ventricular). Approximately 25% of patients requiring significant inotropic support prior to organ retrieval will exhibit asystole [6].

Pulmonary

Pulmonary complications are common after severe traumatic brain injury. These can be due to direct lung contusion, aspiration, and cardiogenic and noncardiogenic pulmonary edema.

- The sympathetic surge mentioned above is usually accompanied by a severe systemic inflammatory response, both of which may lead to increased permeability of pulmonary capillary beds and subsequent pulmonary edema [7].
- Therefore, higher values of inspired oxygen (FiO_2) and positive end-expiratory pressure (PEEP) are required to achieve optimal tissue oxygenation [8].

Endocrine

Significant reduction of hormonal levels is generally observed following severe brain injury, reflecting the effect on both anterior and posterior pituitary function.

- Approximately 80% of cases develop diabetes insipidus due to loss of secretion of antidiuretic hormone (ADH) from the hypothalamus.
- Partial preservation of perfusion of the posterior hypothalamus is maintained in approximately 20% of patients via the inferior hypophyseal artery (extradural circulation) [5].
- Reduced thyroid stimulating hormone (TSH) levels impair the synthesis of triiodothyronine (T3), an effect that is potentiated by reduced peripheral conversion of tetraiodothyronine [9].
- Insulin levels also decrease after NDD, and reduced intracellular glucose levels result in anaerobic metabolism and lactic acidosis.
- Systemic hyperglycemia can potentially lead to hypovolemia via osmotic diuresis, particularly after administering glucose- containing solutions and/or other hyperosmotic agents administered to reduce cerebral edema [4].
- Decreased production of adrenocorticotropic hormone (ACTH) from the anterior pituitary results in decreased serum cortisol levels. This, along with the hypothyroid state that occurs after NDD may cause further hemodynamic compromise.

Hypothermia

With the loss of hypothalamic control following NDD, body temperature regulation becomes markedly impaired and hypothermia ensues. The loss of sympathetic tone and peripheral vasodilation increase heat loss. Furthermore, heat production is reduced due to the fall in metabolic rate and the loss of muscle activity.

- Hypothermia carries detrimental consequences, including arrhythmias, myocardial depression, hypotension, left-shift of the oxygen dissociation curve, reduced GFR, nephrogenic diabetes insipidus (NDI) – also called "cold diuresis"– coagulopathy, hemolysis and pancreatitis.
- All patients require active warming following NDD.
- It is important to maintain core temperatures above 34 °C, which is a criterion to allow the clinical determination of NDD.

Hepatic

Brainstem death causes activation of leukocytes, platelets and endothelial cells and, along with the upregulation in proinflammatory mediators, the hepatic microcirculation may be compromised. This results in reduced hepatic sinusoidal perfusion and thus variable degrees of liver dysfunction and increases in transaminases.

Coagulation

Nearly 28% of NDD cases develop disseminated intravascular coagulation (DIC), to some degree, due to the increased production of tissue thromboplastin by the necrotic brain cells. Bleeding is aggravated by the concomitant occurrence of hypothermia and hepatic dysfunction.

Immunological

The sera of brain-dead donors have been shown to have elevated levels of proinflammatory cytokines, chemokines and adhesion molecules due to brain injury, circulatory dysfunction and cellular activation [10]. This renders transplanted organs more immunogenic, and therefore more susceptible to the recipient's immune system, which may affect rejection.

Organ monitoring

Clinical monitoring of the organ donor should include checking the vital signs hourly to assess for hypotension, bradycardia and hypothermia.

- Blood pressure should be monitored using an intra-arterial catheter to follow accurately the mean arterial pressure (MAP).
- A central venous catheter should be placed to monitor the central venous pressure (CVP) and facilitate administration of vasoactive drugs.
- A urinary catheter is required for accurate hourly fluid balance assessment.

Under special circumstances, pulmonary artery catheter (PAC) insertion is recommended, to distinguish between pump versus resistance failure, as a cause of hypotension.

- Criteria for PAC insertion include reduced left ventricular ejection fraction (below 40%) and/or severe hemodynamic instability requiring escalation of inotropic or vasopressor support.
- Therapy is titrated to target a pulmonary capillary wedge pressure (PCWP) of 8–12 mmHg and it is recommended to keep the PCWP/CVP on the lower side for lung transplant, to reduce the severity of pulmonary edema [11].
- As well, a normal cardiac index and mixed venous oximetry (SvO_2) over 60–70% is recommended, with the judicious use of fluid resuscitation and intropic therapy to maintain these parameters, which should be checked once every 2–4 hours, guided by ongoing hemodynamic therapy.

Investigations

Initial laboratory investigations include:

- Arterial blood gas, serum electrolytes (including Mg, Ca and PO_4) and serum lactate every 4 hours and post-electrolyte replacement as required
- Capillary blood glucose every 2 hours
- Complete blood count every 8 hours
- Troponin and CK every 6 hours
- Creatinine and blood urea nitrogen every 6 hours
- Urine analysis
- AST, ALT, alkaline phosphatase, total and fractionated bilirubin, LDH, GGT, PTT, INR, total protein and albumin every 6 hours
- Serum lipase and amylase every 6 hours
- Blood, urine and endotracheal tube Gram stain and cultures daily
- Transplant serology (prior to methyl prednisolone): hepatitis B and C serology, HIV-1 and -2, CMV, EBV, HSV and VZV.
- Chest X-ray
- Potential lung donors should undergo bronchoscopic evaluation to assess for evidence of gastric aspiration, endotracheal lesions or presence of purulent secretions. Bronchoscopy is also necessary to ensure either normal anatomy or the presence of an aberrant right upper lobe bronchus, which will determine whether lung donation is feasible.
- Potential heart transplant donors require 12-lead ECGs and echocardiograms at baseline and following hemodynamic resuscitation. Coronary angiography is also indicated as per the criteria established by the heart transplant programs.

Therapeutic interventions

Healthcare professionals managing donors from NDD should anticipate the physiological responses that we previously discussed. This should enable them to provide the appropriate therapeutic measures in order to:

1. Maintain optimal circulatory and metabolic states
2. Maintain adequate organ perfusion and tissue oxygenation
3. Maximize the number of organs recovered and transplanted
4. Improve transplanted graft function.

The following are the recommendations for support of each of the organ systems.

Cardiovascular

Interventions aim to reach a normal cardiac index (CI), MAP >70 mmHg with SBP >100 mmHg, CVP of 8–10 mmHg, PCWP 8–10 mmHg, heart rate >60 and <120 bpm, urine output >0.5 mL/kg/h, mixed venous oximetry >60–70% and normal serum lactate.

Hypotension

Hypotension following determination of NDD often occurs due to various reasons including hypovolemia, hypothermia, myocardial dysfunction, endocrine abnormalities, electrolyte disorders and distributive/neurogenic shock.

Fluid therapy

Treatment usually requires infusing crystalloids to overcome hypotension and aiming for a target CVP. The injudicious use of crystalloids could potentially result in tissue edema, thus the administration of colloids is often employed in donor resuscitation.

- While the use of hydroxyethylstarch reduces the volume required for resuscitation, it has been shown to increase the incidence of acute kidney injury (AKI) and the need for dialysis [12].
- Judicious use of crystalloid/colloid resuscitation, including the use of albumin as a colloid substitute, is recommended.
- Blood transfusion should be considered when hemoglobin drops below 7 g/dL or when there is evidence of inadequate tissue perfusion or oxygen delivery, e.g. a reduction in SvO_2 or an increase in lactic acidosis, respectively.

Vasoactive drug support

- Dopamine has been traditionally used as the inotrope of choice in the brain-dead donor. However, recent studies did not support its beneficial effect on renal or splanchnic circulation, and it may have an inhibitory effect on the anterior pituitary hormones [13,14].
- Vasopressin was found superior to either saline alone or epinephrine in maintaining blood pressure and in reducing inotrope use [15].

Therefore, it is recommended to use vasopressin, norepinephrine and phenylephrine for vasopressor support with milrinone if inotropic support is needed.

Hypertension

Hypertension is common during the evolution of brain ischemia, but it is unusual following NDD. Therapy should be started if the MAP is sustained above 95 mmHg for 30 minutes.

- Therapy should start by weaning inotropes and vasopressors.
- It is recommended, however, to continue a vasopressin infusion to a maximum dose of 2.4 units/h, to provide DI prophylaxis.
- If hypertension persists, the use of short-acting agents, such as esmolol (100–500 µg/kg bolus followed by 100–300 µg/kg/min infusion) or nitropusside (0.5–5 µg/kg/min infusion) is preferred.

Endocrine

Diabetes insipidus

Central diabetes insipidus (CDI) is a common finding and is seen in up to 80% of brain-dead donors, due to reduced production of ADH by the posterior pituitary gland [16].

- The diagnosis of CDI is made when there is hypernatremia (serum Na >145 mmol/L), increased serum osmolality (>300 mOsm/L) and polyuria (urine output >4 mL/kg/h) in the presence of hypotonic urine (urine osmolality <200 mOsm/L; specific gravity <1.005) with low urine sodium (<10 mmol/L).

- Polyuria due to other causes should be distinguished from DI. These include osmotic diuresis (hyperglycemia, hyperosmolar therapy), large intravenous fluid volume resuscitation and uncorrected hypothermia.

- DI results in hypovolemia, hyperosmolar hypernatremia and numerous electrolyte derangements, including hypomagnesemia, hypophosphatemia, hypokalemia and hypoclacemia, due to their urinary losses.

- Once the diagnosis of CDI is established, treatment should be initiated with a bolus of vasopressin (1 unit, IV) followed by a continuous infusion at 0.04 U/min (2.4 U/h).

- Vasopressin exerts its physiological effects through three different receptors V1, V2 and V3. Activation of V2 receptors, which are found on the epithelia of the renal cortical collecting duct [17] results in reabsorption of free water via aquaporin-2 (water channels).

- Additional intermittent intravenous boluses with the V2-selective vasopressin analog, 1-deamino-8-D-arginine vasopressin (dDAVP), may also be required starting with 1–4 µg as an initial bolus followed by 1–2 µg every 6 hours to keep the urine output under 4 mL/kg/h.

- The resulting hypernatremia (serum Na >145 mmol/L) should be treated with intravenous hypotonic solutions such as D5W or 0.45NS, or by enteral free water.

- Electrolytes should be replaced to resume their normal physiological ranges.

Anterior pituitary hormones

In comparison to vasopressin deficiency, which occurs in the majority of cases, variable deficiency of hormones regulated by the anterior pituitary, including T3, thyroxine (T4), ACTH, TSH and growth hormone (GH) have been described.

Replacing these hormones showed inconsistent improvement in physiological parameters in animal and human studies [18,19].

Thyroid hormones

Thyroid hormone administration was shown to improve donor hemodynamics, heart and lung utilization and post-transplant cardiac allograft function [20–23].

Proposed mechanisms include:

1. Augmentation of active ion transport system (i.e. Ca-ATPase, adenylate cyclase, Na-channel activities), thus increasing myocardial calcium/cardiac contractility
2. Sensitization of β-adrenergic pathways
3. Increased diastolic relaxation [24].

The generally recommended doses using T4 include: 100 μg intravenous bolus followed by 50 μg IV every 12 hours, or 20 μg IV bolus followed by 10 μg/h infusion.

Adrenal hormones

Relative adrenal insufficiency has been proposed in brain injury. This occurs following the initial rise in serum cortisol as a result of the stress response to brain ischemia. Hence, the use of corticosteroids has been tried with variable responses. Doses of 15 mg/kg methyl prednisolone IV every 24 hours are recommended; however, this is administered primarily for its immunomodulatory affects.

Although it has not been adequately evaluated, the initiation of triple hormonal therapy with vasopressin (or dDAVP), methyl prednisolone and levothyroxine has been commonly utilized to achieve better hemodynamic stability in NDD cases by most North American transplant centers.

Hyperglycemia

Hyperglycemia after NDD is common, likely due to insulin resistance and the stress response [25]. Target glycemic control ranges are extrapolated from studies done in critically ill patients with acceptable ranges of 4–8 mmol/L.

Hypothermia

Core body temperature should be maintained at 36–37.5 °C (97–99.5 °F) by using active surface warming with heated-liquid or hot-air warming blanket plus insulating thermal blankets. Warm inspired gas can be administered through the ventilator. Body surface exposure to environmental temperatures should be minimized.

Should active external rewarming measures fail, internal rewarming can be utilized to reach target temperatures, but external warming devices usually suffice.

Pulmonary

- Mechanical ventilation should deliver FiO_2 to maintain SaO_2 over 95%.
- Ventilation should be adjusted to target a $PaCO_2$ of 35–40 mmHg with a normal arterial pH (7.35–7.45).
- Positive end-expiratory pressure (PEEP) of 5–10 cmH$_2$O to keep FiO_2 below 0.50.
- Peak airway pressure <30 cmH$_2$O.
- Head of the bed should be kept at 45° to reduce the risk of aspiration.
- Lung-protective strategy with tidal volume of 6–8 mL/kg of predicted body weight and higher PEEP values at 8–10 cmH$_2$O resulted in a higher number of eligible donors and harvested lungs in one study when compared with conventional strategy without exerting an effect on the numbers of harvested hearts, livers and kidneys [8].

Nutritional support

Intravenous dextrose infusions are routinely given, but this should not preclude the administration of enteral feeding. Feeding should be stopped on call to the OR; TPN should be generally avoided.

Hematological support

Disseminated intravascular coagulation in the potential donor can be the result of hypoxia, sepsis, shock and severe multiple trauma. Correcting the underlying cause is the mainstay of treating DIC. The NDD donor should receive red blood cells, platelet transfusion, fresh frozen plasma and cryoprecipitate according to the general guidelines in treating DIC.

Summary

- It is important to take the time necessary in the ICU to optimize organ function for the purpose of improving transplant outcomes.
- Reversible organ dysfunction may be improved with revised resuscitation strategies and frequent re-evaluation.
- Once organ dysfunction is optimized, surgical procurement should be arranged.
- The key to managing organ donors is to anticipate physiological changes post-NDD and to treat expeditiously.

References

1. Shemi SD, Ross H, Pagliarello J et al. Organ donor management in Canada: recommendations of the forum on Medical Management to Optimize Donor Organ Potential. CMAJ. 2006; 174 : S13–32.

2. Rosendale JD, Kauffman HM, McBride MA et al. Aggressive pharmacologic donor management results in more transplanted organs. Transplantation 2003; 75 : 482–87.

3. Salim A, Velmahos GC, Brown C et al. Aggressive organ donor management significantly increases number of organs available for transplantation. J Trauma 2005; 58 : 991–4.

4. Smith M. Physiologic changes during brain stem death–lessons for management of the organ donor. J Heart Lung Transplant 2004; 23(9 Suppl) : S217–22.

5. Wijdicks EFM Atkinson JLD. Pathophysiologic responses to brain death. In: Wijdicks EFM, ed. Brain Death. Philadelphia: Lippincott Williams & Wilkins; 2001 : 29–43.

6. Mackersie RC, Bronsther OL, Shackford SR. Organ procurement in patients with fatal head injuries. Ann Surg 1991; 213 : 143–50.

7. Pennefather SH, Bullock RE, Dark JH. The effect of fluid therapy on alveolar arterial oxygen gradient in brain-dead organ donors. Transplantation 1993; 56 : 1418–22.

8. Mascia L, Pasero D, Slutsky AS et al. Effect of a lung protective strategy for organ donors on eligibility and availability of lungs for transplantation: a randomized controlled trial. JAMA 2010; 304 : 2620–7.

9. Powner DJ, Hendricj A, Lagler RG et al. Hormonal changes in brain dead patients. Crit Care Med 1990; 18 : 702–8.

10. Takada M, Nadeau KC, Hancock WW et al. Effects of explosive brain death on cytokine activation of peripheral organs in the rat. Transplantation 1998; 65 : 1533–42.

11. Tuttle-Newhall JE, Collins BH, Kuo PC, Schoeder R. Organ donation and treatment of the multi-organ donor. Curr Probl Surg 2003; 40 : 266–310.

12. Cittanova ML, Leblanc I, Legendre C et al. Effect of hydroxyethylstarch in brain-dead kidney donors on renal function in kidney transplant recipients. Lancet 1996; 348 : 1620–22.

13. Debaveye YA, Van den Berghe GH. Is there still a place for dopamine in the modern intensive care unit? Anesth Analg 2004; 98 : 461–8.

14. Marik PE, Mohedin M. The contrasting effects of dopamine and norepinephrine on systemic and splanchnic oxygen utilization in hyperdynamic sepsis. JAMA 1994; 272 : 1354–7.

15. Kinoshita Y, Yahata K, Yoshioka T et al. Long-term renal preservation after brain

death maintained with vasopressin and epinephrine. *Transpl Int* 1990; 3 : 15–18.

16. Chen EP, Bittner HB, Kendall SW, Van Trigt P. Hormonal and hemodynamic changes in a validated model of brain death. *Crit Care Med* 1996; 24 : 1352–9.

17. Kutsogiannis DJ, Pagliarello G, Doig C *et al.* Medical management to optimize donor organ potential: review of the literature. *Can J Anaesth* 2006; 53 : 820–30.

18. Howlett TA, Keogh AM, Perry L *et al.* Anterior and posterior pituitary function in brainstem-dead donors. *Transplantation* 1989; 47 : 828–34.

19. Gramm HJ, Meinhold H, Bickel U *et al.* Acute endocrine failure after brain death. *Transplantation* 1992; 54 : 851–7.

20. Orlowski JP, Spees EK. Improved cardiac transplant survival with thyroxine treatment of hemodynamically unstable donors: 95.2% graft survival at 6 and 30 months. *Transplant Proc* 1993; 25 : 1535.

21. Jeevanandam V. Triiodothyronine: spectrum of use in heart transplantation. *Thyroid* 1997; 7 : 139–45.

22. Zuppa AF, Nadkarni V, Davis L *et al.* The effect of a thyroid hormone infusion on vasopressor support in critically ill children with cessation of neurologic function. *Crit Care Med* 2004; 32 : 2318–22.

23. Nath DS, Ilias Basha H, Liu MH *et al.* Increased recovery of thoracic organs after hormonal resuscitation therapy. *J Heart Lung Transplant* 2010; 29 : 594.

24. Salter DR, Dyke CM, Wechsler AS. Triiodothyronine (T3) and cardiovascular therapeutics: a review. *J Card Surg* 1992; 7 : 363–74.

25. Masson F, Thicoipe M, Gin H *et al.* The endocrine pancreas in brain-dead donors. *Transplantation* 1993; 56 : 363–7.

The patient with cardiac arrest

Osama Al-muslim

Cardiac arrest is cessation in the pumping action of the heart. The diagnosis of cardiac arrest is based on the lack of a palpable central pulse, apnea and unresponsiveness. No oxygen delivery to the vital organs results in catastrophic ischemic brain injury within 5 minutes. Nevertheless, cardiac arrest does not equate with death. Some victims of cardiac arrest can be resuscitated. Besides, post-resuscitation care can mitigate the neuronal injury leading to survival with good neurologic outcome.

For healthcare providers, cardiac arrest represents the most serious medical emergency.

The process of care for cardiac arrest victims is optimized by effective implementation of the chain of survival [1].

The chain of survival links are:

1. Prevention and early recognition of cardiac arrest
2. Early CPR with emphasis on chest compressions
3. Early defibrillation
4. Effective advanced life support
5. Comprehensive post-resuscitation care.

This chapter reviews important classifications and causes of cardiac arrest, the updated resuscitation guidelines, cardiac arrest outcomes, training and quality-improvement issues in this field. The detailed management skills of cardiopulmonary resuscitation (CPR) are best learned during designated courses on basic life support (BLS) and advanced life support (ALS).

Classification

Sudden cardiac arrest and asphyxial arrest

Sudden cardiac arrest (SCA) is a sudden collapse usually due to ventricular fibrillation. Asphyxial arrest follows a period of gradual and progressive vital organ deterioration due to untreated hypoxemia and hypotension.

Shockable and nonshockable rhythms

Based on the need to defibrillate, cardiac arrest is classified into shockable and nonshockable rhythms. The shockable rhythms are ventricular fibrillation and pulseless ventricular tachycardia (VF/pulseless VT). The nonshockable rhythms are asystole and pulseless

Handbook of ICU Therapy, third edition, ed. John Fuller, Jeff Granton and Ian McConachie. Published by Cambridge University Press. © Cambridge University Press 2015.

electrical activity (asystole/PEA). Untreated shockable rhythms degenerate to nonshockable rhythms, which have a worse outcome.

Out-of-hospital and in-hospital cardiac arrest

Out-of-hospital cardiac arrest (OHCA) is usually SCA due to shockable rhythms. In-hospital cardiac arrest (IHCA) is usually asphyxial arrest due to nonshockable rhythms. However, hospitalized patients with acute coronary syndrome or acute electrolyte imbalance could have cardiac arrest caused by shockable rhythms.

Expected death in critically ill patients

Some critically ill patients deteriorate despite extensive monitoring and provision of aggressive artificial life support. For these imminently dying patients, CPR has no benefit, but may merely prolong the dying process. Critical care practitioners should recognize this syndrome to optimize comfort measures and support these patients and their families.

Causes

Sudden cardiac arrest is commonly caused by acute coronary syndrome. Other causes of SCA are cardiomyopathy, valvular disease, congenital heart disease and inherited abnormalities (e.g. long and short QT syndromes, Brugada syndrome). Asphyxial arrest is caused by conditions that lead to progressive shock, hypoxemia and acidosis. The important different cardiac arrest causes can be remembered as the "Hs and Ts":

Hs

- Hypovolemia
- Hypoxia
- Hydrogen ions (acidosis)
- Hyperkalemia or hypokalemia
- Hypothermia.

Ts

- Thrombosis (myocardial infarction)
- Thrombosis (pulmonary embolism)
- Tension pneumothorax
- Tamponade, cardiac
- Toxins
- Trauma.

Prevention of in-hospital cardiac arrest

Early recognition of the deteriorating patient and prevention of cardiac arrest is the first link in the chain of survival. When patients deteriorate, they display common signs that represent failing respiratory, cardiovascular and nervous systems. Several studies have identified abnormalities of heart rate, blood pressure, respiratory rate and conscious level as possible markers of impending cardiac arrest. Medical emergency teams (METs) or rapid response teams (RRTs) are designated to respond to these patients who are critically ill, to prevent cardiac arrest. These teams may replace or coexist with traditional cardiac arrest teams, which typically respond to patients already in cardiac arrest. The METs/RRTs usually include medical and nursing staff from the intensive care team and respond to specific calling criteria; interventions often involve simple tasks such as starting oxygen therapy and intravenous fluids. The implementation of METs/RRTs has been shown to be effective in reducing in-hospital cardiac arrests, hospital mortality and morbidities [2]. This is further discussed in the chapter on Recognizing and responding to the deteriorating patient.

Basic life support

The updated *Resuscitation Guidelines* continue to emphasize the importance of high-quality CPR [1].

The components of high-quality CPR for adults are:

- Compress the chest at a rate of 100–120 per minute
- Compression depth of 5–6 cm
- Allow for complete chest recoil after each compression
- Minimize interruptions in chest compression
- Avoid excessive ventilation
- Compression-to-ventilation ratio of 30:2
- Avoiding fatigue by switching the compressing rescuer every 2 minutes.

Adult BLS sequence

For adults, CPR should start with chest compressions rather than ventilations. The healthcare provider checks the victim simultaneously for response and breathing, before activating the emergency response system. After activation of the emergency response system, the rescuer delivers 30 compressions followed by 2 breaths. Uninterrupted CPR continues until the victim starts to move or the ALS team arrives [1].

Team resuscitation

Healthcare providers commonly provide CPR as a team with rescuers performing several actions simultaneously. In hospital settings, the BLS rescuers should be trained in multi-rescuer CPR and defibrillation use. This BLS team coordinates chest compressions, airway management, rescue breathing, rhythm detection and shocks (if appropriate) [1].

Alternative CPR techniques

Interposed abdominal compression-CPR (IAC-CPR) is an alternative CPR technique that may be considered during in-hospital resuscitation when sufficient trained personnel are available. The rescuer who provides manual abdominal compressions will compress the abdomen mid-way between the xiphoid and the umbilicus during the relaxation phase of chest compression. The use of IAC-CPR improves coronary perfusion pressure and blood flow to other vital organs by increasing diastolic aortic pressure and venous return and can improve survival to hospital discharge compared with conventional CPR [3].

CPR devices

An impedance threshold device (ITD) limits air entry into the lungs during the decompression phase of CPR, creating negative intrathoracic pressure. This improves venous return to the heart and cardiac output during CPR. It does so without impeding positive-pressure ventilation or passive exhalation. The ITD improved short-term survival when used in adults with out-of-hospital cardiac arrest, but no significant improvement in survival to hospital discharge [4].

Advanced life support

Although drugs and advanced airways are still included among ALS interventions, they are of secondary importance to early defibrillation, high-quality chest compressions and effective resuscitation teamwork.

Rhythm-based management

Advanced life support is based on rhythm assessment and appropriate action. The ALS team has to connect the cardiac monitor to start this rhythm-based management. For patients in VF/pulseless VT, shocks should be delivered promptly, with minimal interruptions in chest compressions. Subsequently, the resuscitation efforts must be organized around 2 minutes of uninterrupted CPR. Every 2 minutes the team has to stop CPR to analyze the rhythm and switch the compressing rescuer. Except for delivering defibrillation, resuscitation interventions should be done while CPR is ongoing [5].

Electrical therapies

The high first-shock efficacy of newer biphasic defibrillators has led to the recommendation of a single shock protocol. Rescuers must coordinate high-quality CPR with defibrillation to minimize interruptions to chest compressions and to ensure immediate resumption of chest compressions after shock delivery. Familiarity with the available defibrillator machine will avoid unnecessary delay or errors in operation. If the machine-specific defibrillation dose is unknown, it is recommended to use the maximum available dose. Pacing is not generally recommended for patients in asystolic cardiac arrest [6].

Monitoring and optimization of CPR quality

Current guidelines emphasize the use of objective monitoring parameters to optimize CPR quality and to detect the return of spontaneous circulation (ROSC). The quantitative waveform capnography target should be above 10 mmHg at end expiration to indicate high-quality CPR. When invasive arterial pressure monitoring is available, the relaxation phase should be above 20 mmHg. Abrupt elevation of end-tidal CO_2 and invasive arterial pressure are markers of ROSC [5].

Effective teamwork and leadership

Advanced resuscitation requires medical expertise and organized team approach. The team leader and members need to use effective communication with clear messages, and clear roles and responsibilities.

- The team leader guides the resuscitation and makes clinical decisions without directly performing specific procedures.
- The team leader assigns the team members, monitors individual performance and provides assistance and guidance to the team members.

- The team leader ensures high-quality CPR and early appropriate defibrillation.
- The team members help in providing high-quality CPR, early appropriate defibrillation, drug administrations and recording of the CPR event.

It is appropriate for the ALS team leader to invite suggestions from other team members, to ensure that all members are comfortable with the decisions and resuscitation interventions. Team debriefing of actual resuscitation events can be a useful strategy to improve future performance.

Drugs

Despite no evidence of long-term survival advantage, vascular access and drug administration continue to be part of ALS. Either intravenous (IV) access or the intraosseous (IO) route is used to give drugs during the CPR. Delivery of drugs via a tracheal tube is no longer recommended. When treating VF/VT cardiac arrest, adrenaline (epinephrine) 1 mg is given once chest compressions have restarted after the second shock and then every 3–5 minutes. Amiodarone 300 mg could be given after the third shock. For the nonshockable rhythms (asystole/PEA), adrenaline (epinephrine) 1 mg is given initially and then every 3–5 minutes. Atropine is no longer recommended in the management of cardiac arrest [7].

Advanced airway management

Adequate airway management can often be obtained with a bag-mask device. However, endotracheal intubation is preferred for airway control, if it does not lead to prolonged interruptions in chest compressions. A laryngeal mask airway is an acceptable alternative. Advanced airway insertion should be confirmed and monitored by a quantitative waveform capnography. After placement of a laryngeal mask airway or an endotracheal tube, chest compressions are continuous at a rate of 100 to 120 per minute without pauses for ventilations. The ventilation rate is 1 breath every 6 to 8 seconds (8–10 breaths per minute). Excessive ventilation rates should be avoided [8].

Cardiac arrest in special circumstances
Asthma

Significant air-trapping (dynamic hyperinflation) in asthma may lead to severely reduced venous return and subsequent cardiac arrest. The air-trapping may be relieved by actively compressing the chest wall during a brief cessation of the ventilation.

Pulmonary embolism

Emergency echocardiography may be helpful to support this diagnosis. In patients with cardiac arrest due to presumed or known PE, it is reasonable to administer fibrinolytics.

Hyperkalemia

Hyperkalemia can be confirmed rapidly using a blood gas analyzer if available. It is recommended to give 10 mL 10% calcium chloride by rapid bolus injection, to stabilize myocardial cell membrane.

Cardiac arrest following cardiac surgery

For shockable rhythms (VF/pulseless VT) in the early post-operative period, the use of up to three-stacked shocks may be considered. For nonshockable rhythms (asystole/PEA), emergency resternotomy and cardiopulmonary bypass (CPB) are essential for successful resuscitation, especially in the context of tamponade or hemorrhage, where external chest compressions may be ineffective.

Cardiac arrest associated with pregnancy

After 20 weeks gestation, the pregnant woman's uterus can press down against the inferior vena cava and the aorta, impeding venous return and cardiac output. This aortocaval compression may precipitate arrest in the critically ill patient. To relieve aortocaval compression during chest compressions and optimize the quality of CPR, it is reasonable to perform manual left uterine displacement in the supine position. If this technique is unsuccessful, providers may consider placing the patient in a left-lateral tilt of 30°, using a firm wedge to support the pelvis and thorax. If chest compressions remain inadequate after lateral uterine displacement or left-lateral tilt, perimortem cesarean delivery (PMCD) should be considered. This should be done after 4 minutes of CPR, aiming for delivery within 5 minutes from onset of cardiac arrest and can save the life of both the mother and the infant [9].

Post-resuscitation care

The primary goal of resuscitating victims of cardiac arrest is survival with the best neurologic function. The initial anoxic neuronal injury is followed by post-resuscitation cerebral syndrome. This syndrome results in the activation of destructive pathways which further damage the cerebral neurons. Managing this reperfusion injury by the implementation of a structured post-resuscitation treatment protocol may improve survival and neurologic outcome in cardiac arrest victims. This requires a comprehensive therapeutic plan delivered in an multidisciplinary environment. This post-resuscitation care should include optimizing cardiopulmonary function, therapeutic hypothermia and treating the cause of the arrest [10].

Avoiding hyperoxia

There is potential harm caused by hyperoxemia when return of spontaneous circulation (ROSC) is achieved [11]. The beneficial effect of high FiO_2 on systemic oxygen delivery should be balanced with the deleterious effect of generating oxygen-derived free radicals during the reperfusion phase. Provided appropriate equipment is available, inspired oxygen is titrated to achieve an SaO_2 of 94–98%. The goal is avoiding hyperoxia, while ensuring adequate oxygen delivery.

Induced hypothermia

Induced hypothermia is a helpful therapeutic approach in patients who remain comatose (defined as a lack of meaningful response to verbal commands) after ROSC.

- Two prospective clinical trials demonstrated better neurologic outcome by inducing mild therapeutic hypothermia for 12 or 24 hours in comatose survivals of out-of-hospital VF arrest.

- Induced hypothermia may be also considered for asystole/PEA in OHCA, or after in-hospital cardiac arrest of any initial rhythm [12,13].

For inducing hypothermia, 30 mL/kg of iced isotonic fluid can be infused over 30 minutes to initiate core cooling, but must be combined with a follow-up method for maintenance of hypothermia [14]. Clinicians should continuously monitor the patient's core temperature using an esophageal thermometer, bladder catheter or pulmonary artery catheter. The target core temperature is 32–34 °C, for 12 to 24 hours. Active rewarming should be avoided. The potential complications associated with cooling include coagulopathy, arrhythmias, hyperglycemia and sepsis. Blood glucose values >10 mmol/dL should be treated appropriately.

Acute coronary syndrome management

Primary percutaneous coronary intervention (PCI) should be considered in all post-cardiac arrest patients who are suspected of having coronary artery disease. Several studies indicate that the combination of therapeutic hypothermia and PCI is feasible and safe after cardiac arrest caused by acute myocardial infarction.

Survival and neurologic outcomes

The overall survival of victims of cardiac arrest is disappointing. Most adult survivors of cardiac arrest have a witnessed ventricular fibrillation (VF) arrest. Hence, survival is often higher for arrests in public than arrests at home. Survival depends, in part, on the institution of bystander CPR and the time from arrest to defibrillation. A 25% survival rate for out-of-hospital arrests is possible with rapid bystander CPR.

- The Ontario Prehospital Advanced Life Support (OPALS) Study was conducted to assess the effects of comprehensive implementation of the four links in the chain of survival. This study showed that 18% of the victims achieved ROSC, 15% survived to hospital admission and only 5% survived to hospital discharge. Two-thirds of the survivals to hospital discharge had a good neurologic outcome [15].

One might expect survival from arrests in hospital to be better due to rapid availability of trained personnel and equipment, but overall results are equally poor. This is due to the presence of pathology other than ischemic heart disease in many of these patients. The exception is cardiac arrest due to VF in a coronary care unit (CCU) for which survival is high because of immediate defibrillation, though many of these patients will not receive formal CPR.

- The investigators of the American Heart Association recently published a study of in-hospital cardiac arrest victims. This study showed that 50% of these victims achieved ROSC, 30% survived to ICU admission and only 17% survived to hospital discharge. Two-thirds of the survivals to hospital discharge had a good neurologic outcome [16].

Factors increasing survival include:
- Witnessed arrest
- VF as the initial rhythm
- Rapid high-quality CPR
- Rapid defibrillation
- Short duration of CPR.

Prognostication of neurological outcome

Among adult patients who are comatose and have not been treated with hypothermia, the absence of both pupillary light and corneal reflexes at 72 hours after cardiac arrest predicted poor outcome with high reliability.

Physical examination (motor response, pupillary light and corneal reflexes), EEG and imaging studies are less reliable for predicting poor outcome in patients treated with hypothermia. Durations of observation greater than 72 hours after ROSC should be considered before predicting poor outcome in patients treated with hypothermia.

Providing emotional support to the family

The ALS team should provide emotional support to the family during resuscitative efforts. Some family members should be given the opportunity to attend the resuscitation. A recently published randomized clinical trial showed that family presence during CPR did not interfere with the resuscitation efforts and was beneficial to the grieving process. Nevertheless, the resuscitation team should be sensitive to the presence of family members by assigning a trained person to remain with the family to answer questions and offer psychological support [17].

In case of unsuccessful resuscitation, notifying the family members of the death of a loved one should be performed compassionately. It is important to consider the family's culture, values and religious beliefs. Appropriate psychological support should be offered to the family to relieve preconceptions surrounding death and any associated guilt with the event [18].

Education and training

Training intervals

Basic and advanced life support knowledge and skills deteriorate in as little as 3–6 months after training. Hence, resuscitation training and certification standards should be based on competency retention rather than certificate expiration time. The use of frequent assessments will identify those individuals who require refresher training to help maintain their knowledge and skills in resuscitation [19].

Improving communication skills

An increased emphasis on nontechnical skills, such as leadership, teamwork, task management and structured communication, will help to improve the performance of CPR and subsequently patient care. Healthcare providers need to practice multirescuer CPR during BLS training. In ALS courses, the roles of the team leader and members should be simulated to achieve effective teamwork interactions.

Debriefing

Debriefing is a learner-focused, nonthreatening technique to help individual rescuers and teams reflect on and improve performance. Debriefing should be included in ALS courses to facilitate learning. In addition, debriefing is recommended after real resuscitation events in the clinical setting to learn from the actual experience [19].

Quality improvement in resuscitation

Healthcare needs to have quality improvement initiatives in the resuscitation systems, processes and outcomes. This process of quality improvement consists of a repetitious and continuous cycle of:

1. Systematic evaluation of resuscitation care processes and outcomes
2. Benchmarking with stakeholder feedback
3. Strategic efforts to address identified deficiencies
4. Re-evaluation of the effects of implementations on outcomes.

Reviewing the cardiac arrest reports and organizing simulation-based mock codes will help to prioritize gaps in the chain of survival links that need to be strengthened to reduce the variability in survival from cardiac arrest. Higher survival rate with good neurologic outcome is achievable by educating and implementing best practices [20,21].

Further reading

Resuscitation Council (UK). *Resuscitation Guidelines* 2010. http://www.resus.org.uk/pages/guide.htm (accessed July 2014).

References

1. Berg RA, Hemphill R, Abella BS *et al.* Part 5: Adult basic life support 2010 American Heart Association Guidelines for cardiopulmonary resuscitation and emergency cardiovascular care. *Circulation* 2010; 122 : S685–705.

2. Al-Quathani S, Al-Dorzi HM, Tamim HM *et al.* The impact of an intensivist-led multidisciplinary extended rapid response team on hospital-wide cardiopulmonary arrests and mortality. *Crit Care Med* 2013; 41 : 506–17.

3. Shuster M, Lim SH, Deakin CD *et al.* Part 7: CPR techniques and devices 2010 American Heart Association Guidelines for cardiopulmonary resuscitation and emergency cardiovascular care. *Circulation* 2010; 122; S720–8.

4. Aufderheide TP, Nichol G, Rea TD *et al.* A trial of an impedance threshold device in out-of-hospital cardiac arrest. *N Engl J Med* 2011; 365 : 798–806.

5. Neumar RW, Otto CW, Link MS *et al.* Part 8: Adult advanced cardiovascular life support 2010 American Heart Association guidelines for cardiopulmonary resuscitation and emergency cardiovascular care. *Circulation* 2010; 122; S729–67.

6. Link MS, Atkins DL, Passman RS *et al.* Part 6: electrical therapies automated external defibrillators, defibrillation, cardioversion, and pacing 2010 American Heart Association guidelines for cardiopulmonary resuscitation and emergency cardiovascular care. *Circulation* 2010; 122; S706–19.

7. Hagihara A, Hasegawa M, Abe T *et al.* Prehospital epinephrine use and survival among patients with out-of-hospital cardiac arrest. *JAMA* 2012; 307 : 1161–8.

8. Hasegawa K, Hiraide A, Chang Y, Brown DF. Association of prehospital advanced airway management with neurologic outcome and survival in patients with out-of-hospital cardiac arrest. *JAMA* 2013; 309 : 257–66.

9. Vanden Hoek TL, Morrison LJ, Shuster M, *et al.* Part 12: Cardiac arrest in special situations 2010 American Heart Association guidelines for cardiopulmonary resuscitation and emergency cardiovascular care. *Circulation* 2010; 122 : S829–61.

10. Peberdy MA, Callaway CW, Neumar RW *et al.* Part 9: Post-cardiac arrest care 2010 American Heart Association guidelines for cardiopulmonary resuscitation and emergency cardiovascular care. *Circulation* 2010; 122 : S768–86.

11. Kilgannon JH, Jones AE, Shapiro NI *et al.* Association between arterial hyperoxia following resuscitation from cardiac

arrest and in-hospital mortality. *JAMA* 2010; 303 : 2165–171.

12. The Hypothermia after Cardiac Arrest Study Group. Mild therapeutic hypothermia to improve the neurologic outcome after cardiac arrest. *N Engl J Med* 2002; 346 : 549–56.

13. Bernard SA, Gray TW, Buist MD *et al.* Treatment of comatose survivors of out-of-hospital cardiac arrest with induced hypothermia. *New Engl J Med* 2002; 346 : 557–63.

14. Bernard S, Buist M, Monteiro O, Smith K. Induced hypothermia using large volume, ice-cold intravenous fluid in comatose survivors of out-of-hospital cardiac arrest: a preliminary report. *Resuscitation* 2003; 56 : 9–13.

15. Ontario Prehospital Advanced Life Support Study Group. Advanced cardiac life support in out-of-hospital cardiac arrest. *N Engl J Med*. 2004; 351 : 647–56.

16. Girotra S, Nallamothu BK, Spertus JA *et al.* Trends in survival after in-hospital cardiac arrest. *N Engl J Med* 2012; 367 : 1912–20.

17. Jabre P, Belpomme V, Azoulay E *et al.* Family presence during cardiopulmonary resuscitation. *N Engl J Med* 2013; 368 : 1008–18.

18. Morrison LJ, Kierzek G, Diekema DS *et al.* Part 3: Ethics 2010 American Heart Association guidelines for cardiopulmonary resuscitation and emergency cardiovascular care. *Circulation* 2010; 122(suppl 3) : S665– 75.

19. Bhanji F, Mancini ME, Sinz E *et al.* Part 16: Education, implementation, and teams 2010 American Heart Association guidelines for cardiopulmonary resuscitation and emergency cardiovascular care. *Circulation* 2010; 122(suppl 3) : S920–33.

20. Travers AH, Rea TD, Bobrow BJ *et al.* Part 4: CPR overview 2010 American Heart Association guidelines for cardiopulmonary resuscitation and emergency cardiovascular care. *Circulation* 2010; 122(suppl 3) : S676–84.

21. Morrison LJ, Neumar RW, Zimmerman JL *et al.* Strategies for improving survival after in-hospital cardiac arrest in the United States 2013 consensus recommendations: a consensus statement from the American Heart Association. *Circulation* 2013; 127 : 1538–63.

Index

α-receptors, 162
abdominal compartment
    syndrome (ACS), 270,
    354–5, 380–1
abnormal automaticity, 324
acid/base analysis, 107
acute cardiogenic pulmonary
    edema (ACPE), 91
acute colonic pseudo-
    obstruction, 385–8
acute coronary syndromes
    (ACS). See also ischemic
    heart disease
    clinical presentation, 290
    complications, 298–9
    diagnosis, 291
    epidemiology, 290
    management, 291–8, 457
    oxygen therapy, 23
    perioperative management,
        299–300
    risk stratification, 296–7
    spectrum, 290
acute heart failure (AHF)
    chronic care transition,
        315
    classification, 303
    clinical profile, 307
    diagnosis, 304–6
    diuretics/ultrafiltration,
        309–10
    etiology, 304
    inotropes, 311–12
    laboratory testing, 305
    management, 306–9
    MCS, 312–15
    oxygenation/ventilatory
        support, 311
    patient characteristics, 304
    score, 306
    vasodilators, 310
acute kidney injury (AKI), 197,
    348–9
    causes, 348
    diagnosis and assessment,
        350
    impact and outcomes, 350
    incidence, 348
    pathogenesis, 349

post-cardiac surgery, 437
prevention and treatment,
    351–3
staging, 349
syndromes associated with,
    353–8
acute liver failure (ALF),
    356–8
acute lung injury (ALI)
    diagnosis, 361
    ventilation strategies, 148
acute mesenteric ischemia,
    383–5
acute pancreatitis
    etiology, 381
    management, 382
    management controversies,
        383
    scoring systems, 381–2
    surgery, 383
acute renal failure (ARF).
    See acute kidney injury
    (AKI)
acute respiratory distress
    syndrome (ARDS)
    adjuvant therapy, 367–70
    clinical features, 364
    definition, 361
    diagnosis, 361–2
    drug therapies, 370–1
    fluid balance and, 48
    incidence, 363
    management, 364–7
    NIPPV management, 92
    outcome, 371
    oxygen therapy and, 25
    pathophysiology, 363–4
    predispositions, 362–3
    sepsis, 338, 343
    TRALI and, 60
    ventilation strategies, 148,
        362, 365–7
acute respiratory failure, 100
adrenal hormones, 448
adrenal insufficiency, 431
adrenaline (epinephrine), 18,
    164, 167–8, 340
    cardiac arrest, 455
    side effects, 167

adrenergic receptor
    antagonists, 170
adrenoreceptors, 162
advanced life support (ALS)
    guidelines, 454–5
AECC criteria, 361–2
afferent limb, 222, 224–6
afterload, 3–5
airway management
    adjunct devices, 82–3
    algorithm, 80
    assessment and
        documentation, 78
    awake intubation, 82
    cardiac arrest, 455
    failed/difficult airway, 80, 83
    NAP4, 85
    optimization, 79
    post-intubation, 84
    reducing complications, 84
    RSII, 81
    surgical airway, 84
    trauma patient, 262–3
    ventilated patient, 134
airway pressure release
    ventilation (APRV), 146
AKIN criteria, 348–9
albumin, 41, 46–7
albuterol, 418
aldosterone, 110
alfentanil, 190
aminoglycosides, 180–1
amiodarone, 322, 325, 437, 455
amniotic fluid embolism,
    409–10
amphotericin, 178
ampicillin, 176
analgesia
    management, 190–2
    therapeutic agents, 189–90
    trauma patient, 271
anaphylactic shock, 18–19
anemia. See also blood
    transfusion
    epidemiology and etiology,
        53–4
    hemoglobin levels, 53
    management in the critically
        ill, 56–7

Printed in the United States
By Bookmasters